Imaging Brain Diseases

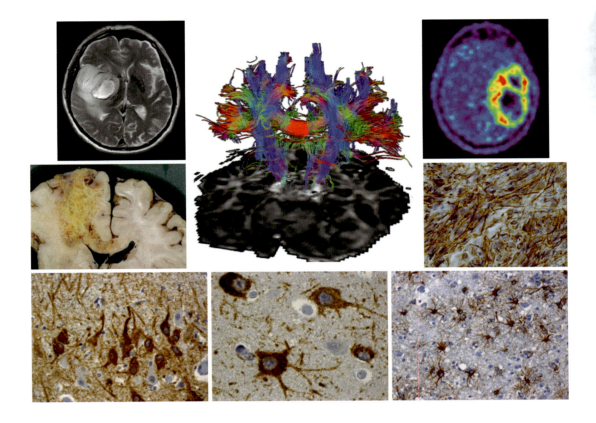

Serge Weis • Michael Sonnberger
Andreas Dunzinger • Eva Voglmayr
Martin Aichholzer • Raimund Kleiser
Peter Strasser

Imaging Brain Diseases

A Neuroradiology, Nuclear Medicine, Neurosurgery, Neuropathology and Molecular Biology-based Approach

Volume II

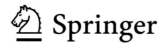

Serge Weis
Division of Neuropathology
Neuromed Campus
Kepler University Hospital
Johannes Kepler University
Linz
Austria

Michael Sonnberger
Department of Neuroradiology
Neuromed Campus
Kepler University Hospital
Johannes Kepler University
Linz
Austria

Andreas Dunzinger
Department of Neuro-Nuclear Medicine
Neuromed Campus
Kepler University Hospital
Johannes Kepler University
Linz
Austria

Eva Voglmayr
Department of Neuroradiology
Neuromed Campus
Kepler University Hospital
Johannes Kepler University
Linz
Austria

Martin Aichholzer
Department of Neurosurgery
Neuromed Campus
Kepler University Hospital
Johannes Kepler University
Linz
Austria

Raimund Kleiser
Department of Neuroradiology
Neuromed Campus
Kepler University Hospital
Johannes Kepler University
Linz
Austria

Peter Strasser
PMU University Institute for Medical &
Chemical Laboratory Diagnostics
Salzburg
Austria

ISBN 978-3-7091-1543-5   ISBN 978-3-7091-1544-2   (eBook)
https://doi.org/10.1007/978-3-7091-1544-2

© Springer-Verlag GmbH Austria, part of Springer Nature 2019

This work is subject to copyright. All rights are reserved by the Publisher, whether the whole or part of the material is concerned, specifically the rights of translation, reprinting, reuse of illustrations, recitation, broadcasting, reproduction on microfilms or in any other physical way, and transmission or information storage and retrieval, electronic adaptation, computer software, or by similar or dissimilar methodology now known or hereafter developed.
The use of general descriptive names, registered names, trademarks, service marks, etc. in this publication does not imply, even in the absence of a specific statement, that such names are exempt from the relevant protective laws and regulations and therefore free for general use.
The publisher, the authors, and the editors are safe to assume that the advice and information in this book are believed to be true and accurate at the date of publication. Neither the publisher nor the authors or the editors give a warranty, expressed or implied, with respect to the material contained herein or for any errors or omissions that may have been made. The publisher remains neutral with regard to jurisdictional claims in published maps and institutional affiliations.

This Springer imprint is published by the registered company Springer-Verlag GmbH, AT part of Springer Nature.
The registered company address is: Prinz-Eugen-Str. 8-10, 1040 Wien, Austria

Dedicated
to my late mother Louise and my Aunt Marie-Antoinette
for their lifelong generous support and
to Denisa for our future adventures

(Serge Weis)

to my brother Geri

(Michael Sonnberger)

Dedicated
to my parents for their support and encouragement and
to my daughter Ella the sunshine of my life

(Andreas Dunzinger)

For my wife, my sons, and my daughter.
Thank you for being here with me, you make my life
worth living …

(Peter Strasser)

Preface

The present book deals with picturing various diseases of the human nervous system using different imaging modalities. The appearances of the diseases are visualized on computerized tomography (CT) scans, magnetic resonance imaging (MRI) scans, nuclear medicine scans, surgical intraoperative pictures, gross anatomy, histology, and immunohistochemistry pictures. It is aimed at attracting the interest of neurologists, neuroradiologists, neurosurgeons, and neuropathologists as well as all allied neuroscientific disciplines. The information provided should facilitate the understanding of the disease processes in their daily routine work.

There exist many good and detailed books on the neuroradiologic aspects of brain diseases. Although these books contain hundreds of CT and MR scans, no histologic picture disclosing the microscopic features of the disorders dealt with is included. On the other hand, there exist excellent books describing the neuropathological features of brain disorders. Again, many light and electron microscopic pictures are included; however, the neuroradiologic scans are sparse or lacking. The correlative combination of nuclear medicine scans with either neuroradiologic scans or neuropathology images is nearly absent. The present book is, hence, an attempt to bridge the gap between neuro-clinicians, neuro-imagers, and neuropathologists.

It is our intention to present the brain disorders in a very systematic way allowing the reader to easily find the topics in which she or he is particularly interested. Although it might be considered monotonous, we feel that this approach is an effective didactic way in presenting data which can quickly be retrieved.

The book starts with a description of the various imaging modalities, i.e. computerized tomography and nuclear magnetic resonance imaging (Chap. 1). Here, the tremendous advances achieved during the last two decades are illustrated with the wealth of new imaging techniques available for daily routine diagnosis like spectroscopy, perfusion imaging, diffusion weighted imaging, and diffusion tensor imaging. Nuclear medicine imaging (Chap. 2) aims at representing the functional/metabolic state of the brain using different techniques (SPECT, PET) and applying various tracers like methionine, fluordeoxyglucose, fluorethyltyrosine, etc. in order to visualize various biochemical pathways (i.e., transmitter, amino acids, glucose). Chapter 3 describes the neuropathological approach for analyzing brain diseases. The cellular and tissue components of the normal nervous system are presented. The immunohistochemical typing of the various cells which make up the nervous system is presented in detail. A detailed description of the normal human brain and its vascular supply is provided in Chaps. 4–14 of Part II.

The subsequent chapters (Chaps. 15–83) of Part III to Part X deal with the various disorders involving the nervous system which can be grouped into the following disorders: hemodynamic (Chaps. 15 and 16), vascular (Chaps. 17–24), infectious (Chaps. 25–29), neurodegenerative (Chaps. 30–40), demyelination (Chaps. 41–43), epilepsy (Chaps. 44 and 45), trauma and intoxication (Chaps. 46–48), and the vast field of tumors (Chaps. 49–83).

The approach in presenting a brain disease entity is in the following order: brief definition of the entity, relative incidence, age incidence, sex incidence, predilection sites of the lesion, description of the characteristic CT findings with representative CT scans, description of the characteristic MRI findings with representative MRI scans, nuclear medicine findings, macroscopic features including intraoperative findings, microscopic features, ultrastructural features, immunohistochemical staining characteristics, spectrum of reactivities to proliferation markers, differential diagnosis, pathogenesis and molecular biological characteristics, treatment, and biologic behavior, prognosis, and prognostic factors.

Although molecular biology was and is undoubtedly the scientific trendsetter during the last decades and for the forthcoming years, however, some doubts about the promises made by medical molecular biologists are appropriate. In the future, people will see bands on blots, but they will not see anymore the cell, the tissue, and the organism and finally not anymore the patient. Okazaki in his *Fundamentals of Neuropathology* expressed the same opinion as follows: "Many residents are intelligent and well versed in the latest molecular biologic concepts or neurochemical advances, but they often have difficulties in recognizing actual brain lesions or interpreting histologic findings."

Furthermore, we want to impart to our young colleagues a sound and comprehensive knowledge on diseases involving the nervous system. Through this schematic, straightforward presentation, the aspiring clinical neuroscientist in training will hopefully not undergo the same frustrations that we experienced.

Special thanks are expressed to Johannes Trenkler, M.D. (Head, Department of Radiology); Robert Pichler, M.D., Ph.D. (Head, Department of Nuclear Medicine); and Prof. Andreas Gruber, M.D., Ph.D. (Head, Department of Neurosurgery), at the Neuromed Campus of the Kepler University Hospital (formerly Landes-Nervenklinik Wagner-Jauregg) for their fruitful collaboration. Dr. Weis thanks his medical team including Ognian Kalev, M.D. (senior consultant); Karoline Ornig, M.D. (trainee); and Dave Bandke, M.D., B.S.A. (trainee), for providing interesting cases. The help of Michaela Gnauer, clinical psychologist, for reviewing Chap. 14 is highly appreciated.

Finally, the authors acknowledge the skillful technical help of the following medical technologists (in alphabetical order):

- In neuropathology: Sabine Engstler, Susanne Fiedler, Gabriele Göberl, Christina Keuch, Anna Kroiss, Monika Lugmayr, and Christa Winter-Schwarz. Special thanks are necessary to appreciate the diligent work of Stefan Pirngruber as best mortuary technician and archivist of the histological blocks and sections. Birgit Kronfuss helped with secretarial work.
- In Neurosurgery: Hans-Peter Dahl, Franz Knogler, and Thomas Wimmer for registering the intraoperative images. Hans-Peter was very helpful with annotating some images.
- In neuroradiology: to the whole team of radiotechnologists (too many to name).
- In neuronuclear medicine: to the whole team of radiotechnologists (especially Silke Kern for her technical knowledge and her good memory of patients).

The authors thank Mag. Barbara Pfeiffer (Vienna), Claus-Dieter Bachem (Heidelberg), Andrea Ridolfi (Turin), Abha Krishnan, Jeyaraj Allwynkingsly, and Shanjini Rajasekaran (Chennai) from Springer-Verlag Wien, New York, for a smooth and perfect collaboration.

Linz, Austria	Serge Weis
Linz, Austria	Michael Sonnberger
Linz, Austria	Andreas Dunzinger
Linz, Austria	Eva Voglmayr
Linz, Austria	Martin Aichholzer
Linz, Austria	Raimund Kleiser
Salzburg, Austria	Peter Strasser

Contents

Volume I

Part I The Techniques

1 Imaging Modalities: Neuroradiology 3
   1.1 Introduction 3
   1.2 CT-Imaging 4
       1.2.1 Equipment 4
       1.2.2 Image Presentation.......................... 5
       1.2.3 Characteristics of CT-Imaging................. 6
       1.2.4 Contrast and Details Resolution................ 6
       1.2.5 Artifacts 6
       1.2.6 Contrast Medium 6
       1.2.7 Recent Developments and Trends 6
       1.2.8 CT-Angiography 7
       1.2.9 CT-Perfusion 7
   1.3 MR Imaging.. 9
       1.3.1 Equipment 9
       1.3.2 Image Presentation.......................... 9
       1.3.3 Characteristics of MR Imaging 11
       1.3.4 Contrast and Details Resolution................ 13
       1.3.5 Imaging Protocols 13
       1.3.6 Artifacts 14
       1.3.7 Contrast Medium 14
       1.3.8 Recent Developments and Trends 15
       1.3.9 MR Spectroscopy........................... 15
       1.3.10 MR Angiography 16
       1.3.11 MR-Perfusion Imaging 18
       1.3.12 MR Diffusion-Weighted Imaging (DWI)......... 19
       1.3.13 MR Diffusion Tensor Imaging (DTI)............ 19
       1.3.14 Functional MRI (fMRI)...................... 20
       1.3.15 Neuronavigation and Intraoperative MRI 22
       1.3.16 Imaging Protocol Lists....................... 27
   Selected References 28

2	**Imaging Modalities: Nuclear Medicine**.	29
	2.1 Introduction	29
	2.2 SPECT: Single Photon Emission Computed Tomography	39
	2.3 PET—Positron Emission Tomography	42
	2.4 FDG-PET.	44
	2.5 Amino Acid PET	48
	2.6 123I-FP-CIT.	49
	2.7 D2 Receptor Ligands	50
	2.8 Brain Perfusion SPECT	51
	2.9 Amyloid Imaging.	53
	2.10 Indications for Nuclear Medicine Examinations	54
	Selected References	55
3	**Imaging Modalities: Neuropathology**	57
	3.1 Introduction	57
	3.2 Removal, Fixation, and Cutting of the Brain and Spinal Cord	58
	3.2.1 Removal and Fixation of the Brain	58
	3.2.2 Removal and Fixation of the Spinal Cord	63
	3.2.3 Brain Cutting	65
	3.2.4 Gross Anatomical Examination of the Cut Brain	74
	3.2.5 Sampling of Brain Regions for Microscopic Examination	75
	3.2.6 Handling of Surgical Specimens	75
	3.3 Fixation and Processing of Tissue	76
	3.3.1 Fixation of Sampled Tissue	76
	3.3.2 Processing of Tissue.	78
	3.4 Staining of Tissue.	79
	3.4.1 Classical Stain	79
	3.4.2 Special Stains.	83
	3.4.3 Special Neuro-stains	84
	3.4.4 Special Stains for Connective Tissue.	87
	3.4.5 Other Special Stains.	89
	3.5 Immunohistochemistry	89
	3.5.1 General Principles	89
	3.5.2 Neuronal Markers	92
	3.5.3 Synaptic Markers.	95
	3.5.4 Astroglial Markers	96
	3.5.5 Oligodendroglial Markers: Myelin Markers	97
	3.5.6 Microglial Markers	99
	3.5.7 Markers for Neurodegeneration	100
	3.5.8 Tumor Markers.	102
	3.5.9 Vascular Markers	103
	3.5.10 Hematopoietic and Lymphatic Markers.	105
	3.5.11 Proliferation Markers in Tumors	105
	3.5.12 Markers for Infectious Agents	107
	3.5.13 Immunohistochemical Panels	108

	3.6	Other Techniques	108
		3.6.1 Electron Microscopy	108
		3.6.2 Fluorescence Microscopy	108
		3.6.3 Enzyme Histochemistry	108
		3.6.4 *In Situ* Hybridization (ISH)	111
		3.6.5 Molecular Biology	111
		3.6.6 Other Imaging Techniques	114
	Selected References		114

Part II The Normal Human Brain

4 Subdivisions of the Nervous System 121
    4.1 Central Nervous System (CNS) and Peripheral Nervous System (PNS) 121
        4.1.1 Central Nervous System (CNS) 121
        4.1.2 Peripheral Nervous System (PNS) 122
    4.2 Cerebrospinal and Autonomic Nervous System 122
        4.2.1 Cerebrospinal Nervous System 122
        4.2.2 Autonomic Nervous System 123
    4.3 Cortical Areas 123
        4.3.1 Somatotopic Organization 123
        4.3.2 Primary Cortical Areas 123
        4.3.3 Secondary Cortical Areas 123
    4.4 Gray and White Matter 125
        4.4.1 Gray Matter 125
        4.4.2 White Matter 125
        4.4.3 Nuclei and Ganglia 125
        4.4.4 Tracts 125
        4.4.5 Neuropil 125
    Selected References 127

5 Gross Anatomy of the Nervous System 129
    5.1 Subdivisions of the Central Nervous System 129
    5.2 Telencephalon 129
        5.2.1 Superolateral Surface 131
        5.2.2 Medial Surface 135
        5.2.3 Inferior Surface 136
    5.3 Limbic System 137
    5.4 Hippocampal Formation 138
    5.5 Amygdala 142
    5.6 Basal Ganglia 143
        5.6.1 Caudate Nucleus 144
        5.6.2 Globus Pallidus 145
        5.6.3 Putamen 145
        5.6.4 Nucleus Accumbens 145
    5.7 White Matter 146
        5.7.1 Projection Fibers 147
        5.7.2 Association Fibers 147
        5.7.3 Commissural Fibers 148

	5.8	Diencephalon	150
		5.8.1 Thalamus	150
		5.8.2 Hypothalamus	153
		5.8.3 Subthalamus	155
		5.8.4 Epithalamus	155
	5.9	Mesencephalon	156
	5.10	Pons	156
	5.11	Medulla Oblongata	160
	5.12	Cerebellum	162
	5.13	Spinal Cord	163
	5.14	Pituitary Gland	164
	5.15	3D Reconstructions of the Brain and Cutplanes	166
		Selected References	168
6	**Ventricular System: Cerebrospinal Fluid (CSF)—Barriers**		169
	6.1	Introduction	169
	6.2	Ventricular System	169
		6.2.1 Lateral Ventricles	169
		6.2.2 Third Ventricle	174
		6.2.3 Fourth Ventricle	174
	6.3	Cerebrospinal Fluid (CSF)	174
	6.4	Choroid Plexus	176
	6.5	Barriers	176
		6.5.1 The Blood–Brain Barrier (BBB)	176
		6.5.2 The Brain–Liquor Barrier (BLB)	176
		6.5.3 The Blood–Liquor Barrier	176
		Selected References	177
7	**Meninges**		179
	7.1	Introduction	179
	7.2	Dura Mater	179
	7.3	Dural Sinuses	182
	7.4	Arachnoidea	186
	7.5	Pia Mater	186
	7.6	The Meningeal Spaces	188
	7.7	Arachnoidal Granulations	188
		Selected References	189
8	**Arterial Supply of the Brain**		191
	8.1	Introduction	191
	8.2	Carotid System	191
	8.3	Vertebro-Basilar System	199
	8.4	Clinical Vascular Syndromes	202
		8.4.1 Anterior Cerebral Artery Syndrome	202
		8.4.2 Middle Cerebral Artery Syndrome	208
		8.4.3 AICA Syndrome (Lateral Pontine Syndrome)	208
		8.4.4 Posterior Inferior Cerebellar Artery Syndrome (PICA Syndrome)	208
		8.4.5 Posterior Cerebral Artery Syndrome	209
		Selected References	209

9	**Venous Drainage of the Brain**		211
	9.1	Introduction	211
	9.2	Venous System	211
	9.3	Dural Venous Sinuses	218
	Selected References		224
10	**Histological Constituents of the Nervous System**		225
	10.1	Neuron	225
		10.1.1 Classification of Neurons	229
		10.1.2 Size of Neurons	231
		10.1.3 Types of Neuronal Connection	231
	10.2	Synapse	232
		10.2.1 The Presynaptic Membrane	232
		10.2.2 The Postsynaptic Membrane	234
		10.2.3 The Synaptic Cleft	234
		10.2.4 Types of synapses	234
		10.2.5 Classification of synapses	235
	10.3	Nerve Fibers and Peripheral Nerve	236
		10.3.1 Morphological Features of Nerve Fibers	236
		10.3.2 Classification of Nerve Fibers	238
		10.3.3 Structure of Peripheral Nerves	238
	10.4	Glial Cells	239
	10.5	Astroglia (Astrocytes)	240
	10.6	Oligodendroglia (Oligodendrocytes)	245
	10.7	Microglia	247
	10.8	Ependymal Cells	249
	10.9	Tanycytes	250
	10.10	Molecular Composition of White Matter Myelin	250
		10.10.1 Lipids	250
		10.10.2 Myelin Basic Protein (MBP)	250
		10.10.3 Proteolipid Protein (PLP)	250
		10.10.4 Myelin-Associated Glycoprotein (MAG)	250
		10.10.5 Myelin Oligodendrocyte Glycoprotein (MOG)	251
		10.10.6 2′,3′-Cyclic Nucleotide 3′-Phosphodiesterase (CNP)	251
		10.10.7 Myelin Oligodendrocyte Basic Protein (MOBP)	251
		10.10.8 Other CNS Myelin Proteins	252
	10.11	Meninges	252
		10.11.1 Dura mater	252
		10.11.2 Arachnoidea	252
		10.11.3 Pia Mater	252
		10.11.4 Sinuses	254
	10.12	Choroid Plexus	254
	10.13	Vessels	254
		10.13.1 Artery	255
		10.13.2 Arteriole	255
		10.13.3 Capillary	256
		10.13.4 Venule and Vein	258

		10.13.5	Endothelium	258
		10.13.6	Glymphatic System	259
	10.14	Neurovascular Unit		259
	Selected References			261

11 Microscopical Buildup of the Nervous System 267
    11.1 Cerebral Cortex 267
           11.1.1 Architectonics 269
           11.1.2 Layers and Networks of the Cerebral Cortex. 282
    11.2 Hippocampus 294
           11.2.1 Cornu Ammonis (Hippocampus Proper) 295
           11.2.2 Gyrus Dentatus (Fascia Dentata,
                      Gyrus Involutus). 299
           11.2.3 Entorhinal Cortex. 300
           11.2.4 Nucleus Basalis Meynert 300
    11.3 Amygdala 300
    11.4 White Matter 301
    11.5 Basal Ganglia 301
           11.5.1 Caudate Nucleus and Putamen. 301
           11.5.2 Globus Pallidus 304
    11.6 Diencephalon 305
           11.6.1 Thalamus 305
           11.6.2 Hypothalamus 306
    11.7 Mesencephalon 306
           11.7.1 Substantia Nigra 307
           11.7.2 Nucleus Ruber 308
    11.8 Pons 310
    11.9 Medulla Oblongata 311
           11.9.1 Area Postrema 312
           11.9.2 Pyramis 312
           11.9.3 Inferior Olivary Complex. 313
    11.10 Cerebellum 313
    11.11 Spinal Cord 318
    11.12 Ventricular System 321
           11.12.1 Ventricular Lining 321
           11.12.2 Choroid Plexus 321
    Selected References 323

12 Functional Systems 325
    12.1 Introduction 325
    12.2 Sensory System: Visual System 325
    12.3 Motor System: Central Motor System 333
           12.3.1 Corticospinal Tract. 333
    12.4 Motor System: Basal Ganglionic System 333
    12.5 Sensory System: Somatosensory System. 333
    12.6 Cerebral Cortex 341
    12.7 Limbic System 342
    12.8 Hippocampal System 345
           12.8.1 Polysynaptic Intrahippocampal Pathway 345
           12.8.2 Direct Intrahippocampal Pathway 348
           12.8.3 Regulatory Circuits 348

	12.9	Amygdalar System.............................	349
	12.10	Cerebellum..................................	349
	12.11	Thalamic System..............................	351
	12.12	Hypothalamus and Hypophyseal System............	351
	12.13	Two-stream Hypothesis.........................	355
		12.13.1 Visual System: Two-Stream Hypothesis.......	355
		12.13.2 Ventral Stream.........................	357
		12.13.3 Dorsal Stream.........................	360
	12.14	The Connectome...............................	360
	12.15	Rich-Club Organization.........................	363
	Selected References..................................		366
13	**Neurotransmitter Systems**............................		369
	13.1	Acetylcholine.................................	373
	13.2	Catecholamines Monoamines.....................	376
		13.2.1 Dopamine.............................	376
		13.2.2 Noradrenaline..........................	381
		13.2.3 Monoamines: Adrenaline..................	384
		13.2.4 Monoamines: Serotonin...................	385
	13.3	Amino Acids..................................	388
		13.3.1 γ-Aminobutyric Acid (GABA)...............	388
		13.3.2 Glutamic Acid (Glu).....................	391
	Selected References..................................		395
14	**Localization of Brain Function**........................		401
	14.1	Frontal Cortex................................	403
		14.1.1 Primary Motor Cortex....................	403
		14.1.2 Supplementary Motor Area.................	403
		14.1.3 Premotor Cortex........................	403
		14.1.4 Prefrontal Cortex (Frontal Association Cortex)...	403
		14.1.5 Frontal Pole: Orbitofrontal Area.............	404
		14.1.6 Mesial Aspect: Cingulate Gyrus.............	404
	14.2	Parietal Cortex................................	404
		14.2.1 Primary Somatosensory Cortex..............	404
		14.2.2 Secondary Somatosensory Cortex............	405
		14.2.3 Somatosensory Association Area.............	405
		14.2.4 Postcentral Gyrus.......................	405
		14.2.5 Superior and Inferior Parietal Lobules.........	405
		14.2.6 Supramarginal and Angular Gyri............	405
		14.2.7 Angular Gyrus..........................	406
		14.2.8 Mesial Aspect: Cuneus....................	406
	14.3	Occipital Cortex...............................	406
		14.3.1 Primary Visual Cortex....................	406
		14.3.2 Visual Association Cortex.................	406
		14.3.3 Mesial Aspect..........................	406
		14.3.4 Lateral Aspect.........................	407
	14.4	Temporal Cortex...............................	408
		14.4.1 Primary Auditory Cortex..................	408
		14.4.2 Auditory Association Cortex...............	408

		14.4.3	Inferomedial Aspect (Amygdala and Hippocampus)	408
		14.4.4	Anterior Tip (Including Amygdala; Bilateral Lesions).........................	408
		14.4.5	Latero-inferior Aspect	408
		14.4.6	Latero-superior Aspect......................	408
		14.4.7	Non-localizing	409
		14.4.8	With Epileptogenic Lesions..................	409
	14.5	Language Areas		409
	14.6	Cortical Syndromes		412
	14.7	Limbic System......................................		413
		14.7.1	Hippocampus...............................	413
		14.7.2	Amygdala..................................	413
		14.7.3	Stria Terminalis	413
		14.7.4	Septal Nuclei	413
		14.7.5	Cingulate Cortex	413
	14.8	Corpus Callosum		413
	14.9	Basal Ganglia......................................		415
	14.10	Thalamus		416
	14.11	Hypothalamus		417
	14.12	Cerebellum..		418
	14.13	White Matter		419
	Selected References			422

Part III The Brain Diseases: Edema and Hydrocephalus

15	**Brain Edema: Intracranial Pressure—Herniation**		427
	15.1	Definition	427
	15.2	Epidemiology......................................	427
	15.3	Localization	428
	15.4	General Imaging Findings	428
	15.5	Neuropathology Findings............................	434
		15.5.1 Microscopic Features........................	439
		15.5.2 Ultrastructural Features	440
	15.6	Molecular Neuropathology	440
	15.7	Treatment and Prognosis	441
	Selected References		441

16	**Hydrocephalus**..		443
	16.1	Definition	443
	16.2	Clinical Signs and Symptoms	443
	16.3	Epidemiology......................................	443
	16.4	General Imaging Findings	444
	16.5	Neuropathology Findings............................	449
	16.6	Molecular Neuropathology	451
	16.7	Treatment and Prognosis	451
	Selected References		451

Part IV The Brain Diseases: Vascular system

17 Vascular Disorders: Hypoxia 455
    17.1   Introduction 455
    17.2   Clinical Signs....................................... 456
    17.3   Epidemiology....................................... 456
    17.4   Neuroimaging Findings 456
    17.5   Neuropathology Findings............................. 463
    17.6   Molecular Neuropathology 466
    17.7   Treatment and Prognosis 470
    Selected References 470

18 Vascular Disorders: Ischemia–Infarction–Stroke 473
    18.1   Introduction 473
    18.2   Clinical Signs and Symptoms 473
    18.3   Epidemiology....................................... 474
    18.4   Neuroimaging Findings 477
    18.5   Neuropathology Findings............................. 484
    18.6   Molecular Neuropathology 489
    18.7   Treatment and Prognosis 496
    Selected References 496

19 Vascular Disorders: Hemorrhage 499
    19.1   General Considerations 499
    19.2   Intracerebral Hemorrhage 500
            19.2.1   Clinical Signs and Symptoms 500
            19.2.2   Epidemiology............................... 500
            19.2.3   Neuroimaging Findings 500
            19.2.4   Neuropathology Findings..................... 501
            19.2.5   Molecular Neuropathology 501
            19.2.6   Treatment and Prognosis 503
    19.3   Subarachnoid Hemorrhage (SAH)..................... 505
            19.3.1   Clinical Signs and Symptoms 505
            19.3.2   Epidemiology............................... 505
            19.3.3   Neuroimaging Findings 505
            19.3.4   Neuropathology Findings..................... 510
            19.3.5   Molecular Neuropathology 514
            19.3.6   Treatment and Prognosis 514
    19.4   Subdural Hemorrhage 520
            19.4.1   Clinical Signs and Symptoms 520
            19.4.2   Epidemiology............................... 520
            19.4.3   Neuroimaging Findings 520
            19.4.4   Neuropathology Findings..................... 521
            19.4.5   Molecular Neuropathology 522
            19.4.6   Treatment and Prognosis 524
    19.5   Epidural Hemorrhage (EDH)......................... 529
            19.5.1   Clinical Signs and Symptoms 529
            19.5.2   Localization 529
            19.5.3   Neuroimaging Findings 529

	19.5.4	Neuropathology Findings.	530
	19.5.5	Molecular Neuropathology	530
	19.5.6	Treatment and Prognosis	533
	Selected References		533

20 Vascular Disorders: Arteriosclerosis ... 537
- 20.1 Introduction ... 537
- 20.2 Epidemiology ... 537
- 20.3 Neuroimaging Findings ... 538
- 20.4 Neuropathology Findings ... 538
- 20.5 Molecular Neuropathology ... 540
- 20.6 Treatment and Prognosis ... 542
- Selected References ... 548

21 Vascular Disorders: Aneurysms ... 551
- 21.1 Definition ... 551
- 21.2 Epidemiology ... 551
- 21.3 Neuroimaging Findings ... 551
- 21.4 Neuropathology Findings ... 552
- 21.5 Molecular Neuropathology ... 558
- 21.6 Treatment and Prognosis ... 570
- Selected References ... 576

22 Vascular Disorders: Malformations ... 577
- 22.1 Introduction ... 577
- 22.2 Arteriovenous Malformation (AVM) ... 577
  - 22.2.1 Epidemiology ... 577
  - 22.2.2 Neuroimaging Findings ... 577
  - 22.2.3 Neuropathology Findings ... 578
  - 22.2.4 Molecular Neuropathology ... 584
  - 22.2.5 Treatment and Prognosis ... 585
- 22.3 Cavernous Hemangioma (Cavernoma) ... 585
  - 22.3.1 Epidemiology ... 585
  - 22.3.2 Neuroimaging Findings ... 585
  - 22.3.3 Neuropathology Findings ... 586
  - 22.3.4 Molecular Neuropathology ... 586
  - 22.3.5 Treatment and Prognosis ... 586
- 22.4 Capillary Telangiectasia ... 593
  - 22.4.1 Epidemiology ... 593
  - 22.4.2 Neuroimaging Findings ... 596
  - 22.4.3 Neuropathology Findings ... 596
  - 22.4.4 Molecular Neuropathology ... 596
  - 22.4.5 Treatment and Prognosis ... 596
- 22.5 Dural AV-Fistula ... 599
  - 22.5.1 Neuroimaging Findings ... 599
- Selected References ... 603

23 Vascular Disorders: Angiopathies ... 605
- 23.1 Introduction ... 605
- 23.2 Cerebral Amyloid Angiopathy ... 605
  - 23.2.1 Clinical Signs and Symptoms ... 605
  - 23.2.2 Epidemiology ... 606

		23.2.3	Neuroimaging Findings	606
		23.2.4	Neuropathology Findings.	607
		23.2.5	Molecular Neuropathology	607
		23.2.6	Treatment and Prognosis	615
	23.3	Binswanger Disease...............................		615
		23.3.1	Clincal Signs and Symptoms.................	615
		23.3.2	Epidemiology..............................	616
		23.3.3	Neuroimaging Findings	616
		23.3.4	Neuropathology Findings	616
		23.3.5	Molecular Neuropathology	622
		23.3.6	Treatment and Prognosis	622
	23.4	Fahr Disease......................................		622
		23.4.1	Clinical Signs and Symptoms	622
		23.4.2	Localisation	622
		23.4.3	Neuroimaging Findings	622
		23.4.4	Neuropathology Findings.	622
		23.4.5	Molecular Neuropathology	626
		23.4.6	Treatment and Prognosis	626
	23.5	Cerebral Autosomal Dominant Arteriopathy (CADASIL) ...		626
		23.5.1	Clinical Signs and Symptoms	626
		23.5.2	Epidemiology..............................	627
		23.5.3	Neuroimaging Findings	627
		23.5.4	Neuropathology Findings.	628
		23.5.5	Molecular Neuropathology	632
		23.5.6	Treatment and Prognosis	632
	Selected References			633
24	**Vascular Disorders: Vasculitis**			**635**
	24.1	Definition		635
	24.2	Clinical Signs and Symptoms		636
	24.3	Epidemiology.....................................		637
	24.4	Neuroimaging Findings		637
	24.5	Neuropathology Findings.		641
	24.6	Molecular Neuropathology		641
	24.7	Treatment and Prognosis		649
	Selected References			649

Part V The Brain Diseases: Infections

25	**Infections: Bacteria**.....................................		**653**
	25.1	Clinical Signs and Symptoms	653
	25.2	Classification of Bacteria...........................	653
	25.3	General Aspects	655
	25.4	Epidemiology.....................................	655
	25.5	Imaging Features	657
		25.5.1 Meningitis	657
		25.5.2 Encephalitis	661
		25.5.3 Brain Abscess..............................	661
		25.5.4 Subdural Empyema	663

	25.6	Neuropathology Findings.	666
	25.7	Molecular Neuropathology	687
	25.8	Treatment and Prognosis	690
	Selected References		691
26	**Infections: Viruses**		**693**
	26.1	Clinical Signs and Symptoms	693
	26.2	Classification of Viruses.	693
	26.3	Epidemiology.	693
	26.4	Neuroimaging Findings	696
	26.5	Neuropathology Findings.	697
	26.6	Molecular Neuropathology	698
	26.7	Treatment and Prognosis	699
	26.8	Unspecified Nodular Encephalitis	699
	26.9	RNA Viruses: Human Immunodeficiency Virus (HIV)-1.	700
		26.9.1 HIV-1 Encephalitis (HIVE)	702
		26.9.2 HIV-1 Leukoencephalopathy (HIVL)	703
		26.9.3 Lymphocytic Meningitis (LM) and Perivascular Lymphocytic Infiltration (PLI)	703
		26.9.4 Vacuolar Myelopathy (VM) and Vacuolar Leukoencephalopathy (VL)	706
		26.9.5 Neuropathological Changes in Early Stages of HIV-1 Infection	706
		26.9.6 Neuropathological Changes in HIV-1-Infected Children	708
		26.9.7 Therapy: HAART Effects and Therapy-Induced Immune Restitution Inflammatory Syndrome (IRIS)	710
		26.9.8 The Sequalae of HIV-1 Infection of the Nervous System	715
		26.9.9 Pathogenetic Mechanisms	717
	26.10	DNA-Virus: Cytomegalovirus Infection (CMV)	720
		26.10.1 Neuroradiology Findings	720
		26.10.2 Neuropathology Findings.	720
	26.11	Progressive Multifocal Leukoencephalopathy (PML)	722
		26.11.1 Clinical Signs and Symptoms	722
		26.11.2 Neuroimaging Findings	725
		26.11.3 Neuropathology Findings.	725
		26.11.4 Molecular Nauropathology	730
	26.12	Herpes Simplex Virus (HSV) Encephalitis	731
		26.12.1 Clinical Signs and Symptoms	731
		26.12.2 Neuroimaging Findings	731
		26.12.3 Neuropathology Findings.	736
		26.12.4 Molecular Neuropathology	736
		26.12.5 Treatment and Prognosis	736
	26.13	Tick-Borne Encephalitis	736
		26.13.1 Clinical Signs and Symptoms	736
		26.13.2 Epidemiology.	737
		26.13.3 Neuroimaging Findings	737

		26.13.4	Neuropathology Findings.	739
		26.13.5	Molecular Neuropathology	741
		26.13.6	Treatment and Prognosis	742
	Selected References			742

27 Infections: Parasites 749

- 27.1 Classification of Parasitic Agents. 749
- 27.2 Clinical Signs and Symptoms 749
- 27.3 *Toxoplasma gondii*. 749
  - 27.3.1 Clinical Signs and Symptoms 749
  - 27.3.2 Epidemiology. 751
  - 27.3.3 Neuroimaging Findings 752
  - 27.3.4 Neuropathology Findings. 752
  - 27.3.5 Molecular Neuropathology 752
  - 27.3.6 Treatment and Prognosis 756
- 27.4 Taeniasis: Coenurosis/Cysticercosis 762
  - 27.4.1 Cysticercosis: Clinical Signs and Symptoms. 762
  - 27.4.2 Coenurosis: Clinical Signs and Symptoms 762
  - 27.4.3 Epidemiology. 763
  - 27.4.4 Neuroimaging Findings 763
  - 27.4.5 Neuropathology Findings. 767
  - 27.4.6 Molecular Neuropathology 768
  - 27.4.7 Treatment and Prognosis 771
- Selected References 771

28 Infections: Fungi 773

- 28.1 General Aspects 773
  - 28.1.1 Clinical Signs and Symptoms 773
  - 28.1.2 Epidemiology. 773
  - 28.1.3 Classification of Fungi. 773
  - 28.1.4 Neuroimaging Findings 775
  - 28.1.5 Neuropathology Stains. 776
  - 28.1.6 Molecular Neuropathology 776
  - 28.1.7 Treatment 776
- 28.2 *Aspergillus Fumigatus* 777
  - 28.2.1 Neuroimaging Findings 777
  - 28.2.2 Neuropathology Findings. 778
  - 28.2.3 Molecular Neuropathology 781
- 28.3 *Cryptococcus Neoformans*. 782
  - 28.3.1 Neuroimaging Findings 782
  - 28.3.2 Neuropathology Findings. 785
  - 28.3.3 Molecular Neuropathology 785
- 28.4 *Candida Albicans*. 787
  - 28.4.1 Neuropathology Findings. 787
  - 28.4.2 Molecular Pathology 787
- Selected References 793

29 Prion Encephalopathies 797

- 29.1 General Aspects 797
  - 29.1.1 Clinical Signs and Symptoms 799
  - 29.1.2 Neuroimaging Findings 799
  - 29.1.3 Neuropathology Findings. 804

		29.1.4	Treatment and Prognosis	816
		29.1.5	Molecular Neuropathology	816
	29.2	Creutzfeldt–Jakob Disease (CJD)		818
		29.2.1	Clinical Signs	818
		29.2.2	Macroscopic Features	819
		29.2.3	Microscopic Features	819
	29.3	Variant CJD		820
		29.3.1	Clinical Signs and Symptoms	820
		29.3.2	Microscopic Features	821
		29.3.3	Molecular Neuropathology	821
	29.4	Gerstmann–Sträussler–Scheinker Disease (GSS)		821
		29.4.1	Clinical signs	821
		29.4.2	Microscopic Features	821
	29.5	Fatal Familial Insomnia (FFI)		822
		29.5.1	Clinical signs	822
		29.5.2	Microscopic Features	822
	29.6	Kuru		822
		29.6.1	Clinical signs	822
		29.6.2	Macroscopical Features	822
		29.6.3	Microscopical Features	822
	Selected References			823

Volume II

Part VI The Brain Diseases: Aging and Neurodegeneration

30 Neurodegeneration: General Aspects 827
- 30.1 Introduction 827
- 30.2 Clinical Signs and Symptoms 827
  - 30.2.1 Dementia 828
  - 30.2.2 Motor Disorders 830
- 30.3 Neuropathologic Changes 830
  - 30.3.1 Gross-anatomical Changes 830
  - 30.3.2 Microscopical Changes 830
  - 30.3.3 Amyloid Deposits 830
  - 30.3.4 Neurofibrillary Changes: Tauopathies 838
  - 30.3.5 Neuropil Threads 839
  - 30.3.6 Lewy Bodies 839
  - 30.3.7 Granulovacuolar Degeneration 840
  - 30.3.8 Ballooned Neurons 840
  - 30.3.9 Histological Visualization of Amyloid Deposits and Tangles 841
  - 30.3.10 Immunohistochemical Pattern in the Differential Diagnosis 844
  - 30.3.11 Frequencies of Neuropathology Diagnoses 844
- 30.4 Comparisons 844
- 30.5 Molecular Neuropathology 844
  - 30.5.1 Concepts of Neurodegenerative Diseases 844
  - 30.5.2 Relevant Proteins 846

		30.5.3	Amyloid and the Amyloid Cascade Hypothesis................................	847
		30.5.4	Tau...	849
		30.5.5	Synuclein (α-Syn).........................	849
		30.5.6	TDP-43......................................	851
		30.5.7	FUS...	851
		30.5.8	Nucleotide Repeat Diseases.................	853
	30.6	Biomarkers...		853
	30.7	Brief Sketch of the Differential Diagnoses.............		856
	30.8	Differential Diagnoses: Lobar Atrophies................		856
		30.8.1	Pick Disease................................	856
		30.8.2	Primary Progressive Aphasia (PPA)............	856
		30.8.3	Motor Neuron Disease with Dementia..........	857
		30.8.4	Dementia Lacking Distinctive Histopathology (DLDH).....................................	857
	30.9	Differential Diagnoses: Subcortical Dementias..........		857
		30.9.1	Progressive Subcortical Gliosis (PSG).........	857
		30.9.2	Parkinson Disease with Dementia.............	857
	30.10	Differential Diagnoses: Rare Cortical Dementias........		857
		30.10.1	Chromosome 17-Associated Dementia.........	857
		30.10.2	Familial Presenile Dementia with Tangles (FPDT)............................	858
		30.10.3	Meso-Limbo-Cortical Dementia..............	858
	30.11	Differential Diagnoses: Down Syndrome..............		858
	30.12	Differential Diagnoses: Diffuse Neurofibrillary Tangles with Calcifications (DNTC)...................		859
	30.13	Differential Diagnoses: Rare Neurodegenerative Disorders..		859
		30.13.1	Thalamic Degeneration.....................	859
		30.13.2	(Non) Hereditary Bilateral Striatal Necrosis.....	860
		30.13.3	Neuroacanthocytosis........................	860
		30.13.4	Pallidal Degenerations......................	860
		30.13.5	Dentato-Rubro-Pallido-Luysi an Degeneration...	860
		30.13.6	Substantia Reticularis degeneration.............	861
	30.14	Differential Diagnoses: Argyrophilic Grain Disease (AG)..		861
	30.15	Differential Diagnoses: Adult Polyglucosan Body Disease (APBD)......................................		863
	30.16	Differential Diagnoses: Normal Pressure Hydrocephalus (NPH).................................		863
	30.17	Differential Diagnoses: Mitochondrial Encephalomyopathies.................................		864
		30.17.1	Clinical Signs of Mitochondrial Encephalopathies...........................	864
		30.17.2	Neuropathology Findings....................	864
	30.18	Differential Diagnoses: Metabolic and Traumatic Disorders..................................		866
		30.18.1	Hallervorden-Spatz Disease..................	866
		30.18.2	Leukodystrophies...........................	866

		30.18.3	Wilson Disease: Hepato-Lenticular Degeneration	867
		30.18.4	Dementia Pugilistica	867
	Selected References			867

31 Normal Aging Brain … 871
- 31.1 Introduction … 871
  - 31.1.1 WHO Definition of Well-Being … 871
- 31.2 Clinical Signs and Symptoms … 872
- 31.3 Epidemiology … 872
- 31.4 Neuroimaging Findings … 872
- 31.5 Neuropathology Findings … 874
- 31.6 Incidental White Matter Changes … 877
- 31.7 Molecular Neuropathology … 881
  - 31.7.1 Astrocytes … 882
  - 31.7.2 Microglia … 882
  - 31.7.3 Autophagy … 883
  - 31.7.4 Unfolded Protein Response (UPR): Endoplasmic Reticulum Stress—Stress Response Pathways … 883
  - 31.7.5 Mitochondria … 884
  - 31.7.6 Advanced Glycation End-Product (AGE) … 885
  - 31.7.7 cAMP Response Element Binding Protein (CREB) … 885
  - 31.7.8 Ion Channels and ROS … 885
  - 31.7.9 Sirtuins … 885
  - 31.7.10 Translocator Protein (TSPO) … 886
  - 31.7.11 Cathepsins … 886
  - 31.7.12 Ghrelin … 886
  - 31.7.13 Klotho … 886
  - 31.7.14 Iron … 886
  - 31.7.15 Insulin … 887
  - 31.7.16 Signaling … 887
- 31.8 Genetics of Successful Aging … 887
- 31.9 Non-coding RNAs … 888
- 31.10 DNA Damage … 890
- 31.11 Treatment and Prognosis … 890
- Selected References … 892

32 Neurodegenerative Diseases: Alzheimer Disease (AD) … 897
- 32.1 Clinical Signs and Symptoms … 897
- 32.2 International Working Group (IWG) Clinical Criteria … 897
- 32.3 Early-Onset AD Versus Late-Onset AD … 900
- 32.4 Neuroimaging Findings … 900
- 32.5 Neuropathology Findings … 903
- 32.6 The Proposed Diagnostic Criteria … 903
  - 32.6.1 Ball Criteria: The Hippocampal Criteria … 903
  - 32.6.2 Newcastle Criteria (Tomlinson, Roth, Blessed) … 915
  - 32.6.3 NIH Criteria (Khachaturian) … 915

		32.6.4	NINCDS-ADRA	916
		32.6.5	CERAD Criteria	917
		32.6.6	NIH/Reagan	918
	32.7	Staging of Neurofibrillary Tangle Development		919
	32.8	Phases of Aß-deposition by Thal et al. (2002)		923
	32.9	Molecular Neuropathology		923
		32.9.1	Genetics	923
		32.9.2	Aberrations in Mitochondrial DNA (mtDNA)	926
		32.9.3	Epigenetics	927
	32.10	Treatment and Prognosis		928
	Selected References			928
33	**Neurodegenerative Diseases: Lewy Body Dementia**			**933**
	33.1	Clinical Signs and Symptoms		933
	33.2	Epidemiology		933
	33.3	Neuroimaging Findings		935
	33.4	Neuropathology Findings		939
	33.5	Molecular Neuropathology		939
	33.6	Treatment and Prognosis		939
	Selected References			943
34	**Neurodegenerative Diseases: Fronto-temporal Lobar Degeneration**			**945**
	34.1	Clinical Signs and Symptoms		945
	34.2	Epidemiology		945
	34.3	Neuroimaging Findings		945
	34.4	Neuropathology Subgroups		953
	34.5	Types of FTLD		954
		34.5.1	Fronto-temporal Lobar Degeneration with TDP-43 Proteinopathy	954
		34.5.2	Fronto-temporal Lobar Degeneration with Motor Neuron Disease Type Inclusions	956
		34.5.3	Fronto-temporal Lobar Degeneration with *GRN* Mutation	958
		34.5.4	Fronto-temporal Lobar Degeneration with *VCP* Mutation	959
		34.5.5	Fronto-temporal Lobar Degeneration with *C9ORF* Mutation	959
		34.5.6	Fronto-temporal Lobar Degeneration with Ubiquitin-Positive Inclusions (FTLD/UPS)	960
		34.5.7	Fronto-temporal Lobar Degeneration with Tauopathy	960
		34.5.8	Pick Disease	960
		34.5.9	Cortico-basal Degeneration	962
		34.5.10	Progressive Supranuclear Palsy	962
		34.5.11	Argyrophilic Grain Disease	962
		34.5.12	Sporadic Multiple System Tauopathy with Dementia	962

		34.5.13	White Matter Tauopathy with Globular Glial Inclusions	964
		34.5.14	Tangle-Only Dementia	964
		34.5.15	Fronto-temporal Lobar Degeneration with *MAPT* Mutation	965
		34.5.16	Fronto-temporal Lobar Degeneration with FUS Proteinopathy	965
		34.5.17	Neuronal Intermediate Filament Inclusion Disease (NIFID)	966
		34.5.18	Basophilic Inclusion Body Disease (BIBD)	966
		34.5.19	Atypical Fronto-temporal Lobar Degeneration with Ubiquitin-Positive Inclusions (FTLD-U)	967
		34.5.20	Fronto-temporal Lobar Degeneration with No Inclusions	967
	34.6	Molecular Neuropathology		968
	34.7	Treatment and Prognosis		968
	Selected References			968
35	**Neurodegenerative Diseases: Progressive Supranuclear Palsy (PSP)–Cortico-Basal Degeneration (CBD)**			**973**
	35.1	Introduction		973
	35.2	Progressive Supranuclear Palsy (PSP)		973
		35.2.1	Clinical Signs	973
		35.2.2	Epidemiology	973
		35.2.3	Neuroimaging Findings	974
		35.2.4	Neuropathology Findings	976
		35.2.5	Molecular Neuropathology	978
		35.2.6	Treatment and Prognosis	978
	35.3	Cortico-Basal Degeneration (CBD)		978
		35.3.1	Clinical Signs	978
		35.3.2	Neuroimaging Findings	978
		35.3.3	Neuropathology Findings	981
		35.3.4	Molecular Neuropathology	984
		35.3.5	Treatment and Prognosis	984
	Selected References			984
36	**Neurodegenerative Diseases: Vascular Dementia**			**987**
	36.1	Introduction		987
	36.2	Clinical Signs and Symptoms		988
	36.3	Diagnostic Criteria		989
	36.4	Epidemiology		989
	36.5	Neuroimaging Findings		989
	36.6	Neuropathology Findings		991
	36.7	Leuko-araiosis		995
	36.8	Morbus Binswanger		995
	36.9	Cerebral Amyloid Angiopathy		995
	36.10	CADASIL		995
	36.11	Molecular Neuropathology		995
	36.12	Treatment and Prognosis		995
	Selected References			1000

37	**Neurodegenerative Diseases: Parkinson Disease** 1001
	37.1 Clinical Signs and Symptoms 1001
	37.2 Epidemiology................................... 1003
	37.3 Neuroimaging Findings 1003
	37.4 Neuropathology Findings.......................... 1007
	37.5 Molecular Neuropathology 1012
	37.5.1 Pathogenesis............................ 1012
	37.5.2 Genetics............................... 1013
	37.5.3 Epigenetics............................ 1017
	37.6 Treatment and Prognosis.......................... 1018
	Selected References 1019

38	**Neurodegenerative Diseases: Multiple System Atrophy (MSA)** 1021
	38.1 Introduction 1021
	38.2 Clinical Signs and Symptoms 1021
	38.3 Epidemiology................................... 1022
	38.4 Neuroimaging Findings 1022
	38.5 Neuropathology Findings.......................... 1027
	38.6 Molecular Neuropathology 1034
	38.7 Treatment and Prognosis 1034
	Selected References 1035

39	**Neurodegenerative Diseases: Motor Neuron Diseases**........ 1037
	39.1 Introduction 1037
	39.2 Clinical Signs and Symptoms 1037
	39.3 Diagnostic Criteria............................... 1037
	39.4 Epidemiology................................... 1039
	39.5 Neuroimaging Findings 1039
	39.6 Neuropathology Findings.......................... 1042
	39.7 Molecular Neuropathology 1045
	39.7.1 Pathogenetic Mechanisms 1045
	39.7.2 Genes................................. 1050
	39.8 Treatment and Prognosis 1055
	Selected References 1056

40	**Neurodegenerative Diseases: Huntington Disease** 1059
	40.1 Introduction 1059
	40.2 Clinical Signs and Symptoms 1059
	40.3 Epidemiology................................... 1059
	40.4 Neuroimaging Findings 1059
	40.5 Neuropathology Findings.......................... 1063
	40.6 Molecular Neuropathology 1065
	40.6.1 Genetics............................... 1067
	40.6.2 Epigenetics............................ 1067
	40.7 Treatment and Prognosis 1067
	Selected References 1067

Part VII The Brain Diseases: Myelin Disorders

41 Demyelinating Diseases: Multiple Sclerosis 1071
- 41.1 Introduction 1071
- 41.2 Clinical Signs and Symptoms 1071
- 41.3 Epidemiology 1073
- 41.4 Neuroimaging Findings 1073
- 41.5 Neuropathology Findings 1077
- 41.6 Molecular Neuropathology 1087
- 41.7 Treatment and Prognosis 1092
- Selected References 1093

42 Demyelinating Diseases: Neuromyelitis Optica Spectrum Disorder 1097
- 42.1 Clinical Signs and Symptoms 1097
- 42.2 Epidemiology 1098
- 42.3 Neuroimaging Findings 1098
- 42.4 Neuropathology Findings 1101
- 42.5 Molecular Neuropathology 1101
- 42.6 Treatment and Prognosis 1103
- Selected References 1103

43 Demyelinating Diseases: Acute Demyelinating Encephalomyelitis (ADEM) 1105
- 43.1 Introduction 1105
- 43.2 Clinical Signs and Symptoms 1105
- 43.3 Epidemiology 1105
- 43.4 Neuroimaging Findings 1105
- 43.5 Neuropathology Findings 1106
- 43.6 Molecular Neuropathology 1115
- 43.7 Treatment and Prognosis 1115
- Selected References 1115

Part VIII The Brain Diseases: The Epilepsies

44 Epilepsies: General Aspects 1119
- 44.1 Introduction 1119
- 44.2 Definitions 1119
- 44.3 Classification of the Epilepsies 1121
  - 44.3.1 International League Against Epilepsy (ILEA) Classification-1981 1121
  - 44.3.2 International League Against Epilepsy (ILEA) Classification-1989 1121
  - 44.3.3 International League Against Epilepsy (ILEA) Classification-2010 1122
  - 44.3.4 International League Against Epilepsy (ILAE) Classification-2017 1122
  - 44.3.5 International Classification of Diseases Classification (ICD)-2012 1123
  - 44.3.6 Electroclinical Syndromes 1123

	44.4	Neuroimaging Findings 1124
		44.4.1 Transient Seizure Related Imaging Features 1124
	44.5	Etiological Classification of Epilepsies 1129
	44.6	Neuropathological Lesions Associated with the Epilepsies 1129
	44.7	Molecular Neuropathology 1132
	44.8	Malformations Due to Genetic Changes 1135
	44.9	Treatment 1138
		Selected References 1139

45 Epilepsies: Temporal Lobe Epilepsy 1143
- 45.1 Introduction 1143
- 45.2 Clinical Signs 1143
- 45.3 Neuroimaging Findings 1143
- 45.4 Neuropathology Findings 1147
- 45.5 Molecular Neuropathology 1153
- 45.6 Treatment and Prognosis 1154
- Selected References 1154

46 Epilepsies: Malformations of Cortical Development—Focal Cortical Dysplasia (FCD) 1157
- 46.1 Introduction 1157
- 46.2 Neuroimaging Findings 1157
- 46.3 Neuropathology Findings 1158
- 46.4 Historical Classification 1165
- 46.5 Molecular Neuropathology 1168
- Selected References 1168

47 Epilepsies: Malformations of Cortical Development—Heterotopia 1171
- 47.1 Definition 1171
- 47.2 Neuroimaging Findings 1171
- 47.3 Neuropathology Findings 1171
  - 47.3.1 White Matter Heterotopia 1171
  - 47.3.2 Nodular Heterotopia 1175
  - 47.3.3 Periventricular Nodular Heterotopia 1176
  - 47.3.4 Subcortical Laminar Heterotopias 1178
- 47.4 Molecular Neuropathology 1179
- Selected References 1179

Part IX The Brain Diseases: Trauma and Intoxication

48 Trauma 1185
- 48.1 Definition 1185
- 48.2 Epidemiology 1185
- 48.3 Clinical Signs and Symptoms 1185
- 48.4 Classification of TBI 1186
- 48.5 Neuroimaging Findings 1192
  - 48.5.1 Cerebral Contusions 1192
  - 48.5.2 Chronic Traumatic Brain Injury 1192

	48.6	Focal Injuries 1196
	48.7	Diffuse Injuries 1207
	48.8	Chronic Traumatic Encephalopathy................... 1212
	48.9	Molecular Neuropathology 1214
	48.10	Treatment and Prognosis 1218
	Selected References 1220

49 Intoxication: Alcohol............................... 1223
  49.1 Introduction 1223
  49.2 Ethanol: Acute and Chronic Alcoholism 1223
     49.2.1 Clinical Signs and Symptoms 1223
     49.2.2 Epidemiology.............................. 1223
     49.2.3 Neuroimaging Findings 1224
     49.2.4 Neuropathology Findings.................... 1224
  49.3 Wernicke–Korsakoff Encephalopathy 1228
     49.3.1 Clinical Signs............................. 1228
     49.3.2 Neuroimaging Findings 1228
     49.3.3 Neuropathology Findings.................... 1230
     49.3.4 Molecular Neuropathology 1230
  49.4 Cerebellar Degeneration 1230
     49.4.1 Clinical Signs............................. 1230
     49.4.2 Neuropathology Findings.................... 1230
  49.5 Central Pontine Myelinolysis......................... 1233
     49.5.1 Clinical Signs............................. 1233
     49.5.2 Neuroimaging Findings 1233
     49.5.3 Neuropathology Findings.................... 1233
     49.5.4 Molecular Neuropathology 1233
  49.6 Marchiafava–Bignami Disease 1235
     49.6.1 Clinical Signs............................. 1235
     49.6.2 Neuroimaging Findings 1235
     49.6.3 Neuropathology Findings.................... 1238
  49.7 Fetal Alcohol Spectrum Disorders (FASD) 1238
     49.7.1 Clinical Signs............................. 1238
     49.7.2 Neuropathology Findings.................... 1239
     49.7.3 Molecular Neuropathology 1240
  Selected References 1240

50 Intoxication: Street Drugs 1243
  50.1 Introduction 1243
     50.1.1 General Aspects............................ 1243
     50.1.2 Clinical Signs and Symptoms 1243
     50.1.3 Neuroimaging Findings 1244
  50.2 Opiates.. 1244
     50.2.1 Neuroimaging Findings 1244
     50.2.2 Neuropathology Findings.................... 1245
     50.2.3 Molecular Neuropathology 1247
  50.3 Cocaine 1253
     50.3.1 Clinical Signs and Symptoms 1253
     50.3.2 Neuroimaging Findings 1254

		50.3.3	Neuropathology Findings. 1254

- 50.3.3 Neuropathology Findings. 1254
- 50.3.4 Molecular Neuropathology 1254
- 50.4 Cannabis. 1255
  - 50.4.1 CNS Complications of Cannabis 1255
  - 50.4.2 Neuroimaging Findings 1256
  - 50.4.3 Neuropathology Findings. 1256
  - 50.4.4 Molecular Neuropathology 1256
- 50.5 Amphetamine and Methamphetamine 1257
  - 50.5.1 Clinical Signs and Symptoms 1257
  - 50.5.2 Neuroimaging Findings 1257
  - 50.5.3 Neuropathology Findings. 1257
  - 50.5.4 Molecular Neuropathology 1257
- 50.6 Designer Drugs 1258
  - 50.6.1 Substances 1258
  - 50.6.2 Modes of Action. 1258
  - 50.6.3 Molecular Neuropathology 1259
  - 50.6.4 Outcome. 1259
- Selected References 1259

Volume III

Part X The Brain Diseases: Tumors

51 Tumors of the Nervous System: General Considerations 1263
- 51.1 Clinical Signs and Symptoms 1263
- 51.2 Definitions 1264
  - 51.2.1 Neuro-oncology. 1264
  - 51.2.2 Tumor. 1264
  - 51.2.3 Neoplasia 1264
  - 51.2.4 Brain Tumor. 1264
  - 51.2.5 Malignant Versus Benign 1264
  - 51.2.6 Seeding and Metastases 1264
  - 51.2.7 Various Modalities of Therapy. 1265
  - 51.2.8 Endpoints on Clinical Trials 1265
- 51.3 Histologic Tumor Characteristics 1266
  - 51.3.1 Cellularity 1266
  - 51.3.2 Anaplasia 1266
  - 51.3.3 Metaplasia 1266
  - 51.3.4 Pleomorphism 1266
  - 51.3.5 Mitoses. 1266
  - 51.3.6 Reactive Versus Neoplastic 1267
  - 51.3.7 Endothelial Proliferation and Neovascularity 1268
  - 51.3.8 Necrosis 1268
  - 51.3.9 Encapsulation and Invasion 1269
  - 51.3.10 Rosettes 1269
  - 51.3.11 Palisades and Pseudopalisades. 1270
  - 51.3.12 Desmoplasia. 1270
  - 51.3.13 Reactive Astrogliosis 1271
  - 51.3.14 Microglial Activation 1271

		51.3.15	Perivascular Lymphocytic Cuffing..............	1271
	51.4	WHO Classification of Tumors of the Central Nervous System....................................		1271
	51.5	Grading Systems for Brain Tumors....................		1273
		51.5.1	WHO Grading System......................	1273
		51.5.2	Kernohan et al. (1949).....................	1273
		51.5.3	Ringertz (1950)..........................	1273
		51.5.4	St. Anne/Mayo...........................	1274
		51.5.5	Smith Grading for Oligodendroglioma..........	1274
	51.6	Frequencies of Brain Tumors........................		1275
	51.7	Molecular Neuropathology: The Hallmarks of Cancer....		1275
	51.8	Molecular Neuropathology: Cell Cycle.................		1277
		51.8.1	The Cell Cycle in Normal Cells................	1277
		51.8.2	The Cell Cycle in Cancer Cells................	1280
	51.9	Molecular Neuropathology: DNA Damage Response.....		1281
		51.9.1	Mechanisms of DNA Damage Recognition.......	1281
		51.9.2	Mechanisms of DNA Damage Repair...........	1282
	51.10	Molecular Neuro-oncology: Oncogenes.................		1285
	51.11	Molecular Neuropathology: Tumor Suppressors.........		1286
	51.12	Molecular Neuropathology: Cell Death.................		1289
		51.12.1	Apoptosis................................	1289
		51.12.2	Autophagy...............................	1293
		51.12.3	Necroptosis..............................	1296
		51.12.4	Ferroptosis..............................	1296
		51.12.5	Pyroptosis...............................	1296
		51.12.6	Parthanatos..............................	1297
		51.12.7	NETosis.................................	1297
		51.12.8	Caspase-Independent Cell Death................	1297
	51.13	Molecular Neuropathology: Genomic Instability.........		1300
	51.14	Molecular Neuropathology: Signal Transduction Pathways..............................		1302
		51.14.1	PKC....................................	1305
	51.15	Molecular Neuropathology: Epigenetic Changes.........		1305
	51.16	Molecular Neuropathology: Telomeres and Telomerase...		1306
	51.17	Molecular Neuropathology: Angiogenesis..............		1306
		51.17.1	Features of Tumor Endothelial Cells............	1307
	51.18	Molecular Neuro-oncology: Glioma Invasion and Microenvironment..................................		1310
	51.19	Molecular Neuro-oncology: MicroRNAs...............		1315
	51.20	Molecular Neuro-oncology: Stem Cell Hypothesis........		1315
	51.21	Carcinogenic Agents................................		1317
	51.22	Common Molecular Changes in Brain Tumors..........		1318
	51.23	Treatment for Brain Tumors.........................		1325
	Selected References.....................................			1327
52	**Diffuse Astrocytoma WHO Grade II**..........................			**1333**
	52.1	Epidemiology.....................................		1333
	52.2	Neuroimaging Findings.............................		1334
	52.3	Neuropathology Findings...........................		1334

	52.4	Molecular Neuropathology 1344
		52.4.1 Pathogenesis............................. 1344
		52.4.2 Genetics................................. 1344
		52.4.3 Epigenetics.............................. 1344
		52.4.4 Gene Expression 1345
	52.5	Treatment and Prognosis 1345
		Selected References 1345

53 Anaplastic Astrocytoma WHO Grade III 1347
    53.1 Epidemiology.. 1348
    53.2 Neuroimaging Findings 1348
    53.3 Neuropathology Findings............................. 1352
    53.4 Molecular Neuropathology 1358
    53.5 Treatment and Prognosis 1358
    Selected References 1359

54 Glioblastoma 1361
    54.1 Epidemiology.. 1362
    54.2 Neuroimaging Findings 1362
    54.3 Neuropathology Findings............................. 1374
    54.4 Molecular Neuropathology 1389
          54.4.1 Pathogenesis............................. 1389
          54.4.2 Genetics................................. 1390
          54.4.3 Epigenetics.............................. 1395
          54.4.4 Gene Expression 1395
    54.5 Treatment and Prognosis 1398
          54.5.1 Treatment: State of the Art................. 1398
          54.5.2 Treatment: Historical Aspects 1399
    Selected References 1400

55 Gliosarcoma WHO Grade IV-Giant Cell Glioblastoma WHO Grade IV 1403
    55.1 Gliosarcoma WHO Grade IV.......................... 1403
          55.1.1 Epidemiology............................ 1403
          55.1.2 Neuroimaging Findings 1403
          55.1.3 Neuropathology Findings.................. 1406
          55.1.4 Molecular Neuropathology 1406
          55.1.5 Treatment and Prognosis 1410
    55.2 Giant Cell Glioblastoma WHO Grade IV 1410
          55.2.1 Epidemiology............................ 1411
          55.2.2 Neuroimaging Findings 1411
          55.2.3 Neuropathology Findings.................. 1411
          55.2.4 Molecular Neuropathology 1414
          55.2.5 Treatment and Prognosis 1414
    Selected References 1414

56 Gliomatosis Cerebri 1417
    56.1 Epidemiology.. 1417
    56.2 Neuroimaging Findings 1418
    56.3 Neuropathology Findings............................. 1421

	56.4	Molecular Neuropathology 1421
	56.5	Treatment and Prognosis 1421
	Selected References 1423

57 Pilocytic Astrocytoma WHO Grade I 1425
- 57.1 Epidemiology. 1425
- 57.2 Neuroimaging Findings 1426
- 57.3 Neuropathology Findings. 1426
- 57.4 Molecular Neuropathology 1435
  - 57.4.1 Pathogenesis. 1435
  - 57.4.2 Genetics 1435
  - 57.4.3 Epigenetics. 1436
- 57.5 Treatment and Prognosis 1436
- Selected References 1437

58 Oligodendroglioma WHO Grade II-Anaplastic Oligodendroglioma WHO Grade III. 1439
- 58.1 Oligodendroglioma WHO Grade II 1439
  - 58.1.1 Epidemiology. 1439
  - 58.1.2 Neuroimaging Findings 1440
  - 58.1.3 Neuropathology Findings. 1440
  - 58.1.4 Molecular Neuropathology 1446
  - 58.1.5 Treatment and Prognosis 1450
- 58.2 Anaplastic Oligodendroglioma WHO Grade III 1450
  - 58.2.1 Epidemiology. 1451
  - 58.2.2 Neuroimaging Findings 1451
  - 58.2.3 Neuropathology Findings. 1454
  - 58.2.4 Molecular Neuropathology 1454
  - 58.2.5 Treatment and Prognosis 1458
- Selected References 1458

59 Oligo-astrocytoma WHO Grade II-Anaplastic Oligo-astrocytoma WHO Grade III 1461
- 59.1 Oligo-astrocytoma WHO Grade II. 1461
  - 59.1.1 Epidemiology. 1461
  - 59.1.2 Neuroimaging Findings 1461
  - 59.1.3 Neuropathology Findings. 1464
  - 59.1.4 Molecular Neuropathology 1468
  - 59.1.5 Treatment and Prognosis 1468
- 59.2 Anaplastic Oligo-astrocytoma WHO Grade III 1468
  - 59.2.1 Epidemiology. 1469
  - 59.2.2 Neuroimaging Findings 1469
  - 59.2.3 Neuropathology Findings. 1469
  - 59.2.4 Molecular Neuropathology 1478
  - 59.2.5 Treatment and Prognosis 1478
- Selected References 1478

60 Ependymal Tumors. 1481
- 60.1 General Aspects 1481
  - 60.1.1 Clinical Signs and Symptoms 1481
  - 60.1.2 Nuclear Medicine Imaging Findings 1481

		60.1.3	Molecular Neuropathology	1481
	60.2	Ependymoma WHO Grade II		1483
		60.2.1	Epidemiology	1484
		60.2.2	Neuroimaging Findings	1484
		60.2.3	Neuropathology Findings	1486
		60.2.4	Treatment and Prognosis	1491
	60.3	Anaplastic Ependymoma WHO Grade III		1491
		60.3.1	Epidemiology	1492
		60.3.2	Neuroimaging Findings	1492
		60.3.3	Neuropathology Findings	1492
		60.3.4	Treatment and Prognosis	1497
	60.4	Myxopapillary Ependymoma (WHO Grade I)		1497
		60.4.1	Epidemiology	1498
		60.4.2	Neuroimaging Findings	1498
		60.4.3	Neuropathology Findings	1498
		60.4.4	Treatment and Prognosis	1499
	60.5	Subependymoma (WHO Grade I)		1502
		60.5.1	Epidemiology	1503
		60.5.2	Neuroimaging Findings	1503
		60.5.3	Neuropathology Findings	1503
		60.5.4	Treatment and Prognosis	1510
	Selected References			1510
61	**Choroid Plexus Tumors**			1513
	61.1	General Aspects		1513
		61.1.1	Epidemiology	1513
		61.1.2	Nuclear Medicine Imaging Findings	1513
		61.1.3	Differential Diagnosis	1514
		61.1.4	Molecular Neuropathology	1514
		61.1.5	Treatment and Prognosis	1514
	61.2	Choroid Plexus Papilloma WHO Grade I		1514
		61.2.1	Neuroimaging Findings	1515
		61.2.2	Neuropathology Findings	1515
	61.3	Atypical Choroid Plexus Papilloma (WHO Grade II)		1521
		61.3.1	Neuroimaging Findings	1522
		61.3.2	Neuropathology Findings	1522
	61.4	Choroid Plexus Carcinoma WHO Grade III		1522
		61.4.1	Neuroimaging Findings	1526
		61.4.2	Neuropathology Findings	1526
		61.4.3	Molecular Neuropathology	1526
	Selected References			1531
62	**Dysembryoplastic Neuroepithelial Tumor (DNT)**			1533
	62.1	Epidemiology		1533
	62.2	Neuroimaging Findings		1534
	62.3	Neuropathology Findings		1534
	62.4	Molecular Neuropathology		1537
	62.5	Treatment and Prognosis		1542

Selected References 1542

63 Desmoplastic (Infantile) Astrocytoma/Ganglioglioma (DIA/DIG) 1545
63.1 Epidemiology...................................... 1545
63.2 Neuroimaging Findings 1546
63.3 Neuropathology Findings........................... 1546
63.4 Molecular Neuropathology 1549
63.5 Treatment and Prognosis 1551
Selected References 1551

64 Ganglioglioma/Gangliocytoma 1553
64.1 Ganglioglioma 1553
    64.1.1 Epidemiology............................. 1554
    64.1.2 Neuroimaging Findings 1554
    64.1.3 Neuropathology Findings................... 1556
    64.1.4 Molecular Neuropathology 1558
    64.1.5 Treatment and Prognosis 1563
64.2 Anaplastic Ganglioglioma 1563
    64.2.1 Epidemiology............................. 1563
    64.2.2 Neuroimaging Findings 1564
    64.2.3 Neuropathology Findings................... 1564
    64.2.4 Molecular Neuropathology 1564
    64.2.5 Treatment and Prognosis 1565
Selected References 1565

65 Neurocytoma: Central—Extraventricular 1567
65.1 Epidemiology...................................... 1567
65.2 Neuroimaging Findings 1568
65.3 Neuropathology Findings........................... 1570
65.4 Molecular Neuropathology 1572
65.5 Treatment and Prognosis 1574
Selected References 1574

66 Rosette-Forming Glioneuronal Tumor (RGNT) 1575
66.1 Epidemiology...................................... 1575
66.2 Neuroimaging Findings 1575
66.3 Neuropathology Findings........................... 1579
66.4 Molecular Neuropathology 1583
66.5 Treatment and Prognosis 1583
Selected References 1584

67 Pineal Parenchymal Tumors 1587
67.1 General Aspects 1587
    67.1.1 Epidemiology............................. 1587
    67.1.2 Nuclear Medicine Imaging Findings 1587
    67.1.3 Differential Diagnosis 1587
    67.1.4 Molecular Neuropathology 1587
67.2 Pineocytoma....................................... 1588
    67.2.1 Neuroimaging Findings 1588

		67.2.2	Neuropathology Findings. 1591
		67.2.3	Treatment and Prognosis 1595
	67.3	Pineal Parenchymal Tumor of Intermediate Differentiation 1595	
		67.3.1	Neuropathology Findings. 1595
		67.3.2	Treatment and Prognosis 1597
	67.4	Pineoblastoma 1597	
		67.4.1	Neuroimaging Findings 1597
		67.4.2	Neuropathology Findings. 1599
		67.4.3	Treatment and Prognosis 1599
	Selected References 1601		
68	**Medulloblastoma** 1605		
	68.1	Epidemiology 1606	
	68.2	Neuroimaging Findings 1606	
	68.3	Neuropathology Findings. 1609	
	68.4	Molecular Neuropathology 1621	
		68.4.1	Pathogenesis. 1621
		68.4.2	Molecular Classification of Medulloblastomas . . . 1621
		68.4.3	Epigenetics. 1623
	68.5	Treatment and Prognosis 1623	
	Selected References 1626		
69	**Embryonal Tumors: Other CNS Embryonal Tumors** 1629		
	69.1	General Aspects 1629	
	69.2	CNS Embryonal Tumor, NOS 1630	
		69.2.1	Epidemiology 1631
		69.2.2	Neuroimaging Findings 1631
		69.2.3	Neuropathology Findings. 1631
		69.2.4	Molecular Neuropathology 1636
		69.2.5	Treatment and Prognosis 1636
	69.3	Embryonal Tumors with Multilayered Rosettes, C19MC-Altered 1636	
		69.3.1	Epidemiology 1636
		69.3.2	Neuropathology Findings. 1636
		69.3.3	Molecular Neuropathology 1638
		69.3.4	Treatment and Prognosis 1639
	69.4	Medulloepithelioma 1639	
		69.4.1	Epidemiology 1639
		69.4.2	Neuropathology Findings. 1639
		69.4.3	Molecular Neuropathology 1640
		69.4.4	Treatment and Prognosis 1640
	Selected References 1640		
70	**Embryonal Tumors: Atypical Teratoid/Rhabdoid Tumor (ATRT)** 1643		
	70.1	Epidemiology 1643	
	70.2	Neuroimaging Findings 1643	

	70.3	Neuropathology Findings. 1645
	70.4	Molecular Neuropathology 1648
	70.5	Treatment and Prognosis 1649
	Selected References 1649	

71 Tumors of the Peripheral Nervous System 1651

- 71.1 General Aspects 1651
  - 71.1.1 Clinical Signs and Symptoms 1651
  - 71.1.2 Classification of Tumors of the Peripheral Nervous System 1651
  - 71.1.3 Nuclear Medicine Imaging Findings 1652
- 71.2 Schwannoma 1654
  - 71.2.1 Epidemiology. 1654
  - 71.2.2 Neuroimaging Findings 1654
  - 71.2.3 Neuropathology Findings. 1657
  - 71.2.4 Molecular Neuropathology 1665
  - 71.2.5 Treatment and Prognosis 1665
- 71.3 Neurofibroma. 1665
  - 71.3.1 Epidemiology. 1665
  - 71.3.2 Neuroimaging Findings 1666
  - 71.3.3 Neuropathology Findings. 1666
  - 71.3.4 Molecular Neuropathology 1668
  - 71.3.5 Treatment and Prognosis 1670
- 71.4 Perineurioma 1670
  - 71.4.1 Epidemiology. 1672
  - 71.4.2 Neuroimaging Findings 1672
  - 71.4.3 Neuropathology Findings. 1674
  - 71.4.4 Molecular Neuropathology 1674
  - 71.4.5 Treatment and Prognosis 1674
- 71.5 Hybrid Nerve Sheath Tumors 1675
  - 71.5.1 Neuropathology Findings. 1675
- 71.6 Malignant Peripheral Nerve Sheath Tumor (MPNST) 1675
  - 71.6.1 Epidemiology. 1678
  - 71.6.2 Neuroimaging Findings 1678
  - 71.6.3 Neuropathology Findings. 1679
  - 71.6.4 Molecular Neuropathology 1681
  - 71.6.5 Treatment and Prognosis 1682
- 71.7 Neurofibromatosis Type 1 (NF1) 1682
  - 71.7.1 Incidence and Diagnostic Criteria 1682
  - 71.7.2 Neuroimaging Findings 1683
  - 71.7.3 Neuropathology Findings. 1683
  - 71.7.4 Molecular Neuropathology 1683
- 71.8 Neurofibromatosis Type 2 (NF2) 1683
  - 71.8.1 Incidence and Diagnostic Criteria 1686
  - 71.8.2 Neuroimaging Findings 1688
- 71.9 Schwannomatosis. 1688
  - 71.9.1 Incidence and Diagnostic Criteria 1688
- 71.10 Molecular Neuropathology 1688

71.10.1 Neurofibromatosis Type 1 (NF1) 1689
71.10.2 Neurofibromatosis Type 2 (NF2) 1689
71.10.3 Schwannomatosis 1690
71.10.4 Malignant Peripheral Nerve Sheath Tumor (MPNST) 1691
71.10.5 Epigenetics 1692
Selected References 1692

72 Tumors of Meningothelial Cells: Meningiomas 1695
72.1 Introduction 1695
72.2 General Aspects 1695
72.2.1 Clinical Signs and Symptoms 1695
72.2.2 Epidemiology 1695
72.2.3 Neuroimaging Features 1696
72.3 Meningioma 1705
72.3.1 Neuropathology Findings 1707
72.4 Atypical Meningioma 1727
72.4.1 Neuropathology Findings 1727
72.5 Anaplastic (Malignant) Meningioma 1729
72.5.1 Microscopic Features 1729
72.6 Common Neuropathology Aspects 1729
72.7 Molecular Neuropathology 1733
72.7.1 Pathogenesis 1733
72.7.2 Genetics 1733
72.7.3 Signaling Pathways 1733
72.7.4 Hh (Hedgehog) Pathway 1733
72.7.5 Wnt (Wingless) Pathway 1734
72.7.6 Chromosomal Aberrations and Mutations 1734
72.7.7 Epigenetics 1735
72.7.8 Gene Expression 1736
72.8 Treatment and Prognosis 1736
Selected References 1738

73 Tumors of the Sellar Region 1741
73.1 Classification of Tumors of the Sellar Region 1741
73.2 Craniopharyngioma 1741
73.2.1 Clinical Signs and Symptoms 1742
73.2.2 Epidemiology 1742
73.2.3 Neuroimaging Findings 1742
73.2.4 Neuropathology Findings 1743
73.2.5 Molecular Neuropathology 1752
73.2.6 Treatment and Prognosis 1753
73.3 Pituicytoma 1753
73.3.1 Epidemiology 1753
73.3.2 Neuroimaging Findings 1753
73.3.3 Neuropathology Findings 1754
73.3.4 Molecular Neuropathology 1755
73.3.5 Treatment and Prognosis 1755

		73.4	Granular Cell Tumor of the Sellar Region............. 1757
			73.4.1 Epidemiology............................. 1758
			73.4.2 Neuroimaging Findings..................... 1758
			73.4.3 Neuropathology Findings.................... 1758
			73.4.4 Molecular Neuropathology 1762
			73.4.5 Treatment and Prognosis 1762
		73.5	Spindle Cell Oncocytoma 1763
			73.5.1 Epidemiology............................. 1763
			73.5.2 Neuroimaging Findings..................... 1763
			73.5.3 Neuropathology Findings.................... 1763
			73.5.4 Molecular Neuropathology 1764
			73.5.5 Treatment and Prognosis 1764
		Selected References 1764

74 Tumors of the Pituitary Gland......................... 1767
    74.1 Epidemiology....................................... 1767
    74.2 Classification of Pituitary Tumors 1767
        74.2.1 Clinical Classification of Pituitary Tumors 1768
        74.2.2 Radiologic Classification of Pituitary Tumors.... 1768
    74.3 Radiological Features of Pituitary Tumors 1769
        74.3.1 Microadenoma............................. 1769
        74.3.2 Macroadenoma............................. 1770
    74.4 Neuropathology Classification of Pituitary Tumors 1774
        74.4.1 Historical Histological Classification
               of Pituitary Tumors 1774
        74.4.2 Immunohistochemical Classification
               of Pituitary Tumors 1774
    74.5 Molecular Neuropathology 1774
    74.6 Treatment... 1780
    74.7 Prognostic Clinicopathological Classification
        of Pituitary Tumors 1781
    74.8 Pituitary Adenomas 1781
        74.8.1 Somatotroph Adenoma...................... 1781
        74.8.2 Lactotroph Adenoma 1785
        74.8.3 Thyrotroph Adenoma....................... 1787
        74.8.4 Corticotroph Adenoma...................... 1789
        74.8.5 Gonadotroph Adenoma 1790
        74.8.6 Null Cell Adenoma 1792
        74.8.7 Plurihormonal and Double Adenoma........... 1794
    74.9 Atypical Pituitary Adenoma.......................... 1796
    74.10 Pituitary Carcinoma................................ 1798
        74.10.1 Clinical Signs and Symptoms 1798
        74.10.2 Epidemiology............................. 1798
        74.10.3 Neuroimaging Findings..................... 1798
        74.10.4 Neuropathology Findings.................... 1798
        74.10.5 Molecular Neuropathology 1800
        74.10.6 Prognosis 1800
    74.11 Pituitary Blastoma 1800

	74.11.1	Clinical Signs and Symptoms	1801
	74.11.2	Epidemiology	1801
	74.11.3	Neuropathology Findings	1801
	74.11.4	Molecular Neuropathology	1801
	74.11.5	Prognosis	1801

74.12 Apoplexia of the Pituitary 1802
    74.12.1 Clinical Signs and Symptoms 1802
    74.12.2 Epidemiology 1802
    74.12.3 Neuroimaging Findings 1802
    74.12.4 Neuropathology Findings 1802
    74.12.5 Molecular Neuropathology 1802
    74.12.6 Treatment and Prognosis 1805

Selected References 1808

75 Cystic Lesions 1811

75.1 Introduction 1811
75.2 General Aspects 1811
75.3 Epidermoid Cyst 1811
    75.3.1 Epidemiology 1811
    75.3.2 Neuroimaging Findings 1812
    75.3.3 Neuropathology Findings 1812
    75.3.4 Molecular Neuropathology 1817
    75.3.5 Treatment and Prognosis 1817
75.4 Dermoid Cyst 1817
    75.4.1 Epidemiology 1819
    75.4.2 Neuroimaging Findings 1821
    75.4.3 Neuropathology Findings 1821
    75.4.4 Molecular Neuropathology 1825
    75.4.5 Treatment and Prognosis 1825
75.5 Rathke's Cleft Cyst 1825
    75.5.1 Epidemiology 1825
    75.5.2 Neuroimaging Findings 1829
    75.5.3 Neuropathology Findings 1829
    75.5.4 Molecular Neuropathology 1833
    75.5.5 Treatment and Prognosis 1833
75.6 Colloid Cyst of the Third Ventricle 1833
    75.6.1 Epidemiology 1834
    75.6.2 Neuroimaging Findings 1834
    75.6.3 Neuropatholog Findings 1834
    75.6.4 Molecular Neuropathology 1838
    75.6.5 Treatment and Prognosis 1838
75.7 Enterogeneous cyst 1841
    75.7.1 Epidemiology 1841
    75.7.2 Neuroimaging Findings 1841
    75.7.3 Neuropathology Findings 1841
    75.7.4 Molecular Neuropathology 1844
    75.7.5 Treatment and Prognosis 1844
75.8 Arachnoidal Cyst 1845

	75.8.1	Epidemiology............................. 1845
	75.8.2	Neuroimaging Findings...................... 1845
	75.8.3	Neuropathology Findings.................... 1845
	75.8.4	Molecular Neuropathology 1849
	75.8.5	Treatment and Prognosis 1849
	Selected References 1851	

76 Germ Cell Tumors.. 1855
- 76.1 General Aspects 1855
  - 76.1.1 Epidemiology............................. 1855
  - 76.1.2 Nuclear Medicine Imaging Findings 1856
  - 76.1.3 Immunophenotype......................... 1856
  - 76.1.4 Differential Diagnosis 1857
  - 76.1.5 Molecular Neuropathology 1857
  - 76.1.6 Treatment and Prognosis 1857
- 76.2 Germinoma 1858
  - 76.2.1 Neuroimaging Findings...................... 1858
  - 76.2.2 Neuropathology Findings.................... 1858
- 76.3 Yolk Sac tumor..................................... 1861
  - 76.3.1 Neuropathology Findings.................... 1863
- 76.4 Embryonal Carcinoma................................ 1865
  - 76.4.1 Neuroimaging Findings...................... 1865
  - 76.4.2 Neuropathology Findings.................... 1865
- 76.5 Choriocarcinoma 1869
  - 76.5.1 Neuroimaging Findings...................... 1870
  - 76.5.2 Neuropathology Findings.................... 1870
- 76.6 Teratoma 1870
  - 76.6.1 Neuroimaging Findings...................... 1872
  - 76.6.2 Neuropathology Findings.................... 1874
- Selected References 1878

77 Lymphomas.. 1881
- 77.1 Introduction 1881
- 77.2 Primary CNS Lymphoma:............................. 1884
  - 77.2.1 Clinical Symptoms and Signs 1884
  - 77.2.2 Epidemiology............................. 1884
  - 77.2.3 Neuroimaging Findings...................... 1884
  - 77.2.4 Neuropathology Findings.................... 1885
  - 77.2.5 Molecular Neuropathology 1894
  - 77.2.6 Treatment and Prognosis 1903
- 77.3 Intravascular Lymphoma 1904
  - 77.3.1 Clinical Signs and Symptoms 1904
  - 77.3.2 Epidemiology............................. 1904
  - 77.3.3 Neuroimaging Findings...................... 1904
  - 77.3.4 Neuropathology Findings.................... 1904
  - 77.3.5 Molecular Neuropathology 1908
  - 77.3.6 Treatment and Prognosis 1908
- 77.4 Post-Transplant Lymphoproliferative Disorder (PTLD) ... 1909
  - 77.4.1 Epidemiology............................. 1909

		77.4.2	Neuroimaging Findings 1909

- 77.4.2 Neuroimaging Findings 1909
- 77.4.3 Neuropathology Findings. 1910
- 77.4.4 Molecular Neuropathology 1910
- 77.4.5 Treatment and Prognosis 1910
- 77.5 Plasmacytoma 1914
  - 77.5.1 Epidemiology............................... 1914
  - 77.5.2 Neuroimaging Findings 1915
  - 77.5.3 Neuropathology Findings. 1915
  - 77.5.4 Molecular Neuropathology 1920
  - 77.5.5 Treatment and Prognosis 1920
- Selected References 1920

78 Histiocytic Tumors 1923
- 78.1 General Considerations 1923
  - 78.1.1 Definitions 1923
  - 78.1.2 Epidemiology............................... 1923
  - 78.1.3 Nuclear Medicine Imaging Findings 1924
- 78.2 Langerhans Cell Histiocytosis (LCH) 1924
  - 78.2.1 Clinical Signs and Symptoms 1924
  - 78.2.2 Epidemiology............................... 1924
  - 78.2.3 Neuroimaging Findings 1925
  - 78.2.4 Neuropathology Findings. 1927
  - 78.2.5 Molecular Neuropathology 1930
  - 78.2.6 Treatment and Prognosis 1930
- 78.3 Non-Langerhans Cell Histiocytoses 1930
  - 78.3.1 Epidemiology............................... 1930
  - 78.3.2 Neuroimaging Findings 1931
  - 78.3.3 Neuropathology Findings. 1931
  - 78.3.4 Molecular Neuropathology 1934
  - 78.3.5 Treatment and Prognosis 1934
- Selected References 1941

79 Soft Tissue Tumors: Mesenchymal, Non-meningothelial Tumors 1943
- 79.1 General Aspects 1943
  - 79.1.1 Classification of Soft tissue tumors 1943
  - 79.1.2 Grading of Soft Tissue Tumors 1943
  - 79.1.3 Incidence 1944
  - 79.1.4 Pathogenesis............................... 1944
- 79.2 Solitary Fibrous Tumor/Hemangiopericytoma 1944
  - 79.2.1 Epidemiology............................... 1945
  - 79.2.2 Neuroimaging Findings 1945
  - 79.2.3 Neuropathology Findings. 1948
  - 79.2.4 Molecular Pathology 1952
  - 79.2.5 Treatment and Prognosis 1952
- 79.3 Hemangioblastoma 1956
  - 79.3.1 Epidemiology............................... 1956
  - 79.3.2 Neuroimaging Findings 1956
  - 79.3.3 Neuropathology Findings. 1959

		79.3.4	Molecular Pathology 1960

        79.3.5   Treatment and Prognosis 1961
  79.4 Lipoma. 1961
        79.4.1   Definition. 1961
        79.4.2   Neuroimaging Findings. 1962
        79.4.3   Neuropathology Findings. 1962
  79.5 Undifferentiated High-Grade Pleomorphic Sarcoma:
        Malignant Fibrous Histiocytoma (MFH). 1967
        79.5.1   Neuropathology Findings. 1967
  79.6 Other Mesenchymal Tumors 1967
        79.6.1   Hemangioma 1967
        79.6.2   Epithelioid Hemangioendothelioma 1967
        79.6.3   Angiosarcoma 1970
        79.6.4   Kaposi Sarcoma. 1970
        79.6.5   Ewing Sarcoma/Peripheral Primitive
                    Neuroectodermal Tumor 1970
        79.6.6   Angiolipoma 1972
        79.6.7   Hibernoma 1972
        79.6.8   Liposarcoma. 1972
        79.6.9   Desmoid-Type Fibromatosis 1972
        79.6.10 Myofibroblastoma 1972
        79.6.11 Inflammatory Myofibroblastic Tumor 1973
        79.6.12 Benign Fibrous Histiocytoma 1973
        79.6.13 Fibrosarcoma 1973
        79.6.14 Undifferentiated Pleomorphic
                    Sarcoma/Malignant Fibrous Histiocytoma 1973
        79.6.15 Leiomyoma 1973
        79.6.16 Leiomyosarcoma 1973
        79.6.17 Rhabdomyoma. 1974
        79.6.18 Rhabdomyosarcoma. 1974
  Selected References 1974

80 Bone Tumors 1977
  80.1 General Aspects of Bone Tumors 1977
        80.1.1   Classification of Bone tumors 1977
        80.1.2   Incidence 1977
        80.1.3   Nuclear Medicine Imaging Findings 1977
        80.1.4   Molecular Pathogenesis 1977
        80.1.5   Treatment and Prognosis 1984
  80.2 Osteoma. 1985
        80.2.1   Localization 1985
        80.2.2   Neuroimaging Findings. 1985
        80.2.3   Pathology Findings 1985
  80.3 Osteoid Osteoma 1986
        80.3.1   Localization 1986
        80.3.2   Neuroimaging Findings. 1986
        80.3.3   Pathology Findings 1987
  80.4 Osteoblastoma 1992

		80.4.1	Localization 1992

- 80.4.1 Localization 1992
- 80.4.2 Pathology Findings 1992
- 80.5 Osteosarcoma............................... 1992
  - 80.5.1 Localization 1992
  - 80.5.2 Imaging Findings....................... 1992
  - 80.5.3 Pathology Findings 1994
- 80.6 Chondroma................................. 1996
  - 80.6.1 Localization 1996
  - 80.6.2 Pathology Findings 1996
- 80.7 Chondrosarcoma 1998
  - 80.7.1 Localization 1998
  - 80.7.2 Imaging Findings....................... 1998
  - 80.7.3 Pathology Findings 2000
- 80.8 Fibrous Dysplasia........................... 2005
  - 80.8.1 Localization 2005
  - 80.8.2 Imaging Findings....................... 2005
  - 80.8.3 Pathology Findings 2005
- 80.9 Chordoma.................................. 2005
  - 80.9.1 Localization 2010
  - 80.9.2 Imaging Findings....................... 2010
  - 80.9.3 Pathology Findings 2010
- 80.10 Giant Cell Tumor........................... 2010
  - 80.10.1 Localization 2010
  - 80.10.2 Imaging Findings...................... 2014
  - 80.10.3 Pathology Findings 2014
- 80.11 Aneurysmal Bone Cyst 2016
  - 80.11.1 Localization 2017
  - 80.11.2 Imaging Findings...................... 2017
  - 80.11.3 Pathology Findings 2018
- Selected References 2020

81 Metastatic Tumors 2025
- 81.1 General Aspects 2025
  - 81.1.1 Epidemiology.......................... 2025
  - 81.1.2 Neuroimaging Findings 2025
  - 81.1.3 Neuropathology Findings................ 2038
  - 81.1.4 Histologic Features 2038
  - 81.1.5 Molecular Neuropathology 2041
  - 81.1.6 Treatment and Prognosis 2041
  - 81.1.7 Immunohistochemical Approach 2045
- 81.2 Lung Tumors 2051
  - 81.2.1 General Aspects 2051
  - 81.2.2 Neuropathology Findings................ 2051
  - 81.2.3 Immunophenotype...................... 2051
- 81.3 Breast Tumors 2051
  - 81.3.1 General Aspects 2051
  - 81.3.2 Neuropathology Findings................ 2051
  - 81.3.3 Immunophenotype...................... 2061

81.4	Skin Tumors: Melanoma		2061
	81.4.1	General Aspects	2064
	81.4.2	Neuropathology Findings	2064
	81.4.3	Immunophenotype	2070
81.5	Renal Tumors		2073
	81.5.1	General Aspects	2073
	81.5.2	Neuropathology Findings	2073
	81.5.3	Immunophenotype	2073
81.6	Urinary Tract Tumors		2073
	81.6.1	General Aspects	2073
	81.6.2	Neuroimaging Findings	2073
	81.6.3	Immunophenotype	2073
81.7	Prostate Tumors		2076
	81.7.1	General Aspects	2076
	81.7.2	Neuropathology Findings	2076
	81.7.3	Immunophenotype	2082
81.8	Testicular Tumors		2082
	81.8.1	General Aspects	2082
	81.8.2	Neuropathology Findings	2082
	81.8.3	Immunophenotype	2084
81.9	Gastro-Intestinal Tumors		2084
	81.9.1	General Aspects	2084
81.10	Colon Carcinoma		2085
	81.10.1	Neuropathology Findings	2085
	81.10.2	Immunophenotype	2085
81.11	Esophageal Carcinoma		2085
	81.11.1	Neuropathology Findings	2085
81.12	Gastric Carcinoma		2085
	81.12.1	Neuropathology Findings	2085
	81.12.2	Immunophenotype	2085
81.13	Liver Carcinoma		2085
	81.13.1	Neuropathology Findings	2085
	81.13.2	Immunophenotype	2085
81.14	Pancreas		2093
	81.14.1	Neuropathology Findings	2093
	81.14.2	Immunophenotype	2093
81.15	Female Genital Tract		2093
	81.15.1	General Aspects	2093
81.16	Ovarian Carcinoma		2093
	81.16.1	Neuropathology Findings	2095
	81.16.2	Immunophenotype	2099
81.17	Carcinoma of the Vagina and Cervix		2099
	81.17.1	Neuropathology Findings	2099
	81.17.2	Immunophenotype	2101
81.18	Uterine Carcinoma		2101
	81.18.1	Neuropathology Findings	2101
	81.18.2	Immunophenotype	2101
Selected References			2104

82	**Therapy-Induced Lesions**		2107
	82.1	Introduction	2107
	82.2	General Imaging Findings	2107
	82.3	Radiation Necrosis	2107
		82.3.1 Epidemiology	2108
		82.3.2 Neuroimaging Findings	2108
		82.3.3 Neuropathology Findings	2108
		82.3.4 Molecular Neuropathology	2114
		82.3.5 Treatment and Prognosis	2116
	82.4	Therapy-Induced Leukoencephalopathy	2116
		82.4.1 Clinical Signs	2116
		82.4.2 Neuroimaging Findings	2116
		82.4.3 Neuropathology Findings	2116
		82.4.4 Molecular Neuropathology	2117
	82.5	Therapy-Induced Secondary Neoplasms	2117
		82.5.1 Molecular Neuropathology	2117
	Selected References		2117
83	**Tumor Progression– Pseudoprogression**		2119
	83.1	Introduction	2119
	83.2	Neuroimaging Findings	2119
	83.3	Neuroimaging Criteria for Therapeutic Outcome	2122
		83.3.1 RANO Response Criteria for *Low-Grade Glioma*	2122
		83.3.2 The Immunotherapy Response Assessment in Neuro-Oncology (iRANO) Criteria	2125
	83.4	Nuclear Medicine Findings	2125
	83.5	Molecular Neuropathology	2125
	Selected References		2137
84	**Autoimmune Encephalitis: Paraneoplastic Syndromes**		2139
	84.1	Definitions	2139
	84.2	Epidemiology	2139
	84.3	Clinical Signs	2139
	84.4	Autoimmune Encephalitides	2142
		84.4.1 Limbic Encephalitis (LE)	2142
		84.4.2 Paraneoplastic Limbic Encephalitis (PLE)	2142
		84.4.3 NMDA-R Encephalitis	2142
		84.4.4 Voltage-Gated Potassium Antibody Syndromes	2143
		84.4.5 Morvan Syndrome	2145
		84.4.6 AMPAR (GluR1, GluR2) Antibody Syndrome	2145
		84.4.7 Glycine Receptor Antibody Syndrome	2146
		84.4.8 Dopamine 2 Receptor Antibody Syndrome (D2RA)	2146
		84.4.9 GABA Receptor Ab Syndrome	2146
		84.4.10 Metabotropic Glutamate Receptor Antibody Syndrome	2147
		84.4.11 IgLON5 Ab Syndrome	2147

	84.5	Neuroimaging Findings 2148
		84.5.1 General Imaging Findings 2148
	84.6	Neuropathology Findings............................ 2148
	84.7	Molecular Neuropathology 2151
		84.7.1 Predisposition to Autoimmunity 2153
	84.8	Treatment and Prognosis 2155
	Selected References 2164

**Appendix A: WHO Classification of Tumors of the
Central Nervous System................................ 2167**

Appendix B: WHO Classification of Tumors 2181

References 2209

Index... 2215

About the Authors

Serge Weis is the head of the Division of Neuropathology at the Neuromed Campus of the Kepler University Hospital, Johannes Kepler University, Linz, Austria. He is a native of Luxembourg and studied medicine at the University of Vienna (Austria). He was trained in neuropathology at the Ludwig Maximilians University, Munich, Germany. He was deputy director at the Department of Neuropathology, Otto von Guericke University Magdeburg, (Germany) and director of neuropathology at the Stanley Medical Research Institute, Bethesda, MD, USA. His scientific interests are focused on brain tumors, neurodegeneration, and biological psychiatry. He edited the largest book in German-speaking countries on Alzheimer disease and wrote a book, published in 1993, on 3D reconstruction of the brain (serge.weis@kepleruniklinikum.at).

Michael Sonnberger is a senior consultant in neuroradiology at the Department of Neuroradiology of the Neuromed Campus of the Kepler University Hospital, Johannes Kepler University, Linz, Austria. He studied medicine at the University of Innsbruck (Austria) and was trained in radiology/neuroradiology at the University of Regensburg (Germany) and at the State Neuropsychiatric Hospital Wagner-Jauregg, Linz, Austria. His fields of expertise are interventional neuroradiology and stroke (michael.sonnberger@kepleruniklinikum.at).

Andreas Dunzinger is a senior consultant in nuclear medicine at the Department of Nuclear Medicine of the Neuromed Campus of the Kepler University Hospital, Johannes Kepler University, Linz, Austria. He studied medicine at the University of Vienna (Austria). He was trained as a general physician at the Hospital of the Sisters of Mercy, Linz, Austria, and in nuclear medicine at the Medical University of Graz and at the State Neuropsychiatric Hospital Wagner-Jauregg, Linz, Austria. His field of expertise is neuronuclear medicine and neuroendocrinology (andreas.dunzinger@kepleruniklinikum.at).

Eva Voglmayr is a trainee in radiology and neuroradiology at the Department of Neuroradiology of the Neuromed Campus of the Kepler University Hospital, Johannes Kepler University, Linz, Austria. She studied medicine at the University of Vienna. Her field of interest is neurodegeneration (eva.voglmayr@kepleruniklinikum.at).

Martin Aichholzer is deputy head of the Department of Neurosurgery at the Neuromed Campus of the Kepler University Hospital, Johannes Kepler University, Linz, Austria. He studied medicine at the University of Vienna and was trained at the Department of Neurosurgery of the Medical University of Vienna (Austria). His field of expertise is skull base surgery (martin.aichholzer@kepleruniklinikum.at).

Raimund Kleiser is a medical physicist and is the head of the imaging center at the Institute of Neuroradiology at the Kepler University Hospital in Linz. He studied physics in Freiburg im Breisgau (Germany) and supplemented his training with the specialization in medical physics. His focus is on functional imaging, for which he established fMRT measuring equipment in prestigious institutions in Germany, Switzerland, and Austria (Raimund.kleiser@kepleruniklinikum.at).

Peter Strasser is molecular biologist at the PMU University Institute for Medical & Chemical Laboratory Diagnostics of the Paracelsus Medical University in Salzburg, Austria. He studied general biology at the University of Salzburg and specialized in biochemistry and molecular genetics. Dr. Strasser's current focus of interest lies in the genetic background of neurological diseases (p.strasser@salk.at).

Part VI

The Brain Diseases: Aging and Neurodegeneration

Neurodegeneration: General Aspects

30.1 Introduction

Neurodegenerative disorders are complex, and heterogeneity is the rule, rather than the exception, even within a single disease entity (Lantos 1992).

30.2 Clinical Signs and Symptoms

A clinical classification of neurodegenerative diseases can be done as follows:
- Predominantly cognitive symptoms
- Predominantly motor symptoms

A further subclassification is done as follows:
- Predominantly cognitive symptoms
  - Amnestic
    - Alzheimer dementia
  - Executive functions
    - Non-Alzheimer dementia
      - Fronto-temporal dementia complex
        - FTD-tau, i.e., Pick disease, cortico-basal degeneration, progressive supranuclear palsy
        - FTD-ubiquitin
      - Synucleinopathies
        - Lewy body dementia
        - Multi-system atrophy
        - Dementia in Parkinson disease
- Predominantly motor symptoms
  - Movement disorder
    - Parkinson disease
    - Trinucleotide repeat disorder
      - Friedreich ataxia
      - Huntington disease
      - Spinocerebellar ataxia
  - Ataxia
    - Trinucleotide repeat disorder
      - Friedreich ataxia
      - Huntington disease
      - Spinocerebellar ataxia
  - Weakness
    - Motor neuron disease

Clinical features of neurodegenerative disorders include:
- Clinical course.
  - chronic
  - progressive until death
- Not reversible.
- High phenotypical variability.
- Major risk factor is advancing age.
- Heritable in a small percentage of cases.
  - Onset occurs a decade earlier than in sporadic forms.
- Different clinical manifestations are mediated by dysfunction of different anatomical regions.
- More than one disease may exist in one patient.

- Genetics:
  - Diverse clinical phenotypes share similar genotypes.
  - Similar phenotypes are associated with a variety of genotypes.

30.2.1 Dementia

Most frequent cases of dementia are (Table 30.1):
- Alzheimer disease
- Dementia with Lewy bodies
- Fronto-temporal dementia
  - Behavioral variant fronto-temporal dementia
  - Primary progressive aphasia
  - Non-fluent/agrammatic variant primary progressive aphasia
  - Semantic variant primary progressive aphasia
  - Logopenic variant primary progressive aphasia
- Cortico-basal degeneration and progressive supranuclear palsy
  - Cortico-basal degeneration
  - Progressive supranuclear palsy
- Rapidly progressive dementia

Table 30.1 Causes of dementia

Disease group	Disease entity
Neurodegenerative disorders	• Alzheimer disease • Lewy body dementia • Fronto-temporal dementia • Pick disease • Parkinson disease • Multi-system atrophy • Huntington disease • Progressive supranuclear palsy (PSP) • Cortico-basal degeneration • ALS-parkinsonism-dementia complex of Guam • Neuroaxonal dystrophy
Cerebrovascular	• Multi-infarct dementia • Binswanger disease • Cerebral amyloid angiopathy • Cranial arteritis • Other cranial angiitis • Ischemia following rupture of aneurysma
Infectious–inflammatory	• Neurosyphilis • Lyme disease • Chronic meningitides • Postencephalitic • Limbic encephalitis (paraneoplastic) • Progressive multifocal leukoencephalopathy (PML) • Multiple sclerosis • Acquired immune deficiency syndrome (AIDS) • Whipple disease
Prion-encephalopathies	• Creutzfeldt–Jakob disease • Creutzfeldt–Jakob disease, new variant • Gerstmann–Sträussler–Scheinker syndrome • Kuru • Fatal familial insomnia
Autoimmune diseases	• Multiple sclerosis • Primary CNS angiitis • Lupus and other vasculitides • Sarcoid

Table 30.1 (continued)

Toxic–metabolic	• Alcohol • Hypo-/hyperthyroidism • Hypoglycemia • Chronic hepatic encephalopathy • Chronic uremia • Dialysis • Vitamin B12 deficiency • Pellagra • Malabsorption syndrome • Wilson disease • Metachromatic/adrenoleukodystrophy • GM_2 and other gangliosidoses • Pantothenate kinase deficiency • Metals (arsenic, thallium, lead, manganese) • Industrial agents (CCl_4, Cs_2, TCE, organophosphides) • Radiation encephalopathy
Drug induced–toxic	• Polypharmacy • Anticholinergic • Levodopa • Anticonvulsive • Barbiturates • Neuroleptics
Trauma	• Diffuse and/or focal trauma • Chronic subdural hematoma • Diffuse axonal injury • Dementia pugilistica
Hydrocephalus	• Normal pressure hydrocephalus • Aqueduct stenosis
Brain tumors	• Any neuroglial tumor • Metastases • Paraneoplastic encephalitis • Disseminated intravascular lymphoma
Mitochondrial encephalomyopathies	• KSS: Kearns-Sayre syndrome • MERRF: myoclonus epilepsy with ragged-red fibers • MELAS: mitochondrial encephalopathy, lactate, acidosis, and stroke-like episodes
Rare neurodegenerative disorders	• Thalamic degeneration • (Non) hereditary bilateral striatal necrosis • Neuroacanthocytosis • Pallidal degeneration including • Pure pallidal degeneration • Pallido-luysian degeneration • Pallido-nigral degeneration • Pallido-nigro-luysian degeneration • Pallido-nigro-spinal degeneration • Dentato-rubro-pallido-nigral degeneration • Dentato-rubro-pallido-luysian degeneration • Substantia reticularis Degeneration • Argyrophilic grain dementia • Adult polyglucosan body disease (APBD)

Table 30.2 Classification of movement disorders

Clinical sign	Disease entity
Akinetic-rigid forms	• Parkinsonism: Parkinson disease, Parkinsonian syndrome • Stiff-person syndrome
Hyperkinetic forms	• Chorea syndromes • Tremor syndromes • Dystonias • Myoclonus • Ballism • Tics
Atactic movement disorders	• Cerebellar ataxias • Spinocerebellar degeneration
Motor neuron disorders	• Motor neuron disease • Spinal muscular atrophy and related disorders

Table 30.3 Classification of neurodegenerative parkinsonian disorders by predominant protein pathology

Synucleinopathies	• Parkinson disease • Multiple system atrophy • Dementia with Lewy bodies
Tauopathies	• Cortico-basal degeneration • Progressive supranuclear palsy (PSP) • Fronto-temporal dementia and parkinsonism linked to chromosome 17 • Postencephalic parkinsonism • Dementia pugilistica • Parkinsonism-dementia complex of Guam • Pantothenate kinase-associated neurodegeneration

30.2.2 Motor Disorders

The classification of movement disorders based on clinical and molecular aspects is outlined in Tables 30.2 and 30.3.

30.3 Neuropathologic Changes

30.3.1 Gross-anatomical Changes

Gross-anatomical features of neurodegenerative disorders include:
- Reduced brain weight
- Signs of atrophy with (Fig. 30.1a–f)
    - Widening of the sulci
    - Thinning of the gyri
- Enlargement of the ventricular system (Fig. 30.1g, h)

30.3.2 Microscopical Changes

Histologic features of neurodegenerative disorders include:
- Formation of abnormal structures
    - Extracellular location:
        ○ Amyloid deposits (Fig. 30.2a–n)
    - Intracellular location:
        ○ Intraneuronal (neurofibrillary tangle (NFT)) (Fig. 30.3a–j)
        ○ Intracytoplasmic (Pick body, Lewy body) (Fig. 30.4a–d)
        ○ Oligodendroglial (Papp-Lantos body)
        ○ Other inclusions (Figs. 30.5a–d and 30.6a–d)
- Loss of neurons
- Loss of synapses
- Glial changes
- Vascular changes

Neurodegenerative disorders are characterized by selective vulnerability of specific neuronal and transmitter-related systems (Table 30.4) (Byrne et al. 2011).

30.3.3 Amyloid Deposits

The following types of amyloid deposits can be described (Fig. 30.2a–n):
- Parenchymal deposits
    - Stellate deposits
    - Diffuse deposits
    - Focal deposits
        ○ Neuritic plaque
        ○ Primitive plaque
        ○ Compact plaque
    - Fleecy, lake-like deposits
    - Subpial deposits
- Cotton whool and inflammatory plaques
- Intracellular deposits
- Perivascular deposits

30.3 Neuropathologic Changes

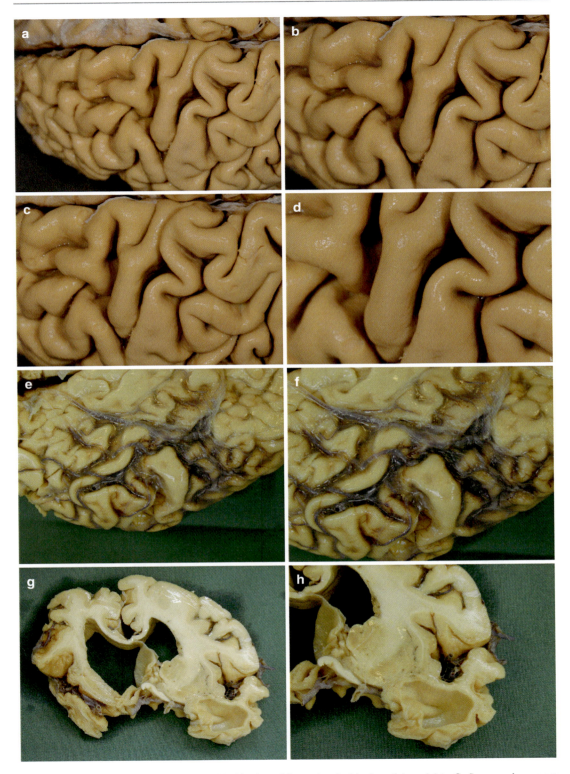

Fig. 30.1 Atrophy of the cerebral cortex with thinning of the gyri and widening of the sulci (**a–f**). Severe enlargement of the ventricular system (**g, h**)

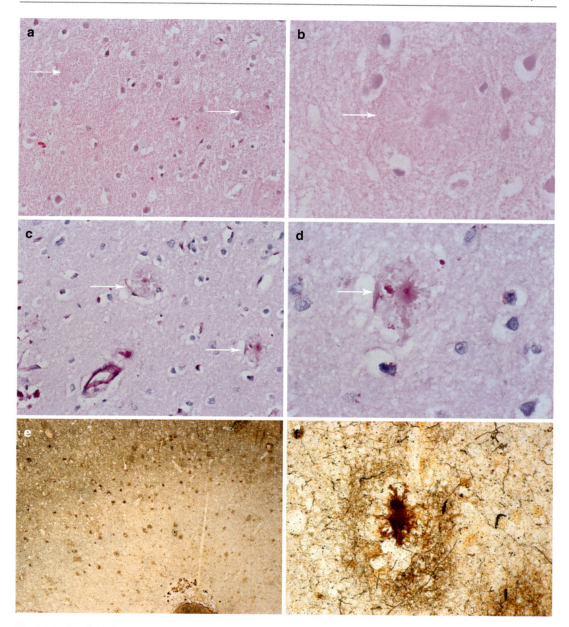

Fig. 30.2 Amyloid deposits (**a–n**). Amyloid plaques are seldom seen with classical stains (→) (**a–d**: **a, b**: H&E stain; **c, d**: PAS stain). Amyloid plaques as seen with silver impregnation techniques (**e, f**: Bileschowski stain). Classical plaque with central core and halo (**g, h**: immunohistochemistry for ß-A4 amyloid), diffuse plaques (**i, j**: immunohistochemistry for ß-A4 amyloid), subpial amyloid deposits (**k, l**: immunohistochemistry for ß-A4 amyloid), neuritic plaque (**m**; immunohistochemistry for ubiquitin), perivascular amyloid deposits (**n**: immunohistochemistry for ß-A4 amyloid)

30.3 Neuropathologic Changes

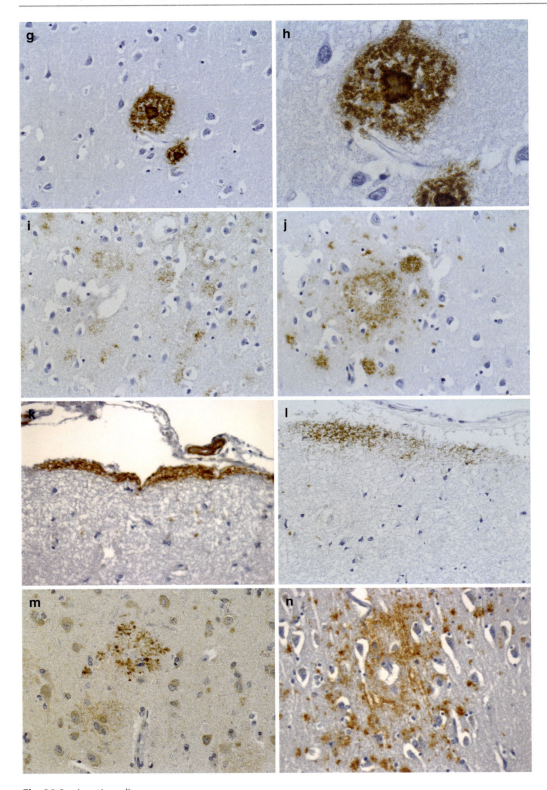

Fig. 30.2 (continued)

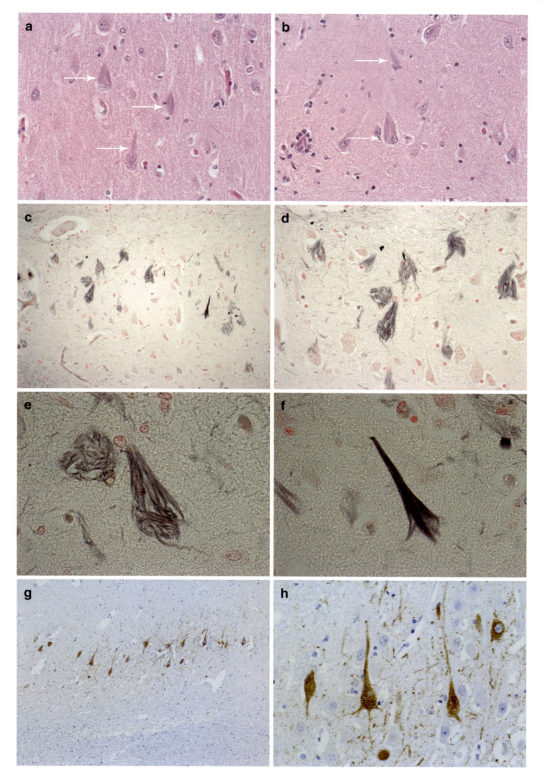

Fig. 30.3 Neurofibrillary tangles (NFTs) (**a–j**). NFTs are seldom seen using H&E stain (→) (**a**, **b**). NFTs visualized with Gallyas silver impregnation technique (**c–f**) and with immunohistochemistry for phosphorylated tau (**g–j**)

30.3 Neuropathologic Changes

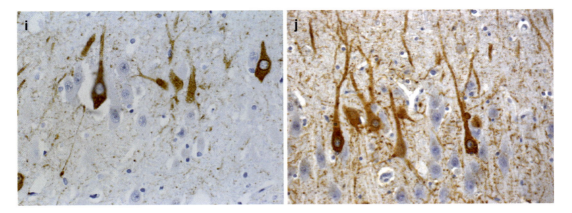

Fig. 30.3 (continued)

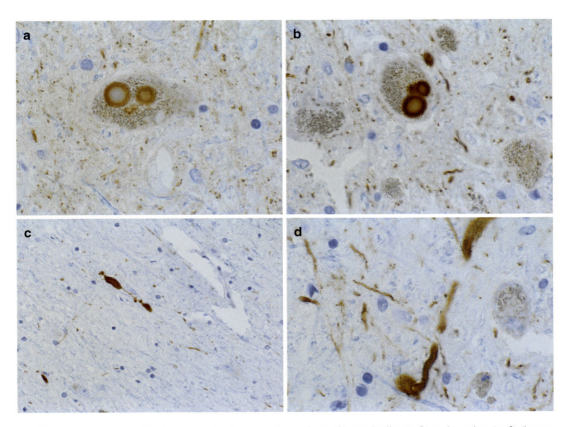

Fig. 30.4 α-synuclein-positive inclusions (**a–d**) as seen in the form of Lewy bodies (**a, b**) and neurites (**c, d**) (immunohistochemistry for α-synuclein)

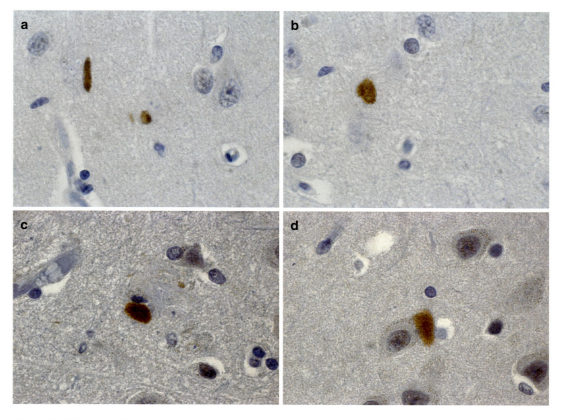

Fig. 30.5 TDP-43-positive inclusions (**a–d**) as seen in fronto-temporal lobe dementia (immunohistochemistry for TDP-43)

- Vascular deposits
  - Angiopathy with capillary involvement (Thal type 1)
  - Angiopathy without capillary involvement (Thal type 2)

Parenchymal deposits—stellate deposits
- small
- irregular
- located at distance from cell bodies
- probably related to astrocytes

Parenchymal deposits—diffuse deposits
- blurred boundaries
- usually large size (50–300 µm)
- absence of neuritis
- microglia
- occur at an early stage of the disease

Parenchymal deposits—focal deposits
- Dense spherical accumulation
  - Neuritic plaque (classical plaque)
    ○ focal deposit as the core of the plaque
    ○ clear halo surrounds core
    ○ light diffuse zone
    ○ neuritic fibers
    ○ surrounded by astrocytes and microglia
  - Primitive plaque
    ○ small and large accumulations of dystrophic neurites without core
  - Compact plaque
    ○ often composed of amyloid only (burnt out plaque)

Parenchymal deposits—fleecy, lake-like deposits

- blurred, ill-defined clouds of amyloid
- the internal layers (pri-alpha, pri-beta, and pri-gamma) of the entorhinal cortex

30.3 Neuropathologic Changes

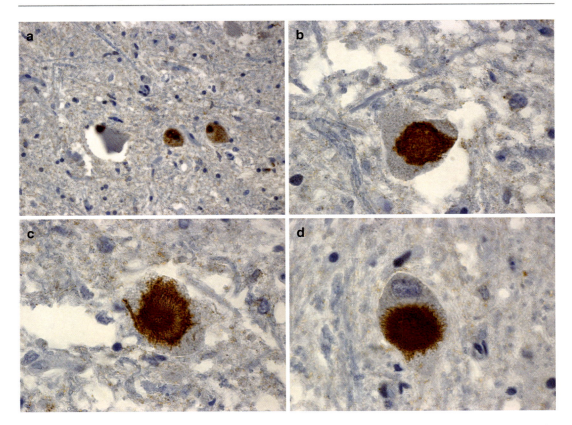

Fig. 30.6 FUS-positive inclusions (**a–d**) as seen in amyotrophic lateral sclerosis (ALS) (immunohistochemistry for FUS)

Table 30.4 Selective vulnerability in neurodegenerative disorders

Disease	Vulnerable neuron
Parkinson disease	Dopaminergic neurons
Amyotrophic lateral sclerosis	Upper and lower motor neurons
Huntington disease	GABA-ergic neurons
Fronto-temporal dementia	Fronto-temporal cortical neurons
Alzheimer disease	Cholinergic neurons

Parenchymal deposits—subpial deposits
- diffuse deposit
- in the subpial region of the isocortex

Cotton whool plaques
- focal deposits of Aß
- identifiable on H&E stained sections
- round homogeneous eosinophilic structures
- made up of Aß42
- not congophilic

Inflammatory plaques
- strong microglial and astrocytic reaction
- amyloid core without Ab reactivity

Intracellular deposits
- intracytoplasmatic

Perivascular deposits
- located at the border of perivascular Robin-Virchow spaces

Vascular deposits
- Angiopathy with capillary involvement (Thal type 1)
- Angiopathy without capillary involvement (Thal type 2)

Within and around amyloid deposits as well as in axonal ending the following neurotransmitter-positive fibers are found:

- Serotonin
- Dopamin
- Somatostatin
- Substance P
- Cholecystokinin
- Neuropeptid Y
- Encephalin
- Vasointestinal peptide (VIP)
- Acetylcholinesterase
- others

Extracellular amyloid is made up of straight fibrils with a diameter of 10 nm. They contain epitopes of paired helical filaments (PHF), tau-protein, microtubule-associated protein-1 (MAP-1), and ubiquitin.

30.3.4 Neurofibrillary Changes: Tauopathies

Neurofibrillary changes include (Fig. 30.3a–j):
- Neurofibrillary tangles (NFT)
- Neuropil threads (see Sect. 30.3.5)

Disorders associated with the presence of *neurofibrillary tangles* (*NFT*)
- Normal aging
- Alzheimer disease
- Progressive supranuclear palsy (PSP)
- Dementia pugilistica
- Subacute sclerosing panencephalitis (SSPE)
- Niemann-Pick disease
- Pb intoxication
- Guam-Parkinson-dementia complex
- Down syndrome
- Postencephalitic parkinsonism
- Myotonic dystrophy
- Congenital muscle dystrophy
- Kufs disease
- Cockayne syndrome
- Hallervorden-Spatz disease
- Gertsmann–Sträussler–Scheinker syndrome
- Dementia with NFT and calcifications

Neurofibrillary tangles are
- Bands of abnormal filamentous material
- Within the perikaryon of neurons
- Extend into the dendrites and axons
- Flame-shaped
- Bundles of fibrils
  - Fibril made from a pair of helically wound filaments, 10–12 nm in diameter, with a periodicity of 160 nm (paired helical filaments)
- Mixed with 10 nm neurofilaments and 15 nm thick filaments
- Neurofilaments are
  - Negative for neurofilament protein and tubulin
  - Positive for tau
- Immunophenotype, positivities for
  - Tau
  - Phosphorylated tau
  - Tau 3R
  - Tau 4R
  - Ubiquitin

Tau is a phosphoprotein containing a tubule-binding domain comprised of three or four repeat regions (tau 3 R and 4 R) depending on the splicing of the RNA.

Tau immunoreactivities can be chararcterized as follows:
- Neuronal cytoplasm
  - Pre-tangle
  - Neurofibrillary tangle (NFT)
  - Pick body
  - Spherical inclusion
  - Other forms
- Neuronal processes
  - Dystrophic neurites
  - Grains
  - Threads
- Astrocytes
  - Tufted astrocyte
  - Astrocytic plaque
  - Thorn-shaped astrocyte
  - Ramified astrocyte

- Globular astroglial inclusions (GAIs)
  - Other types
- Oligodendrocytes
  - Coiled body
  - Globular oligodendroglial inclusions (GOI)

Tauopathies include the following disease entities:
- Pick disease
- Progressive supranuclear palsy (PSP)
- Cortico-basal degeneration (CBD)
- Argyrophilic grain disease
- Neurofibrillary tangle-only dementia
- Globular glial tauopathies
- Tauopathy associated with FTD-17*MAPT*
- Alzheimer disease
- Down syndrome
- Tauopathy in the elderly brain
- Tauopathy in Lewy body disorders
- Tauopathy in chronic traumatic encephalopathy
- Tauopathy in *C9orf72* repeat carriers
- Tauopathy in prion diseases
- Diffuse neurofibrillary tangles with calcification
- Tauopathy in familial British dementia and familial Danish dementia
- Tauopathy in neurodegeneration with brain iron accumulation
- Tauopathy in Niemann-Pick disease type C
- Tauopathy in postencephalic parkinsonism
- Tauopathy in Guadeloupean parkinsonism
- Tauopathy in parkinsonism-dementia complex of Guam
- Tauopathy in subacute sclerosing panencephalitis
- Tauopathy in *SLC9A6* gene-related mental retardation
- Tauopathy in myotonic dystrophy
- Unclassifiable tauopathies

30.3.5 Neuropil Threads

Neuropil threads are:
- small, fragmented, tortuous processes
- weaving between cell bodies
- contain paired helical filaments
- occur at an early stage of neurofibrillary degeneration
- occur in dendrites (apical and basal)
- devoid in axons or glial processes
- located in gray matter of isocortex and allocortex
- first described by Braak and Braak (1988)

30.3.6 Lewy Bodies

Intracytoplasmic inclusion (Fig. 30.4a–d)

Morphologic hallmark of:
- Parkinson disease
- Lewy body dementia (LBD)

Disorders associated with the presence of *Lewy bodies*
- Multi-system atrophy
- Progressive supranuclear palsy
- Cortico-basal degeneration
- Motor neuron disease
- Hallervorden-Spatz disease
- Neuroaxonale dystrophy
- Ataxia telangiectasia
- Subacute sclerosing panencephalitis (SSPE)
- Sporadic Alzheimer disease
- Familial Alzheimer disease
- Down syndrome
- Postpartum

Two types of Lewy bodies are distinguished:
- Classic brain stem LB
- Cortical type LB

Classical brain stem type LB
- Spherical intracytoplasmic neuronal inclusion
- 8–30 μm in diameter
- Hyaline eosinophilic core
- Concentric lamellar bands
- Narrow pale-stained halo
- Ultrastructure:
  - Non-membrane-bound, granulofilamentous structures
  - Composed of radially arranged 7–20 nm intermediate filaments
  - Electron-dense, granular material
  - Vesicular structures

Cortical type LB
- Eosinophilic round structure
- Angular to reniform shape possible
- Lack a halo
- Ultrastructure:
  - Poorly organized granulofibrillary structures
  - Composed of 7–27 nm wide filaments
  - Lack of central core

Immunohistochemical positivity for:
- α-synuclein
- Ubiquitin
- Phosphorylated neurofilaments
- Parkin
- Synphilin-1

Neurodegenerative diseases with concomitant Lewy bodies and/or α-synuclein pathology

- Alzheimer disease
- Down syndrome
- Progressive supranuclear palsy
- Cortico-basal degeneration
- Fronto-temporal dementia
- Essential tremor
- Parkinson-dementia complex of Guam
- Amyotrophic lateral sclerosis
- Dopa-responsive dystonia
- Adult polyglucosan body disease
- Neurodegeneration with iron accumulation due to mutations of the *PLA2G6* gene

30.3.7 Granulovacuolar Degeneration

- First described by Simchowicz (1911)
- Neurons contain 3–5 μm large vacuoles with 1–2 μm dense cores
- Ultrastructure: membrane-bound vacuole with central core (Hirano et al. 1968a, b)

Granulovacuolar degeneration is found in:
- elderly persons
- patients with Down syndrome and Alzheimer disease
- increase with age
- neurons, i.e., pyramidal neurons in the CA regions if the hippocampus
- less frequently anterior olfactory region, basal nucleus Meynert, supraoptic nucleus, amygdala, cingulate gyrus, frontal lobe, corpora mammillaria, basal ganglia, medial geniculate body, wall of the third ventricle

Immunopositivity for:
- Tubulin
- Neurofilament
- Phosphorylated neurofilaments
- Ubiquitin
- Tropomyosin
- Tau (Love et al. 1988; Galloway et al. 1990; Grundke-Iqbal et al. 1986)

30.3.8 Ballooned Neurons

Ballooned neurons are found in various neurodegenerative disorders (Table 30.5).

30.3 Neuropathologic Changes

Table 30.5 Disorders associated with the presence of ballooned neurons

Frequent	• Pick disease with Pick bodies • Cortico-basal degeneration • Creutzfeldt–Jakob disease • Autosomal dominant parkinsonism
Rare	• Alzheimer disease • Lewy body dementia • MND-inclusion dementia
Very rare	• Progressive supranuclear palsy (PSP) • Nasu–Hakola disease

Ballooned neurons are:
- Swollen neurons with large cytoplasm
- Immunophenotype
  - Phosphorylated neurofilaments
  - Alpha ß crystallin

30.3.9 Histological Visualization of Amyloid Deposits and Tangles

Classical histological stains
- Congo red stain
  - visualization of bi-refringent substances using polarized light
  - amyloid deposits in brain and vessel walls

Silver impregnations techniques
- developed at the end of the nineteenth century by:
  - Hortega and Cajal (Spanish School)
  - Golgi (Italian school)
- Classical silver impregnation techniques include those of:
  - Bielschowsky
  - Bodian
  - von Braunmühl
- More recent silver impregnation techniques include those of:
  - Campbell
  - Cross
  - Gallyas

- Further techniques encompass:
  - Methenamine silver
  - Thioflavin S
  - Modified AgNOR method

Immunohistochemical stains
- Beta-amyloid (Kummer and Heneka 2014; Knowles et al. 2014; Hayden and Teplow 2013)
  - Amyloid beta peptide is a 42-amino acid peptide.
  - It is processed from the precursor protein, amyloid beta precursor protein (APP).
  - Amyloid beta precursor protein is a transmembrane glycoprotein that spans the membrane once.
  - The gene for amyloid beta precursor protein is located on chromosome 21.
  - Is found as insoluble aggregates in senile plaques.
- Neurofilament proteins
  - Belong to the class of intermediate filament proteins.
  - consist of 10–12 nm neurofilaments.
  - Three groups are distinguished based on different molecular weights:
    - heavy (NF-H) 200 kDa
    - medium (NF-M) 150 kDa
    - low (NF-L) 68 kDa
    - phosphorylated
- Tau (Spillantini and Goedert 2013; Takashima 2013)
  - microtubule-associated protein
  - sorted into neuronal axons
  - failed sorting mechanisms in Alzheimer disease with missorted tau into the somato-dendritic compartment
- Phosphorylated tau
  - hyperphosphorylated tau
- Tau 3 repeat (tau 3R)
  - 3R Tandem repeat sequence of 31 amino acids defining one tau isoform.

- Expression of the 3R isoform causes more profound axonal transport defects and locomotor impairments, culminating in a shorter life span than the 4R isoform (Di Giorgio et al. 2017).
- Tau 4 repeat
  - 4R Tandem repeat sequence of 32 amino acids defining one tau isoform
  - the 4R isoform leads to greater neurodegeneration and impairments in learning and memory (Di Giorgio et al. 2017).
- Microtubule-associated protein (MAP)
- Tubulin
- Ubiquitin (Atkin and Paulson 2014; Jansen et al. 2014)
  - evolutionary highly conserved protein
  - crucial for intracellular protein homeostasis plays an important role in the degradation of proteins and lysosomal functions ubiquitin-proteasome system (UPS)
  - belongs to the group of heat shock proteins
  - is induced by stress (Lowe and Mayer 1990; Mayer et al. 1991)
- α-B-Crystallin
  - water-soluble protein
  - localized in glial cells (Iwaki et al. 1990)
  - has similarities to heat shock proteins
  - is induced by stress
- P62 (p62/SQSTM1/A170) (Geetha et al. 2012; Komatsu et al. 2012; Salminen et al. 2012)
  - multifunctional protein
  - involved in the regulation of cellular signaling and protein trafficking
  - role in protein degradation and aggregation
  - is a stress-inducible intracellular protein

A comparison among the various staining methods is given in Table 30.6.

Table 30.6 Comparative synopsis of various staining methods for the demonstration of amyloid plaques and neurofibrillary tangles

Thioflavin	VIS	• NFT
		• Plaques
	OST	• Cellular autofluorescence
	SV	• Minimal
	ST	• 1.5 h
	NEP	• Quickly fades out
		• Problems with archiving
		• Fluorescence microscopy is needed
Methenamine	VIS	• Plaques
		• NFT
		• Vascular plaque
	OST	• Cell nuclei
	SV	• Variable between various staining rounds
	ST	• 1.5 h
	NEP	• Faint NFT
Campbell-Switzer-Martin	VIS	• NFT
		• Plaques
	OST	• Nuclei
	SV	• Variable between various batches
	ST	• 1.5 h
	NEP	• Non-uniform staining
		• Weak differentiation

30.3 Neuropathologic Changes

Table 30.6 (continued)

Gallyas	VIS	• NFT • Neuropil threads • Neuritic plaques
	OST	• None
	SV	• Variable between various batches
	ST	• 2.5 h
	NEP	• Some NFT appear pale
Modified AgNOR method (Reusche)	VIS	• NFT • Plaques
	OST	• Nuclei • Blood vessels
	SV	• Minimal
	ST	• 3 h
	NEP	• Artifacts after bad fixation • Bad visualization of cerebral amyloid angiopathy
Garvey's modified Bielschowsky	VIS	• NFT • NT • Plaques
	OST	• Nuclei • Fibers • Blood vessels
	SV	• Variable
	ST	• 1.5 h
	NEP	• Diffuse plaques poorly differentiated • Some NFT are pale
Nickel-Peroxidase	VIS	• NFT • NT • Plaque
	OST	• None
	SV	• Minimal
	ST	• 3 h
	NEP	• No clear staining
Tau-Immunohistochemistry	VIS	• NFT • NT • Neuritic plaques
	OST	• None
	SV	• Minimal
	ST	• 2–4 h
	NEP	• Differentiation between small NFTs and NTs difficult
ß-A4 Immunohistochemistry	VIS	• Plaques • Vascular plaque
	OST	• None
	SV	• Minimal
	ST	• 2–4 h
	NEP	• Strong background on frozen sections

Abbreviations used: *VIS* visualisation of, *OST* other structures stained, *SV* staining variability, *ST* staining time, *NEP* negative properties

30.3.10 Immunohistochemical Pattern in the Differential Diagnosis

An illustration of the immunohistochemical-staining patterns of various neuropathologic changes in different neurodegenerative disorders is given in Table 30.7.

30.3.11 Frequencies of Neuropathology Diagnoses

The frequencies of various neurodegenerative disorders in large autopsy series can be given as follows:

- Alzheimer disease (AD): 30–70%
- Multi-infract dementia (MID): 30–80%
- Mixed (AD)(MID): 7–30%
- Fronto-temporal dementia/Pick: 1–3%

30.4 Comparisons

Comparisons of various clinical, neuroimaging, and neuropathological features between Alzheimer disease, Parkinson disease, and Lewy body dementia are given in Table 30.8.

30.5 Molecular Neuropathology

30.5.1 Concepts of Neurodegenerative Diseases

Concepts of neurodegenerative diseases include (Kovacs 2014):
- Deposition of ß-sheet-rich proteins
- Protein-based molecular classification of neurodegenerative diseases
- Involvement of protein-processing systems
  - Unfolded protein response
  - Ubiquitin-proteasome system
  - Autophagy-lysosome pathway

Table 30.7 Cytoskeletal pathology: immunohistochemical patterns

	PHF	pNF	p-Tau	Ubi	APP	Tub	Crys	ChrA
Alzheimer disease								
NFT	+++	+++	+++	+++	+	–	–	–
Plaque	+++	++	++	+	+++	–	–	–
GVD	+	+	+	–	–	+	–	–
Pick disease								
Pick bodies	++	+++	++	++	+	–	+	++
Ballooned cells	+	+++	++	++	?	–	?	+
Progressive supranuclear palsy								
NFT	+–	+++	+++	++	?	–	–	–
Ballooned cells	–	++	?	+	–	–	–	–
Parkinson disease								
Lewy bodies	+–	+++	+–	+++	–	+	–	+
Pre-Lewy body	?	+	–	++	?	?	?	?
Cortico-basal degeneration								
Inclusions (NFT)	+	++	++	+–	?	?	–	–
Ballooned cells	–	++	+	+–	–	?	+	–
Multi-system atrophy inclusions								
Neuronal	–	+–	–	+++	?	–	?	–
Oligodendroglial	+	–	++	++	?	++	–	–
Other neurodegenerative disorders								
Eosinophilic Granula	–	–	–	–	–	–	–	–
Axonal spheroids	–	++	–	++	–	–	–	–
Hirano-bodies	–	+	–	++	–	–	–	–

PHF paired helical filaments, *PNF* phosphorylated neurofilament epitopes, *p-Tau* phosphorylated tau-protein, *Ubi* ubiquitin, *APP* amyloid precursor protein, *Tub* tubulin, *Crys* α-B-crystallin, *ChrA* chromogranin A

30.5 Molecular Neuropathology

Table 30.8 Comparison AD, PD, LBD, modified after Fong and Press (2011)

	AD	DLB	PD
Cognitive features			
Neuropsychology	Early impairment of declarative memory	Early impairment in attention and visual–spatial skills	Impaired executive functioning
Cognitive fluctuation	+	+++ Can be prominent, severe, and early in disease course	–
Neuropsychiatric features			
Visual hallucinations	+	+++ Persistent and early in disease course	++ Late in disease course
Delusions	++	+++	+
Depression	++	+++	+++
Apathy	++	+++	+
Extrapyramdial motor symptoms			
Tremor	–	++	+++
Rigidity	+	+++	+++
Bradykinesia	+ Rare, usually mild, appears late in disease course	+++ Pronounced rigidity and bradykinesia; may be similar severity to PD	+++ Initial manifestation of disease, often unilateral
Neuroimaging			
Global atrophy	++	++	–
Medial temporal lobe atrophy	+++	–	–
Occipital hypoperfusion	–	+++	+
Impaired dopaminergic activity	–	+++	+++
Neuropathology			
Senile plaque density	+++	++	–
Neurofibrillary tangle density	+++	+	–
Subcortical Lewy bodies	–	++	+++
Cortical Lewy bodies	–	+++	+
Cholinergic deficit	++	+++	++
Dopaminergic deficit	–	++	+++

- Modifications of disease-related proteins
    - Phosphorylation
    - Nitration
    - Oligomer
    - Protease-resistant forms
    - Protein cleavage proteins
- Maturation of protein deposits
    - Non-ubiquinated → ubiquitinated structures
    - Non-argyrophilic → argyrophilic structures
    - Presence or absence of amyloid-staining properties
- Topographical hierarchy of protein deposits in anatomical regions
    - Prion-like cell-to-cell spreading of misfolded proteins
    - Stages or phases of protein deposition
- Neuronal loss due to different pathogenic pathways:
    - Apoptosis
    - Cell cycle disturbances
    - Lipid peroxidation
    - DNA oxidation
    - Energy dysregulation
        ○ Oxidative stress
        ○ Mitochondrial instability
- Metabolic changes

- Ion homeostasis
- Neuro-inflammatory mechanisms:
  - Anti-inflammatory cytokines
  - Microglial activation
  - Anti-apoptotic processes
  - Antioxidant processes
- Tissue reactions:
  - Neuronal loss
  - Synaptic degeneration
  - Reactive astrogliosis
  - Reactive microgliosis
  - Neuronal alterations (ballooned cells, inclusion bodies)
  - Extracellular plaques
  - Absence of inflammatory cell infiltration
  - Spongiform changes

30.5.2 Relevant Proteins

The relevant proteins encountered in neurodegenerative disorders include:
- Amyloid ß
  - Amyloid precursor protein APP
- Tau
  - Phosphorylated tau
  - Tau 3R repeat
  - Tau 4R repeat
- Alpha-synuclein
- Proteasome ubiquitin system
  - Ubiquitin
  - P62
- TDP43
- FET proteins
  - FUS: fused in sarcoma
  - EWSR1: Ewing's saroma RNA-binding protein1
  - TAF15: TATA-binding protein-associated factor 15
- Microtubule-associated proteins tau (MAPT)
- Prion protein (PrP)
- Ubiquilin
- Ubiquilin 2
- Optineurin

Extracellular protein depositions
- ß-Amyloid
  - focal
    - with or without dense core
  - stellate
    - mostly in astrocytes)
  - diffuse
    - fleecy
    - lake-like
    - supial
  - vascular
    - with amyloid features
    - without amyloid features
    - vessel type involved
  - unusual
    - cotton whool plaques
    - inflammatory plaques
- PrP
  - Fine/diffuse—Synaptic
  - Fine or coarse—perineuronal
  - Fine or coarse—axonal
  - Coarse-focal—patchy perivacuolar
  - Focal plaque-like deposit with amyloid characteristics
  - Focal—amyloid plaque
  - Vascular with or without amyloid features

Intracellular protein deposits
- Tau
  - Neuronal cytoplasm
    - neurofibrillary tangle
    - diffuse cytoplasmic granular immunoreactivity (pre-tangle)
    - spherical/globular inclusions
  - Neuronal processes
    - Threads (in axons)
    - Neurites (preplaque)
    - Grains (in dendrites)
  - Astrocyte
    - Tufted
    - Astrocytic plaque
    - Others: ramified, thorny, bush-like, globular
  - Oligodendrocyte
    - Coiled body
    - Globular inclusion
- α-synuclein
  - Neuronal cytoplasm
    - spherical inclusion (Lewy body)

30.5 Molecular Neuropathology

Table 30.9 Deposited proteins in neurodegenerative disorders

Protein deposited	Site of deposition	Disease
α-synuclein	Intracellular Lewy bodies Lewy neurites	Parkinson disease
α-synuclein	Intracellular argyrophilic inclusion in oligodendrocytes and neurons	Multiple system atrophy
Cystatin C	Extracellular	Hereditary cerebral amyloid angiopathy
ß-amyloid	Extracellular	Congophilic amyloid angiopathy
ß-amyloid	Extracellular amyloid plaques	Alzheimer disease
Tau	Intracellular—paired helical filaments	Alzheimer disease
Tau	Intracellular inclusions—paired helical filaments, Pick bodies	Fronto-temporal dementia
ABri	Extracellular amyloid plaques	Familial British dementia
ADan	Extracellular amyloid plaques	Familial British dementia
Prion protein	Extracellular amyloid plaques and/or diffuse plaques	Transmissible spongiform encephalopathies
TDP43-ubiquitin	Cytoplasmic inclusions and ubiquitin-positive neuronal threads	Amyotrophic lateral sclerosis
Mutant huntingtin	Nuclear and cytoplasmic inclusions	Huntington disease
Various proteins with polyglutamine expansions	Nuclear and cytoplasmic inclusions	Inherited spinocerebellar ataxias

- ○ pale body
- ○ granular immunoreativities
- Neuronal nucleus
- Neuronal processes
  - ○ thin and thick Lewy neurites
- Astrocytes
  - ○ Star shaped
  - ○ Crescent shaped
- Oligodendrocytes

Pathogenetic mechanisms at work in neurodegenerative diseases include:
- Aberrant protein structure (Table 30.9)
- more than 20 different proteins can form aberrant structures
- disease-causing mechanism unknown
- loss of vital physiological functions
- acquisition of toxic properties
- Inclusion bodies
  - relatively large electron-dense structures
  - contain membrane-limited protein aggregates
  - contain ubiquitin-positive material (due to impairment of the ubiquitin-proteasome system (UPS))
- Altered RNA metabolism
  - important genes: FUS, TDP-43, progranulin
- Oxidative stress
- Mitochondrial dysfunction
- Excitoxicity
- Disrupted axonal transport
- Neuroinflammation and microglial activation

30.5.3 Amyloid and the Amyloid Cascade Hypothesis
(Fig. 30.2a–n)

Roles of APP in the brain
- Modulation of neurogenesis
- Modulation of Ca2+ homeostasis
- Modulation of synaptic plasticity
- Antioxidant activity
- Modulation of neurotransmission
- Sequestration of metal ions
- Modulation of neurite outgrowth

Roles of APOE in the brain
- Membrane maintenance
- Vascular integrity

- Clearance of Aβ
- Modulation of energy metabolism
- Synaptic repair
- Transport of cholesterol
- Modulation of inflammation

Effects of Aβ on astrocytes
- Release of TNFα, IL-1β, IL-6
- Induction of energetic modifications
- Induction of astrocytic hypertrophy
- Increased expression of calcineurin
- Induction of JAK/STAT pathways
- Participation in astrocyte-neuron shuttle
- Modulation of synaptic plasticity

Hardy and Higgins (1992) postulated in their hypothesis that deposition of amyloid β protein (AβP), the main component of the plaques, is the causative agent of Alzheimer's pathology and that the neurofibrillary tangles, cell loss, vascular damage, and dementia follow as a direct result of this deposition.

The amyloid cascade hypothesis states that
- AβP itself, or APP cleavage products containing APP, are neurotoxic.
- Lead to neurofibrillary tangle formation and cell death.
- Thus, two successive events are needed to produce Alzheimer's pathology:
  - First, APP must be generated as an intact entity, either by accumulation of AβP or as an APP containing fragment of APP.
  - Second, this molecule must facilitate or cause neuronal death and neurofibrillary tangle formation.

The amyloid cascade hypothesis reads as follows:
- All four genes now known to cause AD have been shown to increase Aβ production (APP, PS1, PS2) or Aβ deposition (ApoE4).
- All AD patients have many amyloid deposits containing degenerating nerve endings; their plaque count far exceeds that found in normal aging.
- The amount of Aβ in "thinking" regions of the brain correlates with the degree of impairment.
- Down syndrome patients, who invariably develop classical AD pathology by age 50, produce too much Aβ from birth and begin to get amyloid plaques as early as age 12, long before they get tangles and other AD lesions.
- ApoE4, the major genetic risk factor for AD, leads to excess amyloid buildup in the brain before AD symptoms arise. Thus, Aβ deposition precedes clinical AD.
- Aβ polymers reproducibly damage cultured neurons and activate brain inflammatory cells (microglia). Blocking Aβ polymer formation prevents this toxicity.
- Transgenic mice solely expressing a mutant human APP gene develop first diffuse and the fibrillary Aβ plaques associated with neuronal and microglial changes. Mouse models reproduce the major features of AD.
- In other amyloidosis, blocking the production of the responsible amyloid protein can successfully treat these diseases.
- Rigorous evidence for an alternate basis for AD (virus, toxin, loss of trophic factor, etc.) has not emerged during more than 20 years of intense research on AD.

The cascade hypothesis suggests that other causes of Alzheimer's act by initially triggering APP deposition.

- For example, there is an association between head trauma and AD. Dementia pugilistica, exhibited by boxers, may be thought of as a variant of Alzheimer's disease because these individuals exhibit both AIP deposits and neurofibrillary tangles.
- Furthermore, amyloid deposition occurs as an acute response to neuronal injury in both man and animals. This deposition could be caused by an induction of the APP gene through an interleukin-mediated stress response because APP increases in response to a number of neuronal stresses.

The amyloid cascade hypothesis should be critically evaluated; its strength and weakness at various levels are listed in Table 30.10.

Table 30.10 Strengths and weakness of the amyloid cascade hypothesis (Herrup 2015) reproduced with kind permission by Springer Nature

	Strengths	Weaknesses
Genetics	• fAD: APP and PSEN genes are the only genes identified • sAD: APOE variants affect AD risk and also Aβ clearance • Rare A673T APP mutation lowers Aβ production and protects against AD	• fAD: No α-secretase (ADAM10) or BACE mutations yet found • sAD: APP, PSEN, BACE and MAPT (tau) polymorphisms show little association • MAPT mutations associate with fronto-temporal dementia
Biochemistry	• Amyloid comes from APP after cleavage by γ-secretase (PSEN) • Conditions that favor γ-secretase cleavage to the longer Aβ142 • favor aggregation and AD • APOE4 increases risk of AD and slows clearance of Aβ	• Transgenic mice expressing only Aβ suggest amyloid alone is not sufficient • Other biochemical deficits are present in AD and are sufficient to create dementia
Animal models	• Overexpression of human APP in mouse produces plaques • Mouse transgenics for human APP show memory deficits • Aβ is toxic to neurons in culture. • Overexpression of human APP in fruit flies produces neurodegeneration	• Overexpression of human APP in mouse does not produce tangles, neurodegeneration, or AD-like dementia • PSEN transgenics show neither plaques nor tangles nor neurodegeneration • Memory deficits in transgenics correct quickly and completely
Pathology	• Amyloid plaques are more frequent in AD-affected brains	• Tangles correlate better with neurodegeneration than plaques do • Individuals with substantial plaque burdens can have normal cognition
Clinical findings	• Presence of plaques on imaging associated with increased AD risk • In some subjects with amyloid burdens and early dementia, anti-amyloid therapy improves cognition	• After AD begins, immunoclearing of plaques does not improve cognition • By definition, there is no AD without plaques and plaque deposits without dementia is preclinical AD • No phase 3 clinical trial based on the hypothesis have been successful • Inhibition of γ-secretase increases AD symptoms
Epidemiology		• Certain nonsteroidal anti-inflammatory drugs reduce AD risk by half

30.5.4 Tau (Fig. 30.3a–j)

Roles of Tau in the brain
- Promotion of neurite outgrowth
- Nucleolar organization
- Stabilization of microtubules
- Modulation of axonal transport
- Maintenance of neuronal polarity

The involvement of Tau in various diseases named "Tauopathies" is shown in Table 30.11.

30.5.5 Synuclein (α-Syn)
(Fig. 30.4a–d)

Under physiological conditions (Burre 2015; Burre et al. 2018; Theillet et al. 2016; Valdinocci et al. 2017)

- α-Synuclein (αS) is a neuronal protein that localizes predominantly at the presynaptic terminals.
- In vivo αS is partitioned between water-soluble and membrane-bound states.

Table 30.11 Tauopathies

	Disorder	Affected brain regions	Clinical signs
4R	Progressive supranuclear palsy (PSP)	• Basal ganglia • Brain stem	• Parkinsonism
	Cortico-basal degeneration (CBD)	• Cortex • Basal ganglia	• Parkinsonism • Focal cortical syndromes
	Argyrophilic grain disease	• Limbic	• Amnestic cognitive impairment
3R	Pick disease	• Cortex • Limbic	• Dementia • Focal cortical syndromes
3R + 4R	Tangle predominant dementia	• Limbic	• Dementia
	Guam-Parkinson-dementia complex	• Cortex • Brain stem	• Dementia • Parkinsonism

- α-Syn functions in its native conformation as a soluble monomer.
- α-Syn is a presynaptic protein that binds to small synaptic vesicles.
- α-Syn is a 140 amino acid, soluble protein found predominantly within the central nervous system (CNS).
- Normal role of α-Syn remains unclear; however, high concentrations of the protein exist within neuronal presynaptic terminals, indicating potential function(s) in synaptic transmission.
- Multiple specific roles have been proposed for α-Syn, including soluble NSF attachment protein receptor (SNARE) protein regulation, production of dopamine, and regulation of synaptic vesicle recycling.
- Recombinant α-Syn exists as an unfolded monomer, whereas recent evidence shows that extraction from eukaryotic sources, such as erythrocytes or human brain tissue, produced α-Syn multimers, mostly tetramers, with α-helical content.
- α-Syn normally exists largely as an unfolded monomer in the free cytosolic form while adopting an α-helical conformation once bound or interacting with lipid membranes.

Under neuropathogical conditions (Burre 2015; Burre et al. 2018; Theillet et al. 2016; Valdinocci et al. 2017; Bridi and Hirth 2018)

- α-Syn is found as intracellular inclusions of insoluble fibrils.
- Fibrillar aggregates are the major constituents of Lewy bodies in Parkinson disease.
- Oligomers and protofibrils of α-Syn have been identified to be the most toxic species.

Table 30.12 Synucleinopathies

Disorder	Affected brain regions	Clinical signs
Parkinson disease (PD)	• Brain stem	• Parkinsonism
Dementia with Lewy bodies (DLB)	• Cortex • Limbic • Brain stem	• Dementia • Parkinsonism
Multiple system atrophy (MSA)	• Basal ganglia • Brain stem • Cerebellum	• Parkinsonism • Ataxia

- Accumulation at presynaptic terminals affecting several steps of neurotransmitter release.
- Steps involved in pathogenesis.
  - High levels of α-Syn alter the size of synaptic vesicle pools and impair their trafficking.
  - α-Syn overexpression can either misregulate or redistribute proteins of the presynaptic SNARE complex. This leads to deficient tethering, docking, priming, and fusion of synaptic vesicles at the active zone (AZ).
  - α-Syn inclusions are found within the presynaptic AZ, accompanied by a decrease in AZ protein levels.
  - α-Syn overexpression reduces the endocytic retrieval of synaptic vesicle membranes during vesicle recycling. These presynaptic alterations mediated by accumulation of α-Syn, together impair neurotransmitter exocytosis and neuronal communication.

The involvement of α-synuclein in various diseases named "Synucleinopathies" is shown in Table 30.12.

30.5.6 TDP-43 (Fig. 30.5a–d)

Multifunctional RNA-binding protein involved in (Geser et al. 2009, 2010, 2011):

- Exon skipping of cystic fibrosis transmembrane conductance regulator and apolipoprotein A-II genes
- Exon-inclusion of the survival of motor neuron gene
- Stabilization of low molecular weight neurofilament protein mRNA through a direct interaction with its 3'UTR
- Modulation of cyclin-dependent kinase 6 expression
- Modulation of microRNA biogenesis
- Acting as scaffold for nuclear bodies (i.e., Gemini of coiled bodies) through interaction with survival of motor neuron protein
- Cell cycle regulation and apoptosis
- mRNA transport and regulation of local translation at synapses

The involvement of TDP-43 in various diseases named "TDP-43 proteinopathies" is shown in Tables 30.13 and 30.14.

Genes associated with fronto-temporal lobe degeneration (FTLD), amyotrophic lateral sclerosis (ALS), and FTLD/ALS are shown in Tables 30.15 and 30.16.

30.5.7 FUS

Fused in sarcoma (FUS) (Ishigaki and Sobue 2018; Ling 2018; Mikhaleva and Lemke 2018; Ederle and Dormann 2017; Guerrero et al. 2016; Nolan et al. 2016; Ratti and Buratti 2016)

- Belongs to Ewing's sarcoma breakpoint region 1 (EWS) and TAF15 to the FET family of RNA-binding proteins.
- FUS encodes a 526 amino acid, 15-exon RNA-binding protein of the FET family.
- Normal physiological function of FUS is unclear.
- Known roles include:
  - transcriptional control

Table 30.13 TDP-43 proteinopathies (Geser et al. 2009) reproduced with kind permission from Springer Nature

TDP disease group	Diseases
Major TDP-43 diseases	• Amyotrophic lateral sclerosis with/without dementia • Fronto-temporal degeneration with motor neuron disease • Fronto-temporal degeneration with ubiquitin-positive, tau, and α-synuclein-negative inclusions • Fronto-temporal dementia with inclusion body myopathy • Paget disease of bone • Perry syndrome
Diseases with secondary TDP-43 pathology	• Parkinsonism-dementia complex/amyotrophic lateral sclerosis on geographic isolates • Alzheimer disease/hippocampal sclerosis • Pick disease • Cortico-basal degeneration • Argyrophilic grain disease • Parkinson disease, dementia with Lewy bodies, Parkinson disease dementia • Huntington disease • Myopathies (inclusion body myositis, oculopharyngeal muscular dystrophy, distal myopathies with rimmed vacuoles, polymyositis with mitochondrial pathology, polymyositis)
Diseases with minor or no TDP-43 pathology	• Superoxide dismutase-1 linked amyotrophic lateral sclerosis • Primary lateral sclerosis • TDP-43-negative fronto-temporal lobar degeneration with ubiquitin-positive inclusions • Charged multivesicular body protein 2B linked fronto-temporal dementia • Progressive supranuclear palsy • Multiple system atrophy • Basophilic inclusion body disease/motor neuron disease with basophilic inclusions • Neuronal intermediate filament inclusion disease • Tangle-only dementia • Hereditary diffuse leukoencephalopathy with spheroids • Prion diseases • Schizophrenia • Normal aging • Anoxia • Neoplasm

Table 30.14 TDP-43 proteinopathies

Disorder	Affected brain regions	Clinical signs
Amyotrophic lateral sclerosis (ALS)	• Motor neurons	• Spasticity • Weakness
Fronto-temporal lobar degeneration	• Cortex • Basal ganglia	• Dementia • Focal cortical syndromes

Table 30.15 FTLD-associated genes, modified after Boxer (2011)

Gene	Location	Clinical syndromes	Neuropathology
Tau (MAPT)	Chr 17q21-22	• FTDP-17 (can resemble: bvFTD, tvFTD, CBS, PSP)	Tau (+) inclusions
Progranulin (PGRN)	Chr 17q21	• bvFTD • tvFTD • FTD-ALS PPA • CBS • Rarely ALS alone	FTLD-U/TDP-43(+) inclusions
Valosin-containing protein (VCP)	Chr 9p12-13	• tvFTD • PPA with inclusion body myopathy • Paget disease of bone (IBMPFD)	FTLD-U/TDP-43(+) inclusions; sparing dentate gyrus
Charged multivesicular body protein 2B (CHMP2B)	Pericentromeric Chr 3	• bvFTD • FTD-ALS • Sporadic ALS	FTLD-U; TDP-43(−) inclusions
Presenilin 1 (PSEN1)	Chr 14	• FTD	Pick disease (G183V mutant); most other cases found of harbor PGRN mutations
Unidentified	Chr 9p13.3-21.3	• FTD-ALS	FTLD-U/TDP-43(+) inclusions

Table 30.16 Genes involved in amyotrophic lateral sclerosis (ALS), fronto-temporal dementia (FTD), and FTD/ALS, modified after Thomas et al. (2013) reproduced with kind permission by Oxford University Press

Gene	Function	Clinical phenotype			Mode of inheritance	Neuropathology in mutation cases
		ALS	FTD	FTD-ALS		
C9orf72	Unknown	+++	+++	+++	Dominant	ALS/FTD-TDP
TARDBP	RNA- processing protein	++	+	+	Dominant, recessive	ALS-TDP
VCP	Protein turnover via UPS and autophagy	++/+	+	+	Dominant	ALS/FTD-TDP
FUS	RNA-processing protein	++	Rare		Dominant, recessive	ALS-FUS
UBQLN2	Protein turnover via UPS and autophagy	+		+	Dominant (X-linked) in	ALS-TDP/ALS-FUS
SQSTM1	Autophagy, inflammation, and apoptosis	+	+		ALS unclear, segregation yet to be shown	Unclear

- RNA processing through splicing regulation of pre-mRNAs
- maintenance of cellular RNA homeostasis
- DNA repair
- involved in synaptic transmission and plasticity
- Cellular localization:
  - Physiological conditions: FUS is predominantly localized in the nucleus in neurons, but is exclusively nuclear-based in glia.
  - Pathological conditions: Mislocalization of FUS to the cytoplasm contributes to neurodegeneration by a gain-of-toxicity mechanism.
- FUS mutations significantly alter target gene expression by binding target gene mRNA within the aggregates of transfected human cells.

30.5.8 Nucleotide Repeat Diseases

Nucleotide repeat disease
- Trinucleotide repeat disease
- Tetranucleotide repeat disease
- Pentanucleotide repeat disease

Repeat sequence in either coding or noncoding regions of the gene

Mode of inheritance
- Autosomal recessive
- Autosomal dominant
- X-linked

Diseases
- GAA
  - Friedreich ataxia
- CAG
  - SCA1, SCA2, SCA3, SCA6, SCA7, SCA17
  - Dentate-rubro-pallido-lysian atrophy
  - Huntington disease
  - Kennedy disease
- TGGAA
  - SCA31

30.6 Biomarkers

Biomarker-based diagnostic algorithms for dementia syndromes are shown in Tables 30.17 and 30.18.

- Alzheimer disease
  - MRI to evaluate pattern of atrophy, concomitant vascular disease, and nondegenerative lesions (mimics)
  - Alzheimer disease (AD) molecular biomarkers (cerebrospinal fluid (CSF) or PET) for early-onset AD, atypical clinical features, or possibility of fronto-temporal lobar degeneration; 18F-FDG-PET if patient is amyloid-negative according to CSF or PET studies and MRI is inconclusive
  - Genetic testing: *PSEN1*, *PSEN2*, and *APP* if familial or genetic causes of AD are suspected; *C9orf72* in the case of an amyloid-negative amnestic phenotype
- Fronto-temporal dementia
  - MRI to evaluate pattern of atrophy and nondegenerative lesions (mimics).
  - Amyloid biomarkers (CSF or PET) if AD is included in the differential diagnosis.
  - Can consider genetics in the case of a family history or certain clinical features *C9orf72*: family history of fronto-temporal dementia with or without motor neuron disease (MND), MND, or atypical clinical features (e.g., hallucinations or delusions).
  - *GRN*: extensive white matter damage, striking asymmetry in atrophy, or prominent parietal lobe involvement.
  - *VCP*: if inclusion body myopathy, with or without Paget disease, is present.
  - *MAPT*: family history and extrapyramidal motor dysfunction.
- Lewy body dementia
  - MRI to evaluate pattern of atrophy and nondegenerative lesions (mimics)
  - AD molecular biomarkers (CSF or PET) to test for mixed disease if atrophy patterns or clinical features are suggestive

Table 30.17 Biomarkers of dementia syndromes

Clinical syndrome	Pathology	Cerebrospinal fluid
Alzheimer disease (AD)		
Typical/amnestic AD	• NFTs (3R/4R tau) • amyloid plaques	• Reduced Aβ42 (Aβ42:Aβ40 ratio) • Increased tau and P-tau
Behavioral dysexecutive AD	• NFTs (3R/4R tau) • amyloid plaques	• Reduced Aβ42 (Aβ42:Aβ40 ratio) • Increased tau and P-tau
Posterior cortical atrophy (PCA)	• NFTs (3R/4R tau) • amyloid plaques	• Reduced Aβ42 (Aβ42:Aβ40 ratio) • Increased tau and P-tau
Logopenic variant PPA (lvPPA)	• NFTs (3R/4R tau) • amyloid plaques	• Reduced Aβ42 (Aβ42:Aβ40 ratio) • Increased tau and P-tau
Fronto-temporal dementia (FTD)		
Behavioral variant FTD (bvFTD)	TDP-43 type B > Pick disease (3Rtau)	Nonspecific increase in tau due to neurodegeneration
Non-fluent/agrammatic variant PPA (nfvPPA)	4R tau > TDP-43 type A	Nonspecific increase in tau due to neurodegeneration
Semantic variant PPA (svPPA)	TDP-43 type C	Nonspecific increase in tau due to neurodegeneration
Progressive supranuclear palsy syndrome (PSP-S)	PSP (4R tau)	Nonspecific increase in tau due to neurodegeneration
		Nonspecific increase in tau due to neurodegeneration
Vascular dementia (VaD)		
VaD (small and large vessel disease)	White matter and gray matter lesions, mixed pathology (most commonly AD or LBD)	NA
Prion disease		
Creutzfeldt–Jakob disease (CJD) Scrapie	Prion protein (PrP^{Sc})	RT-QuIC test (most accurate); increased 14-3-3, neuron-specific enolase and tau (specificity increases when more than one cerebrospinal fluid marker is elevated)
Cortico-basal syndrome (CBS)		
Cortico-basal syndrome (CBS)	Cortico-basal degeneration (CBD) and AD most common	Nonspecific increase in tau due to neurodegeneration

Table 30.18 Biomarkers of dementia syndromes

Clinical syndrome	MRI (typical areas of peak atrophy)	Metabolic (18F-FDG-PET) and perfusion (SPECT) imaging	Functional networks (resting state functional MRI)
Alzheimer disease (AD)			
Typical/amnestic AD	MTL (hippocampus and entorhinal cortex), PCC, temporoparietal cortex, precuneus	Reduced perfusion and metabolism in MTL, precuneus, PCC, temporoparietal	Reduced DMN and anterior temporal network activation
Behavioral dysexecutive AD	Temporoparietal cortex > dorsolateral prefrontal cortex	Reduced metabolism in medial and orbital frontal regions	Reduced DMN and frontoparietal network activation

30.6 Biomarkers

Table 30.18 (continued)

Clinical syndrome	MRI (typical areas of peak atrophy)	Metabolic (18F-FDG-PET) and perfusion (SPECT) imaging	Functional networks (resting state functional MRI)
Posterior cortical atrophy (PCA)	MTL, PCC, occipital, and parietal lobes	Reduced signal in parieto-occipital lobes	Reduced DMN and visual network activation
Logopenic variant PPA (lvPPA)	Temporal lobe (superior temporal gyrus), parietal lobe (inferior parietal lobule)	Reduced signal in inferior parietal lobule	Reduced DMN and language network activation
Fronto-temporal dementia (FTD)			
Behavioral variant FTD (bvFTD)	Frontoinsular and anterior temporal lobes right > left	Reduced perfusion and metabolism in frontal and temporal lobes	Reduced salience network and increased DMN activation
Non-fluent/agrammatic variant PPA (nfvPPA)	Gray matter atrophy: left > right posterior frontoinsular cortex, including inferior frontal gyrus; white matter atrophy: aslant tract and arcuate fasciculus	Reduced metabolism in inferior frontal gyrus	Reduced language network activation
Semantic variant PPA (svPPA)	Atrophy of anterior temporal lobe(s) and inferior temporal gyrus	Reduced metabolism in anterior temporal lobe	Reduced language network activation
Progressive supranuclear palsy syndrome (PSP-S)	Classic Richardson: midbrain tegmentum (hummingbird or penguin sign), pons, thalamus, and striatum, with minimal involvement of the frontal lobe	Variable, with reduced metabolism reported in frontal, caudate, midbrain, and thalamic regions in 4R tauopathies	Reduced cerebellothalamocortical network activation
Vascular dementia (VaD)			
VaD (small and large vessel disease)	White matter and gray matter lesions, mixed pathology (most commonly AD or LBD) Frontal subcortical and periventricular white matter hyperintensities, microhemorrhages, lacunar strokes, prominent Virchow-Robin spaces, cortical infarcts and hemorrhage	Reduced perfusion and metabolism in frontal subcortical and periventricular regions	NA
Prion disease			
Creutzfeldt–Jakob disease (CJD)	Diffusion-weighted imaging and T2-hyperintensity in the striatum, hypothalamus, and cortices ("cortical ribboning"), posterior (pulvinar) and medial thalamus ("double hockey stick sign," nonspecific) or pulvinar alone ("pulvinar sign," in variant CJD only)	NA	NA
Cortico-basal syndrome			
Cortico-basal syndrome (CBS)	Perirolandic cortex and posterior extension (AD); perirolandic cortex and prefrontal extension (CBD)	Early changes can be seen typically in the same pattern as the atrophy that follows	NA

MRI (typical areas of peak atrophy), metabolic (18F-FDG-PET), and perfusion (SPECT) imaging, functional networks (resting state functional MRI)

- In-laboratory sleep study to evaluate for REM sleep without atonia; may also find evidence of dream-enactment behavior on video recording
- Prion disease
  - MRI: abnormalities on diffusion-weighted imaging, and apparent diffusion coefficient sequences abnormality; T1-weighted and T2-weighted sequences to test for mimics
  - CSF: real-time quaking-induced conversion (RT-QuIC) preferred; 14-3-3, tau, and neuron-specific enolase (alternative)
  - Paraneoplastic panel (serum and/or CSF) if diagnosis not reached in the first two steps (mimics)
- Vascular dementia
  - MRI for subtype and severity of disease, and atrophy pattern suggestive of mixed disease
  - AD molecular biomarkers (CSF or PET) if clinical features or atrophy patterns suggest mixed disease
  - Genetic testing (e.g., *NOTCH3* for CADASIL) if familial disease suspected, or atypical features are seen, such as white matter disease in anterior temporal lobes

Molecular imaging and emerging techniques
- AD
- 18F-based amyloid tracer (e.g., florbetapir, flutemetamol, and florbetaben) uptake is typically diffuse in the neocortex.
- Tau ligand uptake is closely associated with postmortem NFT distribution and peak areas of atrophy.
- Fronto-temporal dementia (FTD)
  - Ongoing efforts to develop PET tracers that bind the conformations of abnormal tau characteristic of fronto-temporal lobar degeneration tauopathies, while minimizing off-target binding

30.7 Brief Sketch of the Differential Diagnoses

A list of possible disorders leading to dementia is given in Table 30.1. They have to be considered in the differential diagnosis of the major neurodegenerative disorders considered in the subsequent Chaps. 31–40 including AD, PD, LBD, FTLD, PSP, CBD, MSA, and Huntington disease (HD).

In the following subchapters, the neuropathologic changes encountered in other rare dementing disorders are briefly outlined.

30.8 Differential Diagnoses: Lobar Atrophies

30.8.1 Pick Disease

Pick disease is characterized by:
- atrophy of basal parts of the frontal and temporal lobes
- neuronal loss most pronounced in layers IIIA --> IIIB, II and IIIC
- status spongiosus
- reactive astrogliosis
- Pick cells are
  - ballooned neurons with central tigrolysis and excentric nucleus
- Pick bodies are
  - round, intracytoplasmic, argyrophilic inclusions

30.8.2 Primary Progressive Aphasia (PPA)

Primary progressive aphasia (PPA) characterized by:
- fronto-temporal atrophy
- status spongiosus
- neuronal loss in layer II
- reactive astrogliosis

30.8.3 Motor Neuron Disease with Dementia

Motor neuron disease with dementia characterized by:
- Moderate atrophy of the frontal and anterior temporal lobes.
- Moderate neuronal loss.
- Spongiform changes.
- Astrogliosis of layers I-III.
- Loss of motor neurons in spinal cord and rarely in the medulla oblongata.
- Ubiquitin-positive but Tau- and PHF-negative neuronal inclusions in motor neurons, neurons of layer II in the frontal and temporal cortex, dentate gyrus, and hippocampus.
- There exist no neuronal or glial inclusions.

30.8.4 Dementia Lacking Distinctive Histopathology (DLDH)

Dementia lacking distinctive histopathology (DLDH) (Giannakopoulos et al. 1995) characterized by:
- No classical Alzheimer-like changes (amyloid plaques or neurofibrillary tangles) are found.
- Neuronal loss in multiple localizations (frontoparietal cortex, striatum, medial thalamus, substantia nigra, nucleus hypoglossus).
- Astrogliosis is prominent.
- No neuronal inclusions are noted.
- Vacuolization in layer II with marked astrogliosis in the deeper cortical layers.
- Histologic distinction of 4 groups (Giannakopoulos et al. 1995):
  - **Group A:** moderate to severe loss of neurons and astrogliosis in the frontal and/or temporopolar cortex without involvement of subcortical structures
  - **Group B:** severe loss of neurons in the cortex. In the striatum and substantia nigra evidence of astrogliosis, but no neuronal loss
  - **Group C:** similar finding as in group B, in addition severe neuronal loss in at least one subcortical region
  - **Group D:** no evident changes in neocortical pyramidal neurons but various changes in subcortical regions

30.9 Differential Diagnoses: Subcortical Dementias

30.9.1 Progressive Subcortical Gliosis (PSG)

- severe subcortical astrogliosis
- severe involvement of the cortex
- laminar spongiform changes of the cerebral cortex
- no ballooned cell inclusions and argyrophilic plaques (DD: FTD)
- no significant loss of myelin sheaths
- astrocytic and microglial cell proliferation

30.9.2 Parkinson Disease with Dementia

- Subcortical dementia in 15–40% of patients.
- Few plaques and neurofibrillary tangles in the neocortex.
- More tangles in the entorhinal cortex and hippocampus.
- ß-A4 amyloid deposits as diffuse plaques in the neocortex.
- Only patients with Parkinson disease and dementia have numerous Lewy bodies in the cortex, but no plaques or tangles.

30.10 Differential Diagnoses: Rare Cortical Dementias

30.10.1 Chromosome 17-Associated Dementia

Disinhibition-dementia-parkinsonism-amyotrophy complex
- atrophy of gyri in the anterior and inferior regions of the temporal lobe, prefrontal areas, and cingulate gyrus

- pallor of the substantia nigra
- focal neuronal loss
- gliosis and spongiform changes of limbic neocortical regions, association cortex of the frontal, temporal, and occipital lobes
- argyrophilic neuronal inclusions in brain stem nuclei, hypothalamus, and basal ganglia
- Immunopositivity for phosphorylated neurofilament and ubiquitin

30.10.2 Familial Presenile Dementia with Tangles (FPDT)

- numerous neurofibrillary tangles in cortical layers II–V
- no amyloid plaques
- in various regions of the neocortex, amygdala, and parahippocampal gyrus
- hippocampus devoid of neurofibrillary tangles and amyloid plaques

30.10.3 Meso-Limbo-Cortical Dementia

- Predominant involvement of:
  - limbic system
  - caudate nucleus
  - substantia nigra
- Nonspecific neuronal degeneration.
- GFAP-positive astrogliosis.
- Pathologic findings correlate with the topographic distribution of non-striatal dopaminergic tracts.

30.11 Differential Diagnoses: Down Syndrome

Down syndrome (Trisomy 21) is genetically characterized by:
- primary trisomy of chromosome 21 (95% of cases)
- translocation between chromosome 21 and one of group D or group G chromosomes (4% of cases)
- mosaic formation (1% of cases)

Some morphological changes encountered in DS:
- The weight of the brain is lower at birth.
- The weight of the brain is about three-fourth lower in juveniles.
- The form of the skull diverges from the norm.
- The anterior-posterior length of the brain is shorter.
- No signs of atrophy.
- The frontal lobe is shortened.
- The gyri in the occipital lobe are flattened.
- Thinning of the superior temporal gyrus might be evident.
- Histological changes reported include:
  - Abnormal neurons
  - Loss or increase of neurons
  - Delayed myelination
  - Small centrum semiovale
  - Abnormally differentiated Purkinje layer
  - Asymmetry of the inferior olivary nucleus
  - Fusion of both nuclei of the Clark column

Many DS patients develop in old age clinical and neuropathological changes of AD. However, systematic neuropathology analyses of aged DS patients are lacking.

The changes encountered in old DS patients include:

- Atrophy of the cerebral hemispheres
- Loss of pyramidal neurons
- Presence of neuritic plaques
  - Amyloid in DS is similar to the amyloid found in AD.
  - The distribution of plaques differs in the dentate gyrus compared to AD.
- The relationship between the extrachromosomal material and amyloid deposits in DS is unsolved.
  - It is assumed that DS is associated with one-third of the long arm of chromosome 21 (21q).
  - It is assumed that the threefold dosis of this gene product has an effect on accelerated aging in DS.

30.12 Differential Diagnoses: Diffuse Neurofibrillary Tangles with Calcifications (DNTC)

Diffuse neurofibrillary tangles with calcifications (DNTC):
- first described in 1994 by (Kosaka 1994)
- a form of presenile dementia
- ratio male:female: 1:4
- mean age at clinical presentation: 52 years (range: 42–68 years)
- mean duration of disease: 10 years (range: 3–24 years)
- mean age at death: 62.2 years (range: 48–79 years)

Clinical signs:
- slowly progressive cortical dementia
- numerous psychiatric and neurological symptoms
  - verbal dysfunctions (similar to Pick disease)
  - amnestic aphasia
  - sensoric aphasia
  - loss of spontaneity
  - loss of initiative
  - apathia
  - personality changes (similar to Pick disease)
  - parkinsonism
  - Apallic syndrome in final stages

Neuroimaging findings (CT, MRI):
- Temporal or temporo-frontal lobe atrophy
- Calcifications in the globus pallidus and cerebellar dentate nucleus

Neuropathology findings:
- Temporal or temporo-frontal lobe atrophy.
- Numerous neurofibrillary tangles in the whole cerebral cortex.
- The hippocampus and superior temporal gyrus are severely affected.
- Pick bodies are not present.
- The distribution of NFTs resembles that seen in AD.
- Neuritic plaques are never found.
- The involved cortical regions show neuronal loss with accompanying reactive astrogliosis.
- Calcifications, as seen in Fahr disease, are characteristic for DNTC.

30.13 Differential Diagnoses: Rare Neurodegenerative Disorders

30.13.1 Thalamic Degeneration

Thalamic degeneration is a rare disorder.

Clinical signs:
- variable degree of cognitive and behavioral disturbances
- dementia
- akinetic mutism

Three types of selective thalamic degeneration are found:
- In association with other disorders like Friedreich ataxia, spinocerebellar degeneration, multi-system atrophy, Wernicke encephalopathy, Menkes disease, and membranous lipodystrophy
- In association with Creutzfeldt–Jakob disease
- As an isolated degeneration of the thalamus of unknown ethiology

Neuropathologic changes:
- Bilateral symmetrical degeneration of thalamic nuclei.
- Most severe affection of the
  - anterior medial and pulvinar nuclei
  - superficial dorsal dorso-posterior and reticular nuclei
- Preservation of the magnocellular parts of the medial thalamus and the small interneurons (Golgi Type II).
- No signs of
  - infection
  - necrosis
  - vascular lesions
- Cerebral cortex is usually normal.

30.13.2 (Non) Hereditary Bilateral Striatal Necrosis

Rare disorder
Affects children and adults

Clinical signs:
- psychomotor retardation
- apathy
- epileptic seizures
- choreoathetosis
- dystonia
- rigidity
- ataxia
- myoclonus

Neuropathological changes
- isolated bilateral necrosis of the putamen caudate nucleus
- severe neuronal loss
- gliomesenchymal reaction
- vascular endothelial proliferation
- similar changes are encountered in
  - subthalamic nucleus
  - substantia nigra
  - thalamus

30.13.3 Neuroacanthocytosis

Clinical signs and symptoms:
- Dysarthria
- Dystonia
- Motoric and vocal tics
- Seizures
- Parkinsonism
- Signs of dementia (Bird et al. 1978; Hardie 1989; Bruyn 1986)

Macroscopic features:
- severe atrophy of the caudate nucleus caudatus
- moderate atrophy of the putamen

Microscopic features:
- preferential loss of small neurons in the caudate nucleus and putamen
- moderate reactive astrogliosis (Hardie et al. 1991; Alonso et al. 1989)

Mode of inheritance:
- autosomal dominant
- recessive
- X-linked
- sporadic (Critchley et al. 1968; Bird et al. 1978; Sakai et al. 1981; Levine et al. 1968)

30.13.4 Pallidal Degenerations

Pallidal degenerations are extremely rare diseases.

Under the term pallidal degenerations, the following subtypes are grouped:
- pure pallidal degeneration
- pallido-luysian degeneration
- pallido-nigrale degeneration
- pallido-nigro-luysian degeneration
- pallido-nigro-spinal degeneration
- dentato-rubro-pallido-nigral degeneration

Clinical signs:
- motor changes
- development of dementia during the disease course

Neuropathological changes:
- neuronal degeneration affecting the following regions:
  - globus pallidus
  - substantia nigra
  - spinal cord, especially the corticospinal tract
  - dentate nucleus
  - red nucleus
  - Nucleus luysi
- reactive astrogliosis
- myelin pallor

30.13.5 Dentato-Rubro-Pallido-Luysian Degeneration

- Rare disorder.
- Sporadic and familial autosomal dominant disorder.
- Affects the dentato-rubral and the pallido-luysi an circuits (Iizuka and Hirayama 1986; Smith 1975).

Clinical signs
- Ataxo-choreo-athetoid changes are the primary clinical signs.
- Choreo-athetoid or dystonic movement disorders in late stages of the disease.
- Mental dysfunction possible (Iizuka and Hirayama 1986; Smith 1975).

Microscopic features
- Loss of neurons and reactive astrogliosis in:
  - globus pallidus
  - cerebellar nuclei
  - and connections thereof
  - red nucleus
  - subthalamic nucleus Luysi
- Grumouse degeneration in the cerebellar dentate nucleus characterized by deposits of granular argyrophilic material is derived from altered axonal terminals of Purkinje cells (Arai 1989; Arai et al. 1989; Iizuka et al. 1984).

30.13.6 Substantia Reticularis degeneration

- First described by Varela (1969)
- Clinical signs include:
  - cerebellar signs
  - extrapyramidal and pyramidal signs
  - mental deterioration
- Diffuse atrophy of the reticular formation in the spinal cord, brain stem, and thalamus with
- Degeneration of the pallido-subthalamic circuit

30.14 Differential Diagnoses: Argyrophilic Grain Disease (AG)

First described by Braak and Braak (1987, 1989).
Associated with Alzheimer's disease, Pick disease, progressive supranuclear palsy, corticobasal degeneration, dementia with only tangles, Creutzfeldt–Jakob disease, Lewy body disease, and multiple system atrophy.

Clinical signs and symptoms
- Cognitive decline
- Dementia
- Behavioral abnormalities
- Personality changes
- Emotional and mood imbalance
- Episodic memory loss
- Amnesia
- Irritability and agitation
- Delusions
- Dysphoria
- Apathy
- Progressive transcortical sensory aphasia
- Signs of fronto-temporal dementia

Incidence
- AG seen in aged human brain (5–9% in adult autopsies).
- AG increases with age.
- Age onset: 75–80 years.
- Frequency: <60 years: 10%, 61–70 years: 17%; 71–80 years: 30%; >80 years: 43%.

Male:Female ratio: 1:1

Regions involved
- Transentorhinal and entorhinal cortex, layer II
- CA1 of the hippocampus
- Presubiculum
- Temporal cortex
- Orbitofrontal cortex
- Insular cortex
- Basolateral nuclei of the amygdala
- Lateral tuberal nucleus of the thalamus

Macroscopic findings
- Normal appearing.
- Atrophy signs are possible.

Microscopic findings
- Grains (Fig. 30.7a–f)
  - Gallyas silver iodide stain-positive
  - Argyrophilic
  - 4–8 µm in diameter
  - Spindle-shaped, rod-like, button-like, or round bodies
  - Localized in apical, collateral, and basilar dendrites and dendritic branches
- Pre-tangle neurons
  - Same distribution as AGs
  - Anti-phosphorylated tau-positive

- Coiled bodies
  - Same appearance as in other diseases
- Tau-containing astrocytes
  - Granular hyperphosphorylated immunoreactive cytoplasm
  - Bush-like astrocytes appearing in clusters
- Ballooned neurons
  - Gallyas silver iodide stain-negative
  - Express αß-crystallin
  - Large neurons with possible vacuolization

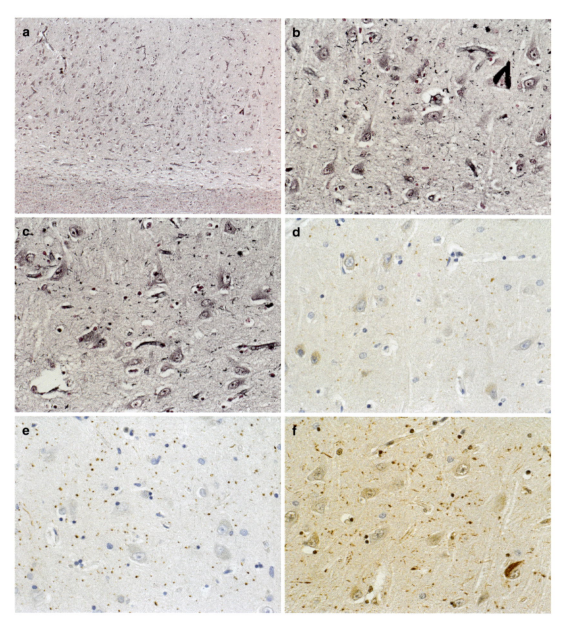

Fig. 30.7 Argyrophilic grain disease: Grains are visualized using Gallyas silver impregnation technique (**a–c**). Note the presence of one neurofibrillary tangle (**b**). Immunophenotype: grains are positive for tauR4 (**d**), p62 (**e**), and ubiquitin (**f**)

Table 30.19 Argyrophilic grain (AG) staging (Ferrer et al. 2008) reproduced with kind permission by Oxford University Press

Stage	Regions involved
Stage I	• Anterior entorhinal cortex • Mild involvement of the cortical and basolateral nuclei of the amygdala • Mild involvement of the hypothalamic lateral tuberal nucleus
Stage II	• Entorhinal cortex; anterior CA1 • Transentorhinal cortex • Cortical and basolateral nuclei of the amygdala • Presubiculum • Hypothalamic lateral tuberal nucleus • Dentate gyrus
Stage III	• Entorhinal cortex • CA1 • Perirhinal cortex • Presubiculum • Amygdala • Dentate gyrus • Hypothalamic lateral tuberal nucleus • Mild involvement of CA2 and CA3 • Mild involvement of the subiculum • Mild involvement of other nuclei of the hypothalamus (i.e., mammillary bodies) • Mild involvement of the anterior temporal cortex, insular cortex, anterior cingulate gyrus, orbitofrontal cortex, nucleus accumbens, septal nuclei • Rare grains in the midbrain
Stage IV	• Moderate to severe additional involvement of the neocortex and brain stem

  – Localized in the amygdale, presubiculum, middle layers of the basal temporal cortex
- Tangles and neuropil threads
  – Variable numbers
- Stages I–IV might be distinguished (Table 30.19).

Immunophenotype
- Phosphorylated tau
- 4R tau (Fig. 30.7d–f)
- αß-crystallin (ballooned neurons)

Ultrastructural features
- AG: Contain straight filaments or tubules (9–25 nm)
- Coiled bodies: Accumulation of filaments (10–13 nm in diameter)

30.15 Differential Diagnoses: Adult Polyglucosan Body Disease (APBD)

Clinical signs
- Motor neuron changes
- Peripheral neuropathy, i.e., with distal sensory loss in the lower extremities
- Neurogenic bladder
- Dementia affecting cortical and subcortical systems

Macroscopic features
- Cortical atrophy
- White matter changes

Microscopic features
- Accumulation of polyglycosan bodies in astrocytes and neuronal processes

30.16 Differential Diagnoses: Normal Pressure Hydrocephalus (NPH)

Normal pressure hydrocephalus is:
- a potentially reversible cause of dementia
- in 2% of all cases of dementia
- communicating and obstructive hydrocephalus

Diagnostic criteria:
- Presence of dementia.
- Urinary bladder incontinence.
- Gait ataxia.
- Typical findings on CT- and MRI scans.
- Intermittent increases of intracranial pressure are possible.

Macroscopic changes:
- enlargement of the entire ventricular system

Microscopic changes:
- focal damage of the ependymal ventricular lining
- subependymal gliosis
- increased number of subependymal glial bumps (i.e., ependymitis granularis)
- fibrosis of the leptomeninges

Pathogenetic mechanism:
- Fibrosis of the leptomeninges leads to an obstruction of the CSF flow through the basal cisterns and at resorptive sites at the cortical convexity into the sinus of the dura mater making NPH to be a communicating and obstructive hydrocephalus.

30.17 Differential Diagnoses: Mitochondrial Encephalomyopathies

Mitochondrial encephalomyopathies include various clinically very hetereogeneous disorders characterized by structural and functional changes of mitochondria encountered in muscle tissue and brain. Besides the affection of the muscles, a certain percentage of patients also develop dementia (Bertini and D'Amico 2009; Chaturvedi et al. 2005; DiMauro 1996; Oldfors and Tulinius 2003; Sarnat and Marin-Garcia 2005).

Under the term of mitochondrial encephalomyopathies, the following entities are grouped:
- Kearns-Sayre syndrome (KSS)
- Myoclonic epilepsy with ragged-red fibers (MERRF)
- Mitochondrial encephalopathy, lactate, acidosis, and stroke-like episodes (MELAS)
- Mitochondrial neurogastrointestinal encephalopathy (MNGIE)

30.17.1 Clinical Signs of Mitochondrial Encephalopathies

Kearns-Sayre syndrome (KSS)
- A mitochondrial myopathy with a typical onset before 20 years of age
- Is a more severe syndromic variant of chronic progressive external ophthalmoplegia
- Cardiac conduction abnormalities
- Weakness of facial, pharyngeal, trunk, and extremity muscles
- Hearing lossw
- Small stature
- Electroencephalographic changes
- Cerebellar ataxia
- Elevated levels of cerebrospinal fluid protein

Myoclonic epilepsy with ragged-red fibers (MERRF)
- Multi-system disorder characterized by myoclonus, which is often the first symptom
- Followed by generalized epilepsy, ataxia, weakness, and dementia

Mitochondrial encephalopathy, lactate, acidosis, and stroke-like episodes (MELAS)
- muscle weakness and pain, recurrent headaches, loss of appetite, vomiting, and seizures
- Most affected individuals experience stroke-like episodes beginning before age 40. These episodes often involve temporary muscle weakness on one side of the body (hemiparesis), altered consciousness, vision abnormalities, seizures, and severe headaches resembling migraines.

Mitochondrial neurogastrointestinal encephalopathy (MNGIE)
- Gastrointestinal dysmotility, in which the muscles and nerves of the digestive system do not move food through the digestive tract efficiently.
- Numbness, and weakness in the limbs (peripheral neuropathy), particularly in the hands and feet.
- Droopy eyelids (ptosis), weakness of the muscles that control eye movement (ophthalmoplegia), and hearing loss.
- Leukoencephalopathy is a hallmark of MNGIE disease.

30.17.2 Neuropathology Findings

Microscopic changes are unspecific and include (Table 30.20):
- spongiform changes
- neuronal degeneration
- astrogliosis
- demyelination
- mineralization
- necroses
- various topographical patterns

30.17 Differential Diagnoses: Mitochondrial Encephalomyopathies

Table 30.20 Presence of neuropathologic changes in KSS, MERRF, and MELAS

Histopathologic changes	KSS	MERRF	MELAS
Spongiform changes	+		+
Neuronal degeneration	+	+ Selective	+
Astrogliosis	+	+	
Demyelination	Rare	+	−
Mineralization	−	−	+
Necroses	−	−	+ Multifocal

Spongiform changes
- Vacuolization of the white matter.
- Vacuoles are ovoid with a major axis oriented parallel to the fiber bundles.
- Diameter of 30–260 μm.
- Vacuoles do not contain any material.
- Oligodendrocytes are present in normal density.
- Myelin breakdown is lacking.
- KSS
  – Typical lesion
  – Gray and white matter affected in various anatomical locations:
    o White matter of telencephalon and cerebellum affected
    o Gray matter of the brain stem
    o Gray and white matter of the spinal cord
- MERRF
  – Seldomly described
- MELAS
  – Cerebral cortex predominantly affected

Neuronal degeneration
- Seen in KSS, MERRF, and MELAS
- Generalized atrophy
- Neuronal loss
- Ballooning of the perikarya and central chromatolysis described in MELAS and MERRF (Mukoyama et al. 1986; Ohama et al. 1987).
- KSS
  – Second most frequent lesion
  – Affects brain stem and cerebellum
- MERRF
  – Affects predominantly the cerebellum, brain stem, and spinal cord
- MELAS
  – Affects predominantly the cerebellum with neuronal loss in the cortex and in the dentate nucleus

Focal necroses
- Characteristic for MELAS
- Also found in MERRF and KSS

Reactive astrogliosis
- Present in KSS, MERRF, and MELAS
- Various degrees of severity

Demyelinization
- KSS
  – White matter of the telencephalon, cerebellum, and posterior fascicles of the spinal cord
- MERRF
  – Superior cerebellar peduncle and posterior columns of the spinal cord
- MELAS
  – Seldomly found

Additional changes
- Pallidal and nigral siderosis in KSS
- Mineralizations
  – KSS: in the globus pallidus and thalamus
  – MERRF: absent
  – MELAS: second most frequent lesions mainly affecting the basal ganglia (globus pallidus), thalamus, cerebellar dentate nucleus, and mesencephalon
- Vascular endothelial cell proliferation
- Axonal spheroids

AD neuropathology
- AD similar changes.
- Primitive diffuse plaques present in the whole brain, predominantly in the frontal and temporal lobes.
- Plaques are positive for ß-A4 and negative for tau-protein, ubiquitin, neurofilaments, α-choline acetyltransferase, and acetylcholinesterase.

- Neurofibrillary tangles found in the parahippocampal gyrus.
- Ischemic lesions not found.

30.18 Differential Diagnoses: Metabolic and Traumatic Disorders

30.18.1 Hallervorden-Spatz Disease

- pantothenate kinase-associated neurodegeneration (PKAN) (Bokhari and Bokhari 2018; Van Craenenbroeck et al. 2010; Gregory and Hayflick 1993; Hartig et al. 2012)
- is a rare autosomal recessive neurodegenerative disorder
- associated with iron accumulation in the brain nuclei
- characterized by progressive extrapyramidal dysfunction and dementia

Macroscopic findings
- Yellowish-brown discoloration of the globus pallidus and substantia nigra

Microscopic findings
- Neuronal loss in the globus pallidus and substantia nigra.
- Astrogliosis.
- Axonal swelling.
- Strong iron deposits as free iron as well as iron continued in neurons and macrophages.

Pathogenesis
- mutation in the *PANK2* gene (band 20p13)
- dysfunction of neuromelanin, respectively, in the dopaminergic system
- resulting from the oxidative effects of elevated iron content

30.18.2 Leukodystrophies

Leukodystrophies are a group of disorders characterized by degeneration of the white matter in the brain caused by imperfect growth or development of the myelin sheath (Boespflug-Tanguy et al. 2008; Costello et al. 2009; Gordon et al. 2014; Kohler 2010; Kohler et al. 2018; Perlman and Mar 2012; van der Knaap and Bugiani 2017).

Leukodystrophies include the following disorders:
- Metachromatic leukodystrophy
- Krabbe disease
- Canavan disease
- X-linked adrenoleukodystrophy
- Alexander disease

Clinical signs
- Vary from one type of leukodystrophy to the next.
- Symptoms are dependent on the age of onset, which is predominant in infancy and early childhood.
- Hyperirritability and hypersensitivity to the environment are common.
- Muscle rigidity.
- Backwards-bent head.
- Spasticity.
- Decrease or loss in hearing and vision.
- Optic and auditory degeneration.
- Progressive ataxia.
- Rapid cognitive deterioration, described as mental retardation.
- Epilepsy.
- Weakness in deglutition, leading to spastic coughing fits due to inhaled saliva.

Macroscopic changes
- moderate to severe atrophy
- hardening of the white matter
- grayish-white discoloration of the white matter

Microscopic changes
- degeneration of the white matter with preservation of the arcuate fibers
- numerical reduction of oligodendrocytes
- severe reactive astrogliosis
- metachromatic keukodystrophy
  - Degeneration of myelin sheaths.
  - Numerous macrophages store the typical cerebroside sulfate metachromatic material.

- This material can also be stored in oligodendrocytes, astrocytes, and surviving neurons of the basal ganglia, brain stem, cerebellar dentate nucleus, and spinal cord.
- Adrenoleukodystrophy
  - Perivascular lymphocytic infiltrates.
  - Macrophages with lipid-containing sudanophilic cytoplasmatic inclusions, i.e., strong PAS-positive granular-vacuolated or ballooned cytoplasm.
  - Granular calcifications are rare.
  - Accumulation of immunglobulins.

30.18.3 Wilson Disease: Hepato-Lenticular Degeneration

Clinical signs and symptoms (Chang and Hahn 2017; Czlonkowska et al. 2017; Kelly and Pericleous 2018; Lo and Bandmann 2017; Poujois et al. 2017; Schilsky 2017; Zimbrean and Seniow 2017):

- Tremor
- Muscular rigidity
- Dysarthria
- Dysphagia
- Dementia
- Psychologic changes

Macroscopic changes
- thinning and brownish discoloration of the putamen

Microscopic changes
- hyperplastic astrocytes with
  - abundant cytoplasm
  - nuclear grooving
- small glial cells with
  - scant cytoplasm
  - fine brown-yellowish cytoplasmic granula
  - pale nucleus with 1–2 nucleoli and PAS-positive and Best-Karmin-positive inclusions
- Opalski cells
  - Spongiform, dull stained cytoplasm
  - Large centrally located nucleus
  - Ultrastructural accumulation of lipofuscin and numerous glycogen granula

30.18.4 Dementia Pugilistica

Repeated exposure to impact on the head leads to the development of dementing symptoms in boxers (Dementia pugilistica).

Macroscopic changes
- no obvious changes
- reduced white matter volume
- thinning of the corpus callosum
- foci of old hemorrhages with necrosis cystic lesions in gray and white matter resulting from tissue tears and vascular occlusions

Microscopic changes
- Neurofibrillary changes.
- Amyloid plaques.
- Congophilic angiopathies.
- Changes can fulfill the criteria of Alzheimer disease.
- Laminar cerebral cortical neuronal loss as a result of ischemia.
- Myelin pallor and nerve fiber loss in white matter including corpus callosum.
- Cystic lesions in gray and white matter.
- Residues of hemorrhages.
- Vascular occlusions.
- Axonal injury.

Neuropathogenesis
- The causal relationship between the occurrence of dementia pugilistica and Alzheimer disease is still unresolved.

Selected References

Alonso ME, Teixeira F, Jimenez G, Escobar A (1989) Chorea-acanthocytosis: report of a family and neuropathological study of two cases. Can J Neurol Sci 16(4):426–431

Arai N (1989) "Grumose degeneration" of the dentate nucleus. A light and electron microscopic study in progressive supranuclear palsy and dentatorubropallidoluysial atrophy. J Neurol Sci 90(2):131–145

Arai N, Yagishita S, Amano N, Iwabuchi K, Misugi K (1989) "Grumose degeneration" of Tretiakoff. J Neurol Sci 94(1-3):319–323

Atkin G, Paulson H (2014) Ubiquitin pathways in neurodegenerative disease. Front Mol Neurosci 7:63. https://doi.org/10.3389/fnmol.2014.00063

Bertini E, D'Amico A (2009) Mitochondrial encephalomyopathies and related syndromes: brief review. Endocr Dev 14:38–52

Bird TD, Cederbaum S, Valey RW, Stahl WL (1978) Familial degeneration of the basal ganglia with acanthocytosis: a clinical, neuropathological, and neurochemical study. Ann Neurol 3(3):253–258. https://doi.org/10.1002/ana.410030312

Boespflug-Tanguy O, Labauge P, Fogli A, Vaurs-Barriere C (2008) Genes involved in leukodystrophies: a glance at glial functions. Curr Neurol Neurosci Rep 8(3):217–229

Bokhari MR, Bokhari SRA (2018) Hallervorden Spatz disease (Pantothenate kinase-associated neurodegeneration, PKAN). In: StatPearls. StatPearls Publishing LLC, Treasure Island, FL

Boxer AL (2011) Frontotemporal dementia. In: Budson AE, Kowall NW (eds) The handbook of Alzheimer's disease and Other dementias. Wiley-Blackwell, Hoboken, NJ, pp 145–178

Braak H, Braak E (1987) Argyrophilic grains: characteristic pathology of cerebral cortex in cases of adult onset dementia without Alzheimer changes. Neurosci Lett 76(1):124–127

Braak H, Braak E (1988) Neuropil threads occur in dendrites of tangle-bearing nerve cells. Neuropathol Appl Neurobiol 14(1):39–44

Braak H, Braak E (1989) Cortical and subcortical argyrophilic grains characterize a disease associated with adult onset dementia. Neuropathol Appl Neurobiol 15(1):13–26

Braak H, Braak E (1998) Argyrophilic grain disease: frequency of occurrence in different age categories and neuropathological diagnostic criteria. J Neural Transm 105(8-9):801–819. https://doi.org/10.1007/s007020050096

Bridi JC, Hirth F (2018) Mechanisms of alpha-Synuclein induced synaptopathy in Parkinson's disease. Front Neurosci 12:80. https://doi.org/10.3389/fnins.2018.00080

Bruyn GW (1986) Choreo-acanthocytosis. In: Vinken PJ, Bruyn GW, Klawans HL (eds) Handbook of clinical neurology, Extrapyramidal disorders, vol 5. Elsevier, Amsterdam, pp 327–334

Burre J (2015) The synaptic function of alpha-synuclein. J Park Dis 5(4):699–713. https://doi.org/10.3233/jpd-150642

Burre J, Sharma M, Sudhof TC (2018) Cell biology and pathophysiology of alpha-synuclein. Cold Spring Harb Perspect Med 8(3). https://doi.org/10.1101/cshperspect.a024091

Byrne SC, Rowland LP, Vonsattel JPG, Welzel AT, Walsh DM, Hardiman O (2011) Common themes in the pathogenesis of neurodegeneration. In: Hardiman O, Doherty CP (eds) Neurodegenerative disorders. Springer, Berlin, pp 1–15

Chang IJ, Hahn SH (2017) The genetics of Wilson disease. Handb Clin Neurol 142:19–34. https://doi.org/10.1016/b978-0-444-63625-6.00002-1

Chaturvedi S, Bala K, Thakur R, Suri V (2005) Mitochondrial encephalomyopathies: advances in understanding. Med Sci Monit 11(7):Ra238–Ra246

Costello DJ, Eichler AF, Eichler FS (2009) Leukodystrophies: classification, diagnosis, and treatment. Neurologist 15(6):319–328. https://doi.org/10.1097/NRL.0b013e3181b287c8

Critchley EM, Clark DB, Wikler A (1968) Acanthocytosis and neurological disorder without betalipoproteinemia. Arch Neurol 18(2):134–140

Czlonkowska A, Litwin T, Chabik G (2017) Wilson disease: neurologic features. Handb Clin Neurol 142:101–119. https://doi.org/10.1016/b978-0-444-63625-6.00011-2

Di Giorgio ML, Esposito A, Maccallini P, Micheli E, Bavasso F, Gallotta I, Verni F, Feiguin F, Cacchione S, McCabe BD, Di Schiavi E, Raffa GD (2017) WDR79/TCAB1 plays a conserved role in the control of locomotion and ameliorates phenotypic defects in SMA models. Neurobiol Dis 105:42–50. https://doi.org/10.1016/j.nbd.2017.05.005

DiMauro S (1996) Mitochondrial encephalomyopathies: what next? J Inherit Metab Dis 19(4):489–503

Ederle H, Dormann D (2017) TDP-43 and FUS en route from the nucleus to the cytoplasm. FEBS Lett 591(11):1489–1507. https://doi.org/10.1002/1873-3468.12646

Ferrer I, Santpere G, van Leeuwen FW (2008) Argyrophilic grain disease. Brain 131(Pt 6):1416–1432. https://doi.org/10.1093/brain/awm305

Fong TG, Press DZ (2011) Dementia with Lewy bodies. In: Budson AE, Kowall NW (eds) The handbook of Alzheimer's disease and other dementias. Wiley-Blackwell, Hoboken, NJ, pp 131–144

Galloway PG, Mulvihill P, Siedlak S, Mijares M, Kawai M, Padget H, Kim R, Perry G (1990) Immunochemical demonstration of tropomyosin in the neurofibrillary pathology of Alzheimer's disease. Am J Pathol 137(2):291–300

Geetha T, Vishwaprakash N, Sycheva M, Babu JR (2012) Sequestosome 1/p62: across diseases. Biomarkers 17(2):99–103. https://doi.org/10.3109/1354750x.2011.653986

Geser F, Martinez-Lage M, Kwong LK, Lee VM, Trojanowski JQ (2009) Amyotrophic lateral sclerosis, frontotemporal dementia and beyond: the TDP-43 diseases. J Neurol 256(8):1205–1214. https://doi.org/10.1007/s00415-009-5069-7

Geser F, Lee VM, Trojanowski JQ (2010) Amyotrophic lateral sclerosis and frontotemporal lobar degeneration: a spectrum of TDP-43 proteinopathies. Neuropathology 30(2):103–112. https://doi.org/10.1111/j.1440-1789.2009.01091.x

Geser F, Prvulovic D, O'Dwyer L, Hardiman O, Bede P, Bokde AL, Trojanowski JQ, Hampel H (2011) On the development of markers for pathological TDP-43 in amyotrophic lateral sclerosis with and without dementia. Prog Neurobiol 95(4):649–662. https://doi.org/10.1016/j.pneurobio.2011.08.011

Giannakopoulos P, Hof PR, Bouras C (1995) Dementia lacking distinctive histopathology: clinicopathological evaluation of 32 cases. Acta Neuropathol 89(4):346–355

Gordon HB, Letsou A, Bonkowsky JL (2014) The leukodystrophies. Acta Neuropathol 34(3):312–320. https://doi.org/10.1007/s00401-017-1739-1

Gregory A, Hayflick SJ (1993) Pantothenate kinase-associated neurodegeneration. In: Adam MP, Ardinger HH, Pagon RA et al (eds) GeneReviews ((R)). University of Washington, Seattle

Grundke-Iqbal I, Iqbal K, Tug YC, Quinlan M, Wisniewski HM, Binder LI (1986) Abnormal phosphorylation of the microtubule-associated protein tau (tau) in Alzheimer cytoskeletal pathology. Proc Natl Acad Sci U S A 83(13):4913–4917

Guerrero EN, Wang H, Mitra J, Hegde PM, Stowell SE, Liachko NF, Kraemer BC, Garruto RM, Rao KS, Hegde ML (2016) TDP-43/FUS in motor neuron disease: complexity and challenges. Prog Neurobiol 145-146:78–97. https://doi.org/10.1016/j.pneurobio.2016.09.004

Hardie RJ (1989) Acanthocytosis and neurological impairment—a review. Q J Med 71(264):291–306

Hardie RJ, Pullon HW, Harding AE, Owen JS, Pires M, Daniels GL, Imai Y, Misra VP, King RH, Jacobs JM et al (1991) Neuroacanthocytosis. A clinical, haematological and pathological study of 19 cases. Brain 114(Pt 1A):13–49

Hardy JA, Higgins GA (1992) Alzheimer's disease: the amyloid cascade hypothesis. Science 256(5054):184–185

Hartig MB, Prokisch H, Meitinger T, Klopstock T (2012) Pantothenate kinase-associated neurodegeneration. Curr Drug Targets 13(9):1182–1189

Hayden EY, Teplow DB (2013) Amyloid beta-protein oligomers and Alzheimer's disease. Alzheimer's Res Ther 5(6):60. https://doi.org/10.1186/alzrt226

Herrup K (2015) The case for rejecting the amyloid cascade hypothesis. Nat Neurosci 18(6):794–799. https://doi.org/10.1038/nn.4017

Hirano A, Dembitzer HM, Kurland LT, Zimmerman HM (1968a) The fine structure of some intraganglionic alterations. Neurofibrillary tangles, granulovacuolar bodies and "rod-like" structures as seen in Guam amyotrophic lateral sclerosis and parkinsonism-dementia complex. J Neuropathol Exp Neurol 27(2):167–182

Hirano A, Tuazon R, Zimmerman HM (1968b) Neurofibrillary changes, granulovacuolar bodies and argentophilic globules observed in tuberous sclerosis. Acta Neuropathol 11(3):257–261

Iizuka R, Hirayama K (1986) Dentato-rubro-pallido-luysian atroph. In: Vinken PJ, Bruyn GW, Klawans HL (eds) Handbook of clinical neurology, vol 5. Elsevier, Amsterdam, pp 437–443

Iizuka R, Hirayama K, Maehara KA (1984) Dentato-rubro-pallido-luysian atrophy: a clinico-pathological study. J Neurol Neurosurg Psychiatry 47(12):1288–1298

Ikeda K, Akiyama H, Arai T, Matsushita M, Tsuchiya K, Miyazaki H (2000) Clinical aspects of argyrophilic grain disease. Clin Neuropathol 19(6):278–284

Ishigaki S, Sobue G (2018) Importance of functional loss of FUS in FTLD/ALS. Front Mol Biosci 5:44. https://doi.org/10.3389/fmolb.2018.00044

Iwaki T, Kume-Iwaki A, Goldman JE (1990) Cellular distribution of alpha B-crystallin in non-lenticular tissues. J Histochem Cytochem 38(1):31–9

Jansen AH, Reits EA, Hol EM (2014) The ubiquitin proteasome system in glia and its role in neurodegenerative diseases. Front Mol Neurosci 7:73. https://doi.org/10.3389/fnmol.2014.00073

Kelly C, Pericleous M (2018) Wilson disease: more than meets the eye. Postgrad Med J 94(1112):335–347. https://doi.org/10.1136/postgradmedj-2017-135381

Knowles TP, Vendruscolo M, Dobson CM (2014) The amyloid state and its association with protein misfolding diseases. Nat Rev Mol Cell Biol 15(6):384–396. https://doi.org/10.1038/nrm3810

Kohler W (2010) Leukodystrophies with late disease onset: an update. Curr Opin Neurol 23(3):234–241. https://doi.org/10.1097/WCO.0b013e328338313a

Kohler W, Curiel J, Vanderver A (2018) Adulthood leukodystrophies. Nat Rev Neurol 14(2):94–105. https://doi.org/10.1038/nrneurol.2017.175

Komatsu M, Kageyama S, Ichimura Y (2012) p62/SQSTM1/A170: physiology and pathology. Pharmacol Res 66(6):457–462. https://doi.org/10.1016/j.phrs.2012.07.004

Kosaka K (1994) Diffuse neurofibrillary tangles with calcification: a new presenile dementia. J Neurol Neurosurg Psychiatry 57(5):594–596

Kovacs GG (2014) Neuropathology of neurodegenerative diseases book and online: a practical guide. Cambridge University Press, Cambridge

Kummer MP, Heneka MT (2014) Truncated and modified amyloid-beta species. Alzheimer's Res Ther 6(3):28. https://doi.org/10.1186/alzrt258

Lantos PL (1992) Neuropathology of unusual dementias: an overview. Baillieres Clin Neurol 1(3):485–516

Levine IM, Estes JW, Looney JM (1968) Hereditary neurological disease with acanthocytosis. A new syndrome. Arch Neurol 19(4):403–409

Ling SC (2018) Synaptic paths to neurodegeneration: the emerging role of TDP-43 and FUS in synaptic functions. Neural Plast 2018:8413496. https://doi.org/10.1155/2018/8413496

Lo C, Bandmann O (2017) Epidemiology and introduction to the clinical presentation of Wilson disease. Handb Clin Neurol 142:7–17. https://doi.org/10.1016/b978-0-444-63625-6.00008-2

Love S, Saitoh T, Quijada S, Cole GM, Terry RD (1988) Alz-50, ubiquitin and tau immunoreactivity of neurofibrillary tangles, Pick bodies and Lewy bodies. J Neuropathol Exp Neurol 47(4):393–405

Lowe J, Mayer RJ (1990) Ubiquitin, cell stress and diseases of the nervous system. Neuropathol Appl Neurobiol 16(4):281–91

Mayer RJ, Lowe J, Landon M (1991) Ubiquitin and the molecular pathology of chronic degenerative diseases. J Pathol 163(4):279–81

Mikhaleva S, Lemke EA (2018) Beyond the transport function of import receptors: what's all the FUS about? Cell 173(3):549–553. https://doi.org/10.1016/j.cell.2018.04.002

Mukoyama M, Kazui H, Sunohara N, Yoshida M, Nonaka I, Satoyoshi E (1986) Mitochondrial myopathy, encephalopathy, lactic acidosis, and stroke-like episodes with acanthocytosis: a clinicopathological study of a unique case. J Neurol 233(4):228–32

Nolan M, Talbot K, Ansorge O (2016) Pathogenesis of FUS-associated ALS and FTD: insights from rodent models. Acta Neuropathol Commun 4(1):99. https://doi.org/10.1186/s40478-016-0358-8

Ohama E, Ohara S, Ikuta F, Tanaka K, Nishizawa M, Miyatake T (1987) Mitochondrial angiopathy in cerebral blood vessels of mitochondrial encephalomyopathy. Acta Neuropathol 74(3):226–33

Oldfors A, Tulinius M (2003) Mitochondrial encephalomyopathies. J Neuropathol Exp Neurol 62(3):217–227

Perlman SJ, Mar S (2012) Leukodystrophies. Adv Exp Med Biol 724:154–171. https://doi.org/10.1007/978-1-4614-0653-2_13

Poujois A, Mikol J, Woimant F (2017) Wilson disease: brain pathology. Handb Clin Neurol 142:77–89. https://doi.org/10.1016/b978-0-444-63625-6.00008-2

Ratti A, Buratti E (2016) Physiological functions and pathobiology of TDP-43 and FUS/TLS proteins. J Neurochem 138(Suppl 1):95–111. https://doi.org/10.1111/jnc.13625

Sakai T, Mawatari S, Iwashita H, Goto I, Kuroiwa Y (1981) Choreoacanthocytosis. Clues to clinical diagnosis. Arch Neurol 38(6):335–338

Salminen A, Kaarniranta K, Haapasalo A, Hiltunen M, Soininen H, Alafuzoff I (2012) Emerging role of p62/sequestosome-1 in the pathogenesis of Alzheimer's disease. Prog Neurobiol 96(1):87–95. https://doi.org/10.1016/j.pneurobio.2011.11.005

Sarnat HB, Marin-Garcia J (2005) Pathology of mitochondrial encephalomyopathies. Can J Neurol Sci 32(2):152–166

Schilsky ML (2017) Wilson disease: diagnosis, treatment, and follow-up. Postgrad Med J 21(4):755–767. https://doi.org/10.1136/postgradmedj-2017-135381

Simchowicz T (1911) Histologische Studien über die senile Demenz. Histol Histopathol Arb Grosshirnrinde 4:267–444

Smith JK (1975) Dentatorubropallidoluysian atrophy. In: Vinken PJ, Bruyn GW (eds) Handbook of clinical neurology, vol 21. Elsevier-North Holland, Amsterdam, pp 519–534

Spillantini MG, Goedert M (2013) Tau pathology and neurodegeneration. Lancet Neurol 12(6):609–622. https://doi.org/10.1016/s1474-4422(13)70090-5

Takashima A (2013) Tauopathies and tau oligomers. J Alzheimers Dis 37(3):565–568. https://doi.org/10.3233/jad-130653

Theillet FX, Binolfi A, Bekei B, Martorana A, Rose HM, Stuiver M, Verzini S, Lorenz D, van Rossum M, Goldfarb D, Selenko P (2016) Structural disorder of monomeric alpha-synuclein persists in mammalian cells. Nature 530(7588):45–50. https://doi.org/10.1038/nature16531

Thomas M, Alegre-Abarrategui J, Wade-Martins R (2013) RNA dysfunction and aggrephagy at the centre of an amyotrophic lateral sclerosis/frontotemporal dementia disease continuum. Brain 136(Pt 5):1345–1360. https://doi.org/10.1093/brain/awt030

Tolnay M, Clavaguera F (2004) Argyrophilic grain disease: a late-onset dementia with distinctive features among tauopathies. Neuropathology 24(4):269–283

Tolnay M, Probst A (2008) Argyrophilic grain disease. Handb Clin Neurol 89:553–563. https://doi.org/10.1016/s0072-9752(07)01251-1

Tolnay M, Schwietert M, Monsch AU, Staehelin HB, Langui D, Probst A (1997a) Argyrophilic grain disease: distribution of grains in patients with and without dementia. Acta Neuropathol 94(4):353–358

Tolnay M, Spillantini MG, Goedert M, Ulrich J, Langui D, Probst A (1997b) Argyrophilic grain disease: widespread hyperphosphorylation of tau protein in limbic neurons. Acta Neuropathol 93(5):477–484

Tolnay M, Mistl C, Ipsen S, Probst A (1998) Argyrophilic grains of Braak: occurrence in dendrites of neurons containing hyperphosphorylated tau protein. Neuropathol Appl Neurobiol 24(1):53–59

Tolnay M, Monsch AU, Probst A (2001) Argyrophilic grain disease. A frequent dementing disorder in aged patients. Adv Exp Med Biol 487:39–58

Tolnay M, Sergeant N, Ghestem A, Chalbot S, De Vos RA, Jansen Steur EN, Probst A, Delacourte A (2002) Argyrophilic grain disease and Alzheimer's disease are distinguished by their different distribution of tau protein isoforms. Acta Neuropathol 104(4):425–434. https://doi.org/10.1007/s00401-002-0591-z

University of Washington, Seattle (1993–2019). GeneReviews is a registered trademark of the University of Washington, Seattle, WA. All rights reserved

Valdinocci D, Radford RA, Siow SM, Chung RS, Pountney DL (2017) Potential modes of intercellular alpha-synuclein transmission. Int J Mol Sci 18(2):E469. https://doi.org/10.3390/ijms18020469

Van Craenenbroeck A, Gebruers M, Martin JJ, Cras P (2010) Hallervorden-Spatz disease: historical case presentation in the spotlight of nosological evolution. Mov Disord 25(15):2486–2492. https://doi.org/10.1002/mds.23217

van der Knaap MS, Bugiani M (2017) Leukodystrophies: a proposed classification system based on pathological changes and pathogenetic mechanisms. Acta Neuropathol 134(3):351–382. https://doi.org/10.1007/s00401-017-1739-1

Varela JM (1969) Atrophy of the reticular formation of the central nervous system. I. Generalized global reticular atrophy. Syndrome of dyshomeostasis of the central nervous system. Psychiatr Clin 2(1):41–61

Zimbrean P, Seniow J (2017) Cognitive and psychiatric symptoms in Wilson disease. Handb Clin Neurol 142:121–140. https://doi.org/10.1016/b978-0-444-63625-6.00003-3

Normal Aging Brain

31.1 Introduction

31.1.1 WHO Definition of Well-Being

As defined by World Health Organization (WHO), well-being is a "state of complete physical, mental, and social well-being, and not merely the absence of disease or infirmity." Health is a dynamic condition resulting from a body's constant adjustment and adaptation in response to stresses and changes in the environment for maintaining an inner equilibrium called homeostasis.

Age of an organism: the length of time the individual has existed

Aging: encompasses the progressive deteriorative changes, during the adult period of life, which underlie an increasing vulnerability to challenges and thereby decrease the ability of the organism to survive.

Successful aging refers to:
- Physical
- Mental
- Social well-being in older age

Traditional definition emphasized:
- Absence of physical disabilities
- Absence of cognitive disabilities

Characterization of successful aging (Rowe and Kahn 1987):
- Freedom from disease and disability
- High cognitive and physical functioning
- Social and productive engagement

Stigma associated with old age (see ageism):
- Considering older people as a burden on society
- Negative aspects of aging or preventing the decline of youth

Recent definitions:
- There is a growing number of older adults functioning at a high level and contributing to the society.
- Importance of adaptation and emotional well-being in successful aging.
- For most senior citizens, subjective quality of life is more important than the absence of disease and other objective measures relating to physical and mental health.

The model of successful aging (Mather 2016):
- More important aspects to aging successfully include:
  – Optimism
  – Effective coping styles
  – Social and community
- Subjective quality of life is strongly tied with psychosocial protective traits such as
  – Resilience
  – Optimism
  – Mental and emotional status
- Mental and psychosocial functioning often improve with age, even if physical health, and some elements of memory decline.

- Age-related wisdom
  - might serve to compensate for the biological losses in old age, thereby enabling older adults to better utilize their remaining resources and age successfully
  - may help to overcome the negative effects of diseases and stressors that are common in late life and lead to improved mental health and psychosocial functioning

31.2 Clinical Signs and Symptoms

- Declines in physical and cognitive processes.
- Emotional functioning fares relatively well.
  - Processes such as attending to and remembering emotional stimuli
  - Regulating emotion
  - Recognizing emotional expressions
  - Empathy, risk taking, impulsivity, behavior change, and attentional focus

31.3 Epidemiology

Incidence
- The whole population

Age Incidence
- Birth until death

Sex Incidence
- Male:Female ratio: 1:1

Localization
- Cerebral cortex
- White matter

31.4 Neuroimaging Findings

General Imaging Findings
- Generalized brain atrophy

CT non-contrast-enhanced
- Enlargement of outer and inner CSF spaces
- Focal or confluent periventricular hypodensities

CT contrast-enhanced
- No contrast enhancement

MRI-T2/FLAIR (Fig. 31.1a–d)
- Focal or confluent periventricular hyperintensities
- Enlargement of perivascular spaces (isointense to CSF)

MRI-T1
- Generalized brain atrophy

MRI-T1 contrast-enhanced
- No contrast enhancement

MRI-T2∗/SWI
- Iron deposition in globus pallidus possible

MR-Diffusion Tensor Imaging
- Decreased anisotropy

Nuclear Medicine Imaging Findings (Fig. 31.2a, b)
- Functional development of the pediatric brain has been assessed with FDG-PET. It has been shown that the pattern of glucose metabolism correlates with the evolution of infantile behavior. By 1 year of age, the metabolism pattern of FDG becomes similar to those of young adults. The metabolic activity in neonates is approximately 30% that of adults. The metabolic activity increases until the third year and reaches a plateau from the age of 4 to the age of 9 with a value of 1.3 times of a normal young adult. The metabolism declines then to adult rates.
- Studies dealing with CBF showed that cortical CBF tends to decrease with age but they showed no significant reduced blood flow, because there is a wide range of blood flow in the general population. CBF in the white matter is relatively preserved in the aging process.
- FDG-PET studies are inconsistent too. Some report no changes but others showed decrease in the whole brain or regionally. As in CBF studies there is a wide variation across and within age groups. Frontal, parietal, and occipital lobes appeared to be symmetrical but in

31.4 Neuroimaging Findings

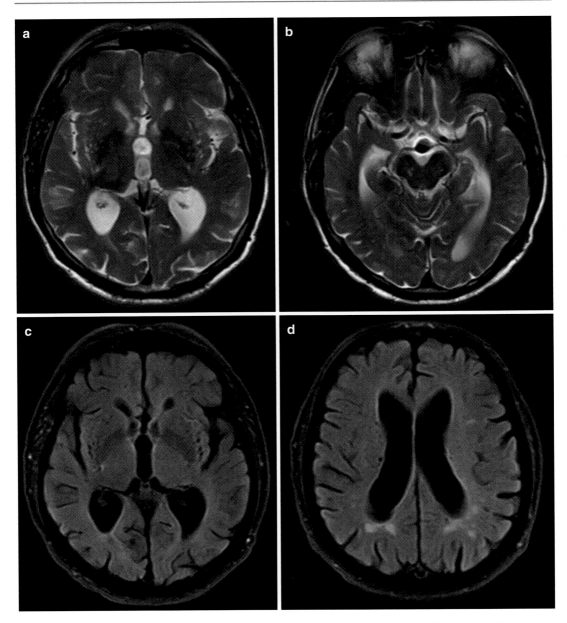

Fig. 31.1 Normal aging brain of an 80-year-old patient—enlarged perivascular spaces in the basal ganglia and brain stem, mild periventricular T2-hyperintensities and only mild brain atrophy; T2 (**a**, **b**), FLAIR (**c**, **d**)

comparison the left temporal lobe appeared to be hypometabolic compared to the right. Basal ganglia, thalamus, cerebellum, and visual cortex were found to be relatively preserved throughout the aging process. But not only the overall or regional FDG uptake is of relevance. The aging brain shows a metabolic pattern corresponding to structural changes and thereby getting more heterogeneous mainly corresponding to small vascular alterations.

- Presynaptic dopamine receptor studies for β-CIT showed a decrease with a normal aging brain of 8% per decade from the age of 18. Studies with FP-CIT showed a mean decrease

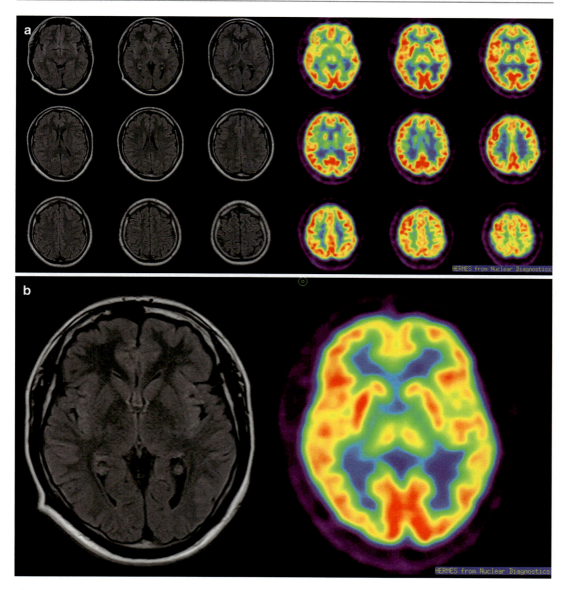

Fig. 31.2 Normal FDG-PET slices (**a**, **b**) combined with MRI scans

of 5.5% per decade with a greater loss in men than in women. Tracer uptake was found to be lesser in the caudate nucleus than in putamen.
- A study with 11C-MET showed an increased brain uptake of this amino acid in pediatric patients compared to adults. This could suggest that the developing brain needs and thereby allows a greater uptake of amino acids in children. Studies in adults are inconclusive—some show a decrease in uptake in older patients, other studies could not verify this results.

31.5 Neuropathology Findings

Macroscopic Features
- Reduction in brain weight
- Signs of minimal to moderate atrophy of the cerebral cortex
- Reduction in the volume of:
    - Telencephalic lobes (Table 31.1)
    - White matter (Fig. 31.3) (Table 31.1)
- Minimal to moderate enlargement of the ventricular system

31.5 Neuropathology Findings

Microscopic Features
- Neurons
  - Shrinkage in size
  - Partial, layer-specific loss of neurons, i.e., layers III and V
- Synapses
  - Loss of synaptophysin-immunoreactivities
- Dendrites
  - Rarefication of the dendritic tree
- White matter
  - Myelin pallor/loss correlated with vascular hyalinosis
- Astroglia
- Oligodendroglia

- Vessels
  - Hyalinosis
- Increased presence of corpora amylacea
- Amyloid deposits
- Neurofibrillary tangles
  - The number of NFTs in the CA1 and the entorhinal cortex seems to be more closely related to cognitive status, compared to the amyloid load (Xekardaki et al. 2015).
- The theory of cognitive reserve has been proposed for further understanding of interindividual differences in terms of compensation despite the presence of pathological lesions (Xekardaki et al. 2015).

Table 31.1 Normal aging: volume (in cm^3) of white matter structures correlated with age in 76 healthy controls (unpublished data from Weis et al. in preparation) (Fig. 31.3)

Brain region	Age—r	Age—p
Frontal lobe	−0.44	0.0001
Parieto-occipital lobe	−0.42	0.0001
Temporal lobe	−0.44	0.0001
Corpus callosum	−0.42	0.0002
Internal capsule	−0.44	0.0001
Capsula externa	−0.34	0.003
Lobar white matter	−0.53	0.0000
Hemispheric white matter	−0.53	0.0000

Corpora amylacea (Fig. 31.4 a–d)
- Round amorphous structures, 5–20 μm in diameter
- Denser staining round core
- Basophilic, argentophilic, PAS-positive
- Localization:
  - Subpial and subependymal regions
  - Median portion of the lentiform nucleus
  - Ammon's horn
  - White matter of spinal cord
- Within astrocytic processes

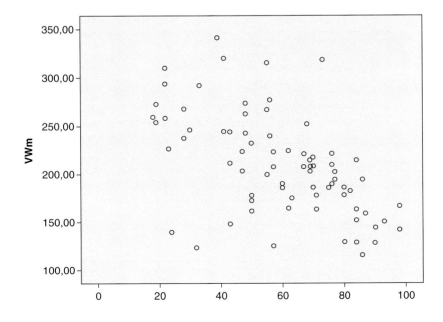

Fig. 31.3 Volume reduction of the white matter during normal aging (Weis: unpublished data)

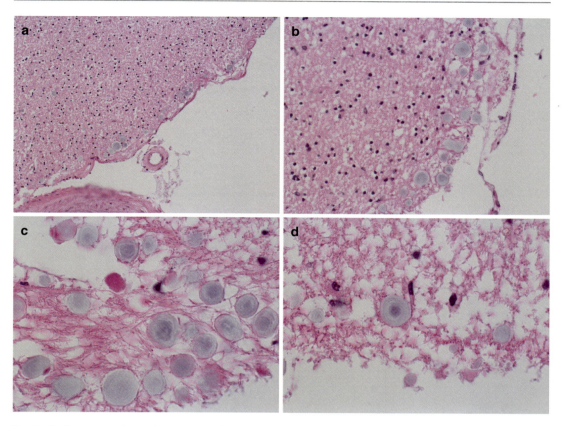

Fig. 31.4 Corpora amylacea: they are very often found in a subpial position (**a–d**)

- EM. 6.5 nm curved and apparently branched filaments arranged in a random fashion
- Composed of glycogen-like carbohydrate mixed with small amounts of protein
- Promiscuous behavior in immunohistochemistry
- Invariably found in aged brains

Region-specific changes of the white matter in the normal aging brain are shown in Table 31.2 (Weis et al. unpublished data).
- Particularly the frontal lobe and medial temporal regions are accompanied by age-related differences in frontal and medial temporal lobe mediated cognitive abilities (Lockhart and DeCarli 2014).
- Degeneration of specific white matter tracts such as those passing through the genu and splenium of the corpus callosum may also be related to age-related differences in cognitive performance (Lockhart and DeCarli 2014).

Hippocampal atrophy rates increase with age with the largest increases occurring from midlife onwards (Fraser et al. 2015).
- Mean total hippocampal atrophy for the entire sample was 0.85% per year (95% CI 0.63, 1.07).
- Age-based atrophy rates were:
  – age <55 years ($n = 413$): 0.38% per year (CI 0.14, 0.62)
  – age 55 to <70 years ($n = 426$): 0.98% per year (CI 0.27, 1.70)
  – age ≥70 years ($n = 2583$): 1.12% per year (CI 0.86, 1.38)
- Meta-regression indicated age was associated with increased atrophy rates of 0.0263% (CI 0.0146, 0.0379) per year and automated

Table 31.2 Region-specific changes encountered in the white matter of aging brain (Weis et al. unpublished data)

Brain region	Correlation with age	r	p
Frontal	Hyalinosis	0.37	0.02
	Corpora amylacea	0.40	0.01
	Myelin pallor	0.37	0.02
	Myelin loss	0.57	0.00
	Myelin (pallor and/or loss)	0.58	0.00
Fronto-orbital	Corpora amylacea	0.59	0.00
	Myelin pallor	0.58	0.00
	Myelin loss	0.45	0.00
	Myelin (pallor and/or loss)	0.70	0.00
Hippocampus	CA: Hyalinosis	0.42	0.02
	Dentate gyrus: Myelin loss	0.40	0.03
Internal capsule	Hyalinosis	0.49	0.00
	Myelin pallor	0.41	0.01
	Myelin loss	0.47	0.00
	Corpora amylacea	0.39	0.01
Anterior commissure	Myelin pallor	0.65	0.01

segmentation approaches were associated with a reduced atrophy rate of −0.466% (CI −0.841, −0.090).

Functional neuroimaging research on normal aging brain (Sugiura 2016)
- Age-related compensatory recruitment of prefrontal cortex, in terms of executive system or reduced lateralization.
- Age-related neural alteration is considered adaptation to the environmental change.
  – The age-related increase in activation of the sensorimotor network may reflect the alteration of the peripheral sensorimotor systems.
  – The increased susceptibility of the network for the mental-state inference to the socio-emotional significance may be explained by the age-related motivational shift due to the altered social perception.
  – The age-related change in activation of the self-referential network may be relevant to the focused positive self-concept of elderly driven by a similar motivational shift.

31.6 Incidental White Matter Changes

Incidental white matter changes (Fig. 31.5a, b)
- Common finding on magnetic resonance imaging (MRI) of the brain in elderly persons
- Synonyms used:
  – White matter lesions
  – White matter hyperintensities
  – Leuko-araiosis
- Hachinski introduced the term leuko-araiosis (from the Greek *leuko* [white] and *araiosis* [rarefaction]) to designate both periventricular or subcortical (centrum semiovale) areas of hypodensity on CT scans or hyperintensity on T2-weighted MRI scans (Hachinski et al. 1986, 1987).
- In population-based studies, the prevalence of any white matter lesion varies between 45 and 95%. Depending on the composition of the investigated cohorts, 12–33% of subjects have severe changes.

MRI classifications of white matter changes usually separate between
- Periventricular
  – Caps around the frontal horns of the lateral ventricles and pencil-thin lining or a smooth halo along the side of the lateral ventricles
- Deep
- Subcortical signal abnormalities
  – Punctate changes
  – Beginning confluent or confluent abnormalities
- Caps/lining and punctate deep subcortical white matter lesions are by far the most common signal changes in elderly subjects and occur in more than half of asymptomatic persons even in age groups below 55 years.
- All other white matter abnormalities are substantially less common, but their frequency increases with age, and in subjects above 75 years old they affect at least one fifth of individuals free of any overt signs of neurologic disease.

Fig. 31.5 Correlation of in vivo magnetic resonance imaging (MRI) and histomorphological features of affected fixed brains in representative cases with white matter lesions (**a**). (*a*) Caps abutt upon the frontal horns of the lateral ventricles, (*b*) gross overview of ventricle, subventricular zone, and partly pale white matter (stain Luxol fast blue), (*c*) multiple punctate white matter hyperintensities in the centrum semiovale bilaterally, (*d*) enlarged cell-free perivascular spaces in the presence of vessel wall hyalinosis. Luxol fast blue periodic acid-Schiff (PAS)-stained whole mount section, (*e*) early confluent and confluent white matter lesions in the deep and periventricular white matter affecting both hemispheres, (*f*) overview picture of severe white matter changes with many large and small white matter lesions of variable shape characterized by patchy myelin loss with some cystic lacunar lesions representing areas of more severe tissue damage (**a**). White matter changes in T2-weighted FLAIR MRI scans. The first column shows periventricular white matter changes: (*a*) caps, (*b*) pencil-thin lining, and (*c*) halo. The second column shows deep or subcortical white matter changes: (*d*) punctate, (*e*) early confluent, and (*f*) confluent lesions (**b**), reproduced with kind permission from Schmidt et al. (2011)

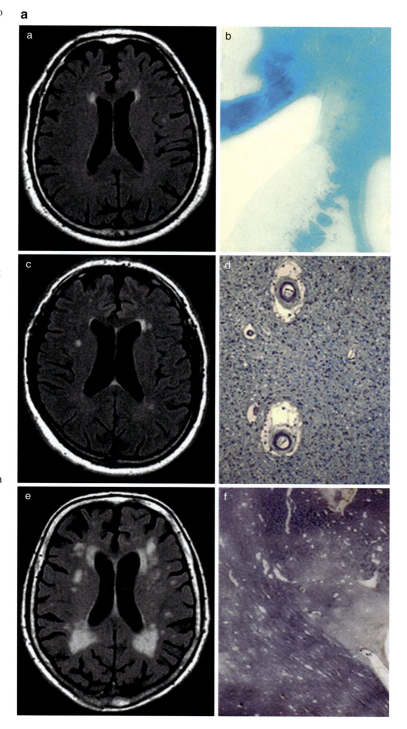

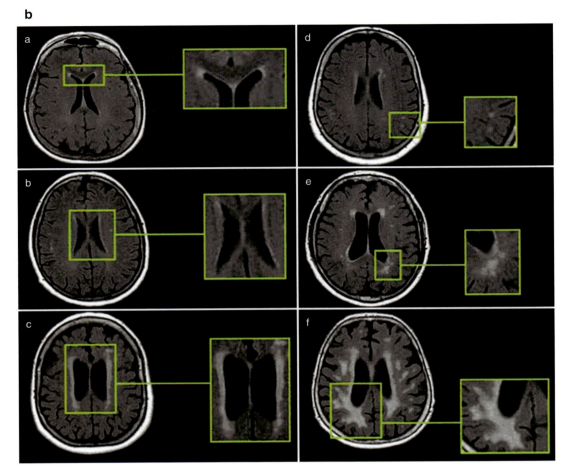

Fig. 31.5 (continued)

White matter lesions affect:
- Executive functions
  - Impair activities of daily life resulting from erroneous goal formation, planning, and organization
- Abstract reasoning
  - From mild memory deficits with slight recognition and cueing difficulties
- Motor disturbances
  - Affect gait, postural control, and urinary continence
- The interindividual variability of the clinical presentation in subjects with white matter changes is high.
  - Clinical sequelae are likely to be influenced by lesion distribution and volume in strategically relevant brain regions.
- In addition, heterogeneity of white matter lesions is another important issue as it influences:
  - The clinical and functional consequences
  - The pace of lesion progression

Neuropathologic correlates of different types of age-related white matter changes
- Partial loss of myelin
- Partial loss of axons
- Astrogliosis in the vicinity of altered small vessel

Pathogenetic mechanisms
- Tissue changes are thought to result from incomplete infarction, although small deep white matter infarcts have been described.

- Non-ischemic as well as ischemic brain changes have been described.
  - Smooth periventricular white matter hyperintensities appear to be of non-vascular origin.
- Bright caps around the frontal horns were consistently found to correspond to a spongiform zone of finely textured myelin.
- Increased periventricular water content, which converges from the surrounding white matter in this area or derives from the intense venous network of this region
- Disruption of the ependymal lining of the lateral ventricle and subependymal gliosis, so-called ependymitis granularis, invariably found with periventricular hyperintense caps.
- Deep and subcortical white matter changes
  - Non-uniform
  - Important to distinguish between the
    - Punctate lesion
    - More widespread early confluent
    - Confluent changes
  - Punctate hyperintensities
    - Commonly of non-ischemic origin
    - Widening of periarteriolar spaces
    - Reduced myelination with atrophy of the neuropil around fibrohyalinotic arteries
  - Early confluent and confluent white matter hyperintensities are:
    - True ischemic lesions
    - Continuum of increasing tissue damage including
      - Widespread perivascular rarefaction of myelin
      - Mild to moderate nerve fiber loss
      - Varying extents of astrogliosis
  - Confluent changes are:
    - Irregular, mostly relatively well demarcated areas of incomplete parenchymal destruction with focal transitions to true infarcts
- Astrocytes
  - Clasmatodendritic astroglia immunoreactive for fibrinogen was more commonly present in periventricular lesions.
  - Platelet-derived growth factor α receptor positive reactive astrocytes increased in periventricular lesions.
- Oligodendrocytes
  - MAP-2-positive remyelinating oligodendrocytes increased in periventricular lesions
- Microglia
  - Periventricular and deep subcortical lesions were associated with severe myelin loss and increased microglia as compared to non-lesional brain tissue.
  - Activated microglia in deep and subcortical abnormalities may rather reflect an innate amoeboid phenotype, which is involved in phagocytosis of myelin breakdown products.
- Blood–brain barrier
  - Periventricular white matter changes contain significantly higher levels of ramified activated microglia which may result from blood–brain barrier disruption

Summary
- Periventricular lesion severity
  - Associated with loss of ventricular ependymal lining
  - Prone to increased fluid accumulation related to the proximity of the ventricles
- Deep and subcortical white matter lesions
  - Arteriolosclerosis was observed.
  - Hypoxia-inducible factors was mainly elevated in deep and subcortical but not in periventricular lesions.
  - Hypoxic environment for deep lesions.

Risk factors and emerging pathways
- Differences in risk factors and clinical consequences of different lesion types, but also in the rate of lesion progression.
- Individuals with coalescent white matter lesions were significantly older, had more frequently hypertension and a history of stroke as compared to subjects with punctate abnormalities.

- The amount of cigarettes smoked, and the interaction between hypercholesterolemia and smoking were associated with confluent white matter changes only.
- Apolipoprotein E genotype: Positive associations between the presence of the epsilon4 allele, and the extent and progression of MRI lesions in the deep and subcortical white matter
- The majority of differentially regulated transcripts in white matter lesions coded for genes associated with:
  - Immune function
  - Cell cycle
  - Proteolysis
  - Ion transport
  - Electron transport
  - Metabolism
  - Cell structure
- Genome-wide association studies
  - Six SNPs mapping to a locus on chromosome 17q25
  - Large cluster of associated SNPs spanning a ~100 kb region, which contains several genes
    ○ Two tripartite motif-containing genes, *TRIM65* and *TRIM47*
    ○ WW domain binding protein 2 gene (*WBP2*)
    ○ Mitochondrial ribosomal protein L38 gene (*MRPL38*)
    ○ Fas-binding factor 1 gene (*FBF1*)
    ○ Acyl-coenzyme A oxidase 1 gene (*ACOX1*)
    ○ Several of these genes are related to apoptosis superfamily and apoptosis-related transcripts.
- Increased production of reactive oxygen species
  - Hemochromatosis gene appears to be a genetic risk factor for severe age-related white matter lesions independently of the APOE ε4 genotype.

Lesion-type-specific clinical consequences and progression rates
- Patients with early confluent and confluent changes show impairment
  - Cognition
  - Depression
  - Gait and balance
  - Urinary incontinence

Immunophenotype
- ß amyloid
- tau, p-tau

Differential Diagnosis
- Neurodegenerative disorder, Alzheimer disease

Pathogenesis
- Increased life expectancy
  - Males: 74.5 years
  - Females: 79.9 years
- Fraction of population above 65 years

31.7 Molecular Neuropathology

- Genes for successful aging
- Sirtuins
- Telomeres
- Damage caused by oxidative stress and other factors
  - Reactive O_2 species
  - Glycation and glycoxidation
  - Mitochondrial damage
  - Somatic mutations
- Inadequate repair of damage
  - DNA repair
  - Protein turnover
  - Membrane deterioration
- Dysregulation of cell number
  - Limitations in cell division
    ○ Telomeres
  - Cell removal
    ○ Apoptosis
- Stress response
- Inflammation
- Signaling: MAPK
- Synaptic transmission
- Axon guidance
- Calcium signaling
- Protein synthesis

31.7.1 Astrocytes

Astrocytes are fundamental for (Rodriguez-Arellano et al. 2016)
- Homeostasis, defense, and regeneration of the central nervous system.
- Loss of astroglial function and astroglial reactivity contributes to the aging of the brain and to neurodegenerative diseases.
- Changes in astroglia in aging and neurodegeneration are highly heterogeneous and region-specific.
- Astrocytes undergo degeneration and atrophy at the early stages of pathological progression, which possibly may alter the homeostatic reserve of the brain and contribute to early cognitive deficits.
- At later stages of AD reactive astrocytes are associated with neurite plaques, the feature commonly found in animal models and in human diseased tissue.

31.7.2 Microglia

- Microglia are highly active and vigilant housekeepers of the central nervous system that function to promote neuronal growth and activity.
- With advanced age, dysregulated inflammatory signaling and defects in phagocytosis impede their ability to perform the most essential of homeostatic functions, including immune surveillance and debris clearance.
- Microglial activation is one of the hallmarks of the aging brain and coincides with age-related neurodegeneration and cognitive decline.
- Age-associated microglial dysfunction leads to cellular senescence and can profoundly alter the response to sterile injuries and immune diseases, often resulting in maladaptive responses, chronic inflammation, and worsened outcomes after injury (Koellhoffer et al. 2017).
- Aging leads to a loss of integrated regulatory networks including aberrant signaling from other brain cells, immune sensors, and epigenetic modifiers. The low-grade chronic neuroinflammation associated with this dysfunctional activity likely contributes to cognitive deficits and susceptibility to age-related pathologies (Matt and Johnson 2016).
- (Dys)regulation of autophagy in microglia affects innate immune functions such as phagocytosis and inflammation, which in turn contribute to the pathophysiology of aging and neurodegenerative diseases (Plaza-Zabala et al. 2017).
- Autophagy may affect microglial phagocytosis of apoptotic cells, amyloid-β, synaptic material, and myelin debris, and regulate the progression of age-associated neurodegenerative diseases.
- Autophagy regulates the microglial inflammatory phenotype, which is known to contribute to age-related brain dysfunction (Plaza-Zabala et al. 2017).
- Macrophages/Microglia:
  - Infiltrating macrophages age differently from central nervous system-intrinsic microglia.
  - Several mechanisms underlie the differential aging process of these two distinct cell types.
  - Therapeutic strategies that selectively target these diverse mechanisms may rejuvenate macrophages and microglia for repair in the aging central nervous system.
  - Most responses of macrophages are diminished with senescence, but activated microglia increase their expression of pro-inflammatory cytokines while diminishing chemotactic and phagocytic activities.
  - The senescence of macrophages and microglia has a negative impact on several neurological diseases, and the mechanisms underlying their age-dependent phenotypic changes vary from extrinsic microenvironmental changes to intrinsic changes in genomic integrity.
  - Rejuvenation of aging macrophage/microglia may preserve neurological integrity and promote regeneration in the aging central nervous system (Rawji et al. 2016).

The roles of microglia in phagocytosis and inflammation during aging and in Alzheimer disease, Parkinson disease, Huntington disease, and stroke are illustrated in Table 31.3.

31.7.3 Autophagy

- Core regulator of central nervous system (CNS) aging and neurodegeneration (Table 31.4).
- Delivers toxic molecules and organelles to the lysosome.
- (Dys)regulation of autophagy in microglia also affects innate immune functions such as phagocytosis and inflammation, which in turn contribute to the pathophysiology of aging and neurodegenerative diseases (Plaza-Zabala et al. 2017).

31.7.4 Unfolded Protein Response (UPR): Endoplasmic Reticulum Stress—Stress Response Pathways

The unfolded protein response (UPR)
- operates as central player to maintain ER homeostasis or the induction of cell death of chronically damaged cells.
- A reduction in the buffering capacity of the proteostasis network occurs during aging.
- The accumulation of misfolded proteins is enhanced.
- As almost one-third of the proteome is synthetized at the endoplasmic reticulum (ER), maintenance of its proper function is fundamental to sustain neuronal function.

Table 31.3 Roles of microglia in phagocytosis and inflammation during aging and in Alzheimer disease, Parkinson disease, Huntington disease, and stroke (modified after Plaza-Zabala et al. (2017) reproduced with kind permission by MDPI, open access)

Disease	Phagocytosis		Inflammation	
	Function	Role of autophagy	Function	Role of autophagy
Aging	Clearance of apoptotic cells, Aß, synaptic material, and myelin debris	Autophagy inhibition (by MTORC1 activation or ATG1 inhibition) prevents neurodegeneration	Inflammation-aging	Unknown
Alzheimer Disease (AD)	Clearance of apoptotic cells, synaptic debris, and Aß	• Autophagy inhibition (by BECN-1 downregulation) reduces Aß phagocytosis and/or degradation. • Autophagy inhibition (by ATG-7 and LC3 deletion) reduces Aß clearance	NLRP3 inflammasome activation and inflammatory mediator production	Autophagy inhibition (by LC3 and ATG-7 deletion) activates NLRP3 inflammasome and inflammatory mediator production
Parkinson Disease (PD)	Clearance of apoptotic cells	Unknown	Inflammatory mediator production	• Baicalein increases LC3-II expression and attenuates inflammation. • Autophagy activation (MTORC1 inhibition) reduces inflammatory mediators
Huntington Disease (HD)	Clearance of apoptotic cells	Unknown	Inflammatory mediator production	Unknown
Ischemia/stroke (I/S)	• Clearance of apoptotic cells • Phagocytosis of live cells	Unknown	Inflammatory mediator production	GSK-3ß blockade increases LC3-II expression and reduces inflammatory mediator release

Table 31.4 Summary of the role that autophagy plays in neurons and microglia during aging, ischemia/stroke, AD, PD, and HD (modified after Plaza-Zabala et al. (2017) reproduced with kind permission by MDPI, open access)

	Status	Role
Aging	• Downregulation of autophagy genes and proteins • Increased MTORC1 activity	• Autophagy inhibition (by ATG-5/7 deletion) results in spontaneous neurodegeneration • Autophagy activation (by caloric restriction) prevents brain atrophy and enhances learning/memory
Alzheimer Disease (AD)	• Defects in autophagy flux	• Autophagy activation (by cystatin b deletion) reduces Aß load, and reduces learning/memory deficits • Autophagy inhibition (by ATG-7 deletion) reduces extracellular Aß deposition, and increases learning/memory deficits • Autophagy activation (by trehalose) decreases tau inclusions and neurodegeneration
Parkinson Disease (PD)	• Blockade of autophagy flux	• Autophagy activation (by TFEB activation) reduces neurodegeneration and improves motor performance
Huntington Disease (HD)	• Defects in autophagosome loading and/or maturation	• Autophagy activation (by MTORC1 inhibition and others) reduces neurodegeneration and improves motor performance
Ischemia/stroke	• Increased autophagy markers and mitophagy	• Autophagy activation (by MTORC1 inhibition) decreases neurodegeneration • Autophagy (by TSC1 deletion and 3-MA) and mitophagy (by mdivi-1) inhibition increases neurodegeneration • Autophagy inhibition (by chloroquine, 3-MA, and BECN-1 deletion) decreases neurodegeneration

- ER stress is a common feature of aging and of most neurodegenerative diseases.
- ER stress as a driver of brain aging.
- ER stress impacts on neuronal UPR in controlling global proteostasis at the whole organismal level (Martinez et al. 2017).
- Aging is associated with a broad induction of stress response pathways.
- The specific genes and pathways involved differ depending on cell type and species.
- A wide variety of functional classes of genes are downregulated with age, often including tissue-specific genes.
- The upregulation of age-regulated genes is likely to be governed by stress-responsive transcription factors.
- Why are particular genes susceptible to age-related transcriptional decline?
- Splicing is misregulated with age.
    - Defects in splicing lead to changes in protein isoform levels.
    - Affects gene expression through nonsense-mediated decay of intron-retained transcripts.
    - Transcription elongation, termination, and polyadenylation are other mechanisms of age-related changes at the transcript levels (Stegeman and Weake 2017).
- Interventions that can modulate life span encompass the activation of cellular stress responses, including the unfolded protein response in the endoplasmic reticulum (UPR^{ER}). The ability to activate the UPR^{ER} declines with age, while its constitutive activation can extend longevity (Taylor 2016).

31.7.5 Mitochondria

- Mitochondria were placed at the center of the "free-radical theory of aging," because these paramount organelles are not only the main producers of energy in the cells, but also the main source of reactive oxygen species (Grimm and Eckert 2017).
- Mitochondrial dysfunction is evident in numerous neurodegenerative and age-related disorders. It has also been linked to:
    - Cellular aging
    - Reduced respiration
    - Dynamic structural modifications
    - Loss of membrane potential (Ingram and Chakrabarti 2016)

31.7 Molecular Neuropathology

- Age and cell-type specific mitochondrial changes in energy metabolism, antioxidants, fusion and fission machinery, chaperones, membrane proteins, and biosynthesis pathways (Ingram and Chakrabarti 2016).
- During aging, damaged mitochondria that produce less ATP and more reactive oxygen species (ROS) accumulate. The current consensus is that ROS cause oxidative stress, damaging mitochondria and resulting in an energetic crisis that triggers neurodegenerative diseases and accelerates aging (Stefanatos and Sanz 2017).
- "Normal brain aging" and AD may represent different pathways of successful or failed capability to adapt brain structures and cerebral functions (Boccardi et al. 2017).
- Cellular senescence and age-related changes (ARCs) affecting the brain may be considered as biologic manifestations of increasing entropy.
- Aging as well as late-onset AD may be regarded as the final effect of a reduced energy production, due to exhausted mitochondria, and an increased entropy in the brain (Boccardi et al. 2017).

31.7.6 Advanced Glycation End-Product (AGE)

- The accumulation of advanced glycation end-product (AGE) and their derivatives promotes accelerated aging by leading to protein modifications and activating several inflammatory signaling pathways via AGE-specific receptors (Frimat et al. 2017).

31.7.7 cAMP Response Element Binding Protein (CREB)

- The transcription factor cAMP response element binding protein (CREB)
- Dysfunction in CREB signaling with aging (Yu et al. 2017)

31.7.8 Ion Channels and ROS

- Ion channels are integral membrane proteins that allow passive diffusion of ions across membranes (Patel and Sesti 2016).
- Increased accumulation of reactive oxidative species (ROS), and subsequent oxidation of proteins, including ion channels, is a hallmark feature of aging and contributes to cell failure as a result.
- Involved ion channels include the potassium (K(+)), calcium (Ca(2+)), and sodium (Na(+)) channels.
- Two general mechanisms through which ROS affect ion channels
  - Via direct oxidation of specific residues
  - Via indirect interference of pathways that regulate the channels (Patel and Sesti 2016)

31.7.9 Sirtuins

Sirtuins (SIRT1–SIRT7) are (Satoh et al. 2017):

- Unique histone deacetylases (HDACs).
- Silent mating type information regulation 2 proteins (sirtuins) 1 of class III histone deacetylases (HDACs).
- Activity depends on NAD+ levels and thus on the cellular metabolic status.
- Regulate energy metabolism and circadian rhythm through its activity in the hypothalamic nuclei (SIRT1 and SIRT3, SIRT6) (Masri 2015).
- Regulate mitochondrial function.
- Orchestrate the stress response and damage repair.
- Modulate the course of aging and affect neurodegenerative diseases
- SIRTSs interact with multiple signaling proteins, transcription factors (TFs), and poly(ADP-ribose) polymerases (PARPs), another class of NAD+-dependent post-translational protein modifiers (Jesko et al. 2017).
- SIRT1 is a crucial component of multiple interconnected regulatory networks that

modulate dendritic and axonal growth, as well as survival against stress.
- This neuronal cell autonomous activity of SIRT1 is also important for neuronal plasticity, cognitive functions, as well as protection against aging-associated neuronal degeneration and cognitive decline (Ng et al. 2015).

31.7.10 Translocator Protein (TSPO)

- TSPO regulates mitochondrial-mediated apoptotic death through the release of cytochrome c.
- Increased expression of TSPO in both elderly people and in patients with Alzheimer disease.
- TSPO forms and mediates opening of the mitochondrial membrane pore, mPTP and oxidizes cardiolipin; these events lead to the leakage of apoptotic death mediators, such as cytochrome c, resulting in cell death.
- TSPO can also increase steroid synthesis, which leads to inhibition of inflammation and inhibition of the release of apoptotic factors, thereby decreasing cell damage and promoting cell survival (Repalli 2014).

31.7.11 Cathepsins

- Lysosomal proteases (Stoka et al. 2016)
- Have important roles in processing and/or degradation of several important neuronal proteins
- Have either neuroprotective or harmful role.

31.7.12 Ghrelin

Ghrelin takes part in: (Amitani et al. 2017; Muller et al. 2015; Stoyanova 2014; Yin and Zhang 2016)
- Lipid and glucose metabolism
- Higher brain functions such as sleep-wake state
- Learning and memory consolidation

- It influences mitochondrial respiration and shows neuroprotective effect.
- Growth hormone (GH) secretagogue (GHS) and appetite stimulator.
- Within the brain: in neurons of the hypothalamic arcuate nucleus (ARC), ventromedial hypothalamic nucleus (VMN), and paraventricular nucleus (PVN).

31.7.13 Klotho

Klotho regulates the activity of (Boksha et al. 2017):
- Protein factors
- Enzymes
- Receptors
- Glycosidase activity

Effects of Klotho on components of the:
- Glutamatergic neurotransmitter system
- Signal cascades involving protein kinases and protein phosphorylation
- Oligodendrocyte differentiation and myelination

31.7.14 Iron

Iron in several proteins is involved in the CNS (Ward et al. 2014)

- Oxygen transportation
- Oxidative phosphorylation
- Myelin production
- Synthesis and metabolism of neurotransmitters
- Abnormal iron homoeostasis can induce cellular damage through
  - hydroxyl radical production
  - which can cause the oxidation and modification of lipids, proteins, carbohydrates, and DNA
- During aging, different iron complexes accumulate in brain regions associated with motor and cognitive impairment.
- Iron accumulation is reduced by the use of iron chelators that are able to cross the blood–

31.7.15 Insulin

- Brain aging is associated with a decrease of central insulin concentration as well as impairment of insulin receptor binding ability (Baranowska-Bik and Bik 2017).
- The above result in deterioration of glucose homeostasis in the brain.
- Peripheral insulin resistance is a typical feature of older age.
- High circulating insulin and insulin resistance are important contributors to progressive cognitive impairment and neurodegenerative processes.

Insulin-like Growth Factor 1 (IGF-1) and its signaling pathway (Frater et al. 2017)
- Play a primary role in normal growth and aging.
- Serum IGF-1 is known to reduce with advancing age.
- Is essential for neurogenesis in the adult brain.
- This reduction of IGF-1 with aging may contribute to age-related cognitive decline.
- Manipulation of the GH/GF-1 axis can slow rates of cognitive decline in animals, making IGF-1 a potential biomarker of cognition, and/or its signaling pathway a possible therapeutic target to prevent or slow age-related cognitive decline.

31.7.16 Signaling

- Aging-induced impairments of the GABAergic system lead to an inhibitory/excitatory imbalance, thereby decreasing neuron's ability to respond with plastic changes to environmental and cellular challenges, leaving the brain more vulnerable to cognitive decline and damage by synaptopathic diseases (Rozycka and Liguz-Lecznar 2017).

- Cyclic nucleotide signaling changes include (Kelly 2017):
  - elevated circulating atrial natriuretic peptide (ANP) and brain natriuretic peptide (BNP) levels being associated with cognitive dysfunction or dementia independent of cardiovascular effects
  - reduced basal and/or NMDA-stimulated $3',5'$-guanosine monophosphate (cGMP) levels in brain with aging or Alzheimer disease (AD)
  - reduced adenylyl cyclase activity in hippocampus and specific cortical regions with aging or AD
  - reduced phosphorylation of cAMP response element binding protein (CREB) in hippocampus with aging or AD
  - reduced expression/activity of the phosphodiesterases (PDE4) family in brain with aging
  - beneficial effects of select phosphodiesterases (PDE) inhibitors, particularly PDE10 inhibitors in HD models and PDE4 and PDE5 inhibitors in aging and AD models

31.8 Genetics of Successful Aging

Genes involved in aging processes include:
- APOE
- GSTT1
- IL6
- IL10
- PON1
- SIRT3
- Genes involved in the maintenance of cholesterol, lipid, or lipoprotein levels.
- Genes related to cytokines.
- Genes involved in drug metabolism and insulin signaling.
- Genes related to age-associated pathological processes (e.g., Alzheimer disease).
- Genes mediating neuroinflammation and immune system activation in particular, show significant age-related upregulation creating a state of vulnerability to neurodegenerative and neuropsychiatric disease in the aging brain (Mohan et al. 2016).

- Cellular ionic dyshomeostasis and age-related decline in a host of molecular influences on synaptic efficacy may underlie neurocognitive decline in later life.
- Critically, these investigations have also shed light on the mobilization of protective genetic responses within the aging human brain that help determine health and disease trajectories in older age.
- Expression levels of genes and length of chromosomal telomeres.
- Genetic variation in maintenance of genome stability is emerging as an important determinant of aging pace. Genome instability is also closely associated with a broad spectrum of conditions involving brain degeneration. Similarities and differences can be found between aging-associated decline of brain functionality and the detrimental effect of genome instability on brain functionality and development (Barzilai et al. 2017).

The *genetic switch model of aging* (Van Raamsdonk 2017) proposes that
- aging is caused by
  - a genetically programmed turning off of survival pathways and
  - a genetically programmed turning off of maintenance pathways after reproduction
  - finally leading to a progressive functional decline
- If this model is correct, it may be possible to extend life span and healthspan by identifying the molecular pathways involved and simply turning the switch back on.

Biological pathways and genes involved in brain aging are listed in Table 31.5.

31.9 Non-coding RNAs

The links between different genetic models such as yeast, fly, mouse, and human systems with regard to aging process implicate a variety of RNA-regulatory processes (Szafranski et al. 2015):

Table 31.5 Key biological pathways and genes implicated in aging, modified after Mohan et al. (2016) reproduced with kind permission by Wolters Kluver Health

Biological pathways implicated	Top genes of significance
• Oxidative stress • Inflammation	• *BMI1* • *IL-6*
• Synaptic function—vesicle trafficking and release • Postsynaptic density scaffolding and synaptic stability • Neurotransmitter receptors and receptor trafficking • Neuromodulatory systems	• *Synaptobrevin 2* • *VAMP2* • *SNAP-25* • *Synapsin I* • *PSD93* • *PSD95* • *Lin7B* • *Shank2* • *AMPA receptors (GRIA2, GRIA3, GRIA4)* • *KA receptors (GRIK1, GRIK2)* • *GABA receptors (GABBR1, GABRA4, GABRB3, GABRD)* • *BDNF* • *SST*
• Cell-to-cell signaling • Nervous system development and functioning	• *miR-9* • *miR-17* • *miR-124a* • *miR-128ab* • *miR132*
• Inflammation/immune activation • Complement signaling • Microglial and perivascular • Macrophage activation	• *C1qA* • *C1qB* • *C1qC* • *C1s* • *C3* • *CFHR1* • *CLU* • *TLR2* • *TLR4* • *TLR5* • *TOLLIP* • *CX3CL1* • *CASPASE1*
• Immunoregulation • Microglial activation	• *miRNA 29a* • *miRNA 29b* • *IGF-1* • *CX3CL1*
• Inhibitory neurotransmission • Calcium signaling • Lipid metabolism	• *SST* • *NPY* • *GAD1* • *NRGN* • *SLC32A1* • *ENTPD2* • *DECR1* • *HRSP12* • *PLA2*

(continued)

Table 31.5 (continued)

Biological pathways implicated	Top genes of significance
• Mitochondrial components • Gene expression regulation	• RHBDL3 • NR3C2 • GPX3 • VPS18 • SGSH
• Apoptosis and cell death • Oxidative stress	• REST • MAPK1 • FAS • FADD • TRADD • BAX • BID • DAXX • PUMA • ANT1 • CATALASE • SOD1 • FOXO1
• Cellular chemical homeostasis • Nervous system development • Neurotransmitter receptors	• GLI2 • HES1 • ID4 • PAX6 • SOX2 • YWHAG • YWHAH • AMIGO1 • CD24 • GPR21 • CHRNB2 • GRIN1 • GPR6 • MCH1R/SLC1 • AVPR1A • DRD1
• Inflammation • Complement signaling • Immune activation • RNA catabolism	• C4A (C4B) • ADORA3 • MS4A7 • BCL6 • C1orf162 • SERPINA5 • RNASE6 • CD44 • C3AR1 • HLA-DRB1
• Calcium homeostasis • Neurodegeneration • Oxidative stress • Ubiquitin-proteasome pathway	• GPAFP • SPARCL1 • B2M • CALM1e3 • CLU • PICALM • PTGD2 • CA11 • SOD1 • PSAM1 • PSMA2
• Inflammatory/immune related • Glial activation • Synaptic, myelin integrity • Neurotrophic genes	• GFAP • TSPO • TRAF6 • IL1RN • IL1B • IL1RAP • NGF • BDNF • CX3CL1 • CX3CR1 • NFKB1 • PTGS2 • MOBP • SYP • SNCA • CASP1 • CD68 • AIF1 • MYD88 • PDGFA • DBN1 • BACE1
• Intracellular CA2+ ion • Homeostasis • CA2+ ion channel • Neuronal excitability	• CB • CAMK18 • GAP43 • CACNA1G

- MicroRNA function
- Paraspeckle formation
- RNA–DNA hybrid regulation
- Nucleolar RNAs and toxic RNA clearance

MicroRNAs (miRNAs) have emerged as important regulators in most physiological processes including fine-tuning of the short-term, cellular regulatory functions as well as modulation of long-term organismal life span (Danka Mohammed et al. 2017).
- 50% of all known miRNAs are found in brain including cortex and hippocampus.
- A significant number of expressed miRNAs were differentially regulated during aging, implicating miRNAs as regulators of brain aging.
- miRNA-mediated, brain functional changes are evident in cognition, inflammation, neuroprotection, lipid metabolism, mitochondrial function, and life span.
- Dysregulation of brain miRNAs contributes to accelerated cognitive decline and increased neurological disorders.

31.10 DNA Damage

- Neurons in the brain are postmitotic and are excluded from many forms of DNA repair (Chow and Herrup 2015).
- DNA damage may be particularly prevalent in the central nervous system owing to the low DNA repair capacity in postmitotic brain tissue.
- The cumulative effects of the deleterious changes that occur in aging, mostly after the reproductive phase, contribute to species-specific rates of aging.
- There is also abundant evidence for a causative link between mitochondrial DNA damage and the major phenotypes associated with aging (Maynard et al. 2015).
- Questions:
  - when does neuronal DNA damage accumulate
  - does this loss of genomic integrity serve as a "time keeper" of nerve cell aging
  - why does this process manifest itself as different diseases in different individuals (Chow and Herrup 2015)

31.11 Treatment and Prognosis

Treatment
- Healthy life style
- Cure/stabilize:
  - Atherosclerosis
  - Diabetes mellitus
  - Hypertonus
  - Hyperlipidemia

Biologic Behavior–Prognosis–Prognostic Factors
Successful aging tends to be more dependent on:
- Behavior
- Attitude
- Environment

Current strategies to enhance successful aging include:
- Restricting calories intake.
- Exercising.
- Quitting smoking and substance use.
- Obtaining appropriate health care.
- Eating healthy.
- Seeking help for mental illnesses such as depression is critical.
- Develop cognitive and psychological strategies such as positive attitude, resilience, and reducing stress.
- Cognitive and emotional adaptation to chronic illnesses that often impact older adults is also an important aspect.
- Social strategies
  - Seeking and giving social support through volunteering
  - Working in a group
  - Learning a new skill
  - Mentoring younger individuals

Epigenetics is a quickly growing field encompassing mechanisms regulating gene expression that do not involve changes in the genotype (Lardenoije et al. 2015).
- Epigenetic variability (DNA methylation/demethylation, histone modifications, microRNA regulation) is common in physiological and pathological conditions.
- Epigenetics affect life span and longevity.
- AD-related genes exhibit epigenetic changes, indicating that epigenetics might exert a pathogenic role in dementia.
- Epigenetic modifications are reversible and can potentially be targeted by pharmacological intervention (Cacabelos and Torrellas 2015).
- Epigenetic regulation covers multiple levels of gene expression; from direct modifications of the DNA and histone tails, regulating the level of transcription, to interactions with messenger RNAs, regulating the level of translation (Lardenoije et al. 2015).

Epigenetics can guide age-associated decline in part by (Delgado-Morales et al. 2017)
- Regulating gene expression.
- Modulation of genomic instability and high-order chromatin architecture.
- Epigenetic mechanisms are involved in:
  – regulation of neural differentiation
  – functional processes related to memory consolidation, learning, or cognition during healthy life span.
- Many neurodegenerative diseases are associated with epigenetic dysregulation.

Classification of selected **epigenetic drugs** (Cacabelos and Torrellas 2015)

- DNA methyltransferase inhibitors
- Histone deacetylase (HDAC) inhibitors
- Histone acetyltransferase modulators
- Histone methyltransferase inhibitors
- Histone demethylase inhibitors
- Other potential epigenetic treatments

Classification of selected epigenetic drugs (Cacabelos and Torrellas 2015)

- *DNA methyltransferase inhibitors*
  – Nucleoside analogs:
    ○ 5-Aza-21-deoxycytidine (Decitabine); 5-Azacytidine (Azacitidine)
  – Small molecules:
    ○ Hydralazine; Procainamide; RG108 [2-(1,3-dioxo-1,3-dihydro-2*H*-isoindol-2-yl)-3-(1*H*-indol-3-yl)propanoic acid]
  – Natural products:
    ○ Curcumin derivatives: RG-108, SGI-1027; Psammaplins; Tea polyphenols:Epigallocatechin-3-gallate; Catechins: Catechin, Epicatechin; Bioflavonoids: Quercetin, Genistein, Fisetin
  – Antisense oligonucleotide inhibitors
  – ncRNAs (miRNAs)
- *Histone deacetylase (HDAC) inhibitors*
  – Short-chain fatty acids:
    ○ Sodium butyrate; Sodium phenyl butyrate; Valproic acid; Pivaloyloxymethyl butyrate (AN-9, Pivanex)
  – Hydroxamic acids:
    ○ Suberoylanilide hydroxamic acid (SAHA, Vorinostat); Oxamflatin; Pyroxamide; TSA; CBHA; Derivatives of the marine sponge Psammaplysilla purpurea: NVP-LAQ824, NVP-LBH589; LBH-589 (Panobinostat); ITF2357 (Givinostat); PXD101 (Belinostat); JHJ-26481585; CHR-3996; CHR-2845; PCI-24781
  – Cyclic peptides:
    ○ Romidepsin (Depsipeptide, FR901228); Apicidin; CHAPS; Trapoxin A and B; Chlamydocin; HC toxin; Bacterial FK228
  – Benzamides:
    ○ MS-275 (Entinostat); CI-994; RGFP136; MGCD0103 (Mocetinostat); Compound 60
  – Ketones:
    ○ Trifluoromethyl ketone
  – Sirtuin modulators:
    ○ Sirtuin inhibitors: Nicotinamide/niacinamide, Suramin, AGK-2, Sirtinol, Salermide, MS3, Splitomycin, Cambiol, SEN-196, Dihydrocoumarin, Tenovin,

UVI5008; Sirtuin activators: Resveratrol, SRT-501, SRT-1460, SRT-1720, SRT-2183, GSK-184072, Quercetin, Piceatannol
– Miscellaneous compounds:
  ○ 3-Deazaneplanocin A (DZNep); Tubacin; EVP-0334; 6-([18F]Fluoroacetamido)-1-hexanoicanilide; Quinazolin-4-one derivatives: (E)-3-(2-Ethyl-7-fluoro-4-oxo-3-phenethyl-3,4-dihydroquinazolin-6-yl)-*N*-hydroxyacrylamide, *N*-Hydroxy-3-(2-methyl-4-oxo-3-phenethyl-3,4-dihydro-quinazolin-7-yl)-acrylamide
- *Histone acetyltransferase modulators*
  – Histone acetyltransferase inhibitors:
    ○ Curcumin (Diferuloylmethane); Lys-CoA; H3-CoA-20; Anacardic acid; Garcinol
  – Histone aceyltransferase activators:
    ○ *N*-(4-Chloro-3-trifluoromethyl-phenyl)-2-ethoxy-6-pentadecyl-benzamide; Pentadecylidenemalonate 1b (SPV-106)
- *Histone methyltransferase inhibitors*
  – Lysine methyltransferase inhibitors:
    ○ *S*-Adenosylmethionine (SAMe); SAMe analogs; Chaetocin; BIX-01294; BIX-01338; UNC0224; EZH2 (KMT6) inhibitors: Deazaneplanocin A
  – Arginine methyltransferase inhibitors:
    ○ AMI-1
- *Histone demethylase inhibitors*
  – LSD1 inhibitors: Tranylcypromine; Parnate; (*S*)-4-(2-(5-(Dimethylamino)naphthalene-1-sulfonamido)-2-phenylacetamido)-*N*-hydroxybenzamide (D17)
- *Non-coding RNAs*
  – miRNAs
  – RNAi
- *Other potential epigenetic treatments*
  – Small molecule inhibitors to chromatin-associated proteins:
    ○ DOT1L histone methyltransferase inhibitors: EPZ004777, EPZ-5676, SGC0946; EZH2 histone methyltransferase inhibitors: GSK126, GSK343, EPZ005687, EPZ-6438, EI1, UNC1999; G9A histone methyltransferase inhibitors: BIX1294, UNC0321, UNC0638, NC0642, BRD4770; PRMT3 histone methyltransferase inhibitors: 14u; PRMT4 (CARM1) histone methyltransferase inhibitors: 17b, MethylGene; LSD1 histone demethylase inhibitors: Tranylcypromine, ORY-1001; BET histone demethylase inhibitors: JQ1, IBET762, IBET151, PFI-1; BAZ2B histone demethylase inhibitors: GSK2801; L3MBTL1 chromodomain inhibitors: UNC669; L3MBTL3 chromodomain: UNC1215; Bromodomain inhibitors: LP99, RVX-208; Chromodomain inhibitors
  – Small molecules for somatic cell reprogramming
  – Chaperones (sHSPs)
  – IGFBP7 inhibitors
  – Nutraceuticals
  – Dietary regimes:
    ○ Vitamins: Folic acid, Vitamin B, Vitamin C, Vitamin D, Vitamin E; Natural products (Cacabelos and Torrellas 2015)

Selected References

Akintola AA, van Heemst D (2015) Insulin, aging, and the brain: mechanisms and implications. Front Endocrinol 6:13. https://doi.org/10.3389/fendo.2015.00013

Amitani M, Amitani H, Cheng KC, Kairupan TS, Sameshima N, Shimoshikiryo I, Mizuma K, Rokot NT, Nerome Y, Owaki T, Asakawa A, Inui A (2017) The role of ghrelin and ghrelin signaling in aging. Int J Mol Sci 18(7):1511. https://doi.org/10.3390/ijms18071511

Apple DM, Solano-Fonseca R, Kokovay E (2017) Neurogenesis in the aging brain. Clin Epigenetics 141:77–85. https://doi.org/10.1016/j.bcp.2017.06.116

Baranowska-Bik A, Bik W (2017) Insulin and brain aging. Prz Menopauzalny 16(2):44–46. https://doi.org/10.5114/pm.2017.68590

Barzilai A, Schumacher B, Shiloh Y (2017) Genome instability: linking ageing and brain degeneration. Mech Ageing Dev 161(Pt A):4–18. https://doi.org/10.1016/j.mad.2016.03.011

Boccardi V, Comanducci C, Baroni M, Mecocci P (2017) Of energy and entropy: the ineluctable impact of aging in old age dementia. Int J Mol Sci 18(12). https://doi.org/10.3390/ijms18122672

Boksha IS, Prokhorova TA, Savushkina OK, Tereshkina EB (2017) Klotho protein: its role in aging and central nervous system pathology. Biochem

Biokhim 82(9):990–1005. https://doi.org/10.1134/s0006297917090024

Cacabelos R, Torrellas C (2015) Epigenetics of aging and Alzheimer's disease: implications for pharmacogenomics and drug response. Int J Mol Sci 16(12):30483–30543. https://doi.org/10.3390/ijms161226236

Chandran R, Kumar M, Kesavan L, Jacob RS, Gunasekaran S, Lakshmi S, Sadasivan C, Omkumar RV (2017) Cellular calcium signaling in the aging brain. J Chem Neuroanat 95:95–114. https://doi.org/10.1016/j.jchemneu.2017.11.008

Chow HM, Herrup K (2015) Genomic integrity and the ageing brain. Nat Rev Neurosci 16(11):672–684. https://doi.org/10.1038/nrn4020

Danka Mohammed CP, Park JS, Nam HG, Kim K (2017) MicroRNAs in brain aging. Mech Ageing Dev 168:3–9. https://doi.org/10.1016/j.mad.2017.01.007

Davis PC, Mirra SS, Alazraki N (1994) The brain in older persons with and without dementia: findings on MR, PET, and SPECT images. AJR Am J Roentgenol 162(6):1267–1278. https://doi.org/10.2214/ajr.162.6.8191980

Delgado-Morales R, Agis-Balboa RC, Esteller M, Berdasco M (2017) Epigenetic mechanisms during ageing and neurogenesis as novel therapeutic avenues in human brain disorders. Clin Epigenet 9:67. https://doi.org/10.1186/s13148-017-0365-z

Fenech M (2017) Vitamins associated with brain aging, mild cognitive impairment, and Alzheimer disease: biomarkers, epidemiological and experimental evidence, plausible mechanisms, and knowledge gaps. Adv Nutr 8(6):958–970. https://doi.org/10.3945/an.117.015610

Fidaleo M, Cavallucci V, Pani G (2017) Nutrients, neurogenesis and brain ageing: from disease mechanisms to therapeutic opportunities. Biochem Pharmacol 141:63–76. https://doi.org/10.1016/j.bcp.2017.05.016

Fraser MA, Shaw ME, Cherbuin N (2015) A systematic review and meta-analysis of longitudinal hippocampal atrophy in healthy human ageing. Neuroimage 112:364–374. https://doi.org/10.1016/j.neuroimage.2015.03.035

Frater J, Lie D, Bartlett P, McGrath JJ (2017) Insulin-like growth factor 1 (IGF-1) as a marker of cognitive decline in normal ageing: a review. Ageing Res Rev 42:14–27. https://doi.org/10.1016/j.arr.2017.12.002

Freitas HR, Ferreira GDC, Trevenzoli IH, Oliveira KJ, de Melo Reis RA (2017) Fatty acids, antioxidants and physical activity in brain aging. Nutrients 9(11). https://doi.org/10.3390/nu9111263

Frimat M, Daroux M, Litke R, Neviere R, Tessier FJ, Boulanger E (2017) Kidney, heart and brain: three organs targeted by ageing and glycation. Clin Sci (Lond) 131(11):1069–1092. https://doi.org/10.1042/cs20160823

Galluzzi S, Beltramello A, Filippi M, Frisoni GB (2008) Aging Neurol Sci 29(Suppl 3):296–300. https://doi.org/10.1007/s10072-008-1002-6

Grimm A, Eckert A (2017) Brain aging and neurodegeneration: from a mitochondrial point of view. J Neurochem 143(4):418–431. https://doi.org/10.1111/jnc.14037

Hachinski VC, Potter P, Merskey H (1986) Leuko-araiosis: an ancient term for a new problem. Can J Neurol Sci 13(4 Suppl):533–534

Hachinski VC, Potter P, Merskey H (1987) Leuko-araiosis. Arch Neurol 44(1):21–23

Ingram T, Chakrabarti L (2016) Proteomic profiling of mitochondria: what does it tell us about the ageing brain? Aging 8(12):3161–3179. https://doi.org/10.18632/aging.101131

Jesko H, Wencel P, Strosznajder RP, Strosznajder JB (2017) Sirtuins and their roles in brain aging and neurodegenerative disorders. Neurochem Res 42(3):876–890. https://doi.org/10.1007/s11064-016-2110-y

Kelly MP (2017) Cyclic nucleotide signaling changes associated with normal aging and age-related diseases of the brain. Cell Signal 42:281–291. https://doi.org/10.1016/j.cellsig.2017.11.004

Koellhoffer EC, McCullough LD, Ritzel RM (2017) Old maids: aging and its impact on microglia function. Int J Mol Sci 18(4). https://doi.org/10.3390/ijms18040769

Kuehn E, Perez-Lopez MB, Diersch N, Dohler J, Wolbers T, Riemer M (2017) Embodiment in the aging mind. Neurosci Biobehav Rev 86:207–225. https://doi.org/10.1016/j.neubiorev.2017.11.016

Lardenoije R, Iatrou A, Kenis G, Kompotis K, Steinbusch HW, Mastroeni D, Coleman P, Lemere CA, Hof PR, van den Hove DL, Rutten BP (2015) The epigenetics of aging and neurodegeneration. Prog Neurobiol 131:21–64. https://doi.org/10.1016/j.pneurobio.2015.05.002

Liu H, Yang Y, Xia Y, Zhu W, Leak RK, Wei Z, Wang J, Hu X (2017) Aging of cerebral white matter. Ageing Res Rev 34:64–76. https://doi.org/10.1016/j.arr.2016.11.006

Lockhart SN, DeCarli C (2014) Structural imaging measures of brain aging. Neuropsychol Rev 24(3):271–289. https://doi.org/10.1007/s11065-014-9268-3

Lopez-Leon M, Outeiro TF, Goya RG (2017) Cell reprogramming: therapeutic potential and the promise of rejuvenation for the aging brain. Ageing Res Rev 40:168–181. https://doi.org/10.1016/j.arr.2017.09.002

Machiela MJ, Chanock SJ (2017) The ageing genome, clonal mosaicism and chronic disease. Curr Opin Genet Dev 42:8–13. https://doi.org/10.1016/j.gde.2016.12.002

Maes C, Gooijers J, Orban de Xivry JJ, Swinnen SP, Boisgontier MP (2017) Two hands, one brain, and aging. Neurosci Biobehav Rev 75:234–256. https://doi.org/10.1016/j.neubiorev.2017.01.052

Martinez G, Duran-Aniotz C, Cabral-Miranda F, Vivar JP, Hetz C (2017) Endoplasmic reticulum proteostasis impairment in aging. Aging Cell 16(4):615–623. https://doi.org/10.1111/acel.12599

Masri S (2015) Sirtuin-dependent clock control: new advances in metabolism, aging and cancer. Curr Opin Clin Nutr Metab Care 18(6):521–527. https://doi.org/10.1097/mco.0000000000000219

Mather M (2016) The affective neuroscience of aging. Annu Rev Psychol 67:213–238. https://doi.org/10.1146/annurev-psych-122414-033540

Matt SM, Johnson RW (2016) Neuro-immune dysfunction during brain aging: new insights in microglial cell regulation. Curr Opin Pharmacol 26:96–101. https://doi.org/10.1016/j.coph.2015.10.009

Maynard S, Fang EF, Scheibye-Knudsen M, Croteau DL, Bohr VA (2015) DNA damage, DNA repair, aging, and neurodegeneration. Cold Spring Harb Perspect Med 5(10). https://doi.org/10.1101/cshperspect.a025130

Mohan A, Mather KA, Thalamuthu A, Baune BT, Sachdev PS (2016) Gene expression in the aging human brain: an overview. Curr Opin Psychiatry 29(2):159–167. https://doi.org/10.1097/yco.0000000000000238

Muller TD, Nogueiras R, Andermann ML, Andrews ZB, Anker SD, Argente J, Batterham RL, Benoit SC, Bowers CY, Broglio F, Casanueva FF, D'Alessio D, Depoortere I, Geliebter A, Ghigo E, Cole PA, Cowley M, Cummings DE, Dagher A, Diano S, Dickson SL, Dieguez C, Granata R, Grill HJ, Grove K, Habegger KM, Heppner K, Heiman ML, Holsen L, Holst B, Inui A, Jansson JO, Kirchner H, Korbonits M, Laferrere B, LeRoux CW, Lopez M, Morin S, Nakazato M, Nass R, Perez-Tilve D, Pfluger PT, Schwartz TW, Seeley RJ, Sleeman M, Sun Y, Sussel L, Tong J, Thorner MO, van der Lely AJ, van der Ploeg LH, Zigman JM, Kojima M, Kangawa K, Smith RG, Horvath T, Tschop MH (2015) Ghrelin. Mol Metab 4(6):437–460. https://doi.org/10.1016/j.molmet.2015.03.005

Nagata K, Yamazaki T, Takano D, Maeda T, Fujimaki Y, Nakase T, Sato Y (2016) Cerebral circulation in aging. Ageing Res Rev 30:49–60. https://doi.org/10.1016/j.arr.2016.06.001

Ng F, Wijaya L, Tang BL (2015) SIRT1 in the brain-connections with aging-associated disorders and lifespan. Front Cell Neurosci 9:64. https://doi.org/10.3389/fncel.2015.00064

Nyberg L (2017) Neuroimaging in aging: brain maintenance. F1000Research 6:1215. https://doi.org/10.12688/f1000research.11419.1

Patel R, Sesti F (2016) Oxidation of ion channels in the aging nervous system. Brain Res 1639:174–185. https://doi.org/10.1016/j.brainres.2016.02.046

Plaza-Zabala A, Sierra-Torre V, Sierra A (2017) Autophagy and microglia: novel partners in neurodegeneration and aging. Int J Mol Sci 18(3). https://doi.org/10.3390/ijms18030598

Rawji KS, Mishra MK, Michaels NJ, Rivest S, Stys PK, Yong VW (2016) Immunosenescence of microglia and macrophages: impact on the ageing central nervous system. Brain 139(Pt 3):653–661. https://doi.org/10.1093/brain/awv395

Ren R, Ocampo A, Liu GH, Izpisua Belmonte JC (2017) Regulation of stem cell aging by metabolism and epigenetics. Cell Metab 26(3):460–474. https://doi.org/10.1016/j.cmet.2017.07.019

Repalli J (2014) Translocator protein (TSPO) role in aging and Alzheimer's disease. Curr Aging Sci 7(3):168–175

Rodriguez-Arellano JJ, Parpura V, Zorec R, Verkhratsky A (2016) Astrocytes in physiological aging and Alzheimer's disease. Neuroscience 323:170–182. https://doi.org/10.1016/j.neuroscience.2015.01.007

Rowe JW, Kahn RL (1987) Human aging: usual and successful. Science (New York, NY) 237(4811):143–149

Rozycka A, Liguz-Lecznar M (2017) The space where aging acts: focus on the GABAergic synapse. Aging Cell 16(4):634–643. https://doi.org/10.1111/acel.12605

Satoh A, Imai SI, Guarente L (2017) The brain, sirtuins, and ageing. Nat Rev Neurosci 18(6):362–374. https://doi.org/10.1038/nrn.2017.42

Schmidt R, Schmidt H, Haybaeck J, Loitfelder M, Weis S, Cavalieri M, Seiler S, Enzinger C, Ropele S, Erkinjuntti T, Pantoni L, Scheltens P, Fazekas F, Jellinger K (2011) Heterogeneity in age-related white matter changes. Acta Neuropathol 122(2):171–185. Epub 2011 Jun 2025.

Shwe T, Pratchayasakul W, Chattipakorn N, Chattipakorn SC (2017) Role of D-galactose-induced brain aging and its potential used for therapeutic interventions. Exp Gerontol 101:13–36. https://doi.org/10.1016/j.exger.2017.10.029

Stefanatos R, Sanz A (2017) The role of mitochondrial ROS in the aging brain. FEBS Lett 592(5):743–758. https://doi.org/10.1002/1873-3468.12902

Stegeman R, Weake VM (2017) Transcriptional signatures of aging. J Mol Biol 429(16):2427–2437. https://doi.org/10.1016/j.jmb.2017.06.019

Stoka V, Turk V, Turk B (2016) Lysosomal cathepsins and their regulation in aging and neurodegeneration. Ageing Res Rev 32:22–37. https://doi.org/10.1016/j.arr.2016.04.010

Stoyanova II (2014) Ghrelin: a link between ageing, metabolism and neurodegenerative disorders. Neurobiol Dis 72(Pt A):72–83. https://doi.org/10.1016/j.nbd.2014.08.026

Stroo E, Koopman M, Nollen EA, Mata-Cabana A (2017) Cellular regulation of amyloid formation in aging and disease. Front Neurosci 11:64. https://doi.org/10.3389/fnins.2017.00064

Sugiura M (2016) Functional neuroimaging of normal aging: declining brain, adapting brain. Ageing Res Rev 30:61–72. https://doi.org/10.1016/j.arr.2016.02.006

Swerdlow RH, Koppel S, Weidling I, Hayley C, Ji Y, Wilkins HM (2017) Mitochondria, cybrids, aging, and Alzheimer's disease. Prog Mol Biol Transl Sci 146:259–302. https://doi.org/10.1016/bs.pmbts.2016.12.017

Szafranski K, Abraham KJ, Mekhail K (2015) Non-coding RNA in neural function, disease, and aging. Front Genet 6:87. https://doi.org/10.3389/fgene.2015.00087

Taylor RC (2016) Aging and the UPR(ER). Brain Res 1648(Pt B):588–593. https://doi.org/10.1016/j.brainres.2016.04.017

Torok N, Majlath Z, Fulop F, Toldi J, Vecsei L (2016) Brain aging and disorders of the central nervous system: kynurenines and drug metabolism. Curr Drug Metab 17(5):412–429

Selected References

Van Raamsdonk JM (2017) Mechanisms underlying longevity: a genetic switch model of aging. Exp Gerontol 107:136–139. https://doi.org/10.1016/j.exger.2017.08.005

Ward RJ, Zucca FA, Duyn JH, Crichton RR, Zecca L (2014) The role of iron in brain ageing and neurodegenerative disorders. Lancet Neurol 13(10):1045–1060. https://doi.org/10.1016/s1474-4422(14)70117-6

Xekardaki A, Kovari E, Gold G, Papadimitropoulou A, Giacobini E, Herrmann F, Giannakopoulos P, Bouras C (2015) Neuropathological changes in aging brain. Adv Exp Med Biol 821:11–17. https://doi.org/10.1007/978-3-319-08939-3_6

Yin Y, Zhang W (2016) The role of ghrelin in senescence: a mini-review. Gerontology 62(2):155–162. https://doi.org/10.1159/000433533

Yu XW, Oh MM, Disterhoft JF (2017) CREB, cellular excitability, and cognition: implications for aging. Behav Brain Res 322(Pt B):206–211. https://doi.org/10.1016/j.bbr.2016.07.042

Neurodegenerative Diseases: Alzheimer Disease (AD)

32.1 Clinical Signs and Symptoms

- Progressive dementia with increasing
  - loss of memory
    - working memory
    - anterograde episodic memory
    - remote memory
    - semantic memory
  - intellectual dysfunction
  - disturbances in speech
- Thought is slow.
- Ability to perform in the social and economic spheres is impaired.
- Early symptoms include:
  - disturbance of language functions
  - apraxia
  - agnosia
- Patients with some insight into their deterioration may become depressed.
- Agitation.
- Restlessness also common.
- The clinical picture in the terminal stages shows
  - that the intellectual activity ceases
  - the patient becomes meek and is eventually reduced to a vegetative condition
  - Control of bowel and bladder functions are lost

32.2 International Working Group (IWG) Clinical Criteria

The International Working Group (IWG) and the US National Institute on Aging-Alzheimer Association have contributed criteria for the diagnosis of Alzheimer disease (AD) that better define clinical phenotypes and integrate biomarkers into the diagnostic process, covering the full staging of the disease (Dubois et al. 2014).

Panel 1: IWG-2 criteria for typical AD (A plus B at any stage)
- *Specific clinical phenotype*
  - Presence of an early and significant episodic memory impairment (isolated or associated with other cognitive or behavioral changes that are suggestive of a mild cognitive impairment or of a dementia syndrome) that includes the following features:
    - Gradual and progressive change in memory function reported by patient or informant over more than 6 months
    - Objective evidence of an amnestic syndrome of the hippocampal type, based on significantly impaired performance on an episodic memory test with established specificity for AD, such as cued recall with control of encoding test

- *In vivo evidence of Alzheimer pathology (one of the following)*
  - Decreased Aβ1–42 together with increased T-tau or P-tau in CSF
  - Increased tracer retention on amyloid PET
  - AD autosomal dominant mutation present (in PSEN1, PSEN2, or APP)
- *Exclusion criteria for typical AD*
  - History
    - Sudden onset
    - Early occurrence of the following symptoms: gait disturbances, seizures, major and prevalent behavioral changes
  - Clinical features
    - Focal neurological features
    - Early extrapyramidal signs
    - Early hallucinations
    - Cognitive fluctuations
  - Other medical conditions severe enough to account for memory and related symptoms
    - Non-AD dementia
    - Major depression
    - Cerebrovascular disease
    - Toxic, inflammatory, and metabolic disorders, all of which may require specific investigations
    - MRI FLAIR or T2 signal changes in the medial temporal lobe that are consistent with infectious or vascular insults

Panel 2: IWG-2 criteria for atypical AD (A plus B at any stage)

- *Specific clinical phenotype (one of the following)*
  - Posterior variant of AD (including)
    - An occipito-temporal variant defined by the presence of an early, predominant, and progressive impairment of visuoperceptive functions or of visual identification of objects, symbols, words, or faces
    - A biparietal variant defined by the presence of early, predominant, and progressive difficulty with visuospatial function, features of Gerstmann syndrome, of Balint syndrome, limb apraxia, or neglect
  - Logopenic variant of AD defined by the presence of an early, predominant, and progressive impairment of single-word retrieval and in repetition of sentences, in the context of spared semantic, syntactic, and motor speech abilities.
  - Frontal variant of AD defined by the presence of early, predominant, and progressive behavioral changes including association of primary apathy or behavioral disinhibition, or predominant executive dysfunction on cognitive testing
  - Down syndrome variant of AD defined by the occurrence of a dementia characterized by early behavioral changes and executive dysfunction in people with Down syndrome
- *In vivo evidence of Alzheimer pathology (one of the following)*
  - Decreased Aβ1–42 together with increased T-tau or P-tau in CSF
  - Increased tracer retention on amyloid PET
  - Alzheimer disease autosomal dominant mutation present (in PSEN1, PSEN2, or APP)
- *Exclusion criteria for atypical AD*
  - History
    - Sudden onset
    - Early and prevalent episodic memory disorders
  - Other medical conditions severe enough to account for related symptoms
    - Major depression
    - Cerebrovascular disease
    - Toxic, inflammatory, or metabolic disorders

Panel 3: IWG-2 criteria for mixed AD (A plus B)

- *Clinical and biomarker evidence of AD (both are required)*
  - Amnestic syndrome of the hippocampal type or one of the clinical phenotypes of atypical AD
  - Decreased Aβ1–42 together with increased T-tau or P-tau in CSF, or increased tracer retention on amyloid PET
- *Clinical and biomarker evidence of mixed pathology*

- For cerebrovascular disease (both are required)
  - Documented history of stroke, or focal neurological features, or both
  - MRI evidence of one or more of the following: corresponding vascular lesions, small vessel disease, strategic lacunar infarcts, or cerebral hemorrhages
- For Lewy body disease (both are required)
  - One of the following: extrapyramidal signs, early hallucinations, or cognitive fluctuations
  - Abnormal dopamine transporter PET scan

Panel 4: IWG-2 Criteria for the Preclinical States of AD
IWG-2 criteria for asymptomatic at risk for AD (A plus B)

- A: Absence of specific clinical phenotype (both are required)
  - Absence of amnestic syndrome of the hippocampal type
  - Absence of any clinical phenotype of atypical AD
- B: In vivo evidence of Alzheimer pathology (one of the following)
  - Decreased Aβ1–42 together with increased T-tau or P-tau in CSF
  - Increased retention on fibrillar amyloid PET

IWG-2 criteria for presymptomatic AD (A plus B)
- A: Absence of specific clinical phenotype (both are required)
  - Absence of amnestic syndrome of the hippocampal type
  - Absence of any clinical phenotype of atypical AD
- B: Proven AD autosomal dominant mutation in PSEN1, PSEN2, or APP, or other proven genes (including Down syndrome trisomy 21)

The Reisberg Global Deterioration Scale reads as follows (Reisberg et al. 1982):
- Stage 1: No cognitive decline independent community living
- Stage 2: Very mild cognitive decline independent community living
- Stage 3: Mild cognitive decline independent community living
- Stage 4: Moderate cognitive decline
  - Looks "normal"
  - Has difficulty with complex tasks (finances, shopping)
  - Requires daily support
  - Decreased sense of time
  - Difficulty with cleaning and cooking
  - Withdrawal from complex tasks
  - May repeat themselves
  - Increased irritability and self-absorption
  - Loss of sense of humor
  - Rigid
  - Requires repetition
  - Memory decreasing
  - Denies problems
  - May be depressed
- Stage 5: Moderately severe cognitive decline
  - Can look "unfinished"
  - Needs help to choose clothing (may wear same clothes all the time)
  - Needs prompting to bathe
  - Needs help with grooming
  - Withdrawal from activities
  - No initiation
  - Sensitivity to noise
  - Decreased visual perceptual abilities—tunnel vision, 14″ in front of them
  - Clings to familiar people and places/hates to be alone
  - Hates change
  - Decreased communication abilities
  - May have delusions
  - Perceives he/she is 20–40 years old
  - Cognitive abilities (processing, decision-making, judgment, etc.) similar to those of an 8-year-old to adolescent
  - May feel physically cold
- Stage 6: Severe cognitive decline
  - Looks disheveled
  - Needs help putting on clothing
  - Requires assistance bathing; may have a fear of bathing
  - Has decreased ability to use the toilet or is incontinent
  - Falling more frequently, shuffling gait, deceased posture

- Eating with fingers
- Difficulty transferring or standing up
- Wandering and rummaging
- Cognitive abilities (processing, decision-making, judgment, etc.) similar to those of a 2–5-year-old
- Experiencing cold or pain can facilitate hostility
- Hard time sitting for meals
- May disrobe; won't wear glasses, shoes, dentures, hearing aids
- Decreased communication—yes/no answers/gestures
- Shuffling gait
• Stage 7: Very severe cognitive decline

32.3 Early-Onset AD Versus Late-Onset AD

Differences between early-onset AD and late-onset AD are shown in (Table 32.1)
• Early-onset AD (EOAD):
  - AD diagnosed before the age of 65 years.
  - 5–10% of all AD cases.
  - 13% of EOAD are familial AD cases.
    ○ mutations in presenilin 1, presenilin 2, and amyloid precursor protein
• Late-onset AD (LOAD)
  - AD diagnosed after the age of 65 years
  - 85–90% of all AD cases
  - sporadic cases
• Differences between EOAD and LOAD
  - Neuropsychology (Sa et al. 2012):
    ○ Praxis and orientation are reduced in EOAD.
    ○ Dissociated profiles between early- and late-onset AD
      • Younger patients have a major impairment in Praxis and a tendency for a great impairment in neocortical temporal functions.
      • AD patients with late-onset forms had a tendency for worse performances in visual memory and orientation, suggesting a more localized disease to the limbic structures.
  - Early-onset AD often present with a non-memory phenotype, of which apraxia/visuospatial dysfunction is the most common presenting symptom.
  - The APOE ε4 alleles were more likely to be found among LOAD compared to APOE ε2 or APOE ε3.

32.4 Neuroimaging Findings

General Imaging Findings
• Atrophy of medial temporal lobe and temporo-parietal cortex

CT non-contrast-enhanced (Fig. 32.1e, f)
• Hippocampal atrophy with enlargement of temporal horns
• Temporo-parietal cortical atrophy

CT contrast-enhanced
• No pathological enhancement

Table 32.1 General characteristics of early-onset Alzheimer disease (EOAD) and late-onset Alzheimer disease (LOAD)

	EOAD	LOAD
Age at onset	Younger than 65 years	65 years and older
Form of onset	Nonamnestic (visuospatial dysfunction, apraxias)	Amnestic
Progression	Faster	Slower
Neuropsychology	Poorer executive function, visuospatial skill, and motor skill	Poorer memory
Pathology findings	Senile plaques and neurofibrillary tangles, with better preservation of the hippocampus	Senile plaques and neurofibrillary tangles
Biomarkers in CSF	Lower level of Aβ42 and increase in tau and P-tau	Lower level of Aβ42 and increase in tau and P-tau
APOE genotype	Favored by absence of ε4 alleles	Favored by 1 or 2 ε4 alleles
Structural MRI	Frontal/temporo-parietal atrophy	Hippocampal atrophy
PET-FDG	Decreased metabolism in temporo-parietal cortex	Decreased metabolism in medial temporal lobe
PET 11C-PiB	Increased uptake (more in parietal zone)	Increased uptake

32.4 Neuroimaging Findings

MRI-T2/FLAIR/T1 (Fig. 32.1a–c)
- Atrophy of temporo-parietal cortex
- Atrophy of medial temporal lobe—assessed by a visual rating scale on coronal T1-weighted MR images (Scheltens MTA-score) (Scheltens et al. 1995)
- Scheltens-score:
  - The scale is based on a visual score of
    - the width of the choroid fissure
    - the width of the temporal horn
    - the height of the hippocampal formation
  - Score results:
    - score 0: no atrophy
    - score 1: only widening of choroid fissure
    - score 2: also widening of temporal horn of lateral ventricle
    - score 3: moderate loss of hippocampal volume (decrease in height)
    - score 4: severe volume loss of hippocampus
  - Interpretation:
    - <75 years: score 2 or more is abnormal
    - >75 years: score 3 or more is abnormal

MRI-T1 contrast-enhanced
- No pathological enhancement

MRI-T2∗ (Fig. 32.1d)
- Occasionally microbleeds caused by cerebral amyloid angiopathy

MRI-Perfusion
- Decreased rCBV parietal and temporal

MR-Spectroscopy
- Decreased NAA and elevated myoinositol values in temporo-parietal lobe

Nuclear medicine Imaging Findings (Fig. 32.2a–j)
- CBF-SPECT and FDG-PET are able to demonstrate hypoperfusion/hypometabolism typically temporo-parietal, hippocampal, posterior cingulum and in later stages the frontal cortex.
- Hypometabolism is often bilateral but can be (especially in the beginning) unilateral.
- Typically the sensorimotor cortex, the primary visual cortex, basal ganglia and thalami are preserved.
- The loss of cerebral metabolism does not always correlate with the clinical stage of the patient (i.e., patients with a high intelligence quotient may present with only mild symptoms but an extensive loss of neuronal function seen in PET or SPECT).
- Image interpretation can be done visually or by a voxel-based analysis by automated systems comparing the metabolic pattern with a normalized population. This may be particularly helpful in patients with mild cognitive impairment (MCI).
- A recent systematic review of the diagnostic utility of SPECT imaging in dementia with ECD and HMPAO revealed the usefulness of brain perfusion SPECT in differentiating AD versus fronto-temporal dementia, AD versus vascular dementia, AD versus dementia with Lewy bodies, and AD versus normal controls including 49 studies between January 1985 and May 2012. The study authors pointed out that imaging has to be an adjunct and be interpreted in the context of clinical information and paraclinical test results. These findings can be assumed to be similar or even better in FDG-PET or even in combination with amyloid PET.
- In recent times, more radiotracers are in development or even available to detect amyloid deposits and thereby influencing diagnosis and thereby therapy. The most prominent compound is PiB (Pittsburgh compound B) which is labeled with 11C, but nowadays some 11F labeled compounds are produced and even approved.
- Recently Tau-Tracers are under investigation. First analyses suggested distinct binding to tau in absence of amyloid binding. At the moment, these tracers are not fully comparable in their distribution.

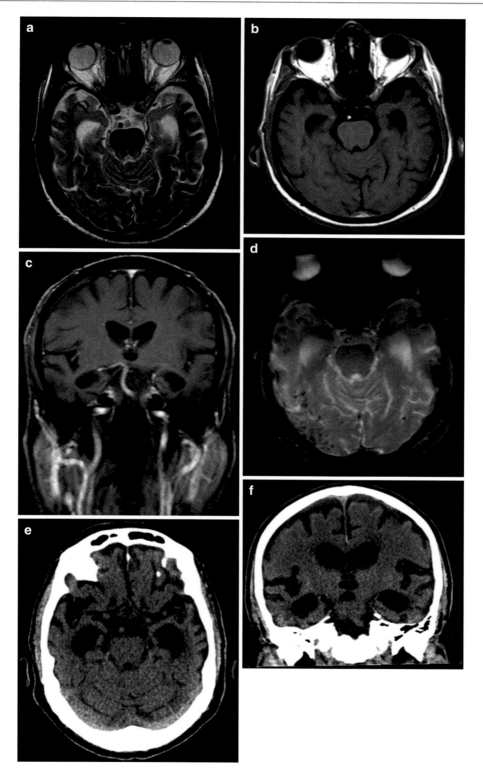

Fig. 32.1 Atrophy of medial temporal lobe with enlargement of temporal horns, temporo-occipital microbleeds; T2 (**a**), T1 (**b**), T1 coronar (**c**), T2* (**d**). Same patient 3 years later with progression of temporo-mesial atrophy; CT non-contrast axial (**e**), coronar (**f**)

32.5 Neuropathology Findings

Macroscopical Findings (Fig. 32.3a–d)
- Reduced brain weight (wide range from 900 to 1400 g)
- Signs of atrophy with
  - smaller gyri
  - enlarged sulci
  - predominantly affecting the frontal, temporal, and parietal lobes
- Enlargement of the ventricular system
- Atrophy of the hippocampal formation

Microscopical findings (Figs. 32.4, 32.5, and 32.6)
The microscopical changes in AD consist of:
- Amyloid deposits (Figs. 32.4c, d and 32.5a–p)
- Neurofibrillary tangles (NFTs) (Figs. 32.4a, b and 32.6a–p)
- Neuropil threads
- Granulovacuolar degeneration
- Loss of neurons
- Loss of synapses

Early-onset AD versus late-onset AD
- The density of amyloid plaques is significantly higher in EOAD
  - in the superior frontal gyrus, inferior frontal gyrus, straight gyrus, cingulate gyrus, superior temporal gyrus, and suprapariteal cortex
- The density of neurofibrillary tangles is significantly higher in EOAD
  - in the superior frontal gyrus, inferior frontal gyrus, straight gyrus, cingulate gyrus, superior temporal gyrus, suprapariteal cortex, and medial temporo-occipital cortex
- The level of significance between EOAD and LOAD was higher for the density of neurofibrillary tangles
  - in the superior frontal gyrus, inferior frontal gyrus, cingulate gyrus, and superior temporal gyrus
- Higher densities of amyloid plaques and neurofibrillary tangles are seen in EOAD.

32.6 The Proposed Diagnostic Criteria

In the following text, the proposed guidelines for the histopathological diagnosis of AD are described, supplemented by some comments illustrating some drawbacks of the criteria.

32.6.1 Ball Criteria: The Hippocampal Criteria

Ball et al. defined AD to be a hippocampal dementia (Ball et al. 1985). The authors did not explicitly characterize the data reported in the paper to be diagnostic criteria for AD but reported on two AD patients in whom only the hippocampal formation was involved showing only neurofibrillary tangles and granulovacuolar degeneration. All other brain regions were unconspicuous.

Based on the results of two previous papers (Ball 1977, 1978), the authors described that in every case diagnosed clinically as Alzheimer disease the hippocampus contains:

- at least 20 tangle-bearing nucleolated neurons per cubic millimeter (the adjusted tangle index) and/or
- at least 55 nucleolated neurons per cubic millimeter showing granulovacuolar degeneration of Simchowicz (the adjusted granulovacuolar index) and/or
- a population of less than 5600 nucleolated neurons per cubic millimeter

Although these data give exact quantitative guidelines, no papers attempting at reproducing these results were published. Furthermore, it seems that these criteria were never applied in daily routine diagnostics. This might be explained by the fact that many morphologists are not familiar with morphometric techniques and that the time spent in data acquisition is not compatible with daily routine.

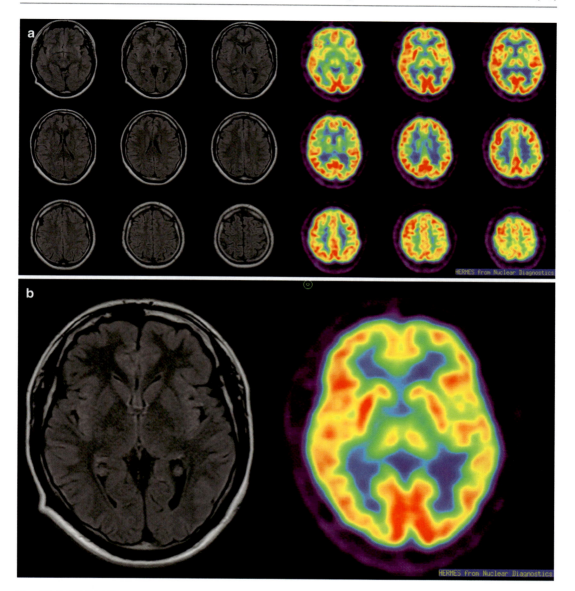

Fig. 32.2 FDG-PET: normal aged brain (**a**, **b**), early phases of Alzheimer disease (**c**, **d**), advanced stage of AD (**e**, **f**), end stage of AD (**g**, **h**). Clinical course of a single patient from 2010 until 2013 (**i**, **j**). Slices of FDG-PET (3 rows left) showing a hypometabolism in the left temporal lobe and amyloid PET (3 rows right) showing pathological uptake especially in the frontal cortex (**k**)

32.6 The Proposed Diagnostic Criteria

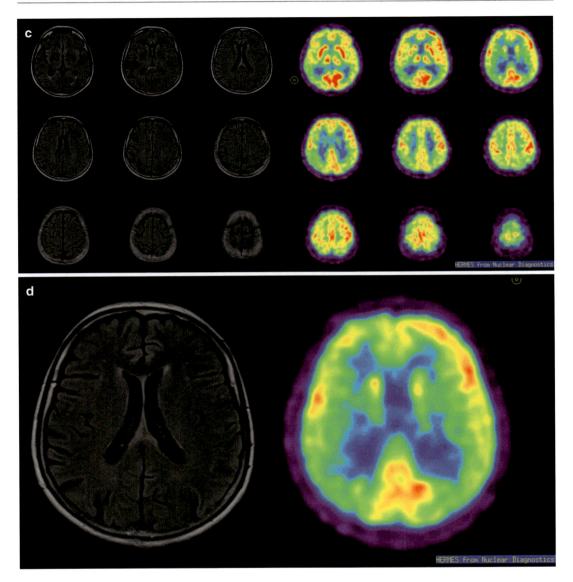

Fig. 32.2 (continued)

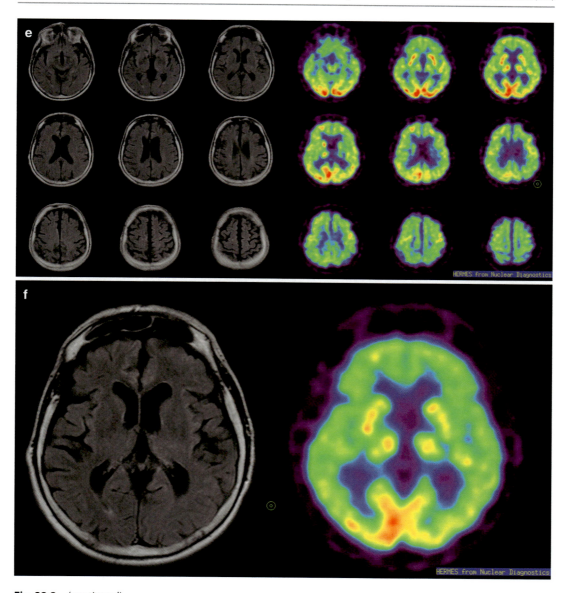

Fig. 32.2 (continued)

32.6 The Proposed Diagnostic Criteria

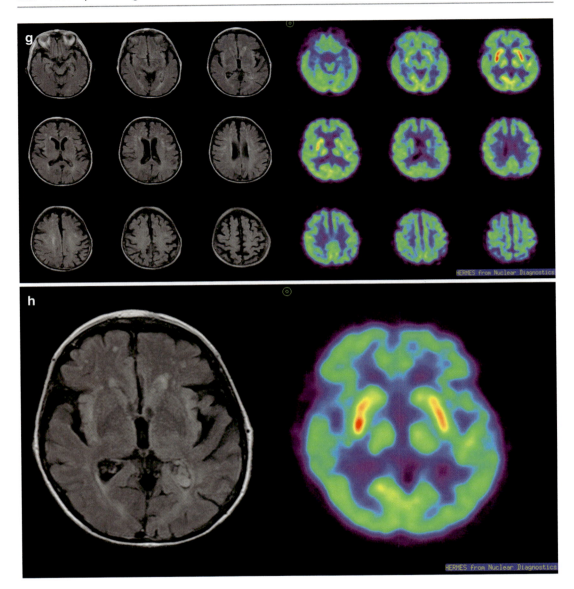

Fig. 32.2 (continued)

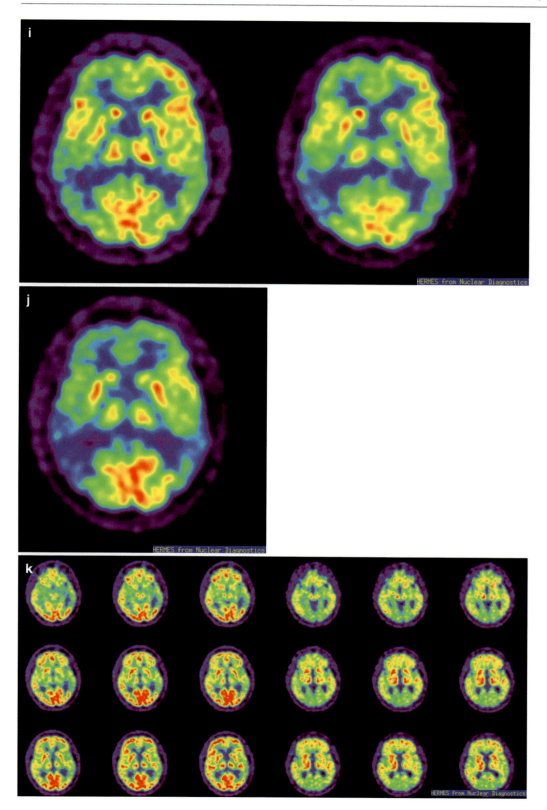

Fig. 32.2 (continued)

32.6 The Proposed Diagnostic Criteria

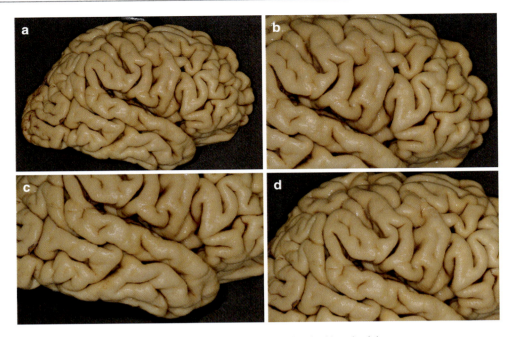

Fig. 32.3 Atrophy of the cerebral cortex (**a–d**) with narrowed gyri and widened sulci

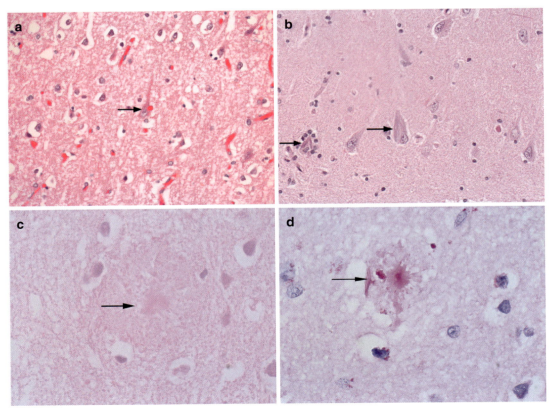

Fig. 32.4 Histological changes include neurofibrillary tangles (**a, b**), amyloid plaques (**c, d**; **d**: stain: PAS) (which are rarely seen on H&E stained sections) as well as hyalinotic vessel wall thickening (**e, f**) with enlargement of the perivascular spaces (**e–h**) and myelin pallor/loss (**g, h**)

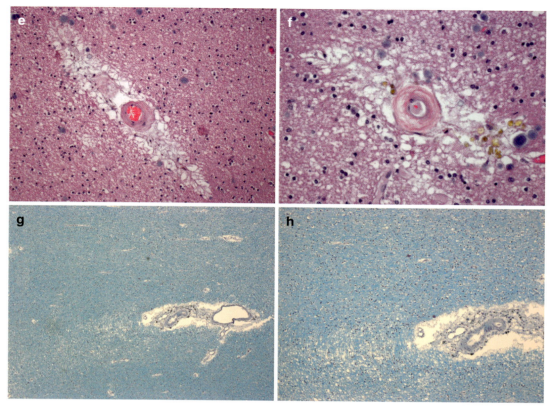

Fig. 32.4 (continued)

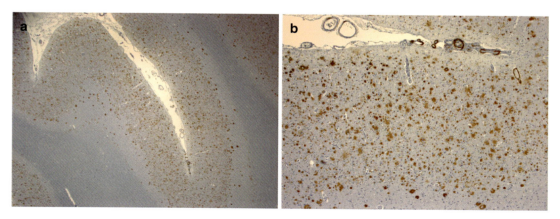

Fig. 32.5 Amyloid deposits: The cerebral cortex can be severely filled with amyloid deposits (**a, b**) in form of classical plaques (**c**) and diffuse plaques (**d**). Amyloid plaques can also be visualized with the Bielschowsky silver impregnation technique (**e, f**). Amyloid is also deposited as subpial accumulation (**g, h**), diffuse deposits (**i**), and perivascular deposits. Neuritic plaques stain for ubiquitin (**k, l**). In approximately 65% of cases with AD, amyloid is also deposited in the vascular walls representing cerebral amyloid angiopathy (CAA) (**m–p**) (Immunohistochemistry for ß-A4: **a–d, m–p**)

32.6 The Proposed Diagnostic Criteria

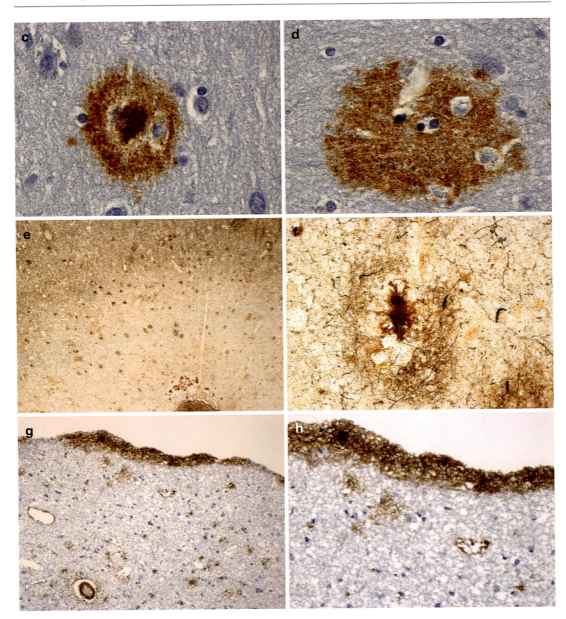

Fig. 32.5 (continued)

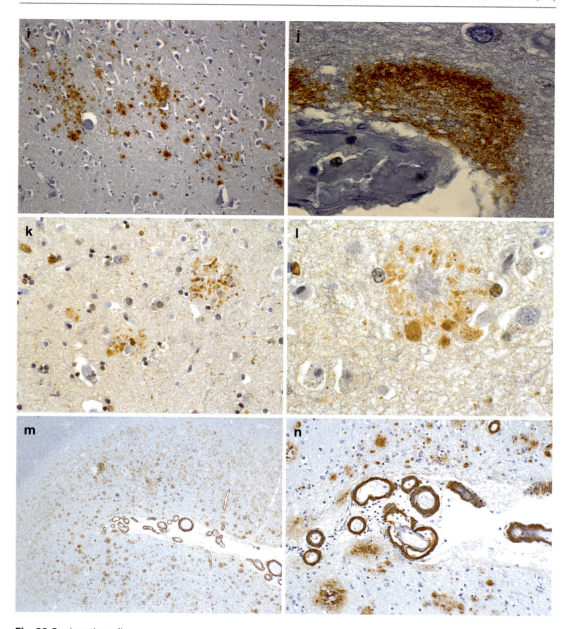

Fig. 32.5 (continued)

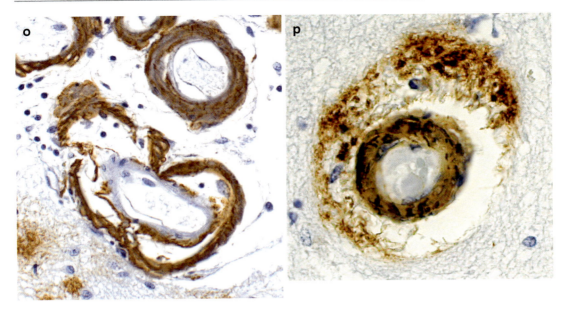

Fig. 32.5 (continued)

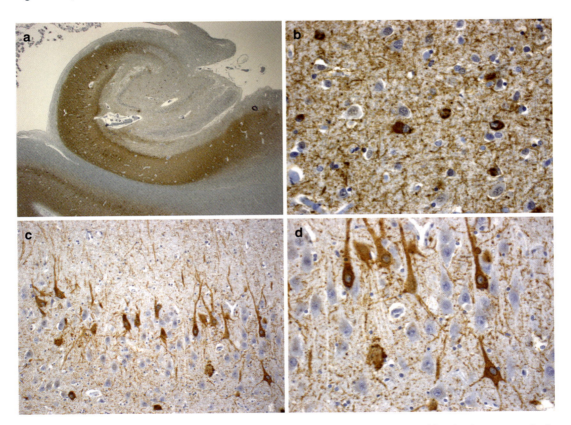

Fig. 32.6 Neurofibrillary changes: The hippocampal formation might be filled with neurofibrillary tangles (NFTs) (**a–d**) in the CA4 region (**b**) and in the CA1-CA2 region (**c, d**) (**a–d**: stain immunohistochemistry for phosphorylated tau). NFTs are visualized by Gallyas silver staining (**e, f**). NFTs are immunopositive for 4 repeat tau (**g–j**). Neuritic plaques stain immunohistochemically for phosphorylated tau (**k, l**) and ubiquitin (**m, n**). Phosphorylated tau deposits are also found in glial cells (**o, p**)

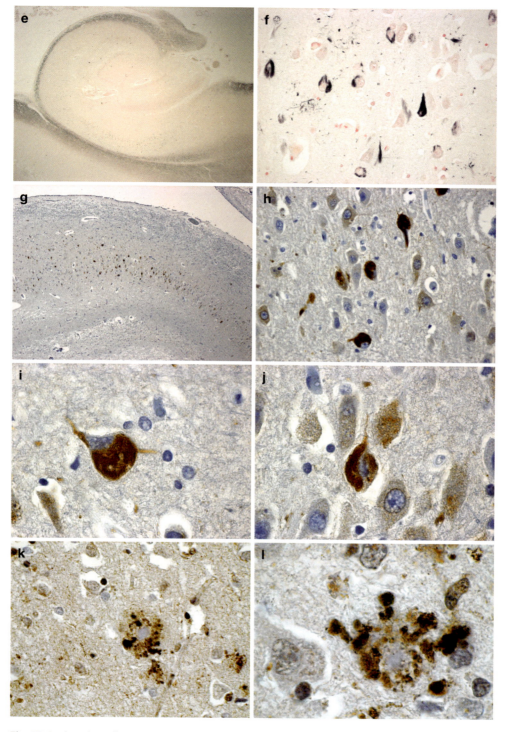

Fig. 32.6 (continued)

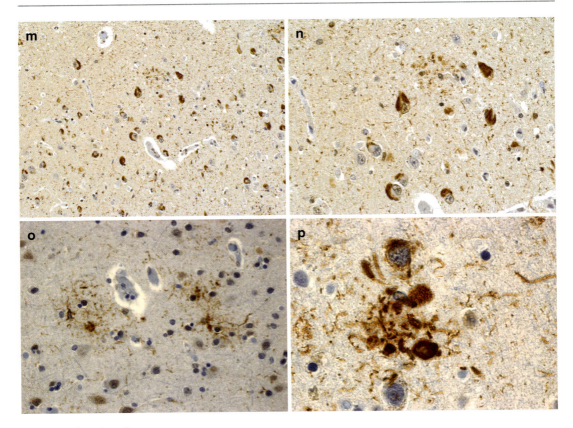

Fig. 32.6 (continued)

32.6.2 Newcastle Criteria (Tomlinson, Roth, Blessed)

The English group from Newcastle headed by the neuropathologist Tomlinson and the psychiatrists Roth and Blessed used the amount of AP as a diagnostic criterion (Tomlinson et al. 1968, 1981; Tomlinson and Henderson 1976).

The group published the following frequencies of control cases and AD patients showing AP in the brain:

- 90% of controls <10 plaques per field
- 70% of controls <5 plaques per field
- 50% of controls <3.3 plaques per field
- 50% of Alzheimer <14.7 plaques per field

Newcastle
- Counting plaques in standardized regions.
- Standardized staining method.
- Rating of neurofibrillary tangles.
- Blessed score assessed 6 month prior to death.
- Correlation between density of senile plaques and cognitive impairment.
- One should not render a neuropathological diagnosis without clinical history.

32.6.3 NIH Criteria (Khachaturian)

During the "Research Workshop on the Diagnosis of Alzheimer Disease," seven neuropathologists as well as representatives from the fields of neuropsychology, neurochemistry, neurology, neuroradiology, and psychiatry convened at the National Institute of Health (NIH) and formulated minimal criteria for the neuropathological diagnosis of AD (Khachaturian 1985).

Since the gross-anatomical changes observed in brains from deceased patients with AD are generally not helpful in this regard, the panel concentrated on the *minimum microscopic criteria* that are necessary to establish a postmortem neuropathological diagnosis.

The following requirements were given:

- The minimum number of areas to be sampled include:
  - three regions of neocortex (frontal, temporal, parietal)
  - amygdala
  - hippocampal formation
  - basal ganglia
  - substantia nigra
  - cerebellar cortex
  - spinal cord
- To establish the presence of pure AD, the following obvious causes of organic dementia should be excluded:
  - chronic subdural hematoma
  - neoplasm
  - Pick disease
  - multi-infarct dementia

The samples for microscopy should be taken
- from paraffin sections
- section thickness between 5 and 15 μm
- Appropriate staining techniques include:
  - Bielschowsky silver technique
  - Thioflavin S method (with ultraviolet illumination)
  - Congo red technique using polarized light
  - Some other staining methods may be insensitive (e.g., the Bodian)

The panel members agreed that in any microscopic field encompassing 1 mm² (microscopic magnification ×200 field) of tissue, the following criteria are necessary for a diagnosis of AD (Table 32.2):

Table 32.2 Summary of the NIH criteria

Patient age (years)	Plaques	NFT
<50	1–5	1–5
50–65	≥8	Some
66–75	>10	
>75	>15	

- Patients younger than 50 years:
  - The number of senile or neuritic plaques and of neurofibrillary tangles anywhere in the neocortex should exceed 2–5 per field.
- Patients aged 50–65 years:
  - There may be some neurofibrillary tangles.
  - The number of senile plaques must be 8 or greater per field.
  - Permit a diagnosis with a very high degree of confidence (±95%).
- Patients aged 66–75 years:
  - Some neurofibrillary tangles may again be present.
  - The number of senile plaques must be greater than 10 per field.
- Patients older than 75 years:
  - Neurofibrillary tangles may sometimes not be found in the neocortex.
  - The number of senile plaques should exceed 15 per microscopic field.

In the presence of a positive clinical history of AD these criteria should be revised downwards, although to what extent remains to be determined by further research.

Critique:

- concentrate on the presence of senile plaques
- only approximative values
- no consideration of normal aging
- considering patients younger than 55 years for the presence of NFT
- no consideration of regional differences

32.6.4 NINCDS-ADRA

Working criteria for the establishment of the clinical diagnosis of AD were established by:

- National Institute of Neurological Communicative Disorders and Stroke (NINCDS)
- Alzheimer and Related Disorders Association (ADRDA) (McKhann et al. 1984)
- Verification of the NINCDS-ADRDA working criteria by Tierney et al. (1988) and estab-

lishment of neuropathologic criteria (Tierney et al. 1988)

The neuropathologic criteria consist of:
- 3 sets of inclusion criteria (A1, A2, and A3).
- 3 sets of vascular exclusion criteria (V1, V2, and V3).
- A total of 9 neuropathologic classifications of pure AD are possible (A1-V1, A1-V2, A1-V3, A2-V1, etc.).

Inclusion criteria:

- A1 one or more NFTs and one or more neuritic plaques per 25×-microscopic field in the hippocampus, independent of changes in the cerebral cortex
- A2 one or more NFTs and one or more neuritic plaques per 25×-microscopic field in the hippocampus as well as in the cerebral cortex
- A3 one or more NFTs and one or more neuritic plaques per 25×-microscopic field in the cerebral cortex independent of the changes in the hippocampus

Exclusion criteria:
Three sets of vascular exclusion criteria were used to exclude cases from pure AD classification as follows:

- V1 one or more ischemic lesions that totaled 50 mL or more of brain tissue in the neocortex, subcortical white matter, and/or hippocampus
- V2 any ischemic lesion irrespective of size or site
- V3 any ischemic lesion in the neocortex, subcortical white matter, and/or hippocampus, irrespective of size

Critique:
- Distinction between pure AD and not pure AD (i.e., vascular disease, Parkinson disease, progressive supranuclear palsy, severe meningeal lymphocytic exudate, combined diseases including mixed AD and Parkinson disease and mixed AD and vascular, and cases with no significant pathology)
- Accuracy: 81–88%
- Sensitivity ranged between 64 and 68%
- Specificity ranged between 89 and 91%
- No weighing for cortical regions
- No specific distinction between plaques and tangles
- No normal aging

32.6.5 CERAD Criteria

The Consortium to Establish a Registry for Alzheimer Disease (CERAD) group proposed in 1991 and 1993 criteria for making the diagnosis of Alzheimer disease (Mirra et al. 1991, 1993). In general, the criteria are based on a semi-quantitative evaluation of plaques and its correlation with the age of the patient resulting in an age-related plaque score. Based on the age-related plaque score and the clinical history of the patient, a certain probability that the symptoms are caused by AD can be estimated.

Regions to be examined:
- superior temporal gyrus
- medial temporal gyrus
- medial frontal gyrus
- inferior parietal lobule

Additional regions to be examined:
- Anterior cingulate gyrus (cortical Lewy body disease)
- Mesencephalon (DD: Parkinson disease, Lewy body disease)

Suggested stains:
- Hematoxylin-Eosin (DD: vascular lesions, spongiform changes, infectious lesions)
- Modified Bielschowsky method
- Thioflavin S method

The CERAD group recommends to look for neuritic plaques at a low magnification (10×) and subsequently rate the amount of neuritic plaques in a 4-tiered system as follows (Table 32.3):
- none
- low
- moderate
- high

Table 32.3 The correspondence between patient age and rating of neuritic plaques is given as follows

Age	Frequencies of plaques			
	None	Low	Moderate	High
<50	0	C	C	C
50–75	0	B	C	C
>75	0	A	B	C

- 0: no histologic evidence of AD
- A: histologic findings are uncertain evidence of AD
- B: histologic findings suggest the diagnosis of AD
- C: histologic findings indicate the diagnosis of AD

Critique:

- The presence and amount of NFTs is completely neglected.
- Very small sample size ($n = 5$) for establishing age-related plaque score (Mirra et al. 1991).
- No data are provided considering normal aging.

32.6.6 NIH/Reagan

Consensus recommendations for the postmortem diagnosis of Alzheimer disease from the National Institute on Aging and the Reagan Institute Working Group on diagnostic criteria for the neuropathological assessment of Alzheimer disease were published in 1997 (Hyman and Trojanowski 1997).

Three levels of likelihood are defined as follows (Table 32.4):

- *High likelihood*
  - High density of neuritic plaques and neurofibrillary tangles
  - High CERAD score
  - Braak & Braak V/VI
- *Intermediate likelihood*
  - Moderate density of neuritic plaques and neurofibrillary tangles
  - Moderate CERAD score
  - Braak & Braak III/IV

Table 32.4 Likelihood that dementia is due to Alzheimer disease following the NIA-Reagan criteria

High likelihood	• High density of neuritic plaques and neurofibrillary tangles • High CERAD score • Braak & Braak V/VI
Intermediate likelihood	• Moderate density of neuritic plaques and neurofibrillary tangles • Moderate CERAD score • Braak & Braak III/IV
Low likelihood	• Limited neuritic plaques and neurofibrillary tangles • Low CERAD score • Braak & Braak I/II

- *Low Likelihood*
  - Limited neuritic plaques and neurofibrillary tangles
  - Low CERAD score
  - Braak & Braak I/II

National Institute on Aging-Alzheimer Association guidelines for the neuropathologic assessment of Alzheimer disease (2012)

In 2012, an update of the NIA-Regan guidelines was proposed (Hyman et al. 2012; Montine et al. 2012) (Table 32.5).

Classification

- A Amyloid β plaque score (modified from Thal et al. (2002), see later)
  - A0:
    - no Aβ or no amyloid plaques
  - A1:
    - Thal phase 1 or 2, i.e., amyloid deposits in the neocortex and allocortical brain regions
  - A2:
    - Thal phase 3, i.e., amyloid deposits in the neocortex, allocortical brain regions, diencephalic nuclei, striatum, and cholinergic neurons of the basal forebrain
  - A3:
    - Thal phase 4 or 5, i.e., amyloid deposits in the neocortex, allocortical brain regions, diencephalic nuclei, striatum, cholinergic neurons of the basal forebrain, brain stem nuclei, and cerebellum

32.7 Staging of Neurofibrillary Tangle Development

Table 32.5 "ABC" score for level of AD neuropathologic change, modified after Hyman et al. (2012) reproduced with kind permission by the Alzheimer Association

AD neuropathologic change		B		
A	C	B0 or B1 (Braak I/II)	B2 (Braak III/IV)	B3 (Braak V/VI)
A0 (0)	C0	Not[a]	Not[a]	Not[a]
A1 (1/2)	C0 or C1	Low	Low	Low[b]
	C2 or C3[c]	Low	Intermediate	Intermediate[b]
A2 (3)	Any C	Low[d]	Intermediate	Intermediate[b]
A3 (4/5)	C0 or C1	Low[d]	Intermediate	Intermediate[b]
	C2 or C3	Low[d]	Intermediate	High

Alzheimer Disease Neuropathologic Change: A1, B0, C0 → no AD or low probability of AD
Alzheimer Disease Neuropathologic Change: A3, B3, C3 → high probability for AD

[a]Medial temporal lobe NFTs in the absence of significant Aβ or neuritic plaques occur in older people and may be seen in individuals without cognitive impairment, with mild impairment, or with cognitive impairment from causes other than AD. Consider other diseases when clinically or pathologically indicated

[b]Widespread NFTs with some Aβ/amyloid plaques or limited neuritic plaques are relatively infrequent and when it occurs, other diseases, particularly tauopathies, should be considered. Such cases may not fit easily into a specific Braak stage, which is intended for categorization of AD-type NFTs

[c]High levels of neuritic plaques in setting of low Thal phase is a rare occurrence and should prompt reconsideration of neuritic vs. diffuse plaques, and the possible contribution of other diseases to cognitive impairment or dementia

[d]Higher levels of Aβ or neuritic plaques with low Braak stage should prompt consideration of contribution by comorbidities like vascular brain injury, Lewy body disease, or hippocampal sclerosis. Also, consider additional sections as well as repeat or additional protocols to demonstrate other non-AD lesions

- B NFT stage (modified from Braak for silver-based histochemistry or phospho-tau immunoreactivity)
  - B0:
    - no NFTs
  - B1:
    - Braak & Braak stages I or II
  - B2:
    - Braak & Braak stages III or IV
  - B3:
    - Braak and Braak stages V or VI
- C Neuritic plaque score (modified from CERAD)
  - C0:
    - no neuritic plaques
  - C1:
    - CERAD score sparse
  - C2:
    - CERAD score moderate
  - C3:
    - CERAD score frequent

32.7 Staging of Neurofibrillary Tangle Development (Braak and Braak 1991)

Braak and Braak (1991) examined the topographical localization of amyloid deposits in the extracellular space and of intraneuronal neurofibrillary changes (including neuritic plaques, neurofibrillary tangles, and neuropil threads). They examined 83 brains from demented and non-demented person. Regions investigated included: frontal, anterior central: uncus level, posterior central: CGL level, occipital.

The topographical distribution and density of amyloid deposits did not allow a good differentiation of stages. It showed a high variation not only within architectonic units but also between individuals.

Based on the topographical localization of neurofibrillary changes, the following NFT stages were described (Table 32.6):

Table 32.6 The operational criteria for Braak & Braak staging as proposed by the BrainNet Europe Consortium reads as follows (Braak et al. 2006)

Stage	Region	Density of neuropil threads
I	• Transentorhinal	+ or ++ or +++
II	• Entorhinal region—outer layers • Entorhinal region—inner layers	++ or +++ + or ++
III	• Occipito-temporal gyrus—superficial and deep layers	++ or +++
IV	• Middle temporal gyrus—superficial and/or deep layers	++ or +++
V	• Peristriate area—superficial and/or deep layers	++ or +++
VI	• Striate area—layer V	++ or +++

- Transentorhinal
  - Stage I: Pre-α cells in the transentorhinal cortex
  - Stage II: Pre-α cells in the entorhinal cortex, CA1 region of the hippocampus
- Limbic
  - Stage III: CA1, subiculum, fusiform gyrus, nucleus basalis of Meynert
  - Stage IV: Severe involvement of the middle temporal gyrus
- Isocortical
  - Stage V: Hippocampus, subiculum, isocortical involvement
  - Stage VI: Isocortical association areas

Stage I—Transentorhinal
- Transentorhinal region (transition zone located between the proper entorhinal region and the adjoining temporal isocortex). The superficial entorhinal cellular layer (Pre-α)
- A few isolated NFT may additionally occur in the proper entorhinal layer Pre-α, in sector CA1, in the magnocellular nuclei of the basal forebrain, and in the antero-dorsal nucleus of the thalamus.

Stage II—Entorhinal
- Aggravation of stage I.
- Exhibits numerous NFT and NT in the transentorhinal Pre-α.
- The hippocampal sector CA1 and in particular the subiculum is affected by modest numbers of NFT.
- The magnocellular forebrain nuclei and the antero-dorsal nucleus of the thalamus remain spared or show only mild changes.
- A few isolated NFT may inconstantly be encountered in isocortical association areas.

Stage III —CA1, subiculum, fusiform gyrus, nucleus basalis of Meinert

- Severe involvement of layer Pre-α, both in the transentorhinal and entorhinal region.
- For the first time, the presence of "ghost tangles" can be observed in the transentorhinal layer Pre-α.
- The hippocampal formation shows an only modest involvement of CA1.
- Pyramidal cells of the subiculum start to develop NFT with far-reaching extensions into the apical dendrite.
- Sectors CA2 to CA4 generally remain devoid of changes except of a few large multipolar nerve cells located close by or within the plexiform layer of the fascia dentata.
- The isocortex remains virtually devoid of changes or is only mildly affected. Some individuals exhibit the presence of a few scattered NFT and NT within layers III and V in basal portions of frontal, temporal, and occipital association areas. Others merely reveal a few irregularly distributed NP in layer III.
- Most cases at this stage display mild changes of magnocellular forebrain nuclei, antero-dorsal nucleus of the thalamus, and amygdala.
- Some isolated NFT may also occur in the reuniens nucleus of the thalamus and in the hypothalamic tuberomammillary nucleus.

32.7 Staging of Neurofibrillary Tangle Development

Stage IV—Middle temporal gyrus—superficial and/or deep layers

- The layer Pre-α is very severely affected.
- Large numbers of ghost tangles are present in both the transentorhinal and entorhinal region.
- There is also a considerable involvement of layers Pri-α and Pre-ß.
- The hippocampal formation contains numerous NFT in CA1.
- The subiculum is only mildly involved.
- In addition, there is a modest affection with star-shaped tangles of the large multipolar CA4-nerve cells close to the fascia dentata.
- The isocortex remains only mildly affected.
- Primary sensory areas and the primary motor field do not show changes or harbor only a few NP in layer III.
- The corticomedial complex of the amygdala reveals the presence of many NE while NFT and NT predominate in the basolateral nuclei.
- Basal portions of the claustrum are mildly affected. NFT may also appear in large neurons located in basal portions of the putamen and the nucleus accumbens.
- The reuniens nucleus and the tuberomammillary nucleus are slightly more intensely affected.
- The antero-dorsal thalamic nucleus is densely filled with NFT and NT.
- The key feature of stages III and IV is that both the entorhinal and transentorhinal layer Pre-α are conspicuously affected and that this is supplemented by a mild to moderate hippocampal and a still-low isocortical involvement. They are, therefore, summarized as "limbic stages."
- Most cases at this stage display mild changes of magnocellular forebrain nuclei, antero-dorsal nucleus of the thalamus, and amygdala.
- Some isolated NFT may also occur in the reuniens nucleus of the thalamus and in the hypothalamic tuberomammillary nucleus.

Stage V—Hippocampus, subiculum, isocortical involvement

- Very large numbers of ghost tangles in layer Pre-α.
- The deep layer Pre-α is severely involved and appears as a band-like structure due to the large number of NT.
- In addition layers Pre-ß and even Pre-γ are also distinctly affected.
- The parvocellular layers of both parasubiculum and transsubiculum show the presence of small NFT and numerous NT.
- Virtually all components of the hippocampal formation are involved.
- Tangles within subicular pyramidal cells have far-reaching extensions into the apical dendrite and can, therefore, easily be distinguished from the flame-shaped type of tangle seen in CA1 pyramidal neurons.
- A circumscribed portion of the uncus is marked by the presence of NFT with long extensions indicating a contribution of the anterior extremity of the subiculum to the formation of the uncus.
- The development of particularly large numbers of NT is a further feature of the subicular pyramidal cell layer. NP occur predominantly in the wedge-shaped portion of CA1 abutting upon the subiculum. They are also found in lower numbers in the pyramidal cell layers of upper portions of CA1, in CA2 and CA3.
- Sector CA1 is infested with NFT-bearing pyramidal cells.
- The outer pyramidal cell layer is more heavily involved than the inner one. In contrast, NFTs are only occasionally observed in the stratum oriens.
- Besides the sparse network of NT seen throughout the pyramidal cell layers, two dense stripes of NT become visible, one accompanying the row of amyloid deposits and NP in the outer half of the stratum radiatum of CA1, the other outlining the stratum oriens.

- NF changes within sector CA2 are subject to considerable interindividual variation.
- Frequently, the sector resists the development of changes but there are also cases with early and severe involvement of CA2.
- NFTs in CA2 are coarse and generate stout extensions into both apical and basal dendrites.
- They, therefore, can readily be differentiated from NFT of CA1 and CA3 pyramidal cells.
- A few compact NFTs occur within CA3 pyramidal cells and the modified pyramidal cells of CA4.
- NFTs located within these cells remain confined to the soma and differ considerably from the star-shaped NFT present in the plexiform layer of the fascia dentate.
- Even the granule cells of the fascia dentate may show a few dot-like NFT.
- The main feature of stage V, however, is that the isocortex is severely affected. In cases in which the isocortex is only mildly affected, changes are confined to the retrosplenial region, the basal portions of the medial facies, and the entire inferior facies of both the temporal and the occipital lobe.
- Antero-basal portions of the insula and orbitofrontal cortex follow. In cases in which the isocortex is more severely affected, these areas tend to show the highest packing density of NFT and NT.
- The temporal isocortex—with the exception of the first temporal gyrus—is characterized by a particularly large number of NP in layer III.
- Virtually all isocortical association areas are affected.
- Primary sensory areas are still more or less resistant to the development of pathological changes showing only modest numbers of NP in layer III with layer V being only initially affected.
- The primary motor field shows sparse numbers of NP in layer III and is the last component of the isocortex affected by the pathological process.
- The subcortical nuclei mentioned in stage IV show a much more pronounced alteration.

Basal portions of the claustrum abutting upon the amygdala are now consistently involved.
- The antero-dorsal nucleus of the thalamus reveals considerable loss of nerve cells and presence of numerous ghost tangles.
- The antero-ventral nucleus displays initial NF changes. Another new component appearing in stage V is a brushwork of argyrophilic cellular processes covering the antero-ventral nucleus.
- A few NFT and NT can also be observed in the lateral tuberal nucleus of the hypothalamus and in pars compacta of the substantia nigra.

Stage VI—Isocortical association areas
- All these changes are even more pronounced.
- Considerable loss of nerve cells in layers Pre-α and Pri-α paralleled by large numbers of ghost tangles.
- Occasionally, even the ghost tangles have been degraded and replaced by glial cell accumulations.
- The parvocellular layers of the parasubiculum and transsubiculum contain many small NFTs and develop a dense web of NT.
- The hippocampal formation is infested with NF changes.
- The large number of NFT-bearing granule cells in the fascia dentata facilitates differentiation of stage V from stage VI.
- CA1 is characterized by severe loss of nerve cells, presence of numerous ghost tangles, and clear-cut stripes of NT within the upper half of the stratum radiatum and within the stratum oriens.
- The subiculum still exhibits an only modest number of NFT but is densely filled with NT.
- All isocortical association areas are very severely affected.
- A special feature of primary sensory areas is the presence of a dense network of NT contrasted by only small numbers of NFT in layer V which thus appears as a darkly stained band with clear-cut boundaries. This pattern can readily be recognized in the narrow fifth layer of the striate area and represents a further difference between stage V and stage VI.

- The primary motor field, in contrast, does not develop a comparable alteration of layer V.
- With the exception of some layer III NP, it remains almost devoid of NF changes.
- Involvement of subcortical nuclei is very severe and does not contribute much to the differentiation of stages.
- The network of pathologically changed cellular processes covering the antero-ventral nucleus now extends into the reticular nucleus of the thalamus. Antero-dorsal portions of this nucleus appear to be particularly affected. The severity of the change gradually decreases when approaching the lateral and posteroventral extremities of the nucleus.
- NFT-bearing neurons can be encountered in the lateral tuberal nucleus of the hypothalamus.
- Stage VI is, furthermore, characterized by the involvement of the extrapyramidal system. Most of the large and quite a number of the medium-sized nerve cells of the striatum contain a NFT.
- In addition, NFT with far-reaching dendritic extensions can be observed in many of the melanin-containing neurons of the substantia nigra.
- The obvious hallmark of stages V and VI is that the isocortex is devastatingly affected. The pathology includes, of course, all the changes noted in earlier stages.
- Stages V and VI are, therefore, denoted as "isocortical stages."

Critique:
- Lack of quantitative data, purely descriptive data
- No reproducible criteria for mild, moderate, or severe load with NFTs
- Lack of statistical evaluation
- No diagnostic criteria, only staging
- Distribution of patients
  - BB I–II non-demented
  - BB III–IV: 50% of cases without dementia
  - BB V–VI: 100% of cases with dementia
  - inclusion of patients with Down syndrome
  - 8 patients with the clinical diagnosis of dementia

- Number of regions investigated
  - Hippocampal region
  - Entorhinal cortex
  - Occipital isocortex

32.8 Phases of Aß-deposition by Thal et al. (2002)

The focus of Thal et al. was the topographical localization of amyloid deposits (Thal et al. 2002).

The following phases were described:

- Phase 1:
  - amyloid deposits exclusively in the neocortex
- Phase 2:
  - Phase 1
  - + allocortical brain regions
- Phase 3:
  - Phase 2
  - + diencephalic nuclei, striatum, cholinergic neurons of the basal forebrain
- Phase 4:
  - Phase 3
  - + brain stem nuclei
- Phase 5:
  - phase 4
  - + cerebellum

Clinically proven AD cases showed
- Phases 3, 4, 5

Non-demented cases with AD-related Aß exhibited:
- Phases 1, 2, 3

32.9 Molecular Neuropathology

32.9.1 Genetics

32.9.1.1 Mutated Genes

The *APOE* Gene
Generally recognized genetic risk markers for developing late-onset (sporadic) Alzheimer dis-

Table 32.7 Estimated population frequencies of *APOE* alleles

APOE allele	Population frequency	
	Worldwide	Frequency range (depending on ethnic group)
ε2	6.7%	0–37.5%
ε3	78.6%	35.6–98.0%
ε4	14.7%	0–49.0%

ease (AD) are germline mutations in the *APOE* gene which codes for apolipoprotein E, an important factor in lipid metabolism. The gene is located at chromosome 19q13.2 and exists in three major allelic variants, ε2, ε3, and ε4. These variants are characterized by combinations of mutated codons at positions 112 and 158 (Table 32.7):

- The wild-type allele *APOE-ε3* encodes cysteine (Cys) at codon 112 and arginine (Arg) at codon 158; homozygous *APOE-ε3/ε3* is the most common genotype in populations worldwide.
- The mutant allele *APOE-ε2* encodes Cys at both codons 112 and 158 (→ Arg158Cys); it correlates with reduced risk of developing sporadic AD. Thus, the presence of the *APOE-ε2* allele appears to confer a protective effect against the disease.
- The mutant allele *APOE-ε4* encodes Arg at both codons 112 (→ Cys112Arg) and 158, and represents an established risk factor for Alzheimer disease. The presence of a single *APOE-ε4* allele increases risk of AD about 2- to 3-fold, the presence of two ε4 alleles even up to 15-fold (in comparison to the most common genotype ε3/ε3).

The original data are available from the **AL**lele **FRE**quency **D**atabase (ALFRED): http://alfred.med.yale.edu/

Given the three existing *APOE* alleles, the following combinations (= genotypes) are possible: ε2/ε2, ε2/ε3, ε3/ε3, ε2/ε4, ε3/ε4, and ε4/ε4. In comparison with the most common genotype, ε3/ε3, homozygous carriers of the ε2 allele have a reduced probability of developing AD, whereas the ε4/ε4 genotype is associated with significantly increased risk, with reported estimated risk factors ranging between 8- and up to 15-fold.

Since the ε4 allele can be observed in ~50% of AD patients (Alonso Vilatela et al. 2012) (as compared to ~15% in control populations; see Table 32.7), it has generally been accepted as the "risk allele." It should be noted, however, that not every individual carrying one or two copies of the ε4 allele develops AD. Thus, its mere presence is not sufficient to cause the disease, it only represents a genetic factor indicating increased risk.

32.9.1.2 Other Mutated Genes

In addition to *APOE*, genome-wide association studies (GWAS) have identified a variety of other genes frequently mutated in AD patients. Table 32.8 depicts a selection of disease-associated candidate genes that have been replicated in several independent studies. The data shown in Table 32.8 were collected and compiled from recent reviews (Reitz 2014; Bettens et al. 2013; Harold et al. 2009).

- It should be noted that causative mutations in the three genes involved in the amyloid pathway, *APP*, *PSEN1*, and *PSEN2*, are typical for early-onset AD. Due to the autosomal dominant inheritance pattern of the mutations, early-onset AD represents the familial form of the disease which, however, accounts for only 5% of the cases.
- In contrast, the vast majority of cases comprise the genetically heterogeneous non-familial, sporadic, late-onset AD. So far, no causative mutations were identified, and the affected genes associated with LOAD (Table 32.8) are considered as "susceptibility loci," merely indicating an increased risk for developing the disease. The observation that different cellular pathways are involved further illustrates the pathogenetic complexity underlying late-onset AD.

32.9 Molecular Neuropathology

Table 32.8 Alzheimer disease-associated candidate genes

Gene symbol	Chromosomal location	Gene product	Putative function(s)/affected pathway(s)	Type of disease
APP	21q21.3	Amyloid beta (A4) precursor protein	• Amyloid-β pathway • Tau pathway • Endocytotic receptor trafficking • GSK 3ß activation	EOAD
PSEN1	14q24.3	Presenilin 1	• Amyloid-β pathway • Neuronal survival • Synaptic plasticity • γ-secretase activity • Transmembrane protein processing • Intracellular signaling	EOAD
PSEN2	1q42.13	Presenilin 2	• Amyloid-β pathway • Neuronal survival • Synaptic plasticity • γ-secretase activity • Transmembrane protein processing • Intracellular signaling	EOAD
CLU	8p21-p12	Clusterin	• Amyloid-β pathway (amyloid-β aggregation, clearance, and toxicity) • Lipid metabolism • Immune system • Inflammation • Apoptosis • Molecular chaperone • Synapse turnover	LOAD
CR1	1q32	Complement component (3b/4b) receptor 1	• Immune system (complement activation) • Amyloid-β pathway (clearance)	LOAD
PICALM	11q14	Phosphatidylinositol binding clathrin assembly protein	• Synaptic cell functioning • Clathrin-mediated endocytosis • Synaptic cell functioning • Amyloid-β toxic effects • Processing of APP	LOAD
BIN1	2q14	Bridging integrator 1	• Synaptic vesicle endocytosis • Caspase-independent apoptosis • Formation of tubular membrane structures	LOAD
EPHA1	7q34	EPH receptor A1	• Synaptic development and plasticity • Immune system	LOAD
ABCA7	19p13.3	ATP binding cassette, subfamily A (ABC1), member 7	• Membrane transport • Immune system • Lipid metabolism • Processing of APP	LOAD
MS4A4A MS4A6E	11q12	Membrane-spanning 4-domains, subfamily A	• Signal transduction • Cell surface signaling • Immune system	LOAD
CD33	19q13.3	CD33 protein	• Clathrin-mediated endocytosis • Immune system • Synaptic cell functioning	LOAD
CD2AP	6p12	CD2-associated protein	• Synaptic cell functioning • Actin remodeling • Receptor-mediated endocytosis	LOAD
SORL1	11q23.2-q24.2	Sortilin-related receptor, L(DLR class) 1	• Endocytosis and sorting • Lipid metabolism • APP binding and processing	LOAD
TOMM40	19q13	Translocase of outer mitochondrial membrane 40 homolog	Mitochondrial protein import	LOAD

Abbreviations used: *EOAD* early-onset Alzheimer disease, *LOAD* late-onset Alzheimer disease

Pathways and related gene products involved in Alzheimer disease have been described and include (Reitz 2014):
- Amyloid
  - APOE—Apolipoprotein E
  - SORL—Sortilin-related receptor
  - CLU—Clusterin
  - CRI—Cribriform degeneration
  - PICALM—Phosphatidylinositol binding clathrin assembly protein
  - BIN1—Bridging integrator 1
  - ABCA7—ATP binding cassette subfamily A member 7
  - CASS4—Cas scaffold protein family member 4
  - PLD3—Phospholipase D family member 3
- Immune system/Inflammation
  - CLU—Clusterin
  - CRI—Cribriform degeneration
  - EPHA1—EPH receptor A1
  - ABCA7—ATP binding cassette subfamily A member 7
  - MS4A4A/MS4A6E—Membrane-spanning 4-domains A4A
  - CD33—CD33 molecule
  - CD2AP—CD2-associated protein
  - HLA-DRB5/DRBI—Major histocompatibility complex, class II, DR beta 5
  - INPP5D—Inositol polyphosphate-5-phosphatase D
  - MEF2C—Myocyte enhancer factor 2C
  - TREM2/TREML2—Triggering receptor expressed on myeloid cells 2
- Lipid transport and metabolism
  - APOE—Apolipoprotein E
  - CLU—Clusterin
  - ABCA7—ATP binding cassette subfamily A member 7
  - SORLI—Sortilin-related receptor
- Synaptic cell funtioning/endocytosis
  - CLU—Clusterin
  - PICALM—Phosphatidylinositol binding clathrin assembly protein
  - BIN I—Bridging integrator 1
  - EPHA I—EPH receptor A1
  - MS4A4A/MS4A6E—Membrane-spanning 4-domains A4A
  - CD33—CD33 molecule
  - CD2AP—CD2-associated protein
  - PTK2B—Protein tyrosine kinase 2 beta
  - SORL I—Sortilin-related receptor
  - SLC24A4/RIN3—Solute carrier family 24 member 4
  - MEF2C—Myocyte enhancer factor 2C
- Tau pathology
  - BIN I—Bridging integrator 1
  - CASS4—Cas scaffold protein family member 4
  - FERMT2—Fermitin family member 2
- Cell migration
  - PTK2B—Protein tyrosine kinase 2 beta
- Hippocampal synaptic function
  - MEF2C—Myocyte enhancer factor 2C
  - PTK2B—Protein tyrosine kinase 2 beta
- Cytoskeletal function and axonal transport
  - CELF I—6-phospho-beta-glucosidase
  - NME8—NME/NM23 family member 8
  - CASS4—Cas scaffold protein family member 4
- Microglial and myeloid cell function
  - INPPD5—Inositol polyphosphate-5-phosphatase D

32.9.2 Aberrations in Mitochondrial DNA (mtDNA)

Impaired cellular energy metabolism has been recognized as a frequent phenomenon in neurodegeneration and in aging brains. In particular, LOAD is often correlated with mitochondrial malfunction, supposedly caused by oxidative damage to the mitochondrial genome. This extrachromosomal double-stranded DNA is a circular molecule of about 16,6 kbp and exists in several copies per mitochondrion.

Mitochondrial DNA (mtDNA) encodes 13 proteins that are crucial for electron transport chain function and oxidative phosphorylation, including several subunits of the respiratory chain complexes I, III, and IV as well as two subunits of the mitochondrial ATP synthase complex. The remaining mitochondrial genes code for 22 tRNAs and 2 ribosomal RNAs.

A commonly observed aberration often associated with normal aging, but also with LOAD, is a 4977bp deletion occurring between two perfect sequence repeats in the mtDNA. In the 4977bp deletion mtDNA, seven protein-coding genes and five tRNA genes are missing. Assuming that the smaller DNA is replicated preferentially to the larger wild-type genome, it becomes amplified in the affected cells which enhance the deleterious effect of the aberrant mtDNA. However, to date it remains unclear to which extent the occurrence of this deletion contributes to LOAD etiology and progression.

32.9.3 Epigenetics

At the epigenetic level, perturbations in the regulatory network controlled by microRNAs (miR-NAs) have been associated with a wide variety of diseases. Aberrant expression of miRNAs affects expression of their target mRNAs with which they interact, thus resulting in altered levels of the respective proteins. In general, upregulation of miRNA expression leads to a reduction of target mRNA translation. It is important to indicate that miRNA expression itself may be subject to altered epigenetic mechanisms such as histone modification (methylation/acetylation) or DNA methylation in miRNA promoter regions.

In Table 32.9, a selection of miRNAs are listed for which a correlation with AD pathology was demonstrated (modified from (Femminella et al. 2015; Van den Hove et al. 2014)): ↑ indicates elevated expression levels, ↓ indicates reduced expression levels

Table 32.9 Selection of miRNAs involved in Alzheimer disease

	Involved in processes	miR expression in AD	Target genes in AD include
let-7b miRNA	Chromatin Structure Cell Cycle	↑	HMAG2 EZH2 DICER1
miR-9	Neural Differentiation Gene Silencing	↓	FOXP2 REST SIRT1
miR-34 (a/b/c)	Apoptosis Neuroplasticity Gene Silencing	↑	BCL2 CREB SIRT1
miR-106	Amyloid β Formation ApoE Expression	↓	APP ABCA1
miR-107	Neuritic Plaque Formation Brain Development Cell Cycle	↓	BACE1 CDK5R1 CDK6
miR-124	Amyloid β Production APP Splicing	↓	BACE1 PTPB1
miR-125b	Hedgehog Pathway Neural Stem Cell Differentiation	↑	SMO NES
miR-132/miR-212	Neuronal Development Neurotransmission/Inflammation	↓	FOXP2 AChE
miR-137	Gene Silencing Neurogenesis	↓	EZH2 CDK6
miR-146a	Inflammatory Response	↑	CFH
miR-148a	Insulin signaling Gene Silencing Cell Cycle	↓	IGF-IR DNMT3b CDK6
miR-181	Notch Signaling Gene Silencing	↓	NOTCH4 SIRT1
miR-200	Cell Adhesion Wnt signaling	↑	ZEB1, ZEB2 CTNNB1

Table 32.10 Biomarkers for AD in CSF (after Farooqui (2017) with kind permission by Elsevier)

Biomarker	Effects
Aß	Decreased
Total tau	Increased
Hyperphosphorylated tau	Increased
APOE4	Increased
TREM2	Increased
Neurogranin	Increased
YKL-40	Increased
VLP1	Increased
Resistin	Increased
Thrombospondin-1	Increased
Growth-associated protein	Increased
F2-isoprostane	Increased
27-Hydroxycholesterol	Increased

Biomarkers measured in the cerebrospinal fluid and its changes in AD are shown in Table 32.10.

32.10 Treatment and Prognosis

Tretament
- Acetylcholine inhibitors
- Try to decrease acetylcholine breakdown at the synapse
- Possible neuroprotective agents
  - Memantine (NMDA antagonist)
  - Selegiline (monoamine oxidase B inhibitor)
  - Vitamin E
  - Muscarinic receptor agonists
  - Nicotinic receptor agonist
- Secretase inhibitors and modulators
- Peroxisome proliferator-activated receptor agonists
- Statins
- Curcumin
- Symptomatic
  - Coexisting depression
    Antidepressant therapy
- Adjunctive—disease modifying
  - Immunotherapy
  - Hormonals
  - NSAIDs
- Antioxidants
- Antipsychotics
- Opioids
- Antiepileptics
- Anxiolytics

Biologic Behavior-Prognosis-Prognostic Factors
- With progression of disease, impairment becomes more generalized.
- Average survival after diagnosis: 5–20 years.

Selected References

Acosta C, Anderson HD, Anderson CM (2017) Astrocyte dysfunction in Alzheimer disease. J Neurosci Res 95(12):2430–2447. https://doi.org/10.1002/jnr.24075

Alonso Vilatela ME, Lopez-Lopez M, Yescas-Gomez P (2012) Genetics of Alzheimer's disease. Arch Med Res 43(8):622–631. https://doi.org/10.1016/j.arcmed.2012.1010.1017. Epub 2012 Nov 1018

Area-Gomez E, Schon EA (2017) Alzheimer disease. Adv Exp Med Biol 997:149–156. https://doi.org/10.1007/978-981-10-4567-7_11

Arnold SE, Arvanitakis Z, Macauley-Rambach SL, Koenig AM, Wang HY, Ahima RS, Craft S, Gandy S, Buettner C, Stoeckel LE, Holtzman DM, Nathan DM (2018) Brain insulin resistance in type 2 diabetes and Alzheimer disease: concepts and conundrums. Nat Rev Neurol 14(3):168–181. https://doi.org/10.1038/nrneurol.2017.185

Ball MJ (1977) Neuronal loss, neurofibrillary tangles and granulovacuolar degeneration in the hippocampus with ageing and dementia. A quantitative study. Acta Neuropathol 37(2):111–118

Ball MJ (1978) Topographic distribution of neurofibrillary tangles and granulovacuolar degeneration in hippocampal cortex of aging and demented patients. A quantitative study. Acta Neuropathol 42(2):73–80

Ball MJ, Fisman M, Hachinski V, Blume W, Fox A, Kral VA, Kirshen AJ, Fox H, Merskey H (1985) A new definition of Alzheimer's disease: a hippocampal dementia. Lancet 1(8419):14–16

Bettens K, Sleegers K, Van Broeckhoven C (2013) Genetic insights in Alzheimer's disease. Lancet Neurol 12(1):92–104. https://doi.org/10.1016/S1474-4422(1012)70259-70254

Bhogal P, Mahoney C, Graeme-Baker S, Roy A, Shah S, Fraioli F, Cowley P, Jager HR (2013) The common dementias: a pictorial review. Eur Radiol 23(12):3405–3417. https://doi.org/10.1007/s00330-013-3005-9

Selected References

Braak H, Braak E (1991) Neuropathological stageing of Alzheimer-related changes. Acta Neuropathol 82(4):239–259

Braak H, Alafuzoff I, Arzberger T, Kretzschmar H, Del Tredici K (2006) Staging of Alzheimer disease-associated neurofibrillary pathology using paraffin sections and immunocytochemistry. Acta Neuropathol 112(4):389–404. https://doi.org/10.1007/s00401-006-0127-z

Calderon-Garciduenas AL, Duyckaerts C (2017) Alzheimer disease. Handb Clin Neurol 145:325–337. https://doi.org/10.1016/b978-0-12-802395-2.00023-7

Caselli RJ, Beach TG, Knopman DS, Graff-Radford NR (2017) Alzheimer disease: scientific breakthroughs and translational challenges. Mayo Clin Proc 92(6):978–994. https://doi.org/10.1016/j.mayocp.2017.02.011

Dubois B, Feldman HH, Jacova C, Hampel H, Molinuevo JL, Blennow K, DeKosky ST, Gauthier S, Selkoe D, Bateman R, Cappa S, Crutch S, Engelborghs S, Frisoni GB, Fox NC, Galasko D, Habert MO, Jicha GA, Nordberg A, Pasquier F, Rabinovici G, Robert P, Rowe C, Salloway S, Sarazin M, Epelbaum S, de Souza LC, Vellas B, Visser PJ, Schneider L, Stern Y, Scheltens P, Cummings JL (2014) Advancing research diagnostic criteria for Alzheimer's disease: the IWG-2 criteria. Lancet Neurol 13(6):614–629. https://doi.org/10.1016/s1474-4422(14)70090-0

Farooqui AA (2017) Neurochemical aspects of Alzheimer's disease. Risk factors, pathogenesis, biomarkers, and potential treatment strategies. Elsevier, San Diego

Femminella GD, Ferrara N, Rengo G (2015) The emerging role of microRNAs in Alzheimer's disease. Front Physiol 6:40. https://doi.org/10.3389/fphys.2015.00040.eCollection02015

Frisoni GB, Fox NC, Jack CR Jr, Scheltens P, Thompson PM (2010) The clinical use of structural MRI in Alzheimer disease. Nat Rev Neurol 6(2):67–77. https://doi.org/10.1038/nrneurol.2009.215

Frisoni GB, Bocchetta M, Chetelat G, Rabinovici GD, de Leon MJ, Kaye J, Reiman EM, Scheltens P, Barkhof F, Black SE, Brooks DJ, Carrillo MC, Fox NC, Herholz K, Nordberg A, Jack CR Jr, Jagust WJ, Johnson KA, Rowe CC, Sperling RA, Thies W, Wahlund LO, Weiner MW, Pasqualetti P, Decarli C (2013) Imaging markers for Alzheimer disease: which vs how. Neurology 81(5):487–500. https://doi.org/10.1212/WNL.0b013e31829d86e8

Gaiteri C, Mostafavi S, Honey CJ, De Jager PL, Bennett DA (2016) Genetic variants in Alzheimer disease—molecular and brain network approaches. Nat Rev Neurol 12(7):413–427. https://doi.org/10.1038/nrneurol.2016.84

Gao F, Barker PB (2014) Various MRS application tools for Alzheimer disease and mild cognitive impairment. AJNR Am J Neuroradiol 35(6 Suppl):S4–S11. https://doi.org/10.3174/ajnr.A3944

Guerriero F, Sgarlata C, Francis M, Maurizi N, Faragli A, Perna S, Rondanelli M, Rollone M, Ricevuti G (2017) Neuroinflammation, immune system and Alzheimer disease: searching for the missing link. Aging Clin Exp Res 29(5):821–831. https://doi.org/10.1007/s40520-016-0637-z

Hardy J, Bogdanovic N, Winblad B, Portelius E, Andreasen N, Cedazo-Minguez A, Zetterberg H (2014) Pathways to Alzheimer's disease. J Intern Med 275(3):296–303. https://doi.org/10.1111/joim.12192

Harold D, Abraham R, Hollingworth P, Sims R, Gerrish A, Hamshere ML, Pahwa JS, Moskvina V, Dowzell K, Williams A, Jones N, Thomas C, Stretton A, Morgan AR, Lovestone S, Powell J, Proitsi P, Lupton MK, Brayne C, Rubinsztein DC, Gill M, Lawlor B, Lynch A, Morgan K, Brown KS, Passmore PA, Craig D, McGuinness B, Todd S, Holmes C, Mann D, Smith AD, Love S, Kehoe PG, Hardy J, Mead S, Fox N, Rossor M, Collinge J, Maier W, Jessen F, Schurmann B, Heun R, van den Bussche H, Heuser I, Kornhuber J, Wiltfang J, Dichgans M, Frolich L, Hampel H, Hull M, Rujescu D, Goate AM, Kauwe JS, Cruchaga C, Nowotny P, Morris JC, Mayo K, Sleegers K, Bettens K, Engelborghs S, De Deyn PP, Van Broeckhoven C, Livingston G, Bass NJ, Gurling H, McQuillin A, Gwilliam R, Deloukas P, Al-Chalabi A, Shaw CE, Tsolaki M, Singleton AB, Guerreiro R, Muhleisen TW, Nothen MM, Moebus S, Jockel KH, Klopp N, Wichmann HE, Carrasquillo MM, Pankratz VS, Younkin SG, Holmans PA, O'Donovan M, Owen MJ, Williams J (2009) Genome-wide association study identifies variants at CLU and PICALM associated with Alzheimer's disease. Nat Genet 41(10):1088–1093. https://doi.org/10.1038/ng.1440. Epub 2009 Sep 1086

Hommet C, Mondon K, Constans T, Beaufils E, Desmidt T, Camus V, Cottier JP (2011) Review of cerebral microangiopathy and Alzheimer's disease: relation between white matter hyperintensities and microbleeds. Dement Geriatr Cogn Disord 32(6):367–378. https://doi.org/10.1159/000335568

Hou Y, Song H, Croteau DL, Akbari M, Bohr VA (2017) Genome instability in Alzheimer disease. Mech Ageing Dev 161. (Pt A:83–94. https://doi.org/10.1016/j.mad.2016.04.005

Hunter S, Brayne C (2018) Understanding the roles of mutations in the amyloid precursor protein in Alzheimer disease. J Neurochem 23(1):81–93. https://doi.org/10.1038/mp.2017.218

Hyman BT, Trojanowski JQ (1997) Consensus recommendations for the postmortem diagnosis of Alzheimer disease from the National Institute on Aging and the Reagan Institute Working Group on diagnostic criteria for the neuropathological assessment of Alzheimer disease. J Neuropathol Exp Neurol 56(10):1095–1097

Hyman BT, Phelps CH, Beach TG, Bigio EH, Cairns NJ, Carrillo MC, Dickson DW, Duyckaerts C, Frosch MP, Masliah E, Mirra SS, Nelson PT, Schneider JA, Thal DR, Thies B, Trojanowski JQ, Vinters HV, Montine TJ (2012) National Institute on Aging-Alzheimer's Association guidelines for the neuropathologic assessment of Alzheimer's disease. Alzheimers Dement 8(1):1–13. https://doi.org/10.1016/j.jalz.2011.10.007

Jack CR Jr, Knopman DS, Chetelat G, Dickson D, Fagan AM, Frisoni GB, Jagust W, Mormino EC, Petersen RC, Sperling RA, van der Flier WM, Villemagne VL, Visser PJ, Vos SJ (2016) Suspected non-Alzheimer disease pathophysiology—concept and controversy. Nat Rev Neurol 12(2):117–124. https://doi.org/10.1038/nrneurol.2015.251

Jevtic S, Sengar AS, Salter MW, McLaurin J (2017) The role of the immune system in Alzheimer disease: etiology and treatment. Ageing Res Rev 40:84–94. https://doi.org/10.1016/j.arr.2017.08.005

Jones SV, Kounatidis I (2017) Nuclear factor-kappa B and Alzheimer disease, unifying genetic and environmental risk factors from cell to humans. Front Immunol 8:1805. https://doi.org/10.3389/fimmu.2017.01805

Kanatsu K, Tomita T (2017) Molecular mechanisms of the genetic risk factors in pathogenesis of Alzheimer disease. Front Biosci (Landmark Ed) 22:180–192

Khachaturian ZS (1985) Diagnosis of Alzheimer's disease. Arch Neurol 42(11):1097–1105

Liu CC, Kanekiyo T, Xu H, Bu G (2013) Apolipoprotein E and Alzheimer disease: risk, mechanisms and therapy. Nat Rev Neurol 9(2):106–118. https://doi.org/10.1038/nrneurol.2012.1263. Epub 2013 Jan 1038

McKhann G, Drachman D, Folstein M, Katzman R, Price D, Stadlan EM (1984) Clinical diagnosis of Alzheimer's disease: report of the NINCDS-ADRDA Work Group under the auspices of Department of Health and Human Services Task Force on Alzheimer's disease. Neurology 34(7):939–944

Medway C, Morgan K (2014) Review: the genetics of Alzheimer's disease; putting flesh on the bones. Neuropathol Appl Neurobiol 40(2):97–105. https://doi.org/10.1111/nan.12101

Mendez MF (2017) Early-onset Alzheimer disease. Neurol Clin 35(2):263–281. https://doi.org/10.1016/j.ncl.2017.01.005

Mirra SS, Heyman A, McKeel D, Sumi SM, Crain BJ, Brownlee LM, Vogel FS, Hughes JP, van Belle G, Berg L (1991) The Consortium to Establish a Registry for Alzheimer's Disease (CERAD). Part II. Standardization of the neuropathologic assessment of Alzheimer's disease. Neurology 41(4):479–486

Mirra SS, Hart MN, Terry RD (1993) Making the diagnosis of Alzheimer's disease. A primer for practicing pathologists. Arch Pathol Lab Med 117(2):132–144

Montine TJ, Phelps CH, Beach TG, Bigio EH, Cairns NJ, Dickson DW, Duyckaerts C, Frosch MP, Masliah E, Mirra SS, Nelson PT, Schneider JA, Thal DR, Trojanowski JQ, Vinters HV, Hyman BT (2012) National Institute on Aging-Alzheimer's Association guidelines for the neuropathologic assessment of Alzheimer's disease: a practical approach. Acta Neuropathol 123(1):1–11. https://doi.org/10.1007/s00401-011-0910-3

Norfray JF, Provenzale JM (2004) Alzheimer's disease: neuropathologic findings and recent advances in imaging. AJR Am J Roentgenol 182(1):3–13. https://doi.org/10.2214/ajr.182.1.1820003

Nucera A, Hachinski V (2017) Cerebrovascular and Alzheimer disease: fellow travelers or partners in crime? J Neurochem 144(5):513–516. https://doi.org/10.1111/jnc.14283

Palop JJ, Mucke L (2016) Network abnormalities and interneuron dysfunction in Alzheimer disease. Nat Rev Neurosci 17(12):777–792. https://doi.org/10.1038/nrn.2016.141

Phillips NR, Simpkins JW, Roby RK (2014) Mitochondrial DNA deletions in Alzheimer's brains: a review. Alzheimers Dement 10(3):393–400

Pierce AL, Bullain SS, Kawas CH (2017) Late-onset Alzheimer disease. J Neurosci Res 35(2):283–293. https://doi.org/10.1016/j.ncl.2017.01.006

Rangachari V, Dean DN, Rana P, Vaidya A, Ghosh P (2018) Cause and consequence of Abeta - lipid interactions in Alzheimer disease pathogenesis. Biochim Biophys Acta 1860:1652. https://doi.org/10.1016/j.bbamem.2018.03.004

Reisberg B, Ferris SH, de Leon MJ, Crook T (1982) The Global Deterioration Scale for assessment of primary degenerative dementia. Am J Psychiatry 139(9):1136–1139. https://doi.org/10.1176/ajp.139.9.1136

Reitz C (2014) Genomic insights into the etiology of Alzheimer's disease: a review. Adv Genom Genet 4:59–66

Ridge PG, Ebbert MT, Kauwe JS (2013) Genetics of Alzheimer's disease. Biomed Res Int 2013:254954. https://doi.org/10.1155/2013/254954. Epub 252013 Jul 254925

Rosenberg RN, Lambracht-Washington D, Yu G, Xia W (2016) Genomics of Alzheimer disease: a review. JAMA Neurol 73(7):867–874. https://doi.org/10.1001/jamaneurol.2016.0301

Sa F, Pinto P, Cunha C, Lemos R, Letra L, Simoes M, Santana I (2012) Differences between early and late-onset Alzheimer's disease in neuropsychological tests. Front Neurol 3:81. https://doi.org/10.3389/fneur.2012.00081

Scheltens P, Launer LJ, Barkhof F, Weinstein HC, van Gool WA (1995) Visual assessment of medial temporal lobe atrophy on magnetic resonance imaging: interobserver reliability. J Neurol 242(9):557–560

Schmidt V, Carlo AS, Willnow TE (2014) Apolipoprotein E receptor pathways in Alzheimer disease. Wiley Interdiscip Rev Syst Biol Med 6(3):255–270. https://doi.org/10.1002/wsbm.1262

Sweeney MD, Sagare AP, Zlokovic BV (2018) Blood-brain barrier breakdown in Alzheimer disease and other neurodegenerative disorders. Nat Rev Neurol 14(3):133–150. https://doi.org/10.1038/nrneurol.2017.188

Thal DR, Rub U, Orantes M, Braak H (2002) Phases of a beta-deposition in the human brain and its relevance for the development of AD. Neurology 58(12):1791–1800

Tierney MC, Fisher RH, Lewis AJ, Zorzitto ML, Snow WG, Reid DW, Nieuwstraten P (1988) The NINCDS-ADRDA Work Group criteria for the clinical diagnosis of probable Alzheimer's disease: a clinicopathologic study of 57 cases. Neurology 38(3):359–364

Tomlinson BE, Henderson G (1976) Some quantitative cerebral findings in normal and demented old people. In: Terry RD, Gershon S (eds) Neurology of aging. Raven Press, New York, pp 183–204

Tomlinson BE, Blessed G, Roth M (1968) Observations on the brains of non-demented old people. J Neurol Sci 7(2):331–356

Tomlinson BE, Irving D, Blessed G (1981) Cell loss in the locus coeruleus in senile dementia of Alzheimer type. J Neurol Sci 49(3):419–428

Tramutola A, Lanzillotta C, Perluigi M, Butterfield DA (2017) Oxidative stress, protein modification and Alzheimer disease. Brain Res Bull 133:88–96. https://doi.org/10.1016/j.brainresbull.2016.06.005

Van den Hove DL, Kompotis K, Lardenoije R, Kenis G, Mill J, Steinbusch HW, Lesch KP, Fitzsimons CP, De Strooper B, Rutten BP (2014) Epigenetically regulated microRNAs in Alzheimer's disease. Neurobiol Aging 35(4):731–745. https://doi.org/10.1016/j.neurobiolaging.2013.1010.1082. Epub 2013 Oct 1018

Verheijen J, Sleegers K (2018) Understanding Alzheimer disease at the interface between genetics and transcriptomics. Trends Genet 34:434. https://doi.org/10.1016/j.tig.2018.02.007

Villemagne VL, Dore V, Burnham SC, Masters CL, Rowe CC (2018) Imaging tau and amyloid-beta proteinopathies in Alzheimer disease and other conditions. Nat Rev Neurol 14(4):225–236. https://doi.org/10.1038/nrneurol.2018.9

Xiao T, Zhang W, Jiao B, Pan CZ, Liu X, Shen L (2017) The role of exosomes in the pathogenesis of Alzheimer' disease. Transl Neurodegener 6:3. https://doi.org/10.1186/s40035-017-0072-x

Neurodegenerative Diseases: Lewy Body Dementia

33.1 Clinical Signs and Symptoms

Lewy body disease (LBD) is a chronic progressive neuropsychiatric disorder characterized by (Table 33.1):

- Parkinsonism with or without dementia.
- Dementia might be the predominant symptom while parkinsonian symptoms occur later during the course of the disease.

Classification of Lewy body disease (Kosaka and Iseki 1996):

- Brain stem type (= Parkinson disease)
- Traditional type
- Diffuse type = diffuse Lewy body disease (frequent form and rare form)
- Cerebral type

33.2 Epidemiology

Incidence
- 0.5–1.6 per 1000 person-years
- 3.2–7.1% of all dementia cases

Dementia Terminology
- **Lewy body dementias**
  - An umbrella term that includes clinically diagnosed dementia with Lewy bodies and Parkinson disease dementia.
- **Dementia with Lewy bodies**
  - Dementia that occurs before or concurrently with parkinsonism or within 1 year of onset of motor symptoms. However, not all patients develop parkinsonism.
  - Second frequent cause of dementia
  - 20% of dementia caused by Lewy body disease
- **Parkinson disease dementia**
  - Dementia starting 1 year or more after well-established Parkinson disease.
- **Mild cognitive impairment in Parkinson disease**
  - Cognitive impairment in patients with Parkinson disease not sufficient to interfere greatly with functional independence.
- **Lewy body disease**
  - Pathological diagnosis. The distribution of Lewy body-type pathology and additional pathologies is often specified.
- **Major and mild neurocognitive disorder with Lewy bodies or due to Parkinson disease**
  - New terms proposed by DSM-5 corresponding to dementia with Lewy bodies and Parkinson disease dementia.

Table 33.1 The Dementia with Lewy bodies Consortium proposed a set of revised criteria for the clinical diagnosis (McKeith et al. 2017) reproduced with kind permission by Wolters Kluwer Health

Central feature (essential for a diagnosis of possible or probable DLB)	• Dementia defined as progressive cognitive decline of sufficient magnitude to interfere with normal social or occupational function or with usual daily activities. • Prominent or persistent memory impairment may not necessarily occur in the early stages but is usually evident with progression. • Deficits on tests of attention, executive function, and visuoperceptual ability may be especially prominent and occur early.
Core clinical features (the first 3 typically occur early and may persist throughout the course)	• Fluctuating cognition with pronounced variations in attention and alertness • Recurrent visual hallucinations that are typically well formed and detailed • REM sleep behavior disorder, which may precede cognitive decline. • One or more spontaneous cardinal features of parkinsonism: these are bradykinesia (defined as slowness of movement and decrement in amplitude or speed), rest tremor, or rigidity.
Supportive clinical features	• Severe sensitivity to antipsychotic agents • Postural instability • Repeated falls • Syncope or other transient episodes of unresponsiveness • Severe autonomic dysfunction, e.g., constipation • Orthostatic hypotension • Urinary incontinence • Hypersomnia • Hyposmia • Hallucinations in other modalities • Systematized delusions • Apathy • Anxiety • Depression
Indicative biomarkers	• Reduced dopamine transporter uptake in basal ganglia demonstrated by SPECT or PET. • Abnormal (low uptake) 123iodine-MIBG myocardial scintigraphy. • Polysomnographic confirmation of REM sleep without atonia.
Supportive biomarkers	• Relative preservation of medial temporal lobe structures on CT/MRI scan. • Generalized low uptake on SPECT/PET perfusion/metabolism scan with reduced occipital activity ± the cingulate island sign on FDG-PET imaging. • Prominent posterior slow-wave activity on EEG with periodic fluctuations in the pre-alpha/theta range.
Probable DLB can be diagnosed if:	• Two or more core clinical features of DLB are present, with or without the presence of indicative biomarkers • Only one core clinical feature is present, but with one or more indicative biomarkers.
Probable DLB should not be diagnosed	• On the basis of biomarkers alone.
Possible DLB can be diagnosed if:	• Only one core clinical feature of DLB is present, with no indicative biomarker evidence • One or more indicative biomarkers are present but there are no core clinical features.
DLB is less likely:	• In the presence of any other physical illness or brain disorder including cerebrovascular disease, sufficient to account in part or in total for the clinical picture, although these do not exclude a DLB diagnosis and may serve to indicate mixed or multiple pathologies contributing to the clinical presentation • If parkinsonian features are the only core clinical feature and appear for the first time at a stage of severe dementia.

33.3 Neuroimaging Findings

General Imaging Findings
- No specific pattern of brain atrophy.
- If signs of atrophy are present, there is a diffuse pattern of global gray matter atrophy (Fig. 33.1a–d).
  - less medial temporal lobe atrophy than Alzheimer disease
  - greater atrophy of medial temporal lobe, frontal lobes, and temporal lobes compared with healthy controls
- Dementia severity correlates with medial temporal lobe atrophy.
- If medial temporal lobe preserved
  - dementia with Lewy bodies diagnosis
- If medial temporal lobe atrophied
  - not diagnostically helpful

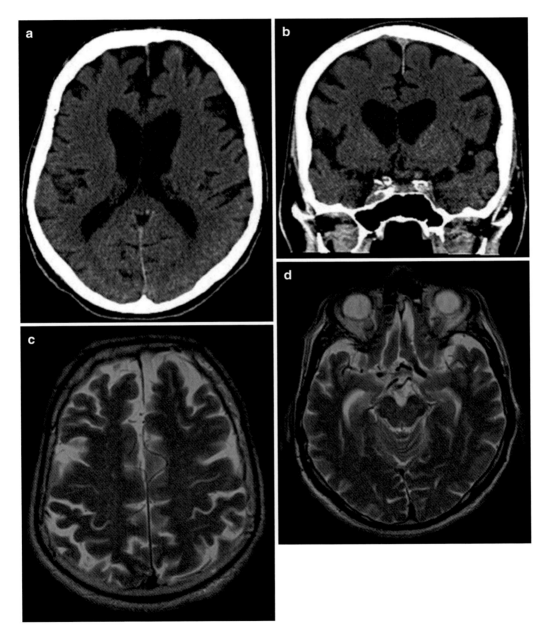

Fig. 33.1 Mild unspecific atrophy in CT ax/cor (**a**, **b**) and MRI-T2 (**c**, **d**)

- Diffusion loss of parieto-occipital white matter integrity compared with healthy controls.
- Changes in frontal, temporal, and occipital white matter diffusivity relative to healthy controls.

Nuclear Medicine Imaging Findings (Fig. 33.2a–e)
- In contrast to Alzheimer dementia, loss of CBF and glucose metabolism is extended to the primary visual occipital cortex.
- Temporo-parietal changes are similar to Alzheimer dementia and allow no differentiation.
- The main point is that in DLB presynaptic dopaminergic changes are present like in patients with Parkinson disease.
- The differentiation of Parkinson-dementia and DLB is made by the clinical symptoms (whether there is the cognitive loss or the movement disorder first).

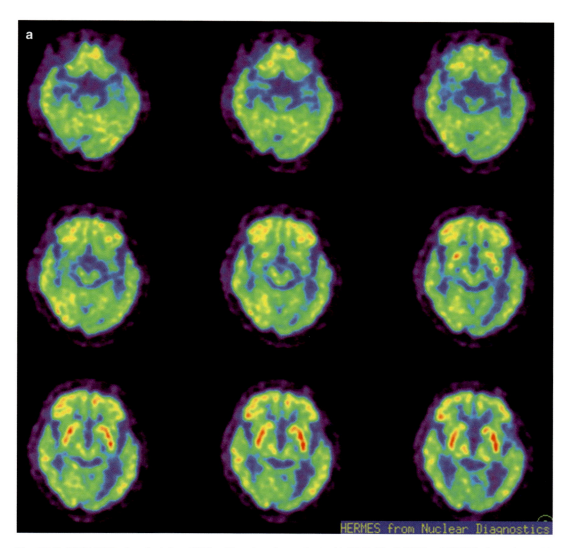

Fig. 33.2 FDG-PET of an incipient DLB with reduced FDG uptake especially occipital (**a**); FDG-PET of an advanced DLB with globally reduced FDG uptake (**b**); FDG-PET (**c**) and corresponding FPCIT SPECT of a patient with DLB (**d**); D-PET and FPCIT of a patient with cortical posterior atrophy (in contrast to DLB there is no reduction in the presynaptic dopaminergic system) (**e**)

33.3 Neuroimaging Findings

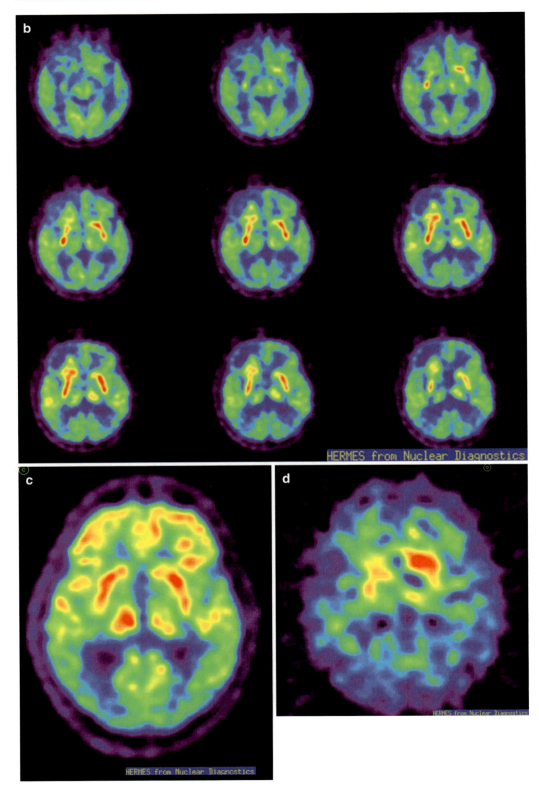

Fig. 33.2 (continued)

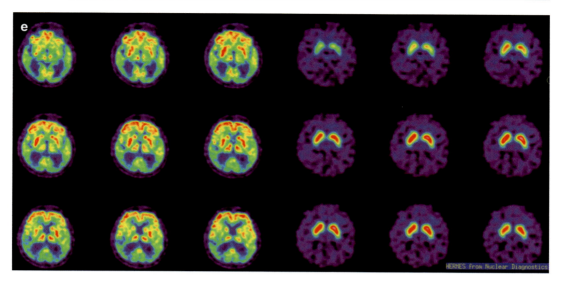

Fig. 33.2 (continued)

- So typically there is performed and FPCIT SPECT showing additional defects in the striatum.
- The differentiation from Alzheimer disease is important because it affects treatment substantially.
- Some reports state a deficit of 123I-MIBG uptake in the myocardium in DLB patients representing cardiac GABA-ergic dysfunction.

SPECT
- Dopamine transporter
  - Significantly reduced uptake in caudate and putamen relative to healthy controls or patients with Alzheimer disease.
  - FPCIT SPECT scan diagnostically useful for distinguishing dementia with Lewy bodies from Alzheimer disease or healthy controls.
  - Dopaminergic dysfunction does not distinguish between Parkinson disease dementia, dementia with Lewy bodies, and other parkinsonian syndromes (cortico-basal degeneration and progressive supranuclear palsy).
- Perfusion
  - Global cortical hypoperfusion relative to healthy controls; some evidence for reduced occipital lobe perfusion relative to Alzheimer disease but findings unreliable.
  - Occipital hypoperfusion a supportive diagnostic feature for dementia with Lewy bodies (common but not specific)

SPECT and PET
- Cholinergic
  - Reduced cortical acetylcholinesterase activity relative to healthy controls or patients with Alzheimer disease.
  - Increased muscarinic and nicotinic receptors in occipital lobe relative to healthy controls
  - Not diagnostically useful; cholinergic dysfunction accounts for effectiveness of acetylcholinesterase inhibitors in Lewy body dementia

PET
- Glucose metabolism
  - Reduced occipital lobe metabolism relative to Alzheimer disease.
  - Occipital hypometabolism predicts development of dementia in Parkinson disease.
  - Supportive diagnostic feature for dementia with Lewy bodies; occipital hypometabolism predicts development of dementia in Parkinson disease; helpful when frontotem-

poral dementia with reduced dopamine transporter uptake is a possibility.
- Amyloid
  - Greater amyloid deposition compared with healthy controls or patients with Parkinson disease dementia, but less than in those with Alzheimer disease
  - Not diagnostically useful; might help identify patients for treatment with antiamyloid drugs in the future

33.4 Neuropathology Findings

Macroscopic Features
- Diffuse brain atrophy
- Substantia nigra and locus coeruleus often depigmented

Microscopic Features (Fig. 33.3a–f)
- Loss of pigmented neurons.
- Aggregation of melanin as free-pigment and in macrophages in the substantia nigra and locus coeruleus.
- Lewy bodies as well as pale inclusions present in high number within the surviving cells.
- Inclusions also present in the substantia reticulata and cerebral cortex with prominent involvement of the anterior temporal and frontal cortex, insula, cingulate gyrus, and entorhinal cortex.
- Density of cortical Lewy bodies is highly variable and shows age dependency.
- Cortical Lewy bodies show immunoreactivities for ubiquitin and seldomly for tau and neurofilament.
- Cortical Lewy bodies are usually found in neurons of layers V and VI.
- In approximately 50% of patients with cortical Lewy body dementia, diffuse ß-A4 amyloid deposits are found.
- Four stages can be defined, i.e., mild, moderate, severe, very severe (Tables 33.2 and 33.3)

The likelihood that the observed neuropathology explains the LBD clinical syndrome is

- directly related to the severity of Lewy-related pathology
- inversely related to the severity of concurrent AD-type pathology

The likelihood that the pathologic findings are associated with a typical, dementia with Lewy Bodies is given in Table 33.4.

Immunophenotype (Fig. 33.3g–r)
- Lewy bodies are positive for:
- α-synuclein
- Phosphorylated α-synuclein

33.5 Molecular Neuropathology

- Associated with intermediate filaments
- Chaperone proteins
- Elements of the ubiquitin-proteasome system
- Downregulation of ACh and hyperactivity of the hypothalamic-pituitary-adrenal axis

33.6 Treatment and Prognosis

Treatment
- Cholinesterase inhibitors (donepezil).
- Neuroleptics (quetiapine).
- Antidepressants (SSRI).
- Dopamine agonists (levodopa).
- Antipsychotic drugs should be avoided.
- Cognition
  - Acetylcholinesterase inhibitors
    o Efficacious
    o Rivastigmine and donepezil class 1 efficacy in dementia with Lewy bodies; Cochrane review of dementia with Lewy bodies, Parkinson disease dementia, and MCI-PD showed overall positive effect
  - Memantine
    o Insufficient evidence
    o Small significant improvement in overall clinical impression

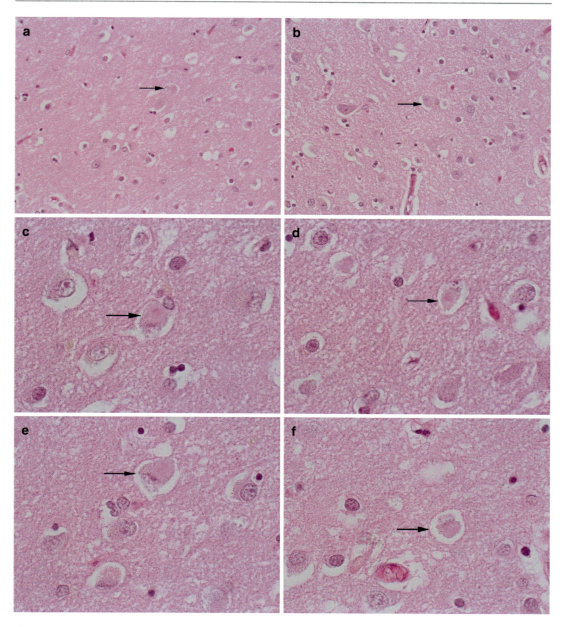

Fig. 33.3 Neurons in the cortex with intracytoplasmic Lewy bodies (arrow) (**a–f**). Lewy bodies stain immunohistochemically for α-synuclein (**g–r**)

33.6 Treatment and Prognosis

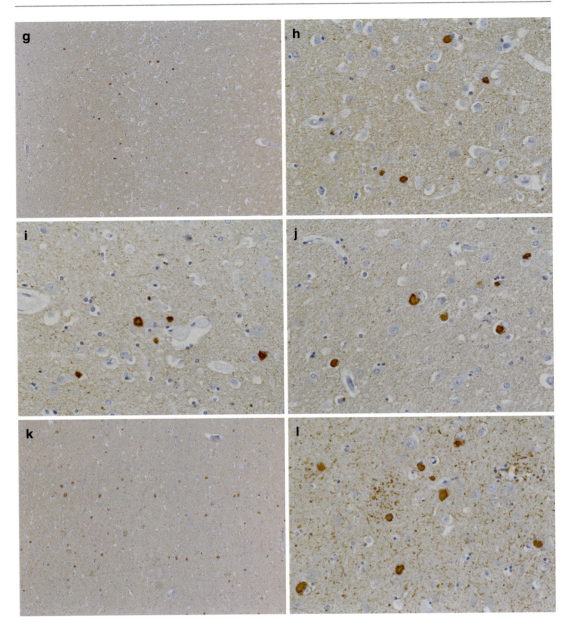

Fig. 33.3 (continued)

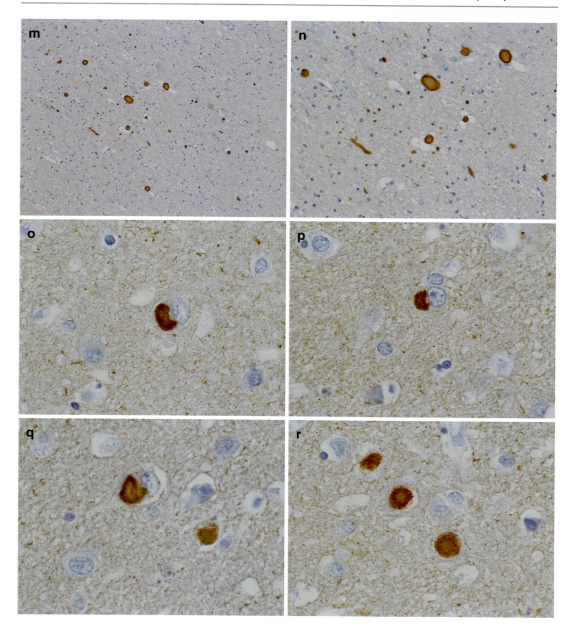

Fig. 33.3 (continued)

Table 33.2 Lesion staging after McKeith et al. (2005) reproduced with kind permission by Wolters Kluwer Health

Stage		LBs	LNs
1	Mild	Sparse	Sparse
2	Moderate	>1 LB per high power field	Sparse
3	Severe	≥4 LBS	Scattered in low power field
4	Very severe	Numerous	Numerous

Table 33.3 Brain structures involved in brain stem, limbic, and neocortical stages of Lewy body pathology (McKeith et al. 2017) reproduced with kind permission by Wolters Kluwer Health

		Lewy body-type pathology		
		Brain stem	Limbic	Neocortical
Brain stem	IX–X	1–3	1–3	1–3
	LC	1–3	1–3	1–3
	SN	1–3	1–3	1–3
Limbic—basal forebrain	nbM	0–2	2–3	2–3
	Amygdala	0–2	2–3	3–4
	Transentorhinal	0–1	1–3	2–4
	Cingulate	0–1	1–3	2–4
Neocortical	Temporal	0	0–2	2–3
	Frontal	0	0–1	1–3
	Parietal	0	0	0–2

Table 33.4 Likelihood that the pathologic findings are associated with a typical, dementia with Lewy Bodies, clinical syndrome (McKeith et al. 2017) reproduced with kind permission by Wolters Kluwer Health

LB pathology	AD pathology		
	NIA-AA none/low Braak 0–II	NIA-AA intermediate Braak III–IV	NIA-AA High Braak V–VI
Diffuse neocortical	High	High	Intermediate
Limbic (transitional)	High	Intermediate	Low
Brain stem-predominant	Low	Low	Low
Amygdala-predominant	Low	Low	Low
Olfactory bulb only	Low	Low	Low

- Parkinsonism
  - Levodopa
    - Insufficient evidence
    - Levodopa replacement less effective in dementia with Lewy bodies than in Parkinson disease
    - Probable increased risk of psychosis in patients with dementia with Lewy bodies
- Hallucinations
  - Acetylcholinesterase inhibitors
    - Insufficient evidence
  - Antipsychotic drugs
    - Unlikely to be efficacious
- Depression or anxiety
  - Antidepressant drugs
    - Insufficient evidence
- Rapid Eye Movement Sleep Behavior Disorder (RBD)
  - Melatonin
    - Insufficient evidence
  - Clonazepam
    - Insufficient evidence
- Excessive daytime sleepiness
  - Modafinil
    - Insufficient evidence
- Urinary symptoms
  - Trospium
    - Insufficient evidence
- Postural hypotension
  - Fludrocortisone
    - Insufficient evidence

Biologic Behavior-Prognosis-Prognostic Factors

- Progressive disease
- Deterioration over 5–8 years

Selected References

Beyer K, Domingo-Sabat M, Ariza A (2009) Molecular pathology of Lewy body diseases. Int J Mol Sci 10(3):724–745. https://doi.org/10.3390/ijms10030724

Bohnen NI, Muller M, Frey KA (2017) Molecular imaging and updated diagnostic criteria in Lewy body dementias. Curr Neurol Neurosci Rep 17(10):73. https://doi.org/10.1007/s11910-017-0789-z

Brigo F, Turri G, Tinazzi M (2015) 123I-FP-CIT SPECT in the differential diagnosis between dementia with Lewy bodies and other dementias. J Neurol Sci 359(1–2):161–171. https://doi.org/10.1016/j.jns.2015.11.004

Cromarty RA, Elder GJ, Graziadio S, Baker M, Bonanni L, Onofrj M, O'Brien JT, Taylor JP (2016) Neurophysiological biomarkers for Lewy body dementias. Clin Neurophysiol 127(1):349–359. https://doi.org/10.1016/j.clinph.2015.06.020

Donaghy P, Thomas AJ, O'Brien JT (2015) Amyloid PET imaging in Lewy body disorders. Am J Geriatr Psychiatry 23(1):23–37. https://doi.org/10.1016/j.jagp.2013.03.001

Galasko D (2017) Lewy body disorders. Neurol Clin 35(2):325–338. https://doi.org/10.1016/j.ncl.2017.01.004

Haller S, Garibotto V, Kovari E, Bouras C, Xekardaki A, Rodriguez C, Lazarczyk MJ, Giannakopoulos P, Lovblad KO (2013) Neuroimaging of dementia in 2013: what radiologists need to know. Eur Radiol 23(12):3393–3404. https://doi.org/10.1007/s00330-013-2957-0

Hogan DB, Fiest KM, Roberts JI, Maxwell CJ, Dykeman J, Pringsheim T, Steeves T, Smith EE, Pearson D, Jette N (2016) The prevalence and incidence of dementia with Lewy bodies: a systematic review. Can J Neurol Sci 43(Suppl 1):S83–S95. https://doi.org/10.1017/cjn.2016.2

Kim WS, Kagedal K, Halliday GM (2014) Alpha-synuclein biology in Lewy body diseases. Alzheimers Res Ther 6(5):73. https://doi.org/10.1186/s13195-014-0073-2

Kosaka K (2014) Latest concept of Lewy body disease. Psychiatry Clin Neurosci 68(6):391–394. https://doi.org/10.1111/pcn.12179

Kosaka K, Iseki E (1996) Dementia with Lewy bodies. Curr Opin Neurol 9(4):271–275

McKeith IG, Dickson DW, Lowe J, Emre M, O'Brien JT, Feldman H, Cummings J, Duda JE, Lippa C, Perry EK, Aarsland D, Arai H, Ballard CG, Boeve B, Burn DJ, Costa D, Del Ser T, Dubois B, Galasko D, Gauthier S, Goetz CG, Gomez-Tortosa E, Halliday G, Hansen LA, Hardy J, Iwatsubo T, Kalaria RN, Kaufer D, Kenny RA, Korczyn A, Kosaka K, Lee VM, Lees A, Litvan I, Londos E, Lopez OL, Minoshima S, Mizuno Y, Molina JA, Mukaetova-Ladinska EB, Pasquier F, Perry RH, Schulz JB, Trojanowski JQ, Yamada M (2005) Diagnosis and management of dementia with Lewy bodies: third report of the DLB consortium. Neurology 65(12):1863–1872. https://doi.org/10.1212/01.wnl.0000187889.17253.b1

McKeith IG, Boeve BF, Dickson DW, Halliday G, Taylor JP, Weintraub D, Aarsland D, Galvin J, Attems J, Ballard CG, Bayston A, Beach TG, Blanc F, Bohnen N, Bonanni L, Bras J, Brundin P, Burn D, Chen-Plotkin A, Duda JE, El-Agnaf O, Feldman H, Ferman TJ, Ffytche D, Fujishiro H, Galasko D, Goldman JG, Gomperts SN, Graff-Radford NR, Honig LS, Iranzo A, Kantarci K, Kaufer D, Kukull W, Lee VMY, Leverenz JB, Lewis S, Lippa C, Lunde A, Masellis M, Masliah E, McLean P, Mollenhauer B, Montine TJ, Moreno E, Mori E, Murray M, O'Brien JT, Orimo S, Postuma RB, Ramaswamy S, Ross OA, Salmon DP, Singleton A, Taylor A, Thomas A, Taraboschi P, Toledo JB, Trojanowski JQ, Tsuang D, Walker Z, Yamada M, Kosaka K (2017) Diagnosis and management of dementia with Lewy bodies: fourth consensus report of the DLB consortium. Neurology 89(1):88–100. https://doi.org/10.1212/wnl.0000000000004058

Mueller C, Ballard C, Corbett A, Aarsland D (2017) The prognosis of dementia with Lewy bodies. Lancet Neurol 16(5):390–398. https://doi.org/10.1016/s1474-4422(17)30074-1

Ramirez EP, Vonsattel JP (2014) Neuropathologic changes of multiple system atrophy and diffuse Lewy body disease. Semin Neurol 34(2):210–216. https://doi.org/10.1055/s-0034-1381732

Spano M, Signorelli M, Vitaliani R, Aguglia E, Giometto B (2015) The possible involvement of mitochondrial dysfunctions in Lewy body dementia: a systematic review. Funct Neurol 30(3):151–158

Taylor JP, O'Brien J (2012) Neuroimaging of dementia with Lewy bodies. Neuroimaging Clin N Am 22(1):67–81. , viii. https://doi.org/10.1016/j.nic.2011.11.001

Velayudhan L, Ffytche D, Ballard C, Aarsland D (2017) New therapeutic strategies for Lewy body dementias. Curr Neurol Neurosci Rep 17(9):68. https://doi.org/10.1007/s11910-017-0778-2

Walker Z, Possin KL, Boeve BF, Aarsland D (2015) Lewy body dementias. Lancet 386(10004):1683–1697. https://doi.org/10.1016/s0140-6736(15)00462-6

Watson R, Colloby SJ (2016) Imaging in dementia with Lewy bodies: an overview. J Geriatr Psychiatry Neurol 29(5):254–260. https://doi.org/10.1177/0891988716654984

34. Neurodegenerative Diseases: Fronto-temporal Lobar Degeneration

Fronto-temporal dementia (FTD) or fronto-temporal lobe dementia (FTLD) includes the following four clinical subgroups (Table 34.1):

- Semantic dementia
- Progressive non-fluent aphasia
- FTD-behavioral variant
- FTD with motor neuron disease/ALS

34.1 Clinical Signs and Symptoms

The diagnostic criteria for semantic dementia, progressive non-fluent aphasia, and FTD-behavioral variant are shown in Table 34.1.

FTD with motor neuron disease/ALS
- Similar behavior and language symptoms as in other FTD syndromes
- Motor symptoms
  - Muscle weakness
  - Clumsiness
  - Muscle atrophy
  - Dysphagia
  - Dysarthria
  - Spasticity
  - Hyper-reflexia

34.2 Epidemiology

Incidence
- 10–20% of all cases with dementia

Age Incidence
- 50–65 years

Sex Incidence
- Male:Female ratio: 1:1

Localization
- Frontal lobe
- Anterior temporal lobe

34.3 Neuroimaging Findings

General Imaging Findings
- Often asymmetric atrophy of (anterior) fronto-temporal lobes

CT non-contrast-enhanced (Fig. 34.1a)
- Fronto-temporal atrophy

CT contrast-enhanced
- No pathological enhancement

Table 34.1 The diagnostic criteria as established in a consensus report of the major clinical subgroups of FTD are given as follows (Neary et al. 1998) (reproduced with kind permission by Springer Nature)

Semantic dementia	

Core diagnostic features	• Insidious onset and gradual progression
	• Language disorder characterized by:
	  – Progressive, fluent, empty spontaneous speech
	  – Loss of word meaning, manifest by impaired naming
	  – Semantic paraphasias and/or
	• Perceptual disorder characterized by:
	  – Prosopagnosia: impaired recognition of identity of familiar faces and/or
	• Associative agnosia: impaired recognition of object identity

Preserved functions	• Perceptual matching and drawing reproduction • Single-word repetition • Ability to read aloud and write to dictation orthographically regular words
Supportive features—Behavior	• Loss of sympathy and empathy • Narrowed preoccupations • Parsimony
Supportive features—Speech and language	• Press of speech • Idiosyncratic word usage • Absence of phonemic paraphasias • Surface dyslexia and dysphagia • Preserved calculation
Supportive features—Physical signs	• Absence of late primitive reflexes • Akinesia • Rigidity • Tremor

Investigations—Neuropsychology	• Profound semantic loss
	  – Failure of world comprehension and naming
	  – Failure of face and object recognition
	• Preserved phonology and syntax, and elementary perceptual processing, spatial skills, and day-to-day memorizing

Investigations—EEG	• Normal
Investigations—Brain Imaging	• Anterior temporal
Progressive non-fluent aphasia	
Core diagnostic features	• Insidious onset and gradual progression • Non-fluent spontaneous speech with at least one of the following: agrammatism, phonemic paraphasias, anomia
Supportive features—Behavior	• Early preservation of social skills • Late behavioral changes similar to FTD
Supportive features—Speech and language	• Stuttering or oral apraxia • Impaired repetition • Alexia, agraphia • Early preservation of word meaning • Late mutism
Supportive features—Physical signs	• Late contralateral primitive reflexes • Akinesia • Rigidity • Tremor
Investigations—Neuropsychology	• Non-fluent aphasia in the absence of severe amnesia or perceptuospatial disorder
Investigations—EEG	• Normal or Minimal asymmetric slowing
Investigations—Brain Imaging	• Asymmetric abnormality Predominantly affecting dominant (usually left) hemisphere

34.3 Neuroimaging Findings

Table 34.1 (continued)

FTD-behavioral variant (bvFTD)	
Core diagnostic features	• Insidious onset and gradual progression • Early decline in social interpersonal conduct • Early impairment in regulation of personal conduct • Early emotional blunting • Early loss of insight
Supportive features—Behavior	• Decline in personal hygiene and grooming • Mental rigidity and inflexibility • Distractibility and impersistence • Hyperorality and dietary changes • Perseveration and stereotyped behavior
Supportive features—Speech and language	• Altered speech output (aspontaneity and economy of speech, press of speech) • Stereotypy of speech • Echolalia • Perseveration • Mutism
Supportive features—Physical signs	• Primitive reflexes • Incontinence • Akinesia, rigidity, and tremor • Low and labile blood pressure
Investigations—Neuropsychology	• Impairment on frontal lobe tests • Absence of severe amnesia, aphasia, or perceptual disorder
Investigations—EEG	• Normal conventional EEG
Investigations—Brain Imaging	• Frontal abnormality • Anterior temporal abnormality

MRI-T2/FLAIR (Fig. 34.1b–g)
- Hyperintense signal in fronto-temporal white matter

MRI-T1
- Fronto-temporal atrophy

MRI-T1 contrast-enhanced
- No pathological enhancement

MR-Spectroscopy
- Decreased NAA/Cr ratio fronto-temporal
- Lactate peak in frontal lobe possible

Nuclear Medicine Imaging Findings (Fig. 34.2a–f)
- In CBF-SPECT and FDG-PET hypoperfusion and hypometabolism in the frontal and anteromedial temporal lobes are observed. Hypometabolism can be seen in subcortical structures too (putamen, globus pallidus, thalamus). Typically the motor cortex and the visual cortex are spared from hypometabolism like in AD. Statistically hypometabolism is more dominant in the left hemisphere. Some studies report that a voxel-based analysis is helpful in distinguishing FTD from AD.
- In contrast to AD amyloid imaging is usually negative in these patients helping differentiate FTD from AD.
- Few reports state a statistically lower uptake of presynaptic dopaminergic tracers in the striatum.
- Semantic dementia has rarely been described as a FDG-PET finding. In early stages, there is a strictly temporal lobe hypometabolism reported which spreads in later stages to other cortical regions.

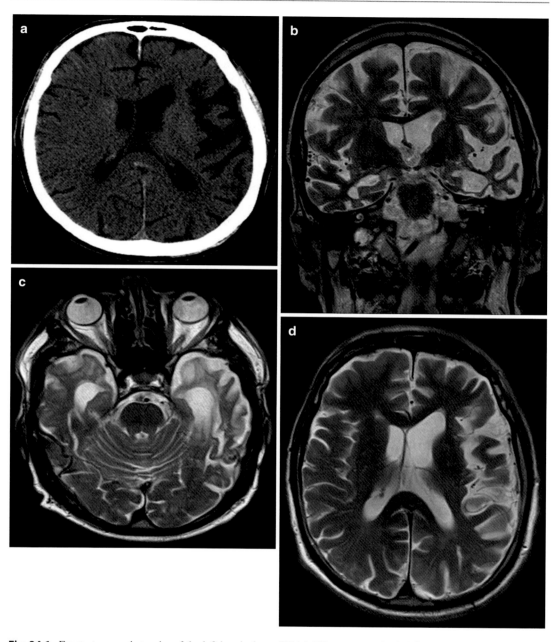

Fig. 34.1 Fronto-temporal atrophy of the left hemisphere; CT (**a**), T2 coronar and axial (**b–e**), FLAIR (**f, g**)

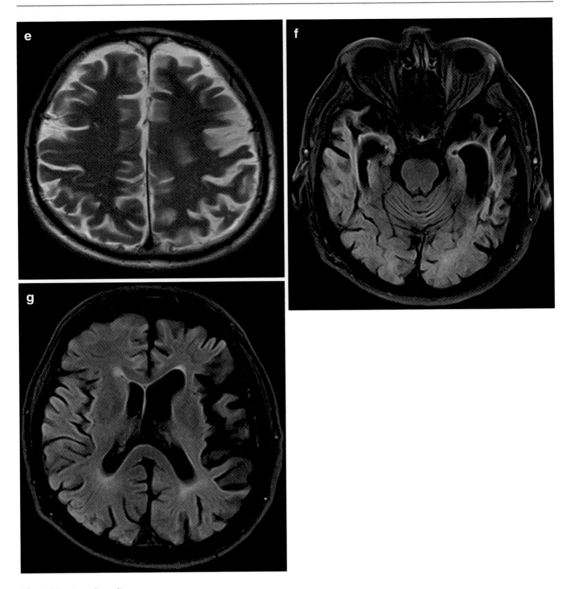

Fig. 34.1 (continued)

- Primary progressive aphasia with the three subtypes of semantic dementia, logopenic aphasia, and progressive non-fluent aphasia have rarely been described as a FDG-PET finding.
  - In early stages, there is a strictly temporal lobe hypometabolism reported in SD which spreads in later stages to other cortical regions, asymmetric left frontal hypometabolism in PNFA and left parietal and posterior temporal lobes in LPA.
  - Patients with LPA are reported to be amyloid positive while in patients with PNFA and SD these finding seems to be rare.
  - Uptake of amyloid tracer is described to be diffuse and similar to the findings in Alzheimer dementia, although some studies describe a statistically more pronounced uptake in the left (dominant) hemisphere.

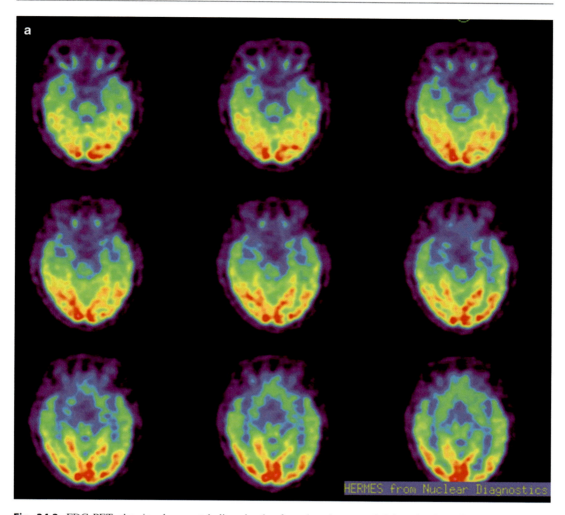

Fig. 34.2 FDG-PET showing hypometabolism in the frontal and temporal lobes (**a–e**); patient with semantic dementia (**f**)

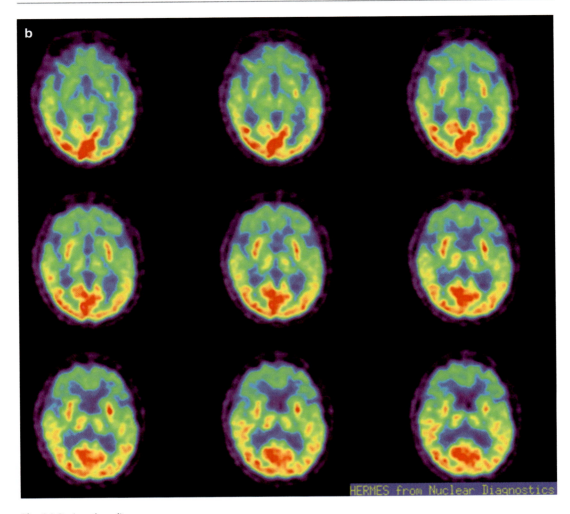

Fig. 34.2 (continued)

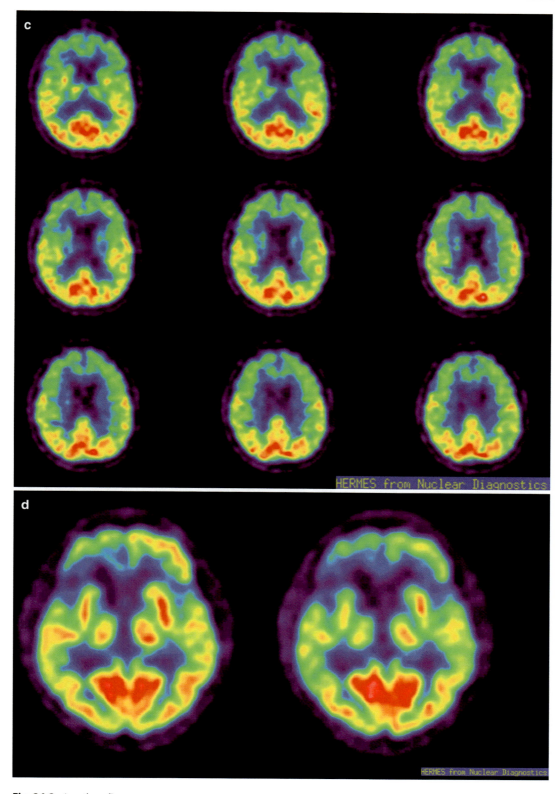

Fig. 34.2 (continued)

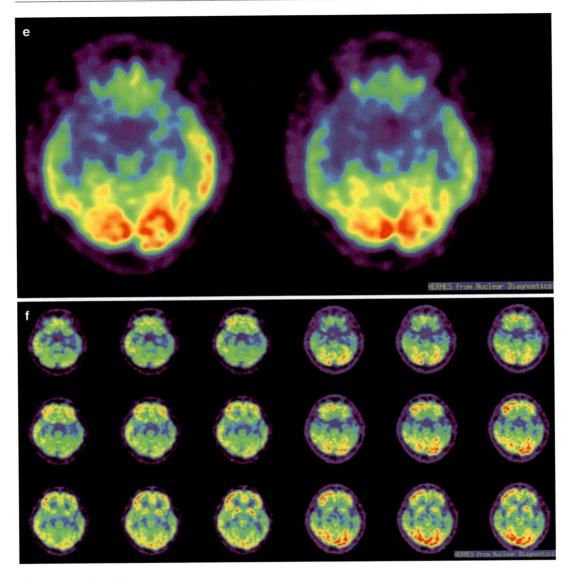

Fig. 34.2 (continued)

34.4 Neuropathology Subgroups

The following neuropathologic subgroups are distinguished:

- Fronto-temporal lobar degeneration with TDP-43 proteinopathy
- Fronto-temporal lobar degeneration with motor neuron disease type inclusions
- Fronto-temporal lobar degeneration with *GRN* mutation
- Fronto-temporal lobar degeneration with *VCP* mutation
- Fronto-temporal lobar degeneration with *C9ORF* mutation
- Fronto-temporal lobar degeneration with tauopathy
- Pick disease
- Cortico-basal degeneration
- Progressive supranuclear palsy
- Argyrophilic grain disease
- Sporadic multiple system tauopathy with dementia
- White matter tauopathy with globular glial inclusions
- Tangle-only dementia

- Fronto-temporal lobar degeneration with *MAPT* mutation
- Fronto-temporal lobar degeneration with FUS proteinopathy
- Neuronal Intermediate Filament Inclusion Disease (NIFID)
- Basophilic Inclusion Body Disease (BIBD)
- Fronto-temporal lobar degeneration with ubiquitin-positive inclusions
- Atypical fronto-temporal lobar degeneration with ubiquitin-positive inclusions
- Fronto-temporal lobar degeneration with no inclusions

Macroscopic features (Fig. 34.3a–h)
- Atrophy of the frontal lobes
- Atrophy of the temporal lobes

The following kinds of inclusions are found:

- Neuronal cytoplasmic inclusions (NCI)
- Neuronal intranuclear inclusions (NII)
- Dystrophic neurites (DN)
- Glial inclusions

A classification of FTLD based on involved proteins is given in Table 34.2 while the updated nomenclature for neuropathologic subtypes of fronto-temporal lobar degeneration is listed in Table 34.3.

A correlation of clinical signs and neuropathological changes is not always straightforward. A list is provided in Table 34.4.

34.5 Types of FTLD

34.5.1 Fronto-temporal Lobar Degeneration with TDP-43 Proteinopathy

TDP-43
- Pathological protein found in ubiquitin-positive inclusions in FTLD-U, FTLD-MND, ALS

- 414 amino acids long
- Predominantly located in the nucleus
- Translocates to the cytoplasm in pathological states
- RNA and DNA splicing, neuronal plasticity
- Insoluble aggregate which is ubiquitinated and hyperphosphorylated
- *TARDBP*: transactive response (TAR) DNA-binding protein of 43 kDA gene encoding for TDP-43
- Mutations sufficient to cause neurodegeneration

Macroscopic Features
- Atrophy variable
- Frontal lobe
- Anterior temporal lobe
- Neocortical thinning
- Atrophy of amygdala and hippocampus

Microscopic Features
- Neuronal loss in layers II and III
- Microvacuolation
- Gliosis
- Swollen achromatic neurons
- TDP-43 positive inclusions
  - Neuronal cytoplasmic inclusions (NCI)
  - Neuronal intranuclear inclusions (NII)
  - Dystrophic neurites (DN)
- Absence of argyrophilic inclusions

FTD-TPD-45 subtypes (Mackenzie 2007):
- Type 1
  - Long DNs in superficial laminae
- Type 2
  - NCI in superficial and deep cortical laminae
- Type 3
  - NCI, DN, and NII
- Type 4
  - Prominence of NII, fewer DN

A new classification system for FTLD-TDP pathology and the comparison with the 2007 system is given in Table 34.5.

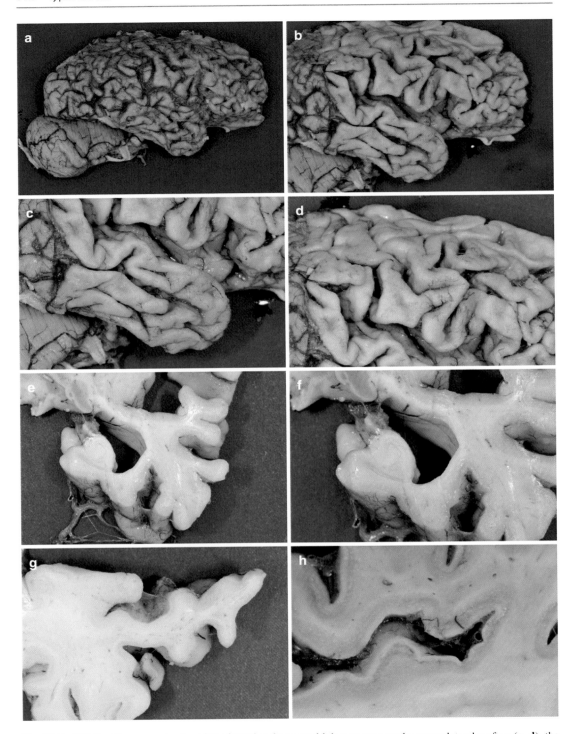

Fig. 34.3 FTLD with severe atrophy of the frontal and temporal lobes as seen on the superolateral surface (**a–d**); the atrophy is also evident on sections of the temporal lobe including the hippocampus (**e, f**) and frontal section (**g, h**)

Table 34.2 Classification of FTLD based on involved proteins

Fronto-temporal lobar degeneration	
Immunoreactivities of inclusions	Disease entities
FTLD-tau—3R tau	• Pick disease • FTLD with MAPT (microtubule-associated protein tau) mutation
FTLD-tau—4R tau	• CBD: cortico-basal degeneration • PSP: progressive supranuclear palsy • AGD: argyrophilic grain disease • GGT: globular glial tauopathy • MSTD: multiple system tauopathy with dementia • WMT-GGI: white matter tauopathy with globular glial inclusions • FTLD with MAPT (microtubule-associated protein tau) mutation
FTLD-tau—3R and 4R tau	• TOD: tangle-only dementia • FTLD with MAPT (microtubule-associated protein tau) mutation • NFT-predominant
FTLD-TDP43	• Type A • Type B • Type C • Type D • FTLD-TDP/FTLD-U sporadic • FTLD with GRN (progranulin) mutation • FTLD with TARDP (transactive response DANN-binding protein of 43 kDa) mutation • FTLD with VCP (valosin-containing protein) mutation • FTLD with c9ORF72 (chromosome 9 open reading frame 72) mutation
FTLD-FUS	• aFTLD-U: atypical FTLD with ubiquitin inclusions • NIFID: neuronal intermediate filament inclusion disease • BIBD: basophilic inclusion body disease • FTLD with FUS (fused in sarcoma) mutation
FTLD-UPS	• FTLD with CHMp2B (charged multivesicular body protein 2B) mutation
FTLD-ni (no inclusions)	

Immunophenotype
- Positivities:
  - Ubiquitin
  - TDP-43
- Negativities:
  - Tau
  - A-synuclein
  - Prion
  - Polyglutamine + FUS

34.5.2 Fronto-temporal Lobar Degeneration with Motor Neuron Disease Type Inclusions

- Clinical and pathological features of classical MND may or may not be present.
- Clinical Signs:
  - cognitive impairment

34.5 Types of FTLD

Table 34.3 Updated nomenclature for neuropathologic subtypes of fronto-temporal lobar degeneration, 2010 recommendation (Mackenzie et al. 2010) reproduced with kind permission by Springer Nature

Major molecular class	Recognized subtypes	Associated genes
FTLD-tau	• Pick disease (PiD) • Cortico-basal degeneration (CBD) • Progressive supranuclear palsy (PSP) • Argyrophilic grain disease (AGD) • Multiple system tauopathy with dementia (MSTD) • Neurofibrillary tangle predominant dementia (NFT dementia) • White matter tauopathy with globular glial inclusions (WMT-GGI) • Unclassifiable	• Microtubule-associated protein tau (MAPT)
FTLD-TDP-43	• Types 1–4 • Unclassifiable	• Progranulin gene (GRN) • Valosin-containing protein (VCP) • Genetic locus on chromosome 9p linked to familial amyotrophic lateral sclerosis and fronto-temporal dementia (9p) • Transactive response DNA binding protein (TARDBP)
FTLD-UPS	• Fronto-temporal dementia linked to chromosome 3 (FTD-3)	
aFTLD-U	• Atypical fronto-temporal lobar degeneration with ubiquitinated inclusions (aFTLD-U) • Neuronal intermediate filament inclusion disease (NIFID) • Basophilic inclusion body disease (BIBD)	
FTLD-ni (no inclusions)		

Table 34.4 Correlation of clinical signs and neuropathological changes

FTLD-Type	NP	bvFTD	nfvPPA	svPPA	CBS	FTD-MND
tau	Pick	+	+	+		
	CBD	+	+		+	
	PSP		+		+	
	GD	+				
	NFT dementia	+				
	MAPT mu	+	+			
TDP-43	Type A	+	+	+	+	+
	Type B	+	+			+
	Type C		+	+		
	Type D					
FUS	aFTLD-U	+				
	NIFID	+				
	BIBD					
FTLD-UPS	FTD-3	+				

Table 34.5 New classification system for FTLD-TDP pathology, compared with existing systems (Mackenzie et al. 2011) reproduced with kind permission by Springer Nature

New system	Mackenzie et al.	Sampathu et al.	Cortical pathology	Common phenotype	Associated genetic defects
Type A	Type 1	Type 3	• Many neuronal cytoplasmic inclusions • Many short dystrophic neurites • Predominantly layer 2	• Behavioral variant fronto-temporal dementia (bvFTD) • Progressive non-fluent aphasia (PNFA)	Progranulin gene GRN mutations
Type B	Type 3	Type 2	• Moderate neuronal cytoplasmic inclusions • Few dystrophic neurites All layers	• Behavioral variant fronto-temporal dementia (bvFTD) • Motor neuron disease (MND) with FTD	Linkage to chromosome 9p
Type C	Type 2	Type 1	• Many long dystrophic neurites DN • Few neuronal cytoplasmic inclusions • Predominantly layer 2	• Semantic dementia (SD) • Behavioral variant fronto-temporal dementia (bvFTD)	
Type D	Type 4	Type 4	• Many short dystrophic neurites • Many lentiform neuronal intranuclear inclusions • Few neuronal cytoplasmic inclusions • All layers	• Familial inclusion body myopathy with Paget disease of bone and fronto-temporal dementia (IBMPFD)	Valosin-containing protein gene VCP mutations

- Starts sixth decade.
- Duration: 2–3 years.

Macroscopic Features
- Moderate atrophy of frontal, anterior temporal, and parietal lobes
- Enlargement of the ventricular system
- Loss of pigment from the substantia nigra

Microscopic Features
- Neuronal loss
- Microvacuolation
- Astrogliosis
- Neuronal loss in the substantia nigra
- Neuronal loss in the anterior horns of the spinal cord, motor nuclei of the brainstem
- Neuronal skein-like inclusions:
  - TDP-43 positive
  - Ubiquitin-positive
  - Non-argyrophilic

Immunophenotype
- Positivities:
  - TDP-43
  - Ubiquitin
- Negativities:
  - Tau

34.5.3 Fronto-temporal Lobar Degeneration with *GRN* Mutation

Progranulin
- ubiquitously expressed secreted precursor protein
- contains tandem repeats of a 10–12 cysteine motif
- proteolytically cleaved to form seven granulin peptides
- functions of progranulin and granulin:
  - cell cycle regulation

- wound repair
- tumor growth
- inflammation
- encoded by *GRN* gene
- loss-of-function mutations

Macroscopic Features
- Moderate atrophy of frontal and anterior temporal lobes

Microscopic Features
- Neuronal loss in layers II and III
- Microvacuolation
- Gliosis
- Swollen achromatic neurons
- TDP-43 positive inclusions
  - Neuronal cytoplasmic inclusions (NCI)
  - Neuronal intranuclear inclusions (NII)
  - Dystrophic neurites (DN)
- Absence of progranulin from ubiquitinated inclusions

Immunophenotype
- Positivities:
  - TDP-43
  - Ubiquitin
- Negativities:
  - Progranulin
  - Tau

34.5.4 Fronto-temporal Lobar Degeneration with *VCP* Mutation

- Lethal, autosomal dominant disease
- Chromosome 9p13.3-p12
- Clinical Signs:
  - adult-onset and distal muscle weakness (hereditary inclusion body myositis)
  - early-onset Paget disease of bone (PDB)
  - fronto-temporal dementia
- Age at onset: 42 years

Valosin-containing protein (VCP)

- 644 amino acid long protein
- Member of the ATPases associated with diverse cellular activities superfamily
- Functions:
  - Vesicle transport and fusion
  - 26S proteasome function
  - Assembly of peroxisomes
  - Assembly of clathrin and heat shock protein HSP70
  - Mitosis (homotypic membrane fusion, spindle pole body function, ubiquitin-dependent protein degradation)

Macroscopic Features
- Atrophy of frontal lobes

Microscopic Features
- Neuronal loss
- Status spongiosus
- Reactive astrogliosis
- Neuronal intranuclear inclusions (NII) positive for ubiquitin and TDP-43

Immunophenotype
- Positivities:
  - TDP-43
  - Ubiquitin

34.5.5 Fronto-temporal Lobar Degeneration with *C9ORF* Mutation

- Gene causing MND, FTLD-MND, FTLD on chromosome 9
- Gene defect: GGGCC hexanucleotide repeat expansion in the first intron of C9ORF72 gene

Macroscopic Features
- Atrophy of frontal lobes

Microscopic Features
- TDP-43 positive NCIs with few DNs
- In the frontal and temporal cortex, hippocampus, and spinal cord

34.5.6 Fronto-temporal Lobar Degeneration with Ubiquitin-Positive Inclusions (FTLD/UPS)

- Limited to a single Danish pedigree
- Mutations in the charged multivesicular body protein 2B (CHMB2B)

Macroscopic Features
- Atrophy of frontal and temporal lobes

Microscopic Features (Fig. 34.4a–j)
- Inclusions negative for TDP-43, tau, or FUS
- Immunopositive for ubiquitin and p62

34.5.7 Fronto-temporal Lobar Degeneration with Tauopathy

Tau-proteins
- Low molecular weight microtubule-associated proteins.
- Expressed in axons.
- Expressed in low levels in astrocytes and oligodendrocytes.
- Encoded by a single-gene chromosome 17q21 with 16 exons.
- CNS isoforms generated by alternative mRNA splicing.
- Alternative splicing of exons 2, 3, and 10 generates 6 tau isoforms (352-441 AA long).
- Presence of either 3 (3R tau) or 4 (4R tau) MT binding repeats encoded by exons 9–12.

Macroscopic Features
- Atrophy of frontal and temporal lobes

Microscopic Features
- Intracellular glial and neuronal inclusions positive for tau

34.5.8 Pick Disease

First described by Arnold Pick in 1892
  Alois Alzheimer described the characteristic histological lesion: Intraneuronal, argyrophilic, globular inclusion

Clinical signs and symptoms
- Sometimes indistinguishable from Alzheimer disease.
- Behavioral features similar to bvFTD.
- Dementia might be present in later stages of the disease.
- Age of onset: 45–65 years, i.e., early-onset dementia
- Duration of disease: 5–10 years
- Male:female ratio: F > M

Macroscopic Features
- Significant atrophy of the basal parts of the frontal and temporal lobes.
- Sparing of the posterior parts of the superior temporal gyrus, parietal and occipital lobes.
- Enlargement of the lateral ventricles.
- Atrophy of the amygdala and hippocampus as well as the basal ganglia.
- The leptomeninges covering the atrophic areas are thickened and fibrosed but not adherent to the brain.
- Brain weight can decrease below 1000 g.

Microscopic Features
- Pick body
  - Spherical, argyrophilic
  - Tau-immunoreactive
  - Neuronal intracytoplasmic inclusion
  - Found in:
    - Granule cells of the dentate gyrus
    - Pyramidal neurons of the frontal and temporal lobes
  - EM:
    - Bundles of disorganized straight fibrils
    - No limiting membrane
- Swollen achromatic, "ballooned" neurons
  - Eccentric nucleus
  - In deep layers of the cortex
  - Immunopositive for ubiquitin and tau
  - EM:
    - Bundles of disorganized straight fibrils
    - Granular material
    - Degenerate organelles
- Neuronal loss
  - Predominantly in layer III
- Status spongiosus
- Astrogliosis

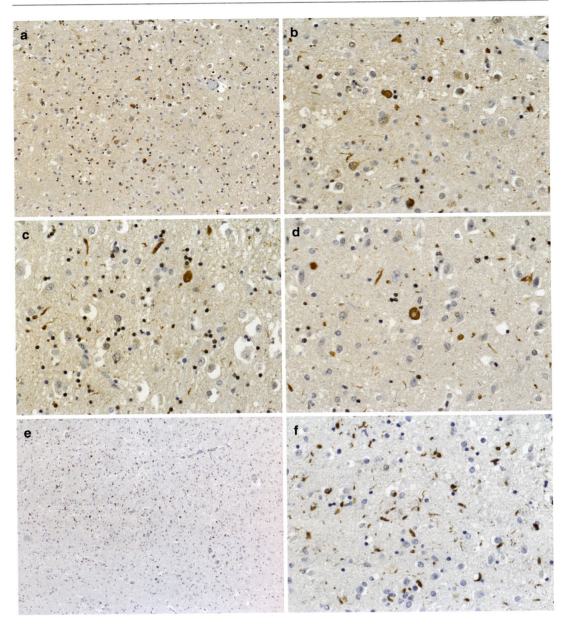

Fig. 34.4 FTLD immunophenotype: inclusions are positive for ubiquitin in FTLD-UPS (**a–d**), and p62 in FTLD-UPS (**e–h**)

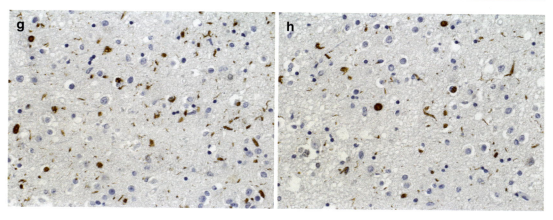

Fig. 34.4 (continued)

Immunophenotype
- Positivities:
  - Tau
  - 3R tau
  - Ubiquitin
  - αB-crystallin

34.5.9 Cortico-basal Degeneration

See Chap. 35.

34.5.10 Progressive Supranuclear Palsy

See chapter 35.

34.5.11 Argyrophilic Grain Disease

First described by Braak and Braak (1987)
   Association with other neurodegenerative disorders (AD, Pick, PSP)

Clinical signs:
- Cognitive decline and dementia
- Episodic memory
- Behavioral abnormalities
- Personality changes
- Emotional and mood disorders

Macroscopic Features
- No visible changes
- Atrophy of frontal and temporal lobes

Microscopic Features (Fig. 34.5a, b)
- Argyrophilic grains
  - found in
    - entorhinal cortex
    - hippocampus
    - amygdala
    - temporal lobe
  - stained on Gallyas silver impregnation
  - small, spindle shaped, rod-like round bodies in the neuropil, 4–8 µm in diameter
  - tau immunopositive
  - 4R tau
  - EM:
    - Straight filaments and tubules 9–25 nm wide
- Coiled bodies
  - 4R tau positive
- Two staging systems, i.e., Saito et al. and Ferrer et al. (Table 34.6)

Immunophenotype (Fig. 34.5c–h)
- Positivities:
  - Tau
  - 4R tau

34.5.12 Sporadic Multiple System Tauopathy with Dementia

Macroscopic Features
- Mild atrophy of the frontal and parietal lobes
- Severe atrophy of the temporal lobe

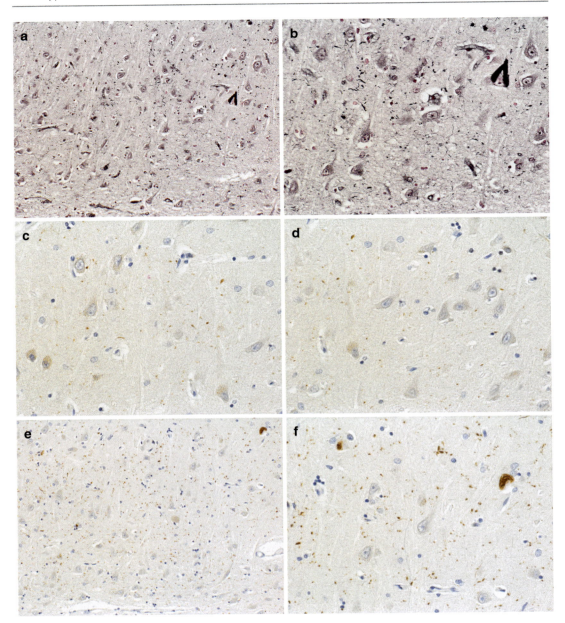

Fig. 34.5 Argyrophilic grain disease: Grains, visualized in Gallyas stain (**a**, **b**), are immunopositive for tauR4 (**c**, **d**), p62 (**e**, **f**), and ubiquitin (**g**, **h**)

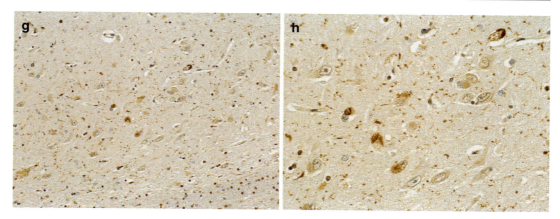

Fig. 35.5 (continued)

Microscopic Features

- Sparse filamentous tau-positive inclusions
- Globular neuronal and glial tau-positive inclusions
- In gray and white matter
- Subcortical regions: substantia nigra, globus pallidus, subthalamic nucleus, dentate nucleus
- 4R tau positivities
- EM:
  - Straight filaments
  - Fingerprint-like bodies

Immunophenotype

- Positivities:
  - Tau
  - 4R tau

34.5.13 White Matter Tauopathy with Globular Glial Inclusions

Clinical Signs

- Behavioral variant of FTD
- Some cases with pyramidal signs

Macroscopic Features

- Slight atrophy of the frontal and temporal lobes

Microscopic Features

- Globular glial inclusions in the white matter
  - With abnormal filaments
  - Mostly in oligodendrocytes
- 4R tau positive
- Neuronal loss
  - Frontal and temporal cortex, subiculum, amygdala

Immunophenotype

- Positivities:
  - Tau
  - 4R tau

34.5.14 Tangle-Only Dementia

Clinical Signs

- Late-onset dementia (mean age: 83 years)
- Memory loss is presenting symptom

Macroscopic Features

- Mild to moderate diffuse atrophy
- With or without atrophy of the hippocampus

Microscopic Features

- Numerous neurofibrillary tangles in the medial temporal lobe
- Few or no tangles in the neocortex
- Absence of Aβ and neuritic plaques

Immunophenotype

- Positivities:
  - Tau
  - 4R tau
  - 3R tau

34.5 Types of FTLD

Table 34.6 Comparison of the two neuropathological staging systems for argyrophilic grain disease, as proposed by Saito et al. (2004) and Ferrer et al. (2008)

Stage	Saito et al. (2004)	Ferrer et al. (2008)
I	• Ambient gyrus and its vicinity	• Anterior entorhinal cortex • Mild involvement of the cortical and basolateral nuclei of the amygdale and of the hypothalamic lateral tuberal nucleus
II	• I + • Anterior and posterior medial temporal lobe, • Including the temporal pole • Subiculum Entorhinal cortex	• More severe involvement of the nuclei involved in stage I + • Entorhinal and transentorhinal cortices • Anterior CA1
III	• II + • Septum • Insular cortex • Anterior cingulate gyrus • Spongy degeneration of the ambient gyrus	• II + • Mild involvement of CA2, CA3, presubiculum • Other nuclei of the amygdala • Dentate gyrus • Other nuclei of the hypothalamus • Temporal, orbitofrontal, and insular cortices • Cingulate gyrus • ncl. accumbens • Septal nuclei • Midbrain
IV		• Moderate to severe additional involvement of the neocortex • Brain stem

34.5.15 Fronto-temporal Lobar Degeneration with *MAPT* Mutation

Macroscopic Features
- Atrophy of frontal and temporal lobes

Microscopic Features
- Neuronal loss
- Astrogliosis
- Microvacuolation
- Swollen neurons
- Inclusions:
  - Intraneuronal NFT-like
  - Neuronal globose tangle-like
  - Pick body-like
  - Astrocytic tangle-like
  - Oligodendroglial coiled bodies-like
  - Presence of NFTs and amyloid plaques to fulfill the criteria of AD

Immunophenotype
- Positivities:
  - Tau
  - 4R tau
  - 3R tau

34.5.16 Fronto-temporal Lobar Degeneration with FUS Proteinopathy

FUS: fused in sarcoma
Associated with heterogeneous ribonucleoprotein

Functions
- DNA repair
- Transcription
- RNA splicing
- RNA translation at the synapse
- microRNA processing

Mutations cause one form of familial ALS.

Macroscopic Features
- Atrophy of the frontal and temporal lobes

Microscopic Features
- Neuronal cytoplasmic inclusions (NCI) positive for FUS
- Negative for TDP-43

FTLD/FUS entities include:

- Neuronal Intermediate Filament Inclusion Disease (NIFID)
- Basophilic Inclusion Body Disease (BIBD)
- Fronto-temporal lobar degeneration with ubiquitin-positive inclusions

34.5.17 Neuronal Intermediate Filament Inclusion Disease (NIFID)

- Rare disease
- Clinical Signs:
  - atypical dementia
  - pyramidal and extrapyramidal signs
  - personality change
  - apathy
  - blunted affect
  - disinhibition
- Age of onset: mean 40 years (range 23–56 years)
- Mean disease duration: 4.5 years
- Male:Female ratio: 2:3

Macroscopic Features
- Severe atrophy of the frontal and temporal lobes
- Mild atrophy of the parietal lobe
- Atrophy of the caudate nucleus
- Thinning of the cortical ribbon
- Brain weight <1000 g

Microscopic Features
- Neuronal loss
- Axonal swelling
- Status spongiosus
- Astrogliosis
- Swollen achromatic neurons
- Hyaline aggregates
- Inclusions variably argyrophilic
- Neuronal inclusions positive for FUS:
  - Neuronal cytoplasmic inclusions (NCI)
  - Neuronal intranuclear inclusions (NII)
  - Glial inclusions
- EM
  - Aggregates of granular filamentous material (10–25 nm diameter)
  - No limiting membrane

Immunophenotype
- Positivities:
  - Neuronal cytoplasmic inclusions (NCI)
    ○ FUS
    ○ Neurofilaments (NF-L, NF-M, NF-l, α-internexin)
    ○ Ubiquitin
  - Neuronal intranuclear inclusions (NII)
    ○ FUS
- Negativities
  - Neuronal intranuclear inclusions (NII) and Glial inclusions
    ○ Neuronal intermediate filaments

34.5.18 Basophilic Inclusion Body Disease (BIBD)

- Rare disease
- Juvenile (29–30 years) or adult (52–58 years) onset MND, FTD; or combined MND/FTD

Macroscopic Features
- Atrophy of the frontal and temporal lobes
- Atrophy of the basal ganglia
- Thinning of caudate nucleus, thalamus, amygdala
- Depigmentation of substantia nigra

Microscopic Features
- Severe neuronal loss
- Superficial microvacuolation
- Reactive astrogliosis
- Swollen achromatic neurons
- Basophilic inclusion body
  - Variably basophilic
  - In the superficial cortical layers, putamen, caudate nucleus, globus pallidus, nucleus basalis Meynert
  - Absent in the hippocampus and dentate gyrus
  - Immunopositive for FUS

34.5 Types of FTLD

- Immunonegative for tau, α-synuclein, neurofilaments
- EM:
  - Made up of fibrils 13–25 nm
  - Granular appearance
  - No limiting membrane

Immunophenotype
- Positivities:
  - FUS
- Negativities
  - Tau
  - α-synuclein
  - Neurofilaments

34.5.19 Atypical Fronto-temporal Lobar Degeneration with Ubiquitin-Positive Inclusions (FTLD-U)

- Early-onset bvFTD
- Psychotic symptoms including eating disorder
- Memory problems appear late in the course of the disease

Macroscopic Features
- Symmetric atrophy of the frontal and temporal lobes and caudate nucleus

Microscopic Features
- Neuronal loss and gliosis in
  - Frontal and temporal neocortex, hippocampus, striatum, globus pallidus, substantia nigra
- Positive for ubiquitin
- Negative for tau and TDP-43

Immunophenotype
- Ubiquitin-positive inclusions
- FUS positive inclusions
  - Neuronal cytoplasmic inclusions, round crescentic
  - Neuronal intranuclear inclusions, vermiform or rod-like
  - Diffuse neurites
- Negative for p62, ß-A4, p-Tau, α-synuclein, neurofilaments, TDP-43, expanded polyglutamine repeats

34.5.20 Fronto-temporal Lobar Degeneration with No Inclusions

Clinical Signs and Symptoms
- First described by Knopman et al. (1990)
- Clinical signs: memory loss, changes in personality, death within 2–7 years
- Dysarthria and dysphagia most prominent signs in the late stages of the disease
- Age at onset: 46–86 years
- In 50% clinical manifestation before 65 years of age
- In a series of 460 patients with dementia, 14 patients (3%) showed only neuronal loss and astrogliosis, no inclusions, no amyloid plaques, no neurofibrillary tangles

Synonyms
- Frontal lobe degeneration of non-Alzheimer type (Brun 1987)
- Dementia of frontal type
- Dementia lacking distinct histopathology
- PiD group C (classification of Constantinidis et al. (1974))

Macroscopic Features
- Atrophy of the frontal and temporal lobes
- Preserved occipital lobe

Microscopic Features
- Neuronal loss.
- Microvacuolation of cortical layer II.
- Diffuse astrocytosis.
- Histological groups as defined by Giannakopoulos et al. (1995):
  - Group A
    - Moderate to severe neuronal loss
    - Gliosis
    - Frontal and/or temporopolar cortex
    - No subcortical involvement
  - Group B
    - Widespread neocortical neuronal loss
    - Striatum and substantia nigra
      - With gliosis of different degrees
      - No neuronal loss
  - Group C
    - Widespread neocortical neuronal loss
    - Severe neuronal loss in at least one subcortical region

Table 34.7 RNA dysfunction and aggrephagy at the center of an amyotrophic lateral sclerosis/fronto-temporal dementia disease continuum (Thomas et al. 2013) reproduced with kind permission by Oxford University Press

Disease subgroup	Genes	Mode of inheritance	Protein species found in inclusions
FTD-FUS	• Unknown	Sporadic	• FUS • P62 • Ubiquitin
FTD-TDP43	• *GRN* • *VCP* • *TDP-43* • *C9ORF72*	Sporadic	• TDP-43 • P62 • Ubiquitin • Ubiquilin • Ubiquilin 2 • Optineurin
FTD-MAPT	• *MAPT*	Sporadic	• Tau • P62 • Ubiquitin

- Group D
  ○ Preserved pyramidal neurons in the neocortex
  ○ Variable subcortical changes
- Despite the topographical differences of the changes, no differences in clinical profile were displayed.

34.6 Molecular Neuropathology

RNA dysfunction and aggrephagy as involved in amyotrophic lateral sclerosis/fronto-temporal dementia disease continuum is shown in Table 34.7.

34.7 Treatment and Prognosis

Treatment
- No specific treatment
- Symptomatic treatment
  - Cholinesterase inhibitors
  - Memantine
  - Selective serotonin reuptake inhibitors
  - L-dopa

Biologic Behavior-Prognosis-Prognostic Factors
- Progressive disease
- Variable end stages
  - Akinetic mutism
- Poor long-term prognosis

Selected References

Al-Mansoori KM, Hasan MY, Al-Hayani A, El-Agnaf OM (2013) The role of alpha-synuclein in neurodegenerative diseases: from molecular pathways in disease to therapeutic approaches. Curr Alzheimer Res 10(6):559–568

Alberici A, Cosseddu M, Padovani A, Borroni B (2011) Chromosome 17 in FTLD: from MAPT tau to progranulin and back. Curr Alzheimer Res 8(3):229–236

Armstrong RA, Gearing M, Bigio EH, Cruz-Sanchez FF, Duyckaerts C, Mackenzie IR, Perry RH, Skullerud K, Yokoo H, Cairns NJ (2011) Spatial patterns of FUS-immunoreactive neuronal cytoplasmic inclusions (NCI) in neuronal intermediate filament inclusion disease (NIFID). J Neural Transm (Vienna, Austria: 1996) 118(11):1651–1657. https://doi.org/10.1007/s00702-011-0690-x

Borroni B, Padovani A (2013) Dementia: a new algorithm for molecular diagnostics in FTLD. Nat Rev Neurol 9(5):241–242. https://doi.org/10.1038/nrneurol.2013.72

Bozzali M, Battistoni V, Premi E, Alberici A, Giulietti G, Archetti S, Turla M, Gasparotti R, Cercignani M, Padovani A, Borroni B (2013) Structural brain signature of FTLD driven by Granulin mutation. J Alzheimers Dis 33(2):483–494. https://doi.org/10.3233/jad-2012-121273

Braak H, Braak E (1987) Argyrophilic grains: characteristic pathology of cerebral cortex in cases of adult onset dementia without Alzheimer changes. Neurosci Lett 76(1):124–127

Brun A (1987) Frontal lobe degeneration of non-Alzheimer type. I. Neuropathology. Arch Gerontol Geriatr 6(3):193–208

Buratti E (2011) TDP-43 and FUS in ALS/FTLD: will common pathways fit all? Neurology 77(17):1588–1589. https://doi.org/10.1212/WNL.0b013e31823433ba

Selected References

Cairns NJ (2008) Neuronal intermediate filament inclusion disease. Handb Clin Neurol 89:443–448. https://doi.org/10.1016/s0072-9752(07)01240-7

Cairns NJ, Grossman M, Arnold SE, Burn DJ, Jaros E, Perry RH, Duyckaerts C, Stankoff B, Pillon B, Skullerud K, Cruz-Sanchez FF, Bigio EH, Mackenzie IR, Gearing M, Juncos JL, Glass JD, Yokoo H, Nakazato Y, Mosaheb S, Thorpe JR, Uryu K, Lee VM, Trojanowski JQ (2004a) Clinical and neuropathologic variation in neuronal intermediate filament inclusion disease. Neurology 63(8):1376–1384

Cairns NJ, Zhukareva V, Uryu K, Zhang B, Bigio E, Mackenzie IR, Gearing M, Duyckaerts C, Yokoo H, Nakazato Y, Jaros E, Perry RH, Lee VM, Trojanowski JQ (2004b) alpha-internexin is present in the pathological inclusions of neuronal intermediate filament inclusion disease. Am J Pathol 164(6):2153–2161

Constantinidis J, Richard J, Tissot R (1974) Pick's disease. Histological and clinical correlations. Eur Neurol 11(4):208–217. https://doi.org/10.1159/000114320

Coulthard E, Firbank M, English P, Welch J, Birchall D, O'Brien J, Griffiths TD (2006) Proton magnetic resonance spectroscopy in frontotemporal dementia. J Neurol 253(7):861–868. https://doi.org/10.1007/s00415-006-0045-y

Dickson DW, Kouri N, Murray ME, Josephs KA (2011) Neuropathology of frontotemporal lobar degeneration-tau (FTLD-tau). J Mol Neurosci 45(3):384–389. https://doi.org/10.1007/s12031-011-9589-0

Fan AC, Leung AK (2016) RNA granules and diseases: a case study of stress granules in ALS and FTLD. Adv Exp Med Biol 907:263–296. https://doi.org/10.1007/978-3-319-29073-7_11

Feneberg E, Gray E, Ansorge O, Talbot K, Turner MR (2018) Towards a TDP-43-based biomarker for ALS and FTLD. Mol Neurobiol 55(10):7789–7801. https://doi.org/10.1007/s12035-018-0947-6

Ferrer I, Santpere G, van Leeuwen FW (2008) Argyrophilic grain disease. Brain 131(Pt 6):1416–1432. https://doi.org/10.1093/brain/awm305

Galimberti D, Scarpini E (2012) Clinical phenotypes and genetic biomarkers of FTLD. J Neural Transm (Vienna, Austria: 1996) 119(7):851–860. https://doi.org/10.1007/s00702-012-0804-0

Gass J, Prudencio M, Stetler C, Petrucelli L (2012) Progranulin: an emerging target for FTLD therapies. Brain Res 1462:118–128. https://doi.org/10.1016/j.brainres.2012.01.047

Gefen T, Ahmadian SS, Mao Q, Kim G, Seckin M, Bonakdarpour B, Ramos EM, Coppola G, Rademakers R, Rogalski E, Rademaker A, Weintraub S, Mesulam MM, Geula C, Bigio EH (2018) Combined pathologies in FTLD-TDP types A and C. J Neuropathol Exp Neurol 77(5):405–412. https://doi.org/10.1093/jnen/nly018

Gelpi E, Llado A, Clarimon J, Rey MJ, Rivera RM, Ezquerra M, Antonell A, Navarro-Otano J, Ribalta T, Pinol-Ripoll G, Perez A, Valldeoriola F, Ferrer I (2012) Phenotypic variability within the inclusion body spectrum of basophilic inclusion body disease and neuronal intermediate filament inclusion disease in frontotemporal lobar degenerations with FUS-positive inclusions. J Neuropathol Exp Neurol 71(9):795–805. https://doi.org/10.1097/NEN.0b013e318266efb1

Giannakopoulos P, Hof PR, Bouras C (1995) Dementia lacking distinctive histopathology: clinicopathological evaluation of 32 cases. Acta Neuropathol 89(4):346–355

Grinberg LT, Heinsen H (2009) Argyrophilic grain disease: an update about a frequent cause of dementia. Dement Neuropsychol 3(1):2–7. https://doi.org/10.1590/s1980-57642009dn30100002

Grinberg LT, Wang X, Wang C, Sohn PD, Theofilas P, Sidhu M, Arevalo JB, Heinsen H, Huang EJ, Rosen H, Miller BL, Gan L, Seeley WW (2013) Argyrophilic grain disease differs from other tauopathies by lacking tau acetylation. Acta Neuropathol 125(4):581–593. https://doi.org/10.1007/s00401-013-1080-2

Haller S, Garibotto V, Kovari E, Bouras C, Xekardaki A, Rodriguez C, Lazarczyk MJ, Giannakopoulos P, Lovblad KO (2013) Neuroimaging of dementia in 2013: what radiologists need to know. Eur Radiol 23(12):3393–3404. https://doi.org/10.1007/s00330-013-2957-0

Heyburn L, Moussa CE (2017) TDP-43 in the spectrum of MND-FTLD pathologies. Mol Cell Neurosci 83:46–54. https://doi.org/10.1016/j.mcn.2017.07.001

Hsu YY, Du AT, Schuff N, Weiner MW (2001) Magnetic resonance imaging and magnetic resonance spectroscopy in dementias. J Geriatr Psychiatry Neurol 14(3):145–166

Hu WT, Wang Z, Lee VM, Trojanowski JQ, Detre JA, Grossman M (2010) Distinct cerebral perfusion patterns in FTLD and AD. Neurology 75(10):881–888. https://doi.org/10.1212/WNL.0b013e3181f11e35

Ikeda K, Akiyama H, Arai T, Matsushita M, Tsuchiya K, Miyazaki H (2000) Clinical aspects of argyrophilic grain disease. Clin Neuropathol 19(6):278–284

Ito H, Fujita K, Nakamura M, Wate R, Kaneko S, Sasaki S, Yamane K, Suzuki N, Aoki M, Shibata N, Togashi S, Kawata A, Mochizuki Y, Mizutani T, Maruyama H, Hirano A, Takahashi R, Kawakami H, Kusaka H (2011) Optineurin is co-localized with FUS in basophilic inclusions of ALS with FUS mutation and in basophilic inclusion body disease. Acta Neuropathol 121(4):555–557. https://doi.org/10.1007/s00401-011-0809-z

Janssens J, Van Broeckhoven C (2013) Pathological mechanisms underlying TDP-43 driven neurodegeneration in FTLD-ALS spectrum disorders. Hum Mol Genet 22(R1):R77–R87. https://doi.org/10.1093/hmg/ddt349

Jellinger KA (1998) Dementia with grains (argyrophilic grain disease). Brain pathology (Zurich, Switzerland) 8(2):377–386

Kim EJ, Kim BC, Kim SJ, Jung DS, Sin JS, Yoon YJ, Chin J, Lee KH, Na DL (2012) Clinical staging of semantic dementia in an FDG-PET study using FTLD-CDR. Dement Geriatr Cogn Disord 34(5–6):300–306. https://doi.org/10.1159/000345506

Knopman DS, Mastri AR, Frey WH 2nd, Sung JH, Rustan T (1990) Dementia lacking distinctive histologic features: a common non-Alzheimer degenerative dementia. Neurology 40(2):251–256

Kovacs GG, Rozemuller AJ, van Swieten JC, Gelpi E, Majtenyi K, Al-Sarraj S, Troakes C, Bodi I, King A, Hortobagyi T, Esiri MM, Ansorge O, Giaccone G, Ferrer I, Arzberger T, Bogdanovic N, Nilsson T, Leisser I, Alafuzoff I, Ironside JW, Kretzschmar H, Budka H (2013) Neuropathology of the hippocampus in FTLD-Tau with Pick bodies: a study of the BrainNet Europe Consortium. Neuropathol Appl Neurobiol 39(2):166–178. https://doi.org/10.1111/j.1365-2990.2012.01272.x

Liscic RM, Grinberg LT, Zidar J, Gitcho MA, Cairns NJ (2008) ALS and FTLD: two faces of TDP-43 proteinopathy. Eur J Neurol 15(8):772–780. https://doi.org/10.1111/j.1468-1331.2008.02195.x

Mackenzie IR (2007) The neuropathology and clinical phenotype of FTD with progranulin mutations. Acta Neuropathol 114(1):49–54. https://doi.org/10.1007/s00401-007-0223-8

Mackenzie IR, Neumann M (2017) Reappraisal of TDP-43 pathology in FTLD-U subtypes. Acta Neuropathol 134(1):79–96. https://doi.org/10.1007/s00401-017-1716-8

Mackenzie IR, Neumann M, Baborie A, Sampathu DM, Du Plessis D, Jaros E, Perry RH, Trojanowski JQ, Mann DM, Lee VM (2011) A harmonized classification system for FTLD-TDP pathology. Acta Neuropathol 122(1):111–113. https://doi.org/10.1007/s00401-011-0845-8

Mackenzie IR, Neumann M, Bigio EH, Cairns NJ, Alafuzoff I, Kril J, Kovacs GG, Ghetti B, Halliday G, Holm IE, Ince PG, Kamphorst W, Revesz T, Rozemuller AJ, Kumar-Singh S, Akiyama H, Baborie A, Spina S, Dickson DW, Trojanowski JQ, Mann DM (2010) Nomenclature and nosology for neuropathologic subtypes of frontotemporal lobar degeneration: an update. Acta Neuropathol 119(1):1–4. https://doi.org/10.1007/s00401-009-0612-2

Majcher V, Goode A, James V, Layfield R (2015) Autophagy receptor defects and ALS-FTLD. Mol Cell Neurosci 66(Pt A):43–52. https://doi.org/10.1016/j.mcn.2015.01.002

Mioshi E, Flanagan E, Knopman D (2017) Detecting clinical change with the CDR-FTLD: differences between FTLD and AD dementia. Int J Geriatr Psychiatry 32(9):977–982. https://doi.org/10.1002/gps.4556

Molina-Porcel L, Llado A, Rey MJ, Molinuevo JL, Martinez-Lage M, Esteve FX, Ferrer I, Tolosa E, Blesa R (2008) Clinical and pathological heterogeneity of neuronal intermediate filament inclusion disease. Arch Neurol 65(2):272–275. https://doi.org/10.1001/archneurol.2007.37

Momeni P, Cairns NJ, Perry RH, Bigio EH, Gearing M, Singleton AB, Hardy J (2006) Mutation analysis of patients with neuronal intermediate filament inclusion disease (NIFID). Neurobiol Aging 27(5):778.e771–778.e776. https://doi.org/10.1016/j.neurobiolaging.2005.03.030

Morris HR, Waite AJ, Williams NM, Neal JW, Blake DJ (2012) Recent advances in the genetics of the ALS-FTLD complex. Curr Neurol Neurosci Rep 12(3):243–250. https://doi.org/10.1007/s11910-012-0268-5

Munoz DG, Neumann M, Kusaka H, Yokota O, Ishihara K, Terada S, Kuroda S, Mackenzie IR (2009) FUS pathology in basophilic inclusion body disease. Acta Neuropathol 118(5):617–627. https://doi.org/10.1007/s00401-009-0598-9

Nagao S, Yokota O, Ikeda C, Takeda N, Ishizu H, Kuroda S, Sudo K, Terada S, Murayama S, Uchitomi Y (2014) Argyrophilic grain disease as a neurodegenerative substrate in late-onset schizophrenia and delusional disorders. Eur Arch Psychiatry Clin Neurosci 264(4):317–331. https://doi.org/10.1007/s00406-013-0472-6

Neary D, Snowden JS, Gustafson L, Passant U, Stuss D, Black S, Freedman M, Kertesz A, Robert PH, Albert M, Boone K, Miller BL, Cummings J, Benson DF (1998) Frontotemporal lobar degeneration: a consensus on clinical diagnostic criteria. Neurology 51(6):1546–1554

Pottier C, Ravenscroft TA, Sanchez-Contreras M, Rademakers R (2016) Genetics of FTLD: overview and what else we can expect from genetic studies. J Neurochem 138(Suppl 1):32–53. https://doi.org/10.1111/jnc.13622

Rabinovici GD, Rosen HJ, Alkalay A, Kornak J, Furst AJ, Agarwal N, Mormino EC, O'Neil JP, Janabi M, Karydas A, Growdon ME, Jang JY, Huang EJ, Dearmond SJ, Trojanowski JQ, Grinberg LT, Gorno-Tempini ML, Seeley WW, Miller BL, Jagust WJ (2011) Amyloid vs FDG-PET in the differential diagnosis of AD and FTLD. Neurology 77(23):2034–2042. https://doi.org/10.1212/WNL.0b013e31823b9c5e

Rodriguez RD, Grinberg LT (2015) Argyrophilic grain disease: an underestimated tauopathy. Dement Neuropsychol 9(1):2–8. https://doi.org/10.1590/s1980-57642015dn91000002

Rodriguez RD, Suemoto CK, Molina M, Nascimento CF, Leite RE, de Lucena Ferretti-Rebustini RE, Farfel JM, Heinsen H, Nitrini R, Ueda K, Pasqualucci CA, Jacob-Filho W, Yaffe K, Grinberg LT (2016) Argyrophilic grain disease: demographics, clinical, and neuropathological features from a large autopsy study. J Neuropathol Exp Neurol 75(7):628–635. https://doi.org/10.1093/jnen/nlw034

Saito Y, Ruberu NN, Sawabe M, Arai T, Tanaka N, Kakuta Y, Yamanouchi H, Murayama S (2004) Staging of argyrophilic grains: an age-associated tauopathy. J Neuropathol Exp Neurol 63(9):911–918

Seilhean D, Bielle F, Plu I, Duyckaerts C (2013) Frontotemporal lobar degeneration: diversity of FTLD lesions. Rev Neurol 169(10):786–792. https://doi.org/10.1016/j.neurol.2013.07.015

Simic G (2002) Pathological tau proteins in argyrophilic grain disease. Lancet Neurol 1(5):276

Strong MJ (2012) Amyotrophic Lateral Sclerosis and Frontotemporal Dementias. Oxford University Press, Oxford

Thal DR, von Arnim CA, Griffin WS, Mrak RE, Walker L, Attems J, Arzberger T (2015) Frontotemporal lobar degeneration FTLD-tau: preclinical lesions, vascular, and Alzheimer-related co-pathologies. J Neural Transm (Vienna, Austria: 1996) 122(7):1007–1018. https://doi.org/10.1007/s00702-014-1360-6

Thomas M, Alegre-Abarrategui J, Wade-Martins R (2013) RNA dysfunction and aggrephagy at the centre of an amyotrophic lateral sclerosis/frontotemporal dementia disease continuum. Brain 136(Pt 5):1345–1360. https://doi.org/10.1093/brain/awt030

Togo T, Sahara N, Yen SH, Cookson N, Ishizawa T, Hutton M, de Silva R, Lees A, Dickson DW (2002) Argyrophilic grain disease is a sporadic 4-repeat tauopathy. J Neuropathol Exp Neurol 61(6):547–556

Tolnay M, Monsch AU, Probst A (2001) Argyrophilic grain disease. A frequent dementing disorder in aged patients. Adv Exp Med Biol 487:39–58

Tolnay M, Probst A (2008) Argyrophilic grain disease. Handb Clin Neurol 89:553–563. https://doi.org/10.1016/s0072-9752(07)01251-1

Trojsi F, Sorrentino P, Sorrentino G, Tedeschi G (2017) Neurodegeneration of brain networks in the amyotrophic lateral sclerosis-frontotemporal lobar degeneration (ALS-FTLD) continuum: evidence from MRI and MEG studies. CNS Spectr 23(6):378–387. https://doi.org/10.1017/s109285291700075x

van der Zee J, Gijselinck I, Dillen L, Van Langenhove T, Theuns J, Engelborghs S, Philtjens S, Vandenbulcke M, Sleegers K, Sieben A, Baumer V, Maes G, Corsmit E, Borroni B, Padovani A, Archetti S, Perneczky R, Diehl-Schmid J, de Mendonca A, Miltenberger-Miltenyi G, Pereira S, Pimentel J, Nacmias B, Bagnoli S, Sorbi S, Graff C, Chiang HH, Westerlund M, Sanchez-Valle R, Llado A, Gelpi E, Santana I, Almeida MR, Santiago B, Frisoni G, Zanetti O, Bonvicini C, Synofzik M, Maetzler W, Vom Hagen JM, Schols L, Heneka MT, Jessen F, Matej R, Parobkova E, Kovacs GG, Strobel T, Sarafov S, Tournev I, Jordanova A, Danek A, Arzberger T, Fabrizi GM, Testi S, Salmon E, Santens P, Martin JJ, Cras P, Vandenberghe R, De Deyn PP, Cruts M, Van Broeckhoven C, van der Zee J, Gijselinck I, Dillen L, Van Langenhove T, Theuns J, Philtjens S, Sleegers K, Baumer V, Maes G, Corsmit E, Cruts M, Van Broeckhoven C, van der Zee J, Gijselinck I, Dillen L, Van Langenhove T, Philtjens S, Theuns J, Sleegers K, Baumer V, Maes G, Cruts M, Van Broeckhoven C, Engelborghs S, De Deyn PP, Cras P, Engelborghs S, De Deyn PP, Vandenbulcke M, Vandenbulcke M, Borroni B, Padovani A, Archetti S, Perneczky R, Diehl-Schmid J, Synofzik M, Maetzler W, Muller Vom Hagen J, Schols L, Synofzik M, Maetzler W, Muller Vom Hagen J, Schols L, Heneka MT, Jessen F, Ramirez A, Kurzwelly D, Sachtleben C, Mairer W, de Mendonca A, Miltenberger-Miltenyi G, Pereira S, Firmo C, Pimentel J, Sanchez-Valle R, Llado A, Antonell A, Molinuevo J, Gelpi E, Graff C, Chiang HH, Westerlund M, Graff C, Kinhult Stahlbom A, Thonberg H, Nennesmo I, Borjesson-Hanson A, Nacmias B, Bagnoli S, Sorbi S, Bessi V, Piaceri I, Santana I, Santiago B, Santana I, Helena Ribeiro M, Rosario Almeida M, Oliveira C, Massano J, Garret C, Pires P, Frisoni G, Zanetti O, Bonvicini C, Sarafov S, Tournev I, Jordanova A, Tournev I, Kovacs GG, Strobel T, Heneka MT, Jessen F, Ramirez A, Kurzwelly D, Sachtleben C, Mairer W, Jessen F, Matej R, Parobkova E, Danel A, Arzberger T, Maria Fabrizi G, Testi S, Ferrari S, Cavallaro T, Salmon E, Santens P, Cras P (2013) A pan-European study of the C9orf72 repeat associated with FTLD: geographic prevalence, genomic instability, and intermediate repeats. Hum Mutat 34(2):363–373. https://doi.org/10.1002/humu.22244

Xi Z, Zhang M, Bruni AC, Maletta RG, Colao R, Fratta P, Polke JM, Sweeney MG, Mudanohwo E, Nacmias B, Sorbi S, Tartaglia MC, Rainero I, Rubino E, Pinessi L, Galimberti D, Surace EI, McGoldrick P, McKeever P, Moreno D, Sato C, Liang Y, Keith J, Zinman L, Robertson J, Rogaeva E (2015) The C9orf72 repeat expansion itself is methylated in ALS and FTLD patients. Acta Neuropathol 129(5):715–727. https://doi.org/10.1007/s00401-015-1401-8

Yokota O, Tsuchiya K, Terada S, Ishizu H, Uchikado H, Ikeda M, Oyanagi K, Nakano I, Murayama S, Kuroda S, Akiyama H (2008) Basophilic inclusion body disease and neuronal intermediate filament inclusion disease: a comparative clinicopathological study. Acta Neuropathol 115(5):561–575. https://doi.org/10.1007/s00401-007-0329-z

Neurodegenerative Diseases: Progressive Supranuclear Palsy (PSP)–Cortico-Basal Degeneration (CBD)

35.1 Introduction

Progressive supranuclear palsy (PSP) and cortico-basal degeneration (CBD) are thought to represent a disease spectrum. The clinical presentation depends on the localization and distribution of the pathological lesions with:

- PSP affects the hindbrain structures.
- CBD affects the forebrain.

35.2 Progressive Supranuclear Palsy (PSP)

- First described by Steele, Richardson, and Olszewski in 1964
- Most frequent tauopathy

35.2.1 Clinical Signs

- Core features (see Table 35.1)
  - Ocular motor dysfunction
  - Postural instability
  - Akinesia
  - Cognitive dysfunction
- Supportive features
  - Levodopa-resistance
  - Hypokinetic, spastic dysarthria
  - Dysphagia
  - Photophobia
- Richardson or PSP syndrome:
  - Progressive supranuclear gaze palsy
  - Postural instability
  - Dysarthria
  - Progressive axial muscle rigidity
- Signs of dementia (mostly of the subcortical type)
- Two variants
  - Cortical-predominant
    - cortico-basal syndrome
    - behavioral variant of fronto-temporal dementia
    - progressive aphasia or speech apraxia
  - Brain stem-predominant
    - asymmetric parkinsonism with tremor, extra-axial dystonia
    - pure akinesia with gait freezing

35.2.2 Epidemiology

Prevalence
- 6.4 per 100,000

Age of onset
- 40–60 years

Gender
- M = F

Table 35.1 Core clinical features and levels of certainty as defined by the Movement Disorder Society (Hoglinger et al. 2017) reproduced with kind permission by Wiley

Levels of certainty	Ocular motor dysfunction	Postural instability	Akinesia	Cognitive dysfunction
Level 1	O1: Vertical supranuclear gaze palsy	P1: Repeated unprovoked falls within 3 years	A1: Progressive gait freezing within 3 years	C1: Speech/language disorder, i.e., non-fluent/agrammatic variant of primary progressive aphasia or progressive apraxia of speech
Level 2	O2: Slow velocity of vertical saccades	P2: Tendency to fall on the pull-test within 3 years	A2: Parkinsonism, akinetic-rigid, predominantly axial, and levodopa resistant	C2: Frontal cognitive/behavioral presentation
Level 3	O3: Frequent macro square wave jerks or "eyelid opening apraxia"	P3: More than two steps backward on the pull-test within 3 years	A3: Parkinsonism, with tremor and/or asymmetric and/or levodopa responsive	C3: Cortico-basal syndrome

35.2.3 Neuroimaging Findings

General Imaging Findings

Atrophy of midbrain and superior cerebellar peduncle

- Morning glory sign—concave lateral margin of tegmentum on axial MRI
- Hummingbird/penguin sign—atrophy of midbrain on midsagittal MRI forming the silhouette of a penguin or hummingbird

CT non-contrast-enhanced
- Atrophy of midbrain and superior cerebellar peduncle with consecutive enlargement of interpeduncular cistern, aqueduct, and third ventricle

CT contrast-enhanced
- No pathological enhancement

MRI-T2/FLAIR (Fig. 35.1a, b, e)
- Atrophy of midbrain and superior cerebellar peduncle—morning glory sign, hummingbird sign/penguin sign
- Hypointensity of putamen (iron deposition)

MRI-T1 (Fig. 35.1c)
- Atrophy of midbrain and superior cerebellar peduncle—morning glory sign, hummingbird sign/penguin sign

MRI-T1 contrast-enhanced
- No pathological enhancement

MRI-T2*/SWI (Fig. 35.1d)
- Hypointensity of putamen (iron deposition)

MR-Diffusion Imaging
- Increased ADC values in superior cerebellar peduncle compared to healthy subjects or Parkinson disease patients

Nuclear Medicine Imaging Findings
- PSP is belonging to the parkinsonian syndromes and thereby showing presynaptic dopamine transporter deficit with SPECT tracers like FP-CIT or β-CIT.
- Some studies suggest a more symmetric loss in contrast to Parkinson disease but there is a large overlap which allows no differentiation.
- Reports state a less evident gradient between the caudate head and putamen in atypical Parkinsonian syndromes than in PD.
- 18F-DOPA PET is used to assess the presynaptic decarboxylase function and dopamine turnover.
- In contrast to Parkinson disease, the postsynaptic dopamine (D2) receptors are affected too, so SPECT studies with IBZM or PET studies with tracers like 11C-raclopride or 18F-fallypride allow a differentiation between PD and atypical Parkinsonian syndromes like PSP by showing the postsynaptic neuronal loss.

35.2 Progressive Supranuclear Palsy (PSP)

- Additional CBF-SPECT and FDG-PET studies reveal hypoperfusion and hypometabolism in the medial frontal cortex, the mesencephalon, and the striatum.
- Myocardial sympathetic innervation can be assessed with 123I-MIBG or 18F-dopamine. Reports state a statistically better uptake in atypical Parkinsonian syndromes than in PD by comparing myocardial and mediastinal uptake.
- Tau-tracers may allow insights in neuropathology and help distinguish tau from non-tau pathologies (CBD and PSP from MSA).
- In classical PSP (Richardson syndrome), amyloid PET is described to be negative, while the other forms are amyloid positive.

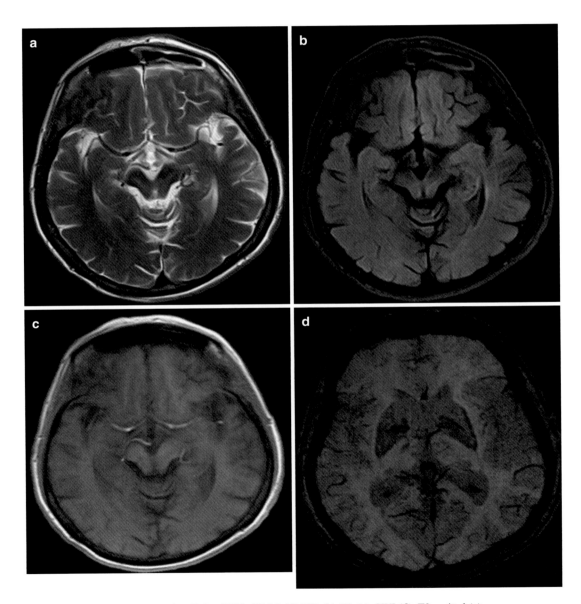

Fig. 35.1 Progressive supranuclear Palsy (PSP): T2 (**a**), FLAIR (**b**), T1 (**c**), SWI (**d**), T2 sagittal (**e**)

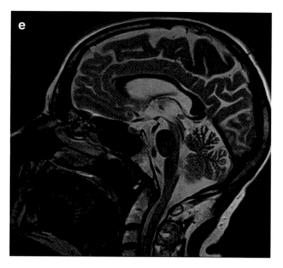

Fig. 35.1 (continued)

35.2.4 Neuropathology Findings

Macroscopic Features
- Reduced brain weight possible
- Signs of fronto-temporal atrophy
- Atrophy of:
  - subthalamic nucleus
  - cerebellar peduncles
  - tectum/tegmentum of mesencephalon
- Depigmentation of the substantia nigra and locus coeruleus

Microscopic Features (Fig. 35.2a–f)
- Neuronal loss.
- Gliosis.
- Globose Neurofibrillary tangles (NFT) positive for tau and 4R tau in:
  - substantia nigra
  - locus coeruleus
  - nucleus basalis Meynert
  - dorsal raphe nucleus
  - pontine nuclei
  - nucleus olivaris inferior
- Additional affected regions include:
  - globus pallidus
  - thalamus
  - subthalamic nuclei
  - dentate nucleus

- Neuropil threads in:
  - cortical regions (precentral gyrus)
  - subcortical regions (globus pallidus, subthalamic nucleus, substantia nigra)
- The cerebral cortex and hippocampus are rarely affected, whereby a single NFT might be found.
- ß-A4 deposits in the cerebral cortex in varying amount.
- Astroglial inclusions
  - tufted astrocytes (precentral gyrus, striatum, superior colliculus)
  - thorn-shaped astrocytes
- Oligodendroglial inclusions
  - coiled bodies (white matter tracts of the basal ganglia, thalamus, and brain stem)

Progression of lesions
- Pallido-luysian-nigral system
- Basal ganglia, pontine nuclei, dentate nucleus
- Frontal and parietal lobes
- Neocortical areas and cerebellum

Immunophenotype (Fig. 35.2g–p)
- NFT are
  - Positive for tau
  - Positive for 4R tau
  - Positive for p62
  - Negative for ubiquitin
  - Negative for 3R tau
- Neuropil threads in cortical regions (predominantly entorhinal cortex) are
  - Positive for tau
  - Negative for ubiquitin
- Tau-positive
  - Astrocytes in the basal ganglia, thalamus and frontal cortex
  - Oligodendrocytes in the white matter, positive for ubiquitin

Ultrastructural Features
- NFTs contain mainly:
  - straight filaments 15 nm in diameter
  - a variable number of 10 nm thick paired helical filaments (PHF)
- Glial cells with
  - tubular profiles
  - straight filaments

35.2 Progressive Supranuclear Palsy (PSP)

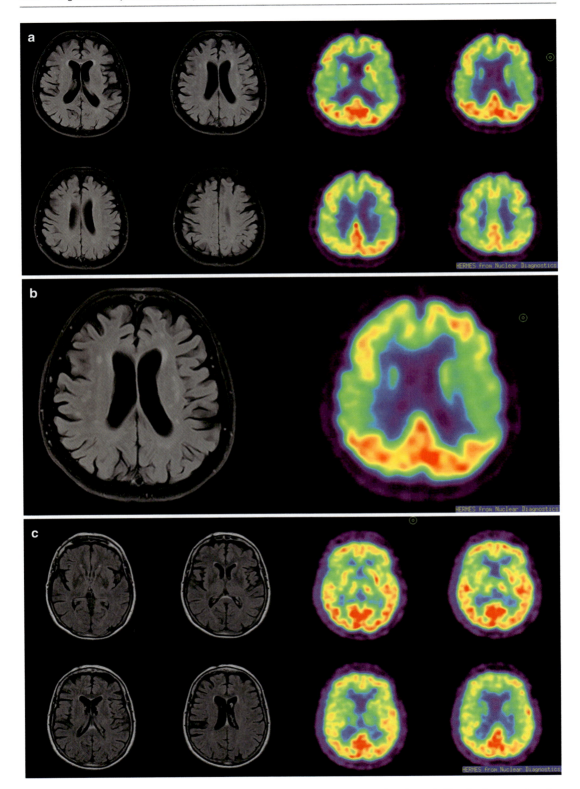

Fig. 35.2 Cortico-basal degeneration (CBD): FGD-PET showing strongly reduced metabolism in the central region (attenuation left > right) (**a–c**)

Diagnostic hints
- Depigmentation of substantia nigra
- NFT in subcortical structures
- Tufted astrocytes
- Oligodendroglial coiled bodies
- Threads 4R tau immunopositive

35.2.5 Molecular Neuropathology

- Hyperphosphorylated tau at 64 and 68 kDa.
- Abnormal tau consists of 4R tau.
- Different proteolytic processing of abnormal tau.
- Mutations in the *MAPT* gene.

35.2.6 Treatment and Prognosis

Treatment
Symptomatic treatment:

- Parkinsonism
- Visual disturbances
- Palliative therapies

Biologic Behavior-Prognosis-Prognostic Factors
- Progressive clinical course
  - immobility
  - anarthria
- Mean disease duration: 5.6 years (range: 3–17 years)
- Predictors of short survival:
  - onset of falls during the first year
  - early dysphagia
  - incontinence

35.3 Cortico-Basal Degeneration (CBD)

Cortico-basal degeneration was first described by Rebeitz (1968) as corticonigral degeneration with neuronal achromasia.

35.3.1 Clinical Signs

Clinical signs and symptoms
- Ideomotor apraxia
- Rigidity
- Dystonia
- Myoclonus
- Cortical sensory signs
- Alien limb phenomenon
- Richardson syndrome

35.3.2 Neuroimaging Findings

General Imaging Findings
- Asymmetric atrophy of frontoparietal cortex (pre- and postcentral gyri)

CT non-contrast-enhanced
- Asymmetric atrophy of pre- and postcentral gyri with consecutive dilatation of central sulcus

CT contrast-enhanced
- No pathological enhancement

MRI-T2/FLAIR:
- Asymmetric atrophy of frontoparietal cortex with dilatation of central sulcus
- Hyperintensity of subcortical white matter of affected gyri (gliosis)
- Midbrain tegmentum atrophy

MRI-T1
- Asymmetric atrophy of frontoparietal cortex
- Midbrain tegmentum atrophy

MRI-T1 contrast-enhanced
- No pathological enhancement

MR-Diffusion Imaging
- Elevated ADC values in putamen compared to healthy subjects or Parkinson disease patients.

35.3 Cortico-Basal Degeneration (CBD)

Nuclear Medicine Imaging Findings (Fig. 35.3)
- In cortico-basal degeneration, FDG hypometabolism is described to be more asymmetrical (especially the contralateral side of the predominant motor symptoms).
- Involved regions: the central region, the contralateral putamen, and the bilateral thalamus.
- Tau-tracers may allow insights in neuropathology and help distinguish tau from non-tau pathologies (CBD and PSP from MSA).

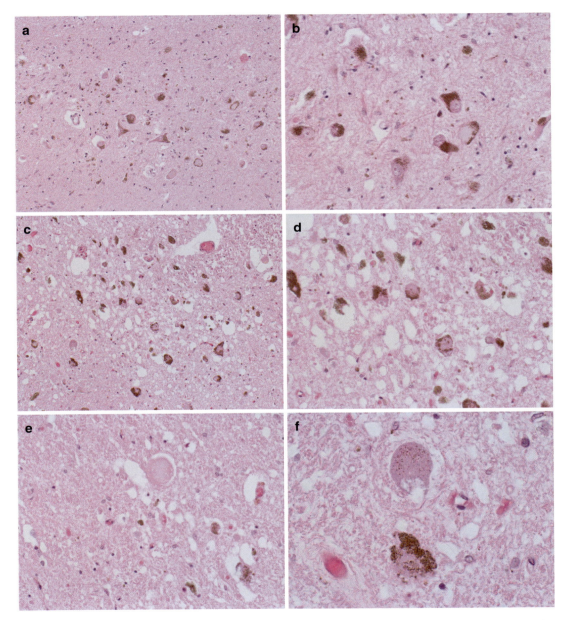

Fig. 35.3 Progressive supranuclear palsy (PSP): substantia nigra shows moderate loss of pigmented neurons (**a–d**); some neurons contain inclusions (**e, f**). The inclusions are positive for four repeat tau (**g, h**). Astrocytes are also positive for four repeat tau (**i–n**). Some of the inclusions are positive for p62 (**o, p**)

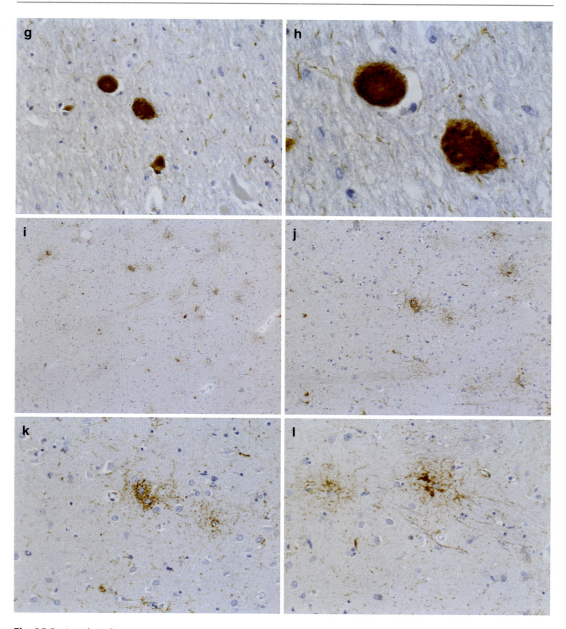

Fig. 35.3 (continued)

35.3 Cortico-Basal Degeneration (CBD)

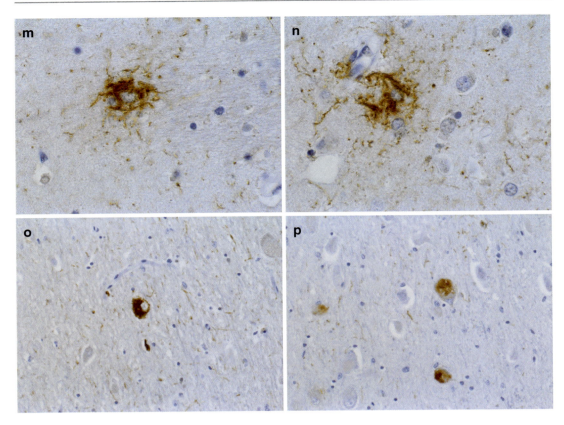

Fig. 35.3 (continued)

35.3.3 Neuropathology Findings

Macroscopic Features
- Diffuse brain atrophy
  - pronounced in the posterior frontal and parietal lobes
  - precentral gyrus and postcentral gyrus
- Secondary asymmetric degeneration of the corticospinal tract and thinning of the corpus callosum
- Flattening of the caudate nucleus
- Depigmentation of the substantia nigra possible

Microscopic Features (Fig. 35.4a, b)
- Neuronal loss
  - substantia nigra pars compacta always shows severe loss of neurons.
  - variable neuronal loss in:
    o lateral thalamus, striatum, globus pallidus, subthalamus, claustrum, amygdala, nucleus basalis Meynert, nucleus ruber, substantia nigra, locus coeruleus and other brain stem nuclei as well as in the anterior horn of the spinal cord
- Reactive astrogliosis
- Pigmentstreuung and pigment-laden macrophages
- Rarely Lewy bodies in surviving neurons especially in elderly patients
- Achromatic or ballooned neurons
- Two different types of inclusions:
  - intraneuronal, cytoplasmatic inclusions, basophilic inclusions, small cortical intraneuronal inclusions, neuropil threads
  - glial inclusions
    o in oligodendrocytes
    o similar to those seen in multi-system atrophy
    o immunoreactive for tau and ubiquitin

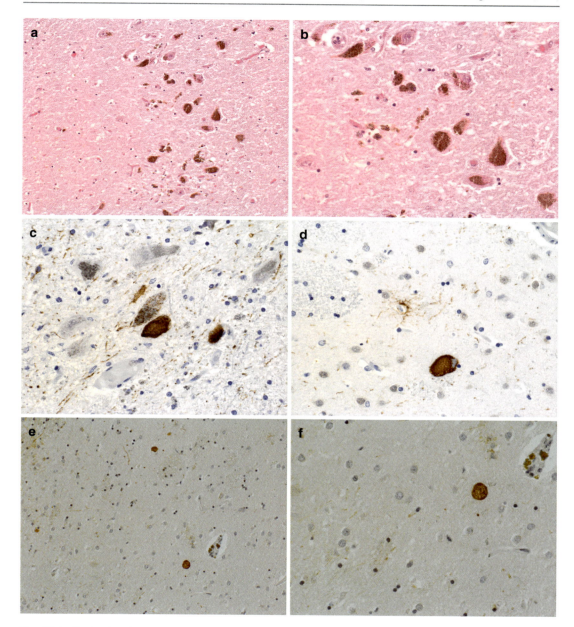

Fig. 35.4 Cortico-basal degeneration (CBD): substantia nigra shows moderate loss of pigmented neurons (**a**, **b**); neuronal inclusions stain positive for phosphorylated tau (**c**, **d**) and α-ß crystalline (**e**, **f**). Astrocytic inclusions (coiled bodies (**g**)) and cytoplasmatic reactivities stain for phosphorylated tau (**g**, **h**) and four repeat tau (**i**) as well as for p62 (**j**)

35.3 Cortico-Basal Degeneration (CBD)

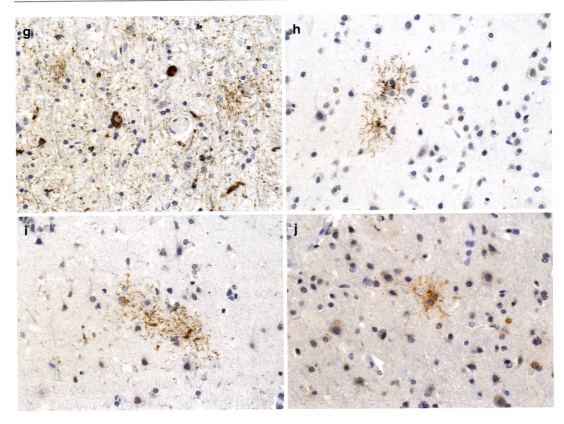

Fig. 35.4 (continued)

Intraneuronal Inclusions
- Round, whorled, weakly basophilic
- Reminiscent of neurofibrillary tangles
- Strongly positive for tau-protein
- No immunoreactivity for ubiquitin
- Immunoreactive for α-B-crystallin

Glial Inclusions
- Oligodendroglial coiled body
  - striatum, globus pallidus
- Astrocytic plaque
  - frontal, motor, and parietal cortex
  - striatum

Immunophenotype (Fig. 35.4a–j)
- tau positivity, 4R tau positivity, and 3R tau negativity in:
  - neurons: granular cytoplasmic
  - thread-like structures (gray and white matter)
  - oligodendroglial coiled bodies
  - astrocytic plaques

Diagnostic hints
- Depigmentation of substantia nigra
- Neurons with diffuse cytoplasmatic immunoreactivity
- Threads in the gray and white matter
- Astrocytic plaques, 4R tau immunopositive in cortex and striatum

Ultrastructural Features
- 20–24 nm twisted ribbons
- Astrocytes with tubular structures and amorphous profiles
- Oligodendrocytes with twisted tubules

35.3.4 Molecular Neuropathology

- Hyperphosphorylated tau at 64 and 68 kDa.
- Abnormal tau consists of 4R tau.
- Different proteolytic processing of abnormal tau.
- Mutations in the *MAPT* gene.

35.3.5 Treatment and Prognosis

Treatment

Symptomatic therapy for:

- Parkinsonism
- Myoclonus/tremor
- Dystonia
- Eyelid movement disorder
- Behavioral abnormalities
- Palliative therapies

Biologic Behavior-Prognosis-Prognostic Factors
- Progressive extrapyramidal disorder
- Poor prognosis
- Mean survival time: 7 years

Selected References

Adachi M, Kawanami T, Ohshima H, Sugai Y, Hosoya T (2004) Morning glory sign: a particular MR finding in progressive supranuclear palsy. Magn Reson Med Sci 3(3):125–132

Boeve BF (2012) Progressive supranuclear palsy. Parkinsonism Relat Disord 18(Suppl 1):S192–S194. https://doi.org/10.1016/s1353-8020(11)70060-8

Borroni B, Agosti C, Magnani E, Di Luca M, Padovani A (2011) Genetic bases of progressive supranuclear palsy: the MAPT tau disease. Curr Med Chem 18(17):2655–2660

Dickson DW, Ahmed Z, Algom AA, Tsuboi Y, Josephs KA (2010) Neuropathology of variants of progressive supranuclear palsy. Curr Opin Neurol 23(4):394–400. https://doi.org/10.1097/WCO.0b013e32833be924

Eusebio A, Koric L, Felician O, Guedj E, Ceccaldi M, Azulay JP (2016) Progressive supranuclear palsy and corticobasal degeneration: diagnostic challenges and clinicopathological considerations. Rev Neurol 172(8-9):488–502. https://doi.org/10.1016/j.neurol.2016.07.009

Hoglinger GU, Respondek G, Stamelou M (2017) Clinical diagnosis of progressive supranuclear palsy: the movement disorder society criteria. Mov Disord 32(6):853–864. https://doi.org/10.1002/mds.26987

Holtbernd F, Eidelberg D (2014) The utility of neuroimaging in the differential diagnosis of parkinsonian syndromes. Semin Neurol 34(2):202–209. https://doi.org/10.1055/s-0034-1381733

Im SY, Kim YE, Kim YJ (2015) Genetics of progressive supranuclear palsy. J Mov Disord 8(3):122–129. https://doi.org/10.14802/jmd.15033

Josephs KA (2015) Key emerging issues in progressive supranuclear palsy and corticobasal degeneration. J Neurol 262(3):783–788. https://doi.org/10.1007/s00415-015-7682-y

Koyama M, Yagishita A, Nakata Y, Hayashi M, Bandoh M, Mizutani T (2007) Imaging of corticobasal degeneration syndrome. Neuroradiology 49(11):905–912. https://doi.org/10.1007/s00234-007-0265-6

Lamb R, Rohrer JD, Lees AJ, Morris HR (2016) Progressive supranuclear palsy and corticobasal degeneration: pathophysiology and treatment options. Curr Treat Options Neurol 18(9):42. https://doi.org/10.1007/s11940-016-0422-5

Ling H (2016) Clinical approach to progressive supranuclear palsy. J Mov Disord 9(1):3–13. https://doi.org/10.14802/jmd.15060

Liscic RM, Srulijes K, Groger A, Maetzler W, Berg D (2013) Differentiation of progressive supranuclear palsy: clinical, imaging and laboratory tools. Acta Neurol Scand 127(5):362–370. https://doi.org/10.1111/ane.12067

Lopez G, Bayulkem K, Hallett M (2016) Progressive supranuclear palsy (PSP): Richardson syndrome and other PSP variants. Acta Neurol Scand 134(4):242–249. https://doi.org/10.1111/ane.12546

Pandey S (2012) Hummingbird sign in progressive supranuclear palsy disease. J Res Med Sci 17(2):197–198

Respondek G, Hoglinger GU (2016) The phenotypic spectrum of progressive supranuclear palsy. Parkinsonism Relat Disord 22(Suppl 1):S34–S36. https://doi.org/10.1016/j.parkreldis.2015.09.041

Rizzo G, Martinelli P, Manners D, Scaglione C, Tonon C, Cortelli P, Malucelli E, Capellari S, Testa C, Parchi P, Montagna P, Barbiroli B, Lodi R (2008) Diffusion-weighted brain imaging study of patients with clinical diagnosis of corticobasal degeneration, progressive supranuclear palsy and Parkinson's disease. Brain J Neurol 131(Pt 10):2690–2700. https://doi.org/10.1093/brain/awn195

Slowinski J, Imamura A, Uitti RJ, Pooley RA, Strongosky AJ, Dickson DW, Broderick DF, Wszolek ZK (2008) MR imaging of brainstem atrophy in progressive supranuclear palsy. J Neurol 255(1):37–44. https://doi.org/10.1007/s00415-007-0656-y

Taki M, Ishii K, Fukuda T, Kojima Y, Mori E (2004) Evaluation of cortical atrophy between progressive supranuclear palsy and corticobasal degeneration by hemispheric surface display of MR images. AJNR Am J Neuroradiol 25(10):1709–1714

Tokumaru AM, O'Uchi T, Kuru Y, Maki T, Murayama S, Horichi Y (1996) Corticobasal degeneration: MR with histopathologic comparison. AJNR Am J Neuroradiol 17(10):1849–1852

Tokumaru AM, Saito Y, Murayama S, Kazutomi K, Sakiyama Y, Toyoda M, Yamakawa M, Terada H (2009) Imaging-pathologic correlation in corticobasal degeneration. AJNR Am J Neuroradiol 30(10):1884–1892. https://doi.org/10.3174/ajnr.A1721

Williams DR, Lees AJ (2009) Progressive supranuclear palsy: clinicopathological concepts and diagnostic challenges. Lancet Neurol 8(3):270–279. https://doi.org/10.1016/s1474-4422(09)70042-0

Neurodegenerative Diseases: Vascular Dementia

36.1 Introduction

Disturbances of the vascular system manifest clinically as:

- Global cerebral ischemia
  - Infarct
- Focal cerebral ischemia
  - Vascular occlusion
  - Multi-infarct dementia
- Chronic hypoperfusion
  - Changes of cerebral microvasculature
  - Binswanger disease
- Cerebral hemorrhage
  - Focal changes of cerebral vessels
  - Intracerebral hemorrhage
  - Cerebral amyloid angiopathy

Vascular dementia (VaD) is defined as a neurocognitive disorder, which is explained by numerous vascular causes in the general absence of other pathologies (Kalaria 2016) (Table 36.1) including:

- Encephalopathy with multiple infarcts: multi-infarct encephalopathy
- Lacunas, lacunar state
- Status cribrosus
- Vascular encephalopathy: Binswanger-type leukoencephalopathy
- Infarcts in strategic areas
- Hippocampal sclerosis
- Granular atrophy of the cerebral cortex
- Infarcts in watershed areas
- Diseases of blood vessels causing cognitive impairment:
  - Atherosclerosis/arteriosclerosis
  - Hypertensive angiopathy
  - Small vessel disease
  - Inflammatory vascular diseases
  - Cerebral amyloid angiopathies
  - Cerebral autosomal dominant arteriopathy with subcortical infarcts and leukoencephalopathy (CADASIL)
  - Cerebral autosomal recessive arteriopathy with subcortical infarcts and leukoencephalopathy (CARASIL)
  - Cerebrovascular occlusive disease with retinal involvement

Table 36.1 Pathological changes seen in cases with clinical VaD (Kalaria 2016), reproduced with kind permission by Springer Nature

Pathological outcomes	Percent
Pure VaD	10
Mixed with small vessel disease	40
Mixed with large vessel disease	8
Alzheimer disease	40
Other types	2

Dementia resulting from vascular changes might be classified as follows:

- Multi-infarct dementia
- Small vessel disease (SVD)
  - "pure SVD"
  - SVD Type "Micro-Infarct-dementia"
  - SVD Type "Subcortical Leukoencephalopathy"
  - SVD Type "Morbus Binswanger"
  - SVD Type "Cerebral Amyloid Angiopathy"
- Strategic infarct dementia
- Hypoperfusion dementia
- Hemorrhagic dementia
- Mixed dementia

36.2 Clinical Signs and Symptoms

Clinical Signs
- Sudden onset of cognitive decline
- History of transient ischemic attacks or strokes
- Focal neurologic deficits
- Gait abnormalities
- Grasp reflexes
- Memory deficits in the form of retrieval deficit
- Depression, apathy, and personality changes
- "Pseudobulbar palsy," including symptoms of emotional incontinence, paradoxical laughter
- Parkinsonism: slowness of movement (bradykinesia), increased rigidity in the arms and/or legs, and problems with walking (short stride length or a "magnetic" gait in which the feet seem glued to the floor)
- Falls
- Weakness or sensory changes affecting one side of the body
- Problems with speech (dysarthria), swallowing (dysphagia), double vision (diplopia), or other "focal" neurologic symptoms
- "Cortical" signs including:
  - Aphasia (impairment of language)
  - Apraxia (loss of ability to perform learned motor movements)
- Visual impairment (loss of attention to part of a visual field, disturbances of visual integration)
- Neglect—inattention to visual or sensory stimuli on one side (e.g., ignoring these things on the left side of the body)
- Hemiparesis—weakness affecting one side of the body

Vascular Cognitive Impairment (VCI)
- encompass all people with cognitive impairment of cerebrovascular origin
- has several clinical presentations, etiologies, and treatment
- forms a spectrum that includes vascular dementia, mixed Alzheimer disease with a vascular component, and VCI that does not meet dementia criteria
- Multiple pathophysiological mechanisms contribute to VCI, accounting for its heterogeneity.
- Although main changes in the brain in VCI include cerebral infarcts, vascular cognitive impairment is thought to be due to factors beyond acute infarcts.
- Cerebral white matter lesions and silent brain infarcts are considered to be risk factors for VCI.

Brain Hemorrhages (Hemorrhagic Dementia)
- Both macroscopic intracerebral hemorrhages (ICH) and microbleeds (MBs) have been associated with cognitive decline or dementia, which may manifest before or after ICH.

Global Hypoperfusion (Hypoperfusion Dementia)
- Global reductions in cerebral perfusion can result in transient or permanent ischemia and, hence, cognitive deficits.

Strategic Infarcts (Strategic Infarct Dementia)
- A single small infarct may cause severe cognitive deficits when located in a strategic brain region. Classical anatomic locations for strategic infarcts include the thalamus, angular gyrus, and basal ganglia, including the caudate nucleus and globus pallidus.

36.3 Diagnostic Criteria

Diagnostic criteria for Vascular Cognitive Impairment (VCI) are as follows (Dichgans and Leys 2017; Gorelick et al. 2011):

- VCI refers to all forms of cognitive deficits of vascular origin ranging from MCI to dementia.
- Diagnosis must be based on cognitive testing involving a minimum of four cognitive domains, including:
  - Executive/attention
  - Memory
  - Language
  - Visuospatial functions
- Vascular dementia (VaD) requires:
  - A decline in cognitive function
  - A deficit in performance in ≥2 cognitive domains that are of sufficient severity to affect activities of daily living.
- Vascular mild cognitive impairment (VaMCI) includes four subtypes:
  - Amnestic
  - Amnestic plus other domains
  - Nonamnestic single domain
  - Nonamnestic multiple domain
- VaMCI should be based on the assumption of a decline in cognitive function. Activities of daily living may be normal or mildly impaired.
- *Probable*: A diagnosis of probable VaD or VaMCI requires the following:
  1. Imaging evidence of cerebrovascular disease and
     (a) a clear temporal relationship between a vascular event (e.g., stroke) and onset of cognitive deficits or
     (b) a clear relationship between the severity and pattern of cognitive impairment and the presence of diffuse subcortical vascular pathology;
  2. Absence of a history of gradually progressive cognitive deficits, suggesting the presence of neurodegenerative disease.
- *Possible*: A diagnosis of possible VaD or VaMCI requires
  - imaging evidence of cerebrovascular disease and
  - should be made if there is no clear relationship between vascular disease and cognitive impairment,
  - if the criteria for probable VaD or VaMCI are not fulfilled,
  - if aphasia precludes proper cognitive assessment, or
  - if there is a history of active cancer or psychiatric or metabolic disorders that may affect cognitive function.
- *Unstable VaMCI:*
  - subjects with probable or possible VaMCI whose symptoms revert to normal

36.4 Epidemiology

Incidence
- 2.5 per 1000 non-demented individuals per year

Prevalence
- 1.5%
- VaD accounts for up to 40% of dementia cases
- Second most common cause of dementia after AD

Onset
- Elderly

Male:Female Ratio
- M > F

36.5 Neuroimaging Findings

General Imaging Findings

Multiple cortical/white matter infarcts, lacunar infarcts in basal ganglia and/or pons

CT Non-Contrast-Enhanced (Fig. 36.1a)
- Multiple hypodensities (cortical/subcortical, periventricular, basal ganglia, pons)
- Diffuse brain atrophy

CT Contrast-Enhanced
- Usually no enhancement

MRI-T2/FLAIR (Fig. 36.1b–d)
- Hyperintense infarcts cortical/subcortical, periventricular, in basal ganglia and/or pons

MRI-T1 (Fig. 36.1e)
- Infarcts hypointense

MRI-T1 Contrast-Enhanced
- Usually no enhancement (except infarction is subacute)

MRI-T2∗/SWI (Fig. 36.1f)
- Detection of hemorrhagic components

MR-Diffusion Tensor Imaging
- Increased diffusivity in infarcts and normal appearing white matter

MR-Spectroscopy
- Low NAA values

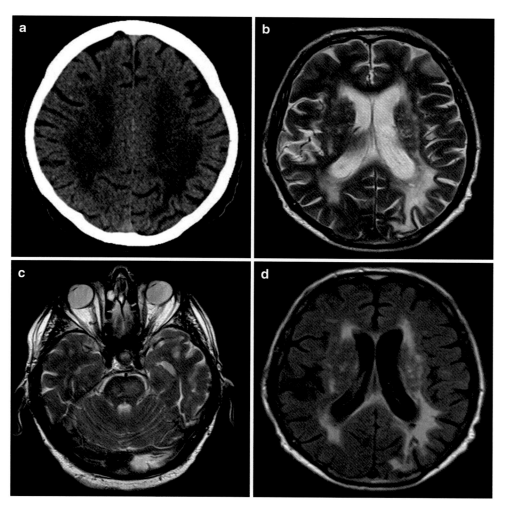

Fig. 36.1 T2-hyperintense gliosis in periventricular white matter, pons and left occipital cortex, microbleeds in left thalamus; CT non-contrast (**a**), T2 (**b**, **c**), FLAIR (**d**), T1 (**e**), T2∗ (**f**)

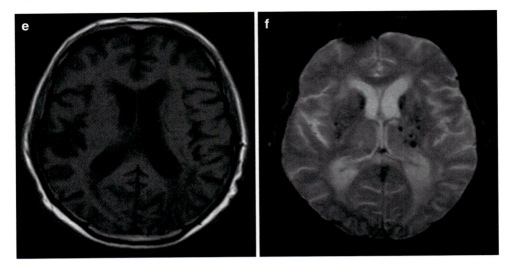

Fig. 36.1 (continued)

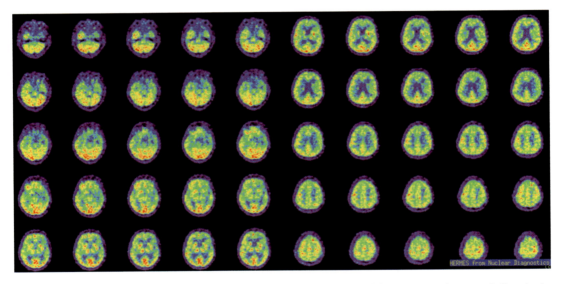

Fig. 36.2 FDG-PET slice of a case with vascular dementia showing diffuse inhomogeneous hypometabolism in the cerebral cortex and basal ganglia

Nuclear Medicine Imaging Findings (Fig. 36.2)
- FDG-PET (and CBF-SPECT) demonstrates an inhomogeneous metabolizing (perfusion) pattern not only in the all cortical regions (also in the motor cortex) but also in basal ganglia—in contrast to AD, FTD, and DLB.
- In regions with a larger infarct area, defects in the metabolizing pattern can be seen.
- Nuclear medicine findings correlate with CT and MRI findings and show hypometabolism in infarct areas.

36.6 Neuropathology Findings

Multi-infarct Dementia (Fig. 36.3a–t)
- Typical ischemic infarcts
  - Various age and size
  - Located in the cerebral cortex, white matter, basal ganglia, and thalamus
  - Regions supplied by large vessels, i.e., arteria cerebri media und posterior
  - Volume of infarct variable 50–100 mL
- Large infarct: >1 cm Ø

- Lacunar infarct: 5–15 mm Ø
- Microinfarct: <1 mm Ø
- Microbleeds: <5 mm Ø
- Pathogenesis
  - Arteriosclerosis of intra- and extracranial blood vessels
  - Thrombus or embolus
  - Cardiac cause (atrial fibrillation, myocardial infarction)
  - Ruptured aneurysm
  - Sickle cell diseases and other hematological disorders predisposing for thrombosis
  - Systemic lupus erythematosus
  - Various forms of arteritis
  - Idiopathic
  - Infection-associated
  - Hereditary cerebrovascular diseases with or without vascular amyloid deposition

Criblures
- Enlarged perivascular spaces around one or more normal appearing arterioles; vessels might have hyalinotic wall thickening.
- They are wrapped by mesenchymal cells derived from the subarachnoid space or by astroglial processes.
- They are round and smooth walled.
- Size: 500–1000 µm.
- Do not contain macrophages or iron.

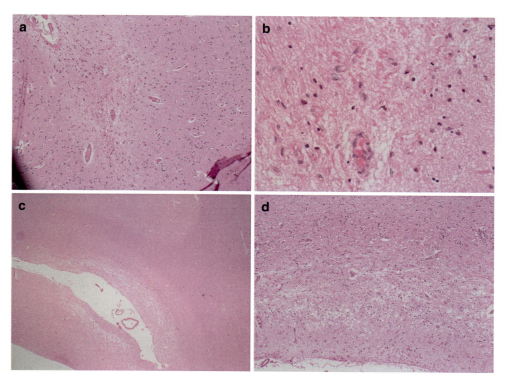

Fig. 36.3 Vascular dementia: small acute infarct (stage I) in the cortical ribbon (**a, b**), larger ischemic infarct (stage II) in the cortical ribbon (**c, d**); GFAP-reactive astrocytes (**e,f**) and reactive microgliosis (IHC: HLA-DRII) (**g,h**) in the infract area. Old infarcts (stage III) with complete tissue loss (**i–n**; **i–l**: cerebral cortex, **m**: subventricular area, **n**: hippocampus). Lacunar state (**o**) with hyalinotic vessels (**p**) enlargement of the perivascular spaces (**p**) and hemosiderinophages (**r**). There is myelin pallor/loss (**s,t**) which is due to vascular hyalinosis (**t**)

36.6 Neuropathology Findings

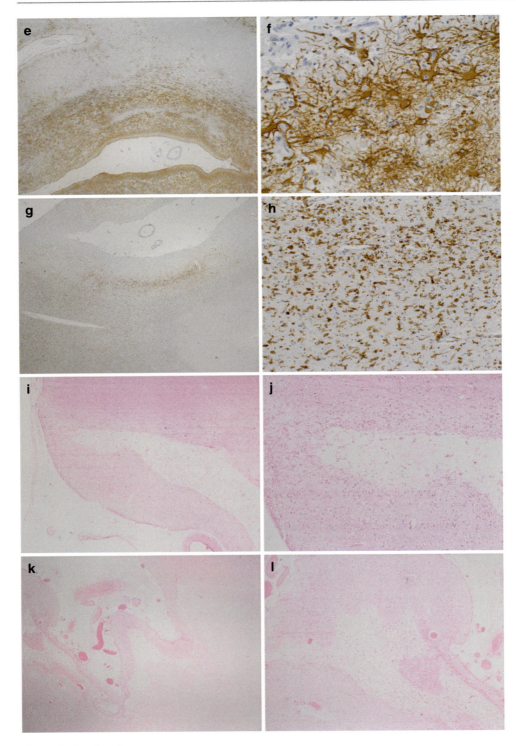

Fig. 36.3 (continued)

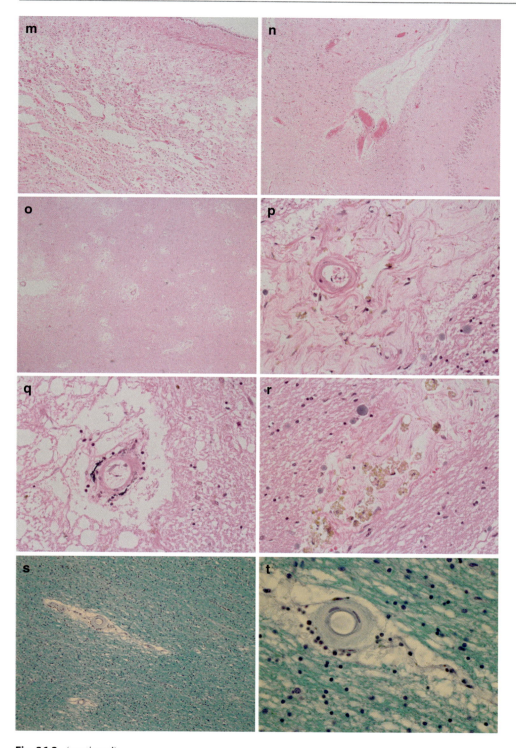

Fig. 36.3 (continued)

Lacunes

- Lacunes or lacunar infarcts are of variable size (can reach several mm) and form.
- Their wall is wrapped by proliferating astrocytes.
- May or may not contain a vessel.
- Contain macrophages.
- Located in the basal ganglia, thalamus, brain stem, and cerebellum; seldomly in cortical and subcortical structures.
- Lacunes are considered to represent infarcts that are related to arteriosclerotic pathology in the long penetrating arteries including the lenticulostriate artery.
- Many of the involved vessels are end arteries.
- Hemosiderin-loaded macrophages.
- Risk factors include atherosclerosis, arteriosclerosis, hypertension, diabetes, and old age.
- Some of the lacunes are clinically asymptomatic.

36.7 Leuko-araiosis

The term "leuko-araiosis" was introduced by Hachinski to define white matter changes in elderly persons and demented patients which are discernible on CT and MRI scans (Hachinski et al. 1986, 1987)

36.8 Morbus Binswanger

See Chap. 23

36.9 Cerebral Amyloid Angiopathy

See Chap. 23

36.10 CADASIL

See Chap. 23

36.11 Molecular Neuropathology

Three major forms can be distinguished:

- Multi-infarct dementia
- Strategic infarct dementia
- Subcortical vascular encephalopathy

Infarct size:

- Large infarct: >1 cm Ø
- Lacunar infarct: 5–15 mm Ø
- Microinfarct: <1 mm Ø
- Microbleeds: <5 mm Ø

A list of selected causes of cognitive impairment related to vascular factors is shown in Table 36.2 while common and uncommon causes of stroke pathophysiology associated with cognitive impairment or dementia are listed in Table 36.3.

A recently updated categorization of different cerebrovascular pathologies associated with dementia is given in Table 36.4.

36.12 Treatment and Prognosis

Treatment
- Control of vascular risk factors
- Long-term antiplatelet therapy
- Physiotherapy
- Speech therapy

Biologic Behavior-Prognosis-Prognostic Factors
- Progressive stepwise decline of cognitive functions
- 50% survival after 6.7 years

Table 36.2 Selected causes of cognitive impairment related to vascular factors, modified after Iadecola (2013) reproduced with kind permission by Elsevier

Condition	Predominant association/cause	Target vessel and vascular pathology	Resulting brain lesions
Hypoperfusion dementia	• Cardiac arrest/failure • Hypotension • Carotid occlusion	• Large vessel atherosclerosis • Vascular stiffening	• "Watershed" infarcts • Cortical laminar necrosis • Incomplete white matter infarcts
"Strategic infarct" dementia	• Arterial occlusion	• Large-medium size arteries	• Infarct in regions involved in cognition, e.g., frontal lobe, thalamus
Multi-infarct dementia	• Multiple arterial occlusions (embolic thrombotic)	• Large-medium size arteries and arterioles	• Multiple large infarcts • Lacunar infarcts • Microinfarcts
White matter lesions (leuko-araiosis) and lacunes	• Vascular risk factors • CADASIL and other genetic cause	• Arterioles (<300 mm Ø) • Small vessel ATS • Arteriolosclerosis • Lipohyalinosis • Venous collagenosis	• Axonal damage • Demyelination • Lacunar infarcts • Microinfarcts • Microbleeds
Microinfarcts	• CADASIL • Cerebral amyloid angiopathy (CAA) • Alzheimer disease (AD) • Vascular risk factors	• Arterioles (<300 mm Ø) • Small vessel atherosclerosis • Arteriolosclerosis	• Infarcts not visible by naked eye
Microbleeds and hemorrhages	• Cerebral amyloid angiopathy (CAA) • Alzheimer disease (AD) • CADASIL • Vascular risk factors	• Arterioles (<300 mm Ø) • Vascular rupture	• Small hemorrhage in perivascular space • Lobar or basal ganglia hemorrhage
CADASIL	• Notch 3 mutations	• Arterioles (<300 mm Ø) • Thickened wall • Smooth muscle cell granular osmiophilic material (GOM) • Pericyte loss	• White matter lesions • Lacunar infarcts • Microinfarcts • Microbleeds • Brain atrophy
Cerebral amyloid angiopathy	• Hereditary • Sporadic • Alzheimer disease	• Amyloid deposits in arteries (<2 mm Ø), arterioles, capillaries • Smooth muscle degeneration • Vascular rupture	• Hemorrhage • White matter lesions • Microinfarcts • Microbleeds
Poststroke dementia	• Ischemic stroke of any cause	• Large-medium size arteries • Perivascular immune cells	• Silent infarcts • White matter lesions • Lacunar infarcts • Neuronal loss • Brain atrophy
Mixed AD vascular dementia	• Sporadic • Vascular risk factors	• Large-medium size arteries and arterioles	• AD pathology • White matter lesions • Lacunar infarcts • Microinfarcts • Microbleeds

Table 36.3 Common and uncommon causes of stroke pathophysiology associated with cognitive impairment or dementia (Kalaria 2016) reproduced with kind permission by Springer Nature

Primary or secondary vascular disorder(s)	Common conditions	Vascular distribution	Predominant tissue changes	Form(s) of vascular dementia (VaD)/major vascular cognitive disorder (VCD)
Atherosclerotic disease	Carotid and cardiac atherosclerosis	• Aorta • Carotid • Intracranial-middle cerebral artery branches	• Cortical and territorial infarcts • White matter lesion • Infarcts • Laminar necrosis • Rarefaction	• Large vessel dementia or • Multi-infarct dementia
		• Aorta, coronary		• Hypoperfusive dementia
Embolic disease	• Cardio or carotid embolism	• Intracranial arteries • Middle cerebral artery	• Large and small infarcts	• Multi-infarct dementia
Arteriolosclerosis	• Sporadic small vessel disease	• Perforating and penetrating arteries • Lenticulostriate arteries	• Cortical infarcts • Lacunar infarcts/lacunes • Microinfarcts • White matter lesion	• Small vessel dementia • Subcortical ischemic vascular dementia • Strategic infarct dementia
		• Hypertensive vasculopathy		• Hypertensive encephalopathy with impairment • Strategic infarct dementia

Non-atherosclerotic non-inflammatory vasculopathies	• Arterial dissections (carotid, vertebral, and intracranial)
	• Fibromuscular dysplasia
	• Dolichoectatic basilar artery
	• Large artery kinking and coiling
	• Radiation-induced angiopathy
	• Moyamoya disease
		• Vertebral basilar
		• Branches of middle cerebral artery
		• Mural hematoma perforating artery
		• Small vessel disease (SVD)
			• No pattern of brain infarctions:
			  – Hemodynamic
			  – Thromboembolic
			  – Due to occlusion of a perforating artery
			• Subarachnoid hemorrhage
			• Lacunar infarcts
			• Perivascular spaces
				• Vascular cognitive impairment

	• Aneurysms—Saccular, berry, fusiform, cerebral	• Circle of Willis • Proximal branches of middle cerebral artery, posterior cerebral artery	• Hemorrhagic infarcts • Herniation	• Hemorrhagic dementia
	• Vascular malformations: cavernous hemangioma, arteriovenous, capillary	• Cortical lobes	• Rarefaction • White matter lesion	• Vascular cognitive impairment
	• Cerebral venous thrombosis	• Venous sinus • Periventricular veins	• Subcortical infarcts (thalamus) • Lobar hemorrhages	

(continued)

Table 36.3 (continued)

Primary or secondary vascular disorder(s)	Common conditions	Vascular distribution	Predominant tissue changes	Form(s) of vascular dementia (VaD)/major vascular cognitive disorder (VCD)
Amyloid angiopathies	• Hereditary CAAs (amyloid β, prion protein, cystatin C, transthyretin, gelsolin)	• Leptomeninges • Intracerebral arteries	• Cortical microinfarcts • Lacunar infarcts • White matter lesion	• Vascular cognitive impairment • Dementia
Monogenic stroke disorders	• CADASIL • CARASIL • Retinal vasculopathy with cerebral leukodystrophies (RVCLs) • Moyamoya disease • Hereditary angiopathy, nephropathy aneurysm and muscle cramps (HANAC)	• Leptomeningeal arteries • Intracerebral subcortical arteries	• Lacunar infarcts/ lacunes • Microinfarcts • White matter lesion	• Vascular cognitive impairment • Dementia
Monogenic disorders involving stroke	• Fabry disease • Familial hemiplegic migraine • Hereditary hemorrhagic telangiectasia • Vascular Ehlers–Danlos syndrome • Marfan syndrome • Pseudoxanthoma elasticum • Arterial tortuosity syndrome • Loeys–Dietz syndrome • Polycystic kidney disease • Neurofibromatosis type 1 (von Recklinghausen disease) • Carney syndrome (facial lentiginosis and myxoma)	• Branching arteries	• Cortical and subcortical infarcts • Hemorrhagic infarcts	• Vascular cognitive impairment • Dementia
Metabolic disorders	• Mitochondrial disorders (MELAS, MERRF, Leigh's disease, MIRAS) • Menkes disease • Homocystinuria • Tangier's disease	• Intracerebral small arteries • Territorial arteries	• Cortical and subcortical stroke-like lesions • Microcystic cavitation • Cortical petechial hemorrhages • Gliosis • White matter lesion	• Vascular cognitive impairment

Table 36.3 (continued)

Primary or secondary vascular disorder(s)	Common conditions	Vascular distribution	Predominant tissue changes	Form(s) of vascular dementia (VaD)/major vascular cognitive disorder (VCD)
Hematological disorders	• Paraproteinemia • Coagulopathies • Antiphospholipid antibodies • Systemic lupus erythematosus (SLE) • Nephrotic syndrome • Sneddon syndrome • Deficiencies in clotting cascade factors, e.g., protein S, C, Z • Antithrombin III • Plasminogen	• Large and intracerebral arteries	• Cortical and subcortical infarcts • Intracerebral hemorrhage • Subarachnoid hemorrhages	• Vascular cognitive impairment
Vasospastic disorders	• Subarachnoid hemorrhage • Migraine-related strokes • Paroxysmal hypertension • Drug-induced vasoconstriction	• Intracranial arteries • Middle cerebral artery	• Cortical and subcortical small infarcts	• Vascular cognitive impairment

CAA cerebral amyloid angiopathy, *CADASIL* cerebral autosomal dominant arteriopathy with subcortical infarcts and leukoencephalopathy, *CARASIL* cerebral autosomal recessive arteriopathy with subcortical infarcts and leukoencephalopathy, *MELAS* mitochondrial myopathy, encephalopathy, lactic acidosis and stroke-like episodes, *MERRF* myoclonic epilepsy with ragged red fibers, *MIRAS* mitochondrial recessive ataxic syndrome

Table 36.4 Newcastle categorization of different cerebrovascular pathologies associated with dementia (Kalaria 2016; Kalaria et al. 2004) reproduced with kind permission by Springer Nature

Subtype				
I	• Large infarcts • Cortical infarcts	• Large vessel disease • Atherosclerosis	• Focal signs • Stepwise progression	• MID • Cortical VaD
II	• Multiple small infarcts • Lacunes	• Small vessel disease • Microvascular changes	• No signs • Slight focal signs • Insidious progression	• Subcortical ischemic vascular dementia
III	• Strategic infarcts • Lacunes	• Embolic disease • Hypertensive disease	• Focal signs • Stepwise progression	• Strategic infarct dementia
IV	• Hypoperfusive lesions • Hippocampal sclerosis	• Cardiac arrest • Myocardial infarction	• Absence of focal signs • Insidious progression	• Vascular cognitive impairment • Vascular dementia
V	• Cerebral hemorrhages	• Different angiopathies	• Focal signs • Stepwise progression	• Vascular cognitive impairment • Dementia with cerebral hemorrhage
VI	• Cerebrovascular disease pathology with Alzheimer disease	• Stroke • Aging-related Alzheimer disease	• Absence of focal signs • Insidious progression	• Vascular dementia with Alzheimer disease pathology

Selected References

Bhogal P, Mahoney C, Graeme-Baker S, Roy A, Shah S, Fraioli F, Cowley P, Jager HR (2013) The common dementias: a pictorial review. Eur Radiol 23(12):3405–3417. https://doi.org/10.1007/s00330-013-3005-9

Dichgans M, Leys D (2017) Vascular cognitive impairment. Circ Res 120(3):573–591. https://doi.org/10.1161/circresaha.116.308426

Du SQ, Wang XR, Xiao LY, Tu JF, Zhu W, He T, Liu CZ (2017) Molecular mechanisms of vascular dementia: what can be learned from animal models of chronic cerebral hypoperfusion? Mol Neurobiol 54(5):3670–3682. https://doi.org/10.1007/s12035-016-9915-1

Gorelick PB, Scuteri A, Black SE, Decarli C, Greenberg SM, Iadecola C, Launer LJ, Laurent S, Lopez OL, Nyenhuis D, Petersen RC, Schneider JA, Tzourio C, Arnett DK, Bennett DA, Chui HC, Higashida RT, Lindquist R, Nilsson PM, Roman GC, Sellke FW, Seshadri S (2011) Vascular contributions to cognitive impairment and dementia: a statement for healthcare professionals from the American Heart Association/American Stroke Association. Stroke 42(9):2672–2713. https://doi.org/10.1161/STR.0b013e3182299496

Guermazi A, Miaux Y, Rovira-Canellas A, Suhy J, Pauls J, Lopez R, Posner H (2007) Neuroradiological findings in vascular dementia. Neuroradiology 49(1):1–22. https://doi.org/10.1007/s00234-006-0156-2

Hachinski VC, Potter P, Merskey H (1986) Leukoaraiosis: an ancient term for a new problem. Can J Neurol Sci 13(4 Suppl):533–534

Hachinski VC, Potter P, Merskey H (1987) Leukoaraiosis. Arch Neurol 44(1):21–23

Iadecola C (2013) The pathobiology of vascular dementia. Neuron 80(4):844–866. https://doi.org/10.1016/j.neuron.2013.10.008

Kalaria RN (2016) Neuropathological diagnosis of vascular cognitive impairment and vascular dementia with implications for Alzheimer's disease. Acta Neuropathol 131(5):659–685. https://doi.org/10.1007/s00401-016-1571-z

Kalaria RN, Kenny RA, Ballard CG, Perry R, Ince P, Polvikoski T (2004) Towards defining the neuropathological substrates of vascular dementia. J Neurol Sci 226(1–2):75–80. https://doi.org/10.1016/j.jns.2004.09.019

Khan A, Kalaria RN, Corbett A, Ballard C (2016) Update on vascular dementia. J Geriatr Psychiatry Neurol 29(5):281–301. https://doi.org/10.1177/0891988716654987

Korczyn AD, Vakhapova V, Grinberg LT (2012) Vascular dementia. J Neurol Sci 322(1–2):2–10. https://doi.org/10.1016/j.jns.2012.03.027

McAleese KE, Alafuzoff I, Charidimou A, De Reuck J, Grinberg LT, Hainsworth AH, Hortobagyi T, Ince P, Jellinger K, Gao J, Kalaria RN, Kovacs GG, Kovari E, Love S, Popovic M, Skrobot O, Taipa R, Thal DR, Werring D, Wharton SB, Attems J (2016) Post-mortem assessment in vascular dementia: advances and aspirations. BMC Med 14(1):129. https://doi.org/10.1186/s12916-016-0676-5

Narayanan L, Murray AD (2016) What can imaging tell us about cognitive impairment and dementia? World J Radiol 8(3):240–254. https://doi.org/10.4329/wjr.v8.i3.240

O'Brien JT, Thomas A (2015) Vascular dementia. Lancet 386(10004):1698–1706. https://doi.org/10.1016/s0140-6736(15)00463-8

O'Sullivan M, Morris RG, Huckstep B, Jones DK, Williams SC, Markus HS (2004) Diffusion tensor MRI correlates with executive dysfunction in patients with ischaemic leukoaraiosis. J Neurol Neurosurg Psychiatry 75(3):441–447

Rohn TT (2014) Is apolipoprotein E4 an important risk factor for vascular dementia? Int J Clin Exp Pathol 7(7):3504–3511

Schmidt H, Freudenberger P, Seiler S, Schmidt R (2012) Genetics of subcortical vascular dementia. Exp Gerontol 47(11):873–877. https://doi.org/10.1016/j.exger.2012.06.003

Sun JH, Tan L, Wang HF, Tan MS, Tan L, Li JQ, Xu W, Zhu XC, Jiang T, Yu JT (2015) Genetics of vascular dementia: systematic review and meta-analysis. J Alzheimers Dis 46(3):611–629. https://doi.org/10.3233/jad-143102

Thal DR, Grinberg LT, Attems J (2012) Vascular dementia: different forms of vessel disorders contribute to the development of dementia in the elderly brain. Exp Gerontol 47(11):816–824. https://doi.org/10.1016/j.exger.2012.05.023

Venkat P, Chopp M, Chen J (2015) Models and mechanisms of vascular dementia. Exp Neurol 272:97–108. https://doi.org/10.1016/j.expneurol.2015.05.006

Vijayan M, Reddy PH (2016) Stroke, vascular dementia, and Alzheimer's disease: molecular links. J Alzheimers Dis 54(2):427–443. https://doi.org/10.3233/jad-160527

Neurodegenerative Diseases: Parkinson Disease

37.1 Clinical Signs and Symptoms

Parkinsonism is a motor syndrome characterized by:
- Bradykinesia/hypokinesia
- Rigidity
- Tremor
- Loss of postural reflexes

Causes of parkinsonism include:
- Primary (idiopathic) parkinsonism: Parkinson disease (PD)
- Multi-system degenerations ("parkinsonism plus" or atypical parkinsonism)
- Heredodegenerative parkinsonism
- Secondary (symptomatic, acquired) parkinsonism

Parkinson disease (PD) is clinically characterized by:
- Tremor
- Bradykinesia
- Rigidity
- Postural instability
- Gait disturbance

Non-motor features of PD include:
- Pain and sensory phenomena
- Anxiety and depression
- Autonomic dysfunction
- Cognitive impairment
- Dementia
- Psychosis and hallucinations

Terminology for the three stages of PD proposed by the MDS task force International Parkinson and Movement Disorder Society are as follows (Berg et al. 2014).

Preclinical PD
- At this stage, neurodegeneration has started, but symptoms are absent
- Diagnosis of this stage consequently requires biomarkers (such as cerebrospinal fluid or imaging markers), but no such markers have yet been validated
- Note that preclinical PD requires neurodegeneration, and does not refer to simply being at risk of PD (for example, people who are carriers of a causative gene but in whom neurodegeneration has not started)

Prodromal PD
- Clinical symptoms or signs of neurodegeneration are evident
- But the patient does not have clinical PD as defined by current diagnostic criteria

Clinical PD
- This stage is defined as the presence of full parkinsonism:
  - Progressive bradykinesia plus either rest tremor, rigidity, or both

- A diagnosis of dementia could also be considered as the end of the prodromal stage, as many markers of prodromal PD are equally predictive of DLB (note that, according to the current MDS definition of PD, diagnosis with DLB does not exclude a diagnosis of PD)

Clinical Symptoms Associated with Parkinson Disease Progression
- Prodromal PD (Table 37.1)
  - REM sleep behavior disorder
  - Depression
  - Constipation
  - Anxiety
  - Hyposmia
- Early-stage PD
  - Excessive daytime sleepiness
  - Bradykinesia
  - Rigidity
  - Tremor
  - Fatigue
  - Apathy
  - Pain
  - Mild cognitive impairment
- Mid-stage PD
  - Fluctuations
  - Dyskinesias
  - Urinary symptoms
  - Orthostatic hypotension
- Late-stage PD
  - Postural instability and gait disorder
  - Dysphagia
  - Axial deformities
  - Falls
  - Dementia
  - Psychotic symptoms (visual hallucinations)

Table 37.1 Markers for prodomal PD, modified after Postuma and Berg (2016) reproduced with kind permission by Springer Nature

Marker	Level of evidence	Approximate relative risk	Estimated lead time (years)
Olfactory loss	High	5	Not estimated
REM sleep behavior disorder	High	50	13
Constipation	High	2.5	>15
Depression and anxiety	High	1.8	Uncertain, possibly biphasic
Somnolence	Moderate	1.8	Not estimated
Orthostatic hypotension	Moderate	2–10 (uncertain)	2–10 years (not directly measured)
Subtle parkinsonism	Moderate	10	4–5
Quantitative motor testing	Moderate	3–4	5
Substantia nigra hyperechogenicity	Moderate	15	Uncertain, possibly a risk marker
Urinary dysfunction	Low to moderate	2.1	>5 years (uncertain)
Erectile dysfunction	Low to moderate	1.2 (mild), 3.8 (severe)	5–10 years
Restless legs syndrome (late onset)	Low	1.5	Probably <4
Color vision loss	Low	2.5	>3 years (uncertain)
Dopaminergic PET/SPECT abnormalities	Low (but high plausibility)	20	5
PD-related pattern on SPECT/PET	Low	Unknown	Not estimated
Hippocampal hyperperfusion	Low	Unknown	Not estimated
Electrocardiogram beat-to-beat variability	Low	2	Up to 20
α-Synuclein gastrointestinal biopsy	Low	3 (uncertain)	Not estimated

37.2 Epidemiology

Incidence
- 16–19 per 100,000 per year

Prevalence
- Increases with age
- 50–59 years: 17.4 in 100,000
- 70–79 years: 93.1 in 100,000

Male-Female
- Male:Female ratio: 3:2

Median Age at Onset
- 60 years

37.3 Neuroimaging Findings

General Imaging Findings
- Atrophy of pars compacta of substantia nigra

CT Non-Contrast-Enhanced
- Normal or non-specific brain atrophy

CT Contrast-Enhanced
- No pathological enhancement

MRI-T2
- Decreased volume or disappearance of pars compacta of substantia nigra
- Hypointensity of putamen, substantia nigra, and caudate nucleus possible (caused by iron accumulation)

MRI-T1
- Non-specific brain atrophy

MRI-T1 Contrast-Enhanced
- No pathological enhancement

MRI-T2*/SWI (Fig. 37.1)
- Depigmentation of substantia nigra possible
- Loss of swallow tail sign of substantia nigra
- Hypointensities due to iron accumulation

MR-Diffusion Imaging
- Normal ADC values compared to healthy subjects
- Increased ADC values in PSP (progressive supranuclear palsy) and CBD (cortico-basal degeneration) compared to PD (Parkinson disease)—may help to distinguish PD from other forms of parkinsonism

MR-Spectroscopy
- Decreased NAA values possible

Nuclear Medicine Imaging Findings (Figs. 37.2, 37.3, and 37.4)
- Parkinson disease is showing presynaptic dopamine transporter deficit with SPECT tracers like FP-CIT or β-CIT.
- There is a more asymmetric loss in contrast to atypical Parkinson syndromes but there is a large overlap which allows no differentiation because of that.
- Symmetric loss of little degree is seen in vascular changes.
- Vascular changes can also result in an accentuated loss of tracer binding in caudate nucleus.

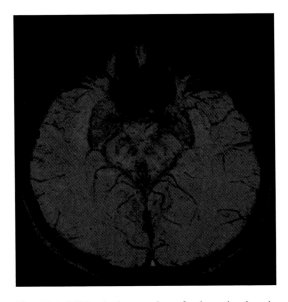

Fig. 37.1 MRI—depigmentation of substantia nigra in SWI

- Reports state a more evident gradient between the caudate head and putamen in Parkinson disease than in atypical parkinsonian syndromes.
- 18F-DOPA PET is used to assess the presynaptic decarboxylase function and dopamine turnover producing similar results than SPECT tracers.
- Semi-quantitative analysis can be performed comparing the tracer uptake of the striatum and the uptake in the occipital cortex or the cerebellum after summing the slices showing the striatum. For this analysis it has to be taken into account, that medication (i.e., serotonin reuptake inhibitors), vascular changes, and normal aging reduce tracer uptake. For each camera system, standardized values have to be established.
- In contrast to atypical parkinsonian syndromes, the postsynaptic dopamine (D2) receptors are not affected.

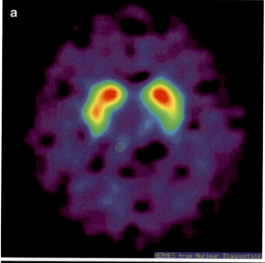

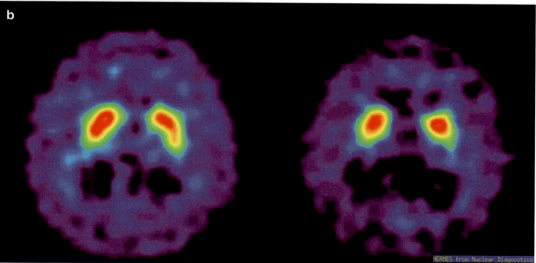

Fig. 37.2 FP-CIT SPECT of a patient with incipient IPS—reduced tracer-uptake in the left putamen correlating to a movement disorder of the right arm (**a**). FP-CIT SPECT of a patient with only minimal reduced uptake in the left putamen in 2012 (left) and distinct loss of tracer-binding in 2013 (right) (**b**). Slices of an FP-CIT SPECT of a 50-year-old patient with advanced IPS (**c**)

37.3 Neuroimaging Findings

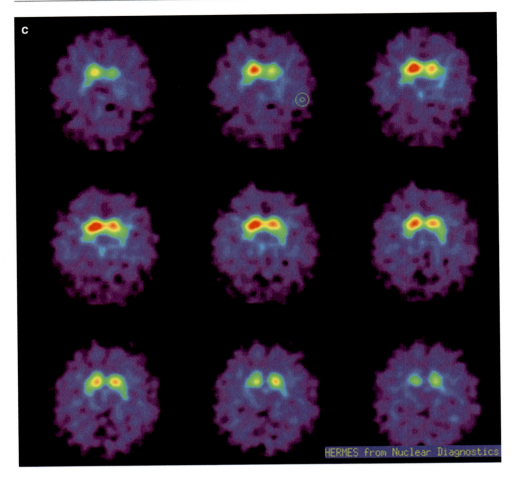

Fig. 37.2 (continued)

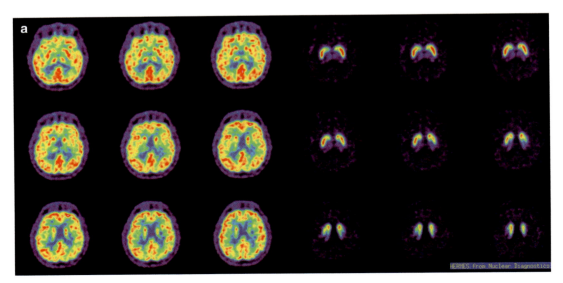

Fig. 37.3 FDG-PET (left) and Fallypride-PET (right) with normal uptake (**a**) and FP-CIT-Pet (left) and DOPA-PET (right) in the same patient with Parkinson disease (**b**). The normal uptake in (**a**) indicates that atypical Parkinson disease can be discarded in the differential diagnosis

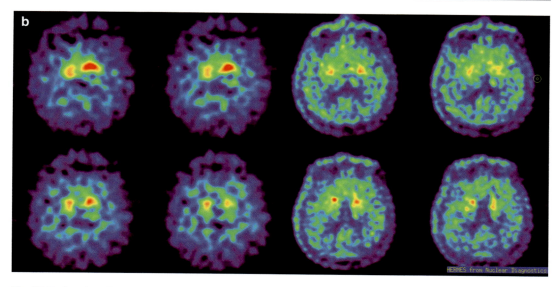

Fig. 37.3 (continued)

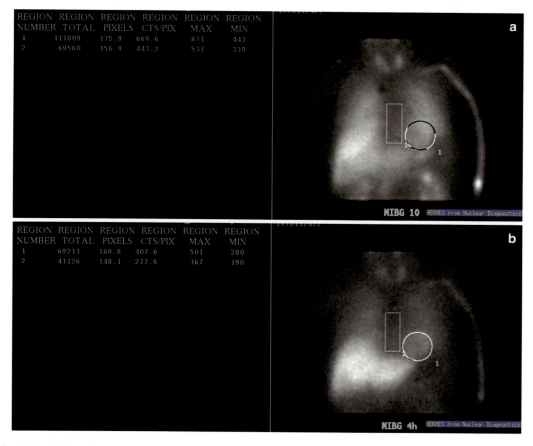

Fig. 37.4 Iodine-123-meta-iodobenzylguanidine (MIBG) scan registered after 10 min (**a**) and 4 h (**b**) comparing activities of the heart and mediastinum in the same patient as shown in Fig. 37.3. The ratio shows reduced cardial uptake which is indicative of sympathomimetic denervation of the heart and supports the diagnosis of Parkinson disease

- In contrast to atypical parkinsonian syndromes, there is an upregulation of the postsynaptic D2 receptors in the first few years of PD.
- SPECT studies with IBZM or PET studies with tracers like 11C-raclopride or 18F-fallypride allow a differentiation between PD and atypical Parkinsonian syndromes.
- Additional CBF-SPECT and FDG-PET studies revealed hypoperfusion and hypometabolism in patients with Parkinson-dementia, which is similar to DLB patients but the motor symptoms occur earlier.
- Myocardial sympathetic innervation can be assessed with 123I-MIBG or 18F-dopamine. Reports state a statistically inferior uptake in PD than in atypical parkinsonian syndromes by comparing myocardial and mediastinal uptake.

- Surviving neurons contain intracytoplasmatic Lewy bodies (LBs)
- Lewy bodies are:
  - Eosinophilic structures with a dense core and a concentric lamellar structure
  - Approximately 15 μm in diameter
  - Immunoreactive for:
    - α-Synuclein (Fig. 37.7a–h)
    - Ubiquitin
    - Neurofilamentprotein
    - Tubulin
    - Microtubule-associated proteins (MAP-1 und MAP-2)
  - Immunonegativity for:
    - Tau-protein
  - Ultrastructurally composed of:
    - Neurofilaments with a diameter of 11 nm
    - Mitochondria
    - Lipofuscin
    - Smooth endoplasmatic reticulum
- Six stages in the evolution of PD-related pathology are defined (Table 37.2).

37.4 Neuropathology Findings

Macroscopical Findings (Fig. 37.5a–d)
- Depigmentation of the substantia nigra
- Depigmentation might sometimes not be so conspicuous

Microscopical Findings (Fig. 37.6a–n)
- Loss of catecholaminergic neurons in the substantia nigra and locus coeruleus
- Deposition of melanin pigment in the neuropil or macrophages

Dementia in Parkinson Disease
- Approximately 15–40% of patients with idiopathic PD develop signs of subcortical dementia
- Occurs late during disease course
- Microscopic changes:
  - Few plaques and neurofibrillary tangles in the neocortex
  - Higher amount of tangles in the entorhinal cortex and hippocampus

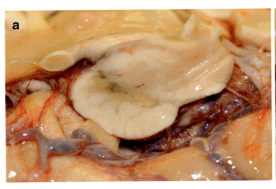
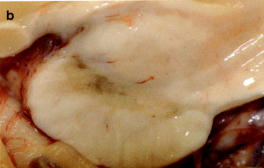

Fig. 37.5 Macroscopic appearance of the pallor of the substantia nigra in the fresh brain (**a**, **b**) and in the fixed brain (**c**, **d**)

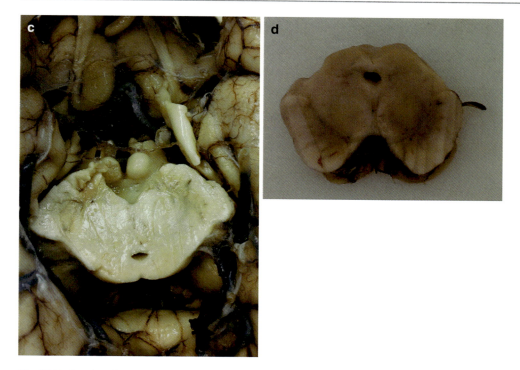

Fig. 37.5 (continued)

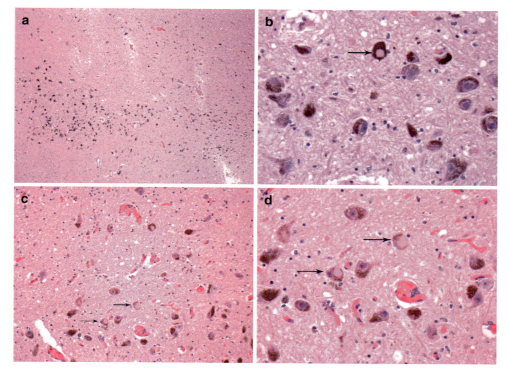

Fig. 37.6 Slight (**a**, **b**) and severe (**c**, **d**) loss of neurons in the substantia nigra. Various appearances (→) of Lewy bodies in nigral neurons (**e–l**). Presence of reactive astrogliosis in proximity of a Lewy body bearing neuron (→) (**m**, **n**)

37.4 Neuropathology Findings

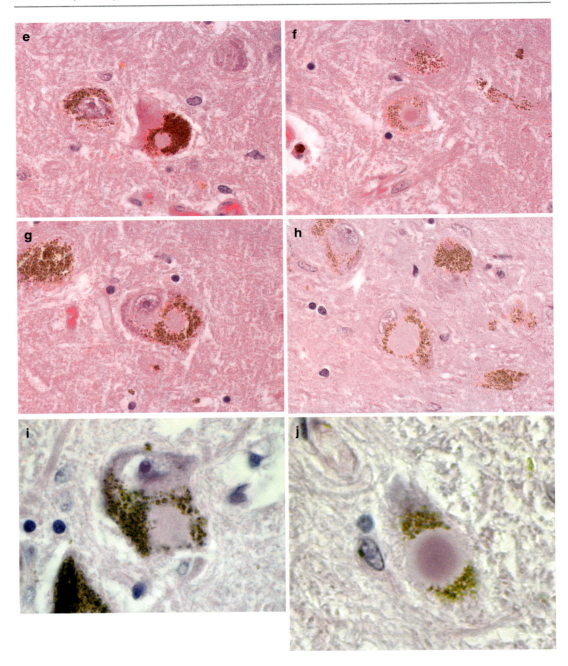

Fig. 37.6 (continued)

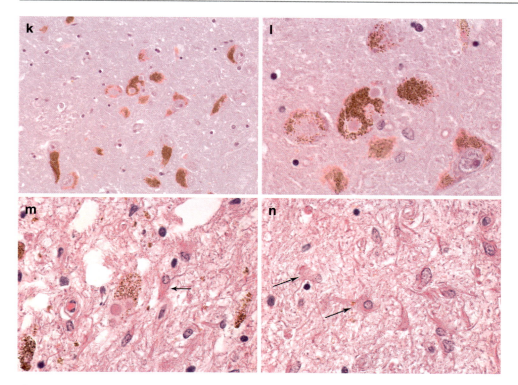

Fig. 37.6 (continued)

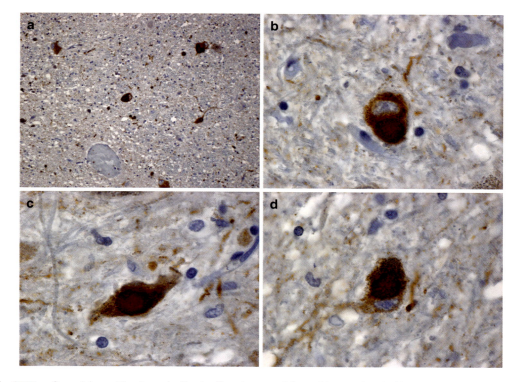

Fig. 37.7 α-Synuclein positive Lewy bodies (**a–d**) and α-synuclein positive neurites (**e–h**)

37.4 Neuropathology Findings

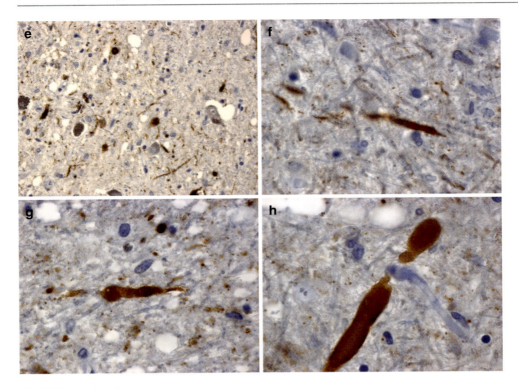

Fig. 37.7 (continued)

Table 37.2 Stages in the evolution of PD-related pathology, modified after Braak et al. (2003) reproduced with kind permission from Elsevier

Stage	Stage name	Involved regions
1	Medulla oblongata	• Dorsal IX/X motor nucleus and/or • Intermediate reticular zone
2	Medulla oblongata + pontine tegmentum	• Stage 1+ • Caudal raphe nuclei • Gigantocellular reticular nucleus • Coeruleus-subcoeruleus complex
3	Midbrain	• Stage 2+ • Midbrain (pars compacta of substantia nigra)
4	Basal prosencephalon + mesocortex	• Stage 3+ • Prosencephalon (temporal mesocortex-transentorhinal region • Allocortex-CA2-plexus
5	Neocortex	• Stage 4+ • High-order sensory association areas of the neocortex and prefrontal neocortex
6	Neocortex	• Stage 5+ • First order sensory association areas of the neocortex • Premotor areas

- High amounts of diffuse plaques in the neocortex
- Other regions usually devoid of these lesions or undistinguishable from normal aging
- Numerous Lewy bodies in the neocortex
- No significant differences of changes in the substantia nigra between non-demented and demented PD patients

37.5 Molecular Neuropathology

37.5.1 Pathogenesis

- Oxidative stress, reactive species production
- Mitochondrial dysfunction
- Excitotoxicity
- Increased intracellular free calcium
- Protein aggregation
- Inflammation
- Hyperactivity in the subthalamic nucleus (STN) and internal globus pallidus (GPi) (Fig. 37.8)

- Loss of dopaminergic neurons in the SN results in dopamine deficiency in the nigrostriatal pathway

Functions of Synuclein
- Physiological
  - Binds to tubulin and enhances microtubule formation
  - Regulates the fusion and clustering of pre-synaptic vesicles
  - Involved in exocytosis and presynaptic dopamine release
- Pathological—Loss-of-function effects
  - Impairs microtubule formation and axonal transport
  - Causes presynaptic dysfunction and abnormal neurotransmitter release
- Pathological—Gain-of-function effects
  - Causes mitochondrial dysfunction, leading to increased oxidative stress
  - Overwhelms the calcium buffering capacity of the cell
  - Induces ER stress

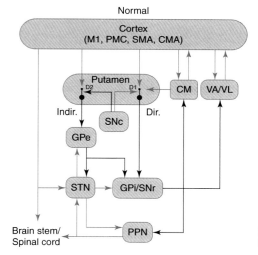
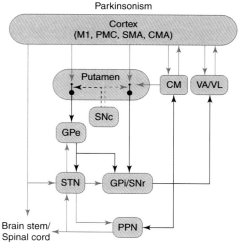

Fig. 37.8 The disturbed basal ganglia-thalamocortical motor circuit in Parkinson disease as compared to normal. Black arrows indicate inhibitory connections; gray arrows indicate excitatory connections. Abbreviations: *CM* centromedian nucleus of thalamus, *CMA* cingulate motor area, *Dir.* direct pathway, *D1, D2* dopamine receptor subtypes, *GPe* external segment of the globus pallidus, *GPi* internal segment of the globus pallidus, *Indir.* indirect pathway, *M1* primary motor cortex, *Pf* parafascicular nucleus of the thalamus, *PMC* premotor cortex, *PPN* pedunculopontine nucleus, *SMA* supplementary motor area, *SNc* substantia nigra pars compacta, *SNr* substantia nigra pars reticulate, *STN* subthalamic nucleus, *VA* ventral anterior nucleus of thalamus, *VL* ventrolateral nucleus of thalamus (reproduced from Galvan and Wichmann (2008) with kind permission by Elsevier, open access)

37.5 Molecular Neuropathology

- Disrupts ER and Golgi trafficking
- Impairs proteostasis, including protein degradation by the ubiquitin-proteasome and autophagy-lysosomal systems
- Facilitates the pathological aggregation of other proteins (e.g., amyloid or tau)
- Promotes neuroinflammation

37.5.2 Genetics

Based on the genetic background, two forms of PD can be distinguished:

- *Familial (monogenic) PD*:
  - This heritable form accounts for only 5–10% of cases
  - Causative mutations in single genes are transmitted in a Mendelian manner in families (autosomal dominant or autosomal recessive)
- *Sporadic (idiopathic) PD*:
  - Various genetic alterations in combination with external factors (lifestyle, environmental influences) are responsible for the disease
  - This "classical" form represents the vast majority of the PD cases

Historically, genomic loci with putative linkage to PD were designated "PARK" and numbered consecutively. Of the more than 20 PARK loci described to date, only a few could be conclusively correlated with PD etiology; so far, mutations causing hereditary PD were definitely confirmed in only six genes. Recently, several more genes have been implicated with the disease, whereas the remaining PD-related loci are suspected genetic risk factors. A short summary is given below and in Table 37.1.

37.5.2.1 Confirmed Causative Genes in PD (Table 37.3)
Autosomal Dominant Gene Alterations
- *SNCA* gene (PARK1, PARK4) (Table 37.3):
  - Located at chromosome region 4q22.1; encodes α-synuclein which appears to be involved in presynaptic neurotransmission.
  - Several missense mutations that alter the protein sequence and cause PD have been identified; the most prominent, A53T (i.e., Ala53Thr), was described in several affected families, whereas the A30P-, E46K-, G51D-, and H50Q variants each were found in single families.
  - In addition to these point mutations, duplication and triplication of the *SCNA* coding region also occurs, resulting in overexpression and increased levels of wild-type α-synuclein.
  - Clinical symptoms of PD as a result of *SCNA* aberrations are heterogeneous, ranging from cognitive impairment/dementia to autonomic dysfunction and seizures. A common feature, however, is the early onset of PD (EOPD) with an average age of ~45 years for A53T carriers and several years later for patients with the A30P-, E46K-, G51D-, and H50Q mutations. Notably, *SNCA* triplication results in a ~10 years earlier onset and rapid progression, as compared to *SCNA* duplication which is associated with milder symptoms and a prolonged life span.
- *LRRK2* gene (PARK8) (Table 37.3):
  - Located at chromosome region 12q12; encodes leucine-rich repeat kinase 2 which is involved in a variety of cellular signaling pathways in neurons.
  - The frequency of *LRRK2* mutations in PD pathology is significantly higher than that reported for *SCNA*. More than 100 missense mutations have been described, many of which are not only linked to familial, but also to sporadic PD. Of those, however, only a few were unequivocally proven as causative agents for the disease.
  - G2019S is the most commonly observed pathogenic mutation in PD patients, albeit with variable prevalence, depending on the population investigated. For instance, the highest numbers are reported for North African Arab patients (~40%), the lowest (less than 1%) for Asian populations. Moreover, G2019S also exhibits increasing penetrance with increasing age (from 28%

Table 37.3 Selected PARK-designated PD-related loci

Locus	Chromosome region	Gene	Protein/proposed function(s)	Inheritance	Phenotype	Aberrations
Confirmed loci						
PARK1 (PARK4)	4q22.1	SNCA	α-Synuclein/presynaptic neurotransmission	AD	EOPD	Missense mutations, genomic multiplications
PARK8	12q12	LRRK2	Leucine-rich repeat kinase 2/vesicular transport, cytoskeleton, mitochondrial function	AD	Classical PD	Missense mutations
PARK17	16q11.2	VPS35	Vacuolar protein sorting 35, retromer complex component/retrograde vesicular transport	AD	Classical PD	Missense mutation
PARK2	6q26	PRKN	Parkin RBR E3 ubiquitin protein ligase/ubiquitination of proteins for proteasomal degradation, mitochondrial quality control	AR	EOPD (juvenile parkinsonism)	Missense/nonsense mutations, exonic rearrangements
PARK6	1p36.12	PINK1	PTEN-induced putative kinase 1/mitochondrial quality control	AR	EOPD	Missense/nonsense mutations, exonic rearrangements
PARK7	1p36.23	DJ-1	DJ-1 (Parkinsonism-associated deglycase)/protection against oxidative stress, transcriptional regulation of PINK1	AR	EOPD	Missense mutations, exonic rearrangements
Unconfirmed loci						
PARK19	1p31.3	DNAJC6	DnaJ heat shock protein family (Hsp40) member C6 (= auxilin)/clathrin-associated endocytosis in neurons	AR	Juvenile parkinsonism, pyramidal signs, dementia	Splice site mutation, nonsense/missense mutations
PARK9	1p36.13	ATP13A2	ATPase 13A2/membrane transport of cations, mitochondrial integrity	AR	Juvenile parkinsonism, Kufor-Rakeb syndrome	Missense/nonsense mutations, deletions
PARK14	22q13.1	PLA2G6	Phospholipase A2 group VI/phospholipid hydrolysis, mitochondrial integrity	AR	Early-onset parkinsonism-dystonia	Missense mutations
PARK15	22q12.3	FBXO7	F-box only protein 7/ubiquitination, mitochondrial integrity	AR	Juvenile parkinsonism and pyramidal signs	Homozygous/compound heterozygous mutations
PARK18	3q27.1	EIF4G1	Eukaryotic translation initiation factor 4 gamma 1/protein synthesis	AD	Classical PD	Missense mutations

AD autosomal dominant, *AR* autosomal recessive, *EOPD* early-onset Parkinson disease

at age 59 to 74% at age 79). The second most frequent mutation is R1441G, the remaining are R1441C/H, Y1699C, S1761R, I2012T, I2020T, and N1437H (Hernandez et al. 2016).
- The clinical manifestation of LRRK2 mutations shows a high resemblance to the classical sporadic PD phenotype, with late onset of the disease at about 60 years of age and slow progression.
- *VPS35* gene (PARK17) (Table 37.3):
  - Located at chromosome region 16q11.2; encodes vacuolar protein sorting 35, retromer complex component, which is involved in cellular retrograde vesicular transport.
  - An autosomal dominant pathogenic mutation in *VPS35*, resulting in a D620N exchange at the protein level, was identified in two independent European families as the causative agent for PD of a classical phenotype, with an average disease onset of slightly over 50 years of age. Several more missense mutations were reported but their pathogenicity could not be established yet.

Autosomal Recessive Gene Alterations
- *PRKN* gene (PARK2) (Table 37.3):
  - Located at chromosome region 6q26; encodes parkin (official full name: parkin RBR E3 ubiquitin protein ligase) which is involved in the ubiquitination of proteins to tag them for degradation in the proteasome. Parkin also is activated by PTEN-induced putative kinase 1 (see below) to counteract mitochondrial dysfunction.
  - Over 100 pathogenic gene alterations, spread across all 12 exons, have been recognized, including not only point mutations but also deletions and multiplications. Parkin aberrations are primarily associated with the rare autosomal recessive juvenile parkinsonism (ARJP) with very early onset (20–30 years of age). Notably, the typical LB pathology is missing in the majority of the observed cases.

- *PINK1* gene (PARK6) (Table 37.3):
  - Located at chromosome region 1p36.12; encodes PTEN-induced putative kinase 1 which phosphorylates ubiquitin and parkin, thereby triggering the degradation process of dysfunctional mitochondria.
  - The first described pathogenic homozygous point mutations were G309D and a nonsense mutation W437X; the latter results in the production of a protein with a C-terminally truncated kinase domain. Later, several more point mutations as well as exonic rearrangements were identified in patients with EOPD. In contrast to the parkin-related phenotype (see above), LB pathology can be observed.
- *DJ-1* gene (PARK7) (Table 37.3):
  - Located at chromosome region 1p36.23; encodes DJ-1 (official full name: Parkinsonism-associated deglycase) which has been implicated to contribute to several cellular processes such as protection against oxidative stress, transcriptional modulation of *PINK1*, and glucose metabolism.
  - Only a minor fraction of EOPD cases (~1%) are caused by mutations in *DJ-1*. The observed homozygous aberrations include missense mutations (E163K, L166P) as well as a deletion of exons 1–5 and a duplication in the promoter region of the gene.

37.5.2.2 Putative Pathogenic Genes in PD

More recently, several other PD candidate genes carrying possible causative mutations were proposed; however, owing to the lack of more supporting data, most of these findings are still unconfirmed to date.

- *DNAJC6* gene (PARK19) (Table 37.3):
  - Located at chromosome region 1p31.3; encodes DnaJ heat shock protein family (Hsp40) member C6 (= auxilin) which is involved in clathrin-mediated endocytosis in neurons.

- So far, a homozygous splice site mutation, nonsense mutations, a missense mutation, and a heterozygous aberration were reported in different unrelated families. The clinical phenotype ranged from juvenile parkinsonism with a very early onset at about 10 years of age to EOPD (mean onset over 30 years).
- *ATP13A2* gene (PARK9) (Table 37.3):
  - Located at chromosome region 1p36.13; encodes ATPase 13A2 which plays a role in cation homeostasis (Zn^{2+}, Mn^{2+}) and mitochondrial integrity.
  - Genetic aberrations have been associated with the rare Kufor-Rakeb disorder.
- *PLA2G6* gene (PARK14) (Table 37.3):
  - Located at chromosome region 22q13.1; encodes phospholipase A2 group VI which participates in phospholipid degradation and mitochondrial integrity.
  - Missense mutations appear to be linked to parkinsonism with dystonia; frequently, iron accumulation in the brain is observed.
- *FBXO7* gene (PARK15) (Table 37.3):
  - Located at chromosome region 22q12.3; encodes F-box only protein 7 which interacts with parkin and PTEN-induced putative kinase 1 in the ubiquitination pathway.
  - Homozygous and compound heterozygous mutations are found in patients with juvenile parkinsonian-pyramidal syndrome.
- *EIF4G1* gene (PARK18) (Table 37.3):
  - Located at chromosome region 3q27.1; encodes eukaryotic translation initiation factor 4 gamma 1, a subunit of the EIF4F complex which participates in protein synthesis.
  - Two missense mutations (R1205H and A502V) were reported in a family with autosomal dominant PD; however, other studies discovered these variants also in healthy controls.

Mitochondrial Dysfunction in PD
- Data currently available on the interplay between *PRKN*, *PINK1*, and *DJ-1* suggest that the three gene products participate in common (or parallel) pathways controlling mitochondria quality, thus protecting cells from damage due to mitochondrial dysfunction and/or oxidative stress (Truban et al. 2017).
- Additionally, recent studies highlighted the involvement of mitochondrial DNA (mtDNA) alterations in PD pathology. Such aberrations include reduced copy number, deletions, and point mutations, frequently observed in dopaminergic neurons of the substantia nigra in PD patients.
- In this context, the most common biochemical manifestation is a deficiency of complex I of the electron transport chain, resulting in impaired mitochondrial function (Giannoccaro et al. 2017).

Genetic Risk Factors for Developing PD
- Advances in molecular techniques have provided new tools to search for associations between genetic traits and the probability of developing a certain disease. For example, genome-wide association studies (GWAS) in sporadic PD have established several genetic risk loci, where variations appear to correlate with increased disease susceptibility. Currently, the most replicated PD risk loci are *SNCA*, *LRRK2*, *MAPT*, and *GBA*.
- *SCNA* and *LRRK2* were discussed earlier in the context of inherited monogenic PD (see above). Apart from the established single nucleotide polymorphisms (SNPs) representing the disease-causing missense mutations in the two genes, several other aberrations, e.g., SNPs in regulatory sequences, were recognized as low- to moderate risk factors for sporadic PD, associated with ~1.2- to ~2.2-fold increase in risk, depending on the ethnic background (Lill 2016).
- The *MAPT* gene encodes the microtubule-associated protein tau which is generally known to be involved in Alzheimer disease. *MAPT* resides at chromosome locus 17q21.31; in Caucasians, a 900 kb inversion of this

region is frequently identified, yielding two distinct haplotypes, H1 and H2. The common *MAPT* haplotype H1 has been associated with increased PD risk.
- *GBA* is located at chromosome region 1q22 and encodes the lysosomal enzyme glucosylceramidase beta which catalyzes the breakdown of glycosylceramide. *GBA* mutations were shown to cause Gaucher disease, a lysosomal storage disorder, which phenotypically is often accompanied by signs of parkinsonism. Based on this notion, large-scale genetic association studies led to the identification of heterozygous *GBA* mutations representing significant risk factors (up to ~fivefold increase) for developing PD, often associated with dementia. The most frequently detected alterations are N370S and L444P.

37.5.3 Epigenetics

Epigenetic regulation, such as DNA-/RNA methylation, changes in histone modification and altered microRNA (miR) levels, appears to play an important role in PD etiology. Epigenetic mechanisms mainly modulate gene expression, thereby affecting cellular protein levels. Reviewed in: Labbe et al. (2016) and Feng et al. (2015).

DNA Methylation
- Two commonly acknowledged PD genes, *SNCA* and *MAPT*, were shown to exhibit different methylation patterns in patients and healthy controls. Generally, a low-methylation status (hypomethylation) correlates with increased protein expression, whereas hypermethylation is associated with reduced protein levels. In several brain regions of PD patients, hypomethylation of the *SNCA*- and *MAPT* loci was observed, yielding higher protein levels in the patients as compared to controls.
- To date, epigenome-wide association studies involving samples from PD patients vs. controls have identified many more differentially methylated genes. Among them, *FANCC* and *TNKS2* should be highlighted since both genes showed significant methylation differences which were confirmed by two independent methodological approaches (Moore et al. 2014). *FANCC* encodes Fanconi anemia complementation group C, a protein involved in DNA repair, and *TNKS2* codes for tankyrase 2, a poly-ADP-ribosyltransferase which regulates telomere length.
- The observed hypermethylation of both genes in PD samples results in underexpression or lack of the gene products, thus compromising chromosomal integrity.

Histone Modification
- Histone methylation and -acetylation are common mechanisms modulating transcription of nuclear genes. For instance, acetylation of histones facilitates gene expression by rendering chromosomal DNA more accessible to the transcriptional machinery. On the other hand, histone de-acetylation is linked to transcriptional repression and gene silencing.
- It has been demonstrated that α-synuclein affects the physiological levels of histone acetylation in the nucleus of neuronal cells. Binding of nuclear α-synuclein to histones prevents acetylation which in turn appears to promote the formation of α-synuclein aggregates. In addition, mutated forms of α-synuclein carrying the PD-related mutations, A53T and A30P, exhibit enhanced nuclear localization as compared to the wild-type protein, which potentiates the pathological process.

Non-coding RNAs
Non-coding RNAs are important modulators of gene expression. In the context of Parkinson disease, long non-coding RNAs (lncRNAs) and small non-coding RNAs (microRNAs; miRs) have been recognized as epigenetic factors. For instance, lncRNA RP11-115D19.1, with a length

of over 500 nucleotides, was identified as an antisense RNA molecule which downregulates α-synuclein expression by binding to the 3′-region of the *SNCA* mRNA. Conversely, downregulated RP11-115D19.1 results in enhanced α-synuclein levels.

Several studies established that microRNAs are also involved in PD-related gene expression. Some of the confirmed miRs are highlighted in the following.

- *miR-133b*:
  - miR-133b is expressed in healthy midbrain dopaminergic neurons but deficient in PD-derived tissues. Its expression is promoted by Pitx3, a transcription factor that plays a crucial role in dopaminergic neuron differentiation. In turn, however, high levels of miR-133b decrease Pitx3 production which may reflect a well-balanced regulatory loop that is malfunctioning in Parkinson disease.
- *miR-7 and miR-153*:
  - Both microRNAs directly bind to SCNA mRNA, thereby reducing α-synuclein expression. This interaction is an important mechanism involved in maintaining physiological concentrations of the protein. Impaired expression of both miR-7 and miR-153 results in increased α-synuclein levels.
- *miR-155*:
  - It has been demonstrated that miR-155 is involved in the modulation of neuroinflammatory responses to α-synuclein. Presence of miR-155 triggers inflammation, whereas its absence reduces inflammatory processes which has a neuroprotective effect.

Finally, a few more microRNAs have been identified that regulate the expression of other PD-related genes:

- miR-205 downregulates LRRK2 expression by binding to *LRRK2* mRNA
- miR-34b and -34c are involved in the regulation of parkin- and DJ-1 expression
- miR-125b and miR-138 have been implicated with tau hyperphosphorylation

37.6 Treatment and Prognosis

Treatment
- Short-term benefit from physical
- Medical therapies
  - Levodopa
  - Anticholinergics
  - Amantadine
  - Dopamine receptor agonists
  - Catechol-O-methyltransferase (COMT) inhibition
  - Monoaminooxidase type B (MAO-B) inhibitors
- Surgical therapies
  - Deep brain stimulation
  - Lesional surgery
    Pallidotomy
    Subthalamotomy
    Thalamotomy
  - Dopamine transplantation

Biologic Behavior–Prognosis–Prognostic Factors
- Slow progression of symptoms over several years
- Average duration until death: 9–15 years
- Side effects from medication:
  - Motor fluctuations occur in 30–80% of patients after 5 years of treatment
  - Dyskinesias
- Prognostic factors:
  - Gait disturbance or postural instability associated with severe disease
  - Cases with tremor-dominant parkinsonism have favorable course and slower progression
  - Onset after age 60 years associated with greater probability of developing dementia

Selected References

Berg D, Postuma RB, Bloem B, Chan P, Dubois B, Gasser T, Goetz CG, Halliday GM, Hardy J, Lang AE, Litvan I, Marek K, Obeso J, Oertel W, Olanow CW, Poewe W, Stern M, Deuschl G (2014) Time to redefine PD? Introductory statement of the MDS Task Force on the definition of Parkinson's disease. Mov Disord 29(4):454–462. https://doi.org/10.1002/mds.25844

Braak H, Del Tredici K, Rub U, de Vos RA, Jansen Steur EN, Braak E (2003) Staging of brain pathology related to sporadic Parkinson's disease. Neurobiol Aging 24(2):197–211

Brooks DJ (2010a) Imaging approaches to Parkinson disease. J Nucl Med 51(4):596–609. https://doi.org/10.2967/jnumed.108.059998

Brooks DJ (2010b) Imaging dopamine transporters in Parkinson's disease. Biomark Med 4(5):651–660. https://doi.org/10.2217/bmm.10.86

Ciurleo R, Di Lorenzo G, Bramanti P (2014) Magnetic resonance spectroscopy: an in vivo molecular imaging biomarker for Parkinson's disease? Biomed Res Int 2014:519816. https://doi.org/10.1155/2014/519816

De Rosa P, Marini ES, Gelmetti V, Valente EM (2015) Candidate genes for Parkinson disease: Lessons from pathogenesis. Clin Chim Acta 449:68–76. https://doi.org/10.1016/j.cca.2015.04.042

van der Merwe C, Jalali Sefid Dashti Z, Christoffels A, Loos B, Bardien S (2015) Evidence for a common biological pathway linking three Parkinson's disease-causing genes: parkin, PINK1 and DJ-1. Eur J Neurosci 41(9):1113–1125. https://doi.org/10.1111/ejn.12872. Epub 2015 Mar 11

Dorszewska J, Kozubski W (2016) Introductory chapter – genetic and biochemical factors in Parkinson's disease. In: Dorszewska J, Kozubski W (eds) Challenges in Parkinson's disease. InTech, Rijeka, pp 1–6. https://doi.org/10.5772/64216

Feng Y, Jankovic J, Wu YC (2015) Epigenetic mechanisms in Parkinson's disease. J Neurol Sci 349(1–2):3–9. https://doi.org/10.1016/j.jns.2014.1012.1017. Epub 2014 Dec 18

Ferreira M, Massano J (2017) An updated review of Parkinson's disease genetics and clinicopathological correlations. Acta Neurol Scand 135(3):273–284. https://doi.org/10.1111/ane.12616. Epub 2016 June 8

Galvan A, Wichmann T (2008) Pathophysiology of parkinsonism. Clin Neurophysiol 119(7):1459–1474. https://doi.org/10.1016/j.clinph.2008.03.017

Giannoccaro MP, La Morgia C, Rizzo G, Carelli V (2017) Mitochondrial DNA and primary mitochondrial dysfunction in Parkinson's disease. Mov Disord 32(3):346–363. https://doi.org/10.1002/mds.26966. Epub 2017 Mar 2

Hernandez DG, Reed X, Singleton AB (2016) Genetics in Parkinson disease: Mendelian versus non-Mendelian inheritance. J Neurochem 139(Suppl 1):59–74. https://doi.org/10.1111/jnc.13593. Epub 2016 Apr 18

Holtbernd F, Eidelberg D (2014) The utility of neuroimaging in the differential diagnosis of parkinsonian syndromes. Semin Neurol 34(2):202–209. https://doi.org/10.1055/s-0034-1381733

Kalia LV, Lang AE (2015) Parkinson's disease. Lancet 386(9996):896–912. https://doi.org/10.1016/S0140-6736(1014)61393-3. Epub 2015 Apr 19

Kalinderi K, Bostantjopoulou S, Fidani L (2016) The genetic background of Parkinson's disease: current progress and future prospects. Acta Neurol Scand 12(10):12563

La Cognata V, D'Agata V, Cavalcanti F, Cavallaro S (2016) Genetics of Parkinson's disease: the role of copy number variations. In: Dorszewska J, Kozubski W (eds) Challenges in Parkinson's disease. InTech, Rijeka, pp 7–38. https://doi.org/10.5772/62881

Labbe C, Lorenzo-Betancor O, Ross OA (2016) Epigenetic regulation in Parkinson's disease. Acta Neuropathol 132(4):515–530. https://doi.org/10.1007/s00401-016-1590-9. Epub 2016 June 29

Lill CM (2016) Genetics of Parkinson's disease. Mol Cell Probes 30(6):386–396. https://doi.org/10.1016/j.mcp.2016.11.001. Epub 2016 Nov 4

Michel PP, Hirsch EC, Hunot S (2016) Understanding dopaminergic cell death pathways in Parkinson disease. Neuron 90(4):675–691. https://doi.org/10.1016/j.neuron.2016.03.038

Moore K, McKnight AJ, Craig D, O'Neill F (2014) Epigenome-wide association study for Parkinson's disease. Neuromolecular Med 16(4):845–855. https://doi.org/10.1007/s12017-014-8332-8. Epub 2014 Oct 11

Obeso JA, Stamelou M (2017) Past, present, and future of Parkinson's disease: a special essay on the 200th anniversary of the Shaking Palsy. Mov Disord 32(9):1264–1310. https://doi.org/10.1002/mds.27115

Oertel W, Schulz JB (2016) Current and experimental treatments of Parkinson disease: a guide for neuroscientists. J Neurochem. https://doi.org/10.1111/jnc.13750

Pihlstrom L, Morset KR, Grimstad E, Vitelli V, Toft M (2016) A cumulative genetic risk score predicts progression in Parkinson's disease. Mov Disord 8(10):26505

Postuma RB, Berg D (2016) Advances in markers of prodromal Parkinson disease. Nat Rev Neurol 12(11):622–634. https://doi.org/10.1038/nrneurol.2016.152

Rizzo G, Martinelli P, Manners D, Scaglione C, Tonon C, Cortelli P, Malucelli E, Capellari S, Testa C, Parchi P, Montagna P, Barbiroli B, Lodi R (2008) Diffusion-weighted brain imaging study of patients with clinical diagnosis of corticobasal degeneration, progressive supranuclear palsy and Parkinson's disease. Brain 131(Pt 10):2690–2700. https://doi.org/10.1093/brain/awn195

Savoiardo M (2003) Differential diagnosis of Parkinson's disease and atypical parkinsonian disorders by magnetic resonance imaging. Neurol Sci 24(Suppl 1):S35–S37. https://doi.org/10.1007/s100720300036

Trinh J, Farrer M (2013) Advances in the genetics of Parkinson disease. Nat Rev Neurol 9(8):445–454. https://doi.org/10.1038/nrneurol.2013.132. Epub 2013 July 16

Truban D, Hou X, Caulfield TR, Fiesel FC, Springer W (2017) PINK1, parkin, and mitochondrial quality control: what can we learn about Parkinson's disease pathobiology? J Park Dis 7(1):13–29. https://doi.org/10.3233/JPD-160989

Wallis LI, Paley MN, Graham JM, Grunewald RA, Wignall EL, Joy HM, Griffiths PD (2008) MRI assessment of basal ganglia iron deposition in Parkinson's disease. J Magn Reson Imaging 28(5):1061–1067. https://doi.org/10.1002/jmri.21563

Zhang H, Duan C, Yang H (2015) Defective autophagy in Parkinson's disease: lessons from genetics. Mol Neurobiol 51(1):89–104. https://doi.org/10.1007/s12035-014-8787-5. Epub 2014 July 4

Neurodegenerative Diseases: Multiple System Atrophy (MSA)

38.1 Introduction

The following subtypes of Multiple System Atrophy (MSA) were previously distinguished:

- Olivo-Ponto-Cerebellar Atrophy (OPCA)
- Striato-Nigral Degeneration (SND)
- Autonomic dysregulation (Shy–Drager syndrome)

The most recent classification of multiple system atrophy, based on clinical presentation, is:

- MSA-P: predominantly parkinsonism subtype
- MSA-C: predominantly cerebellar subtype

80% of the cases show the MSA-P subtype.

38.2 Clinical Signs and Symptoms

- Major clinical signs
  - Parkinsonism
  - Cerebellar ataxia
  - Autonomic failure
- Signs of autonomic dysfunction:
  - Orthostatic hypotension (such as systolic RR drop >20 mmHg or diastolic RR drop >10 mmHg)
  - Impotence erectile dysfunction in males
  - Urinary incontinence
- Possible MSA-P or MSA-C
  - Babinski sign with hyper-reflexia
  - Stridor
- Predominantly cerebellar signs (MSA-C):
  - Dysarthria
  - Gait ataxia
  - Oculomotor dysfunction
  - Possible MSA-C
    - Parkinsonism (bradykinesia and rigidity)
    - Atrophy of putamen, middle cerebellar peduncle, or pons on MRI
    - Hypometabolism in putamen on 18F-FDG–PET
    - Presynaptic nigrostriatal dopaminergic denervation on SPECT or PET
- Predominantly parkinsonism (MSA-P):
  - Poor, mild, or transient response to levodopa therapy
  - Possible MSA-P
    - Rapidly progressive parkinsonism
    - Poor response to levodopa
    - Gait ataxia, cerebellar dysarthria, limb ataxia, or cerebellar oculomotor dysfunction
    - Dysphagia within 5 years of motor onset
    - Atrophy of putamen, middle cerebellar peduncle, pons, or cerebellum on MRI
    - Hypometabolism in putamen, brainstem, or cerebellum on 18F-FDG–PET

- Olivo-Ponto-Cerebellar Atrophy (OPCA)
  - Cerebellar signs
  - Dysautonomia
  - Development of parkinsonism
  - Pyramidal signs
- Striato-Nigral Degeneration (SND)
  - Parkinsonism
  - Brisk reflexes
  - Autonomic failure
  - Cerebellar signs
- Autonomic dysregulation (Shy–Drager syndrome)
  - Progressive orthostatic hypotension
  - Extrapyramidal dysfunction
  - Pyramidal dysfunction
  - Cerebellar dysfunction

38.3 Epidemiology

Prevalence
- 0.6–5 per 100,000
- Dependent on age and region

Age at Onset
- 60 years (35–85 years)

Sex Incidence
- Male:Female: 1:1

38.4 Neuroimaging Findings

General Imaging Findings
- MSA-P: Atrophy of putamen
- MSA-C: Atrophy of pons, cerebellum, and middle cerebellar peduncles

CT Non-Contrast-Enhanced
- Atrophy of involved brain areas with consecutive enlargement of fourth ventricle

CT Contrast-Enhanced
- No pathological enhancement

MRI-T2/FLAIR (Figs. 38.1a, b, d and 38.2a, b)
- MSA-P:
  - Atrophy of putamen
  - Putaminal rim sign: hyperintense signal in dorsolateral rim of putamen at 1.5 T MRI
- MSA-C:
  - "Hot cross bun" sign—cruciform hyperintensity in pons
  - Hyperintensity in middle cerebellar peduncles and cerebellum
  - Atrophy of brain stem and cerebellum

MRI-T1 (Figs. 38.1c and 38.2c)
- Atrophy of putamen (MSA-P)
- Atrophy of brain stem and cerebellum (MSA-C)

MRI-T1 Contrast-Enhanced
- No pathological enhancement

MRI-T2*/SWI (Fig. 38.2d)
- Hypointensity in dorsolateral putamen caused by iron deposition

MR-Diffusion Imaging (Fig. 38.2e, f)
- Elevated ADC values in putamen

MR-Diffusion Tensor Imaging
- Decreased fractional anisotropy in pons, cerebellum, and putamen

MR-Spectroscopy
- Decreased NAA/Cr ratio in pontine base

Nuclear Medicine Imaging Findings (Fig. 38.3a–d)
- MSA belongs to the parkinsonian syndromes and thereby shows presynaptic dopamine transporter deficits with SPECT tracers like FP-CIT or β-CIT
- MSA-C shows FDG hypometabolism in the cerebellum
- MSA-P shows FDG hypometabolism in the striatum
- Some studies suggest a more symmetric loss in contrast to Parkinson's disease but there is a large overlap which allows no differentiation
- Reports state a less evident gradient between the caudate head and putamen in atypical parkinsonian syndromes than in PD
- 18F-DOPA PET is used to assess the presynaptic decarboxylase function and dopamine turnover

38.4 Neuroimaging Findings

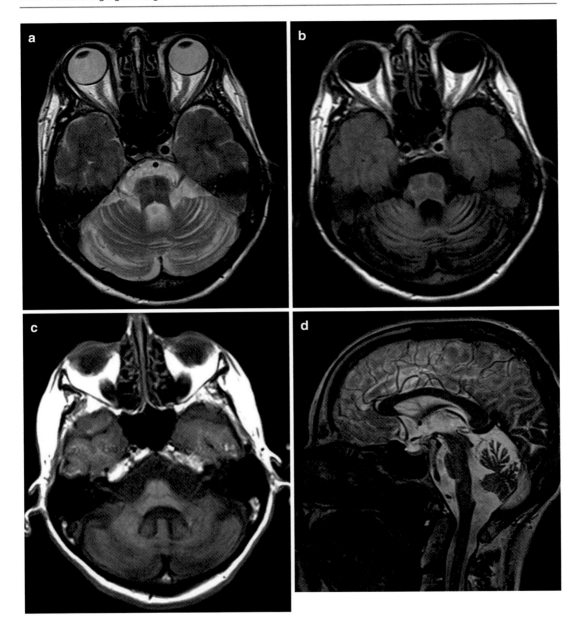

Fig. 38.1 MSA-C—Atrophy of the pons, cerebellum, and middle cerebellar peduncle with pontine "hot cross bun" sign; T2 (**a**), FLAIR (**b**), T1 non-contrast (**c**), T2 sagittal (**d**)

- In contrast to Parkinson's disease, the postsynaptic dopamine (D2) receptors are affected too, so SPECT studies with IBZM or PET studies with tracers like 11C-raclopride or 18F-fallypride allow a differentiation between PD and atypical Parkinsonian syndromes like PSP by showing the postsynaptic neuronal loss.
- Additional CBF-SPECT and FDG-PET studies reveal hypoperfusion and hypometabolism in the medial frontal cortex, the mesencephalon, and the striatum
- Myocardial sympathetic innervation can be assessed with 123I-MIBG or 18F-dopamine. Reports state a statistically better uptake in atypical parkinsonian syndromes than in PD by comparing myocardial and mediastinal uptake

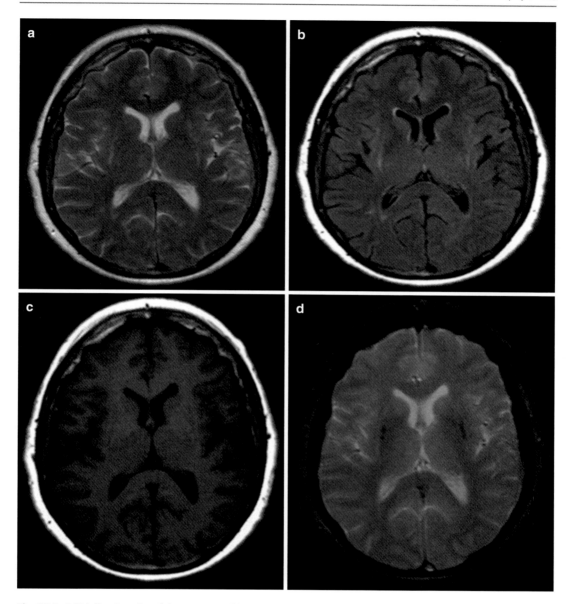

Fig. 38.2 MSA-P—Atrophy of the putamen with T2-hypertintense putaminal rim sign and iron deposition in dorsolateral putamen; T2 (**a**), FLAIR (**b**), T1 (**c**), T2* (**d**), DWI (**e**), ADC (**f**)

38.4 Neuroimaging Findings

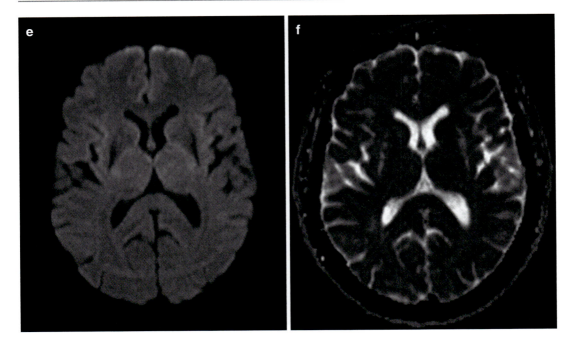

Fig. 38.2 (continued)

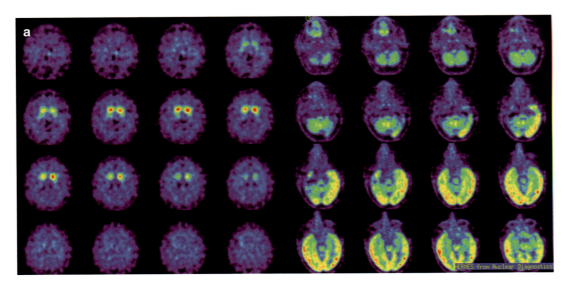

Fig. 38.3 MSA-C FP-CIT (the four rows to the left) showing pathological signal in the basal ganglia, FDG-PET (the four rows to the right) showing a reduced cerebellar uptake (**a**). MSA-P FP-CIT left pictures showing pathological signal in the basal ganglia, rows right IBZM scan showing a pathological postsynaptic uptake (**b**). Fallypride postsynaptic D2 receptor PET showing normal and initial pathological uptake (interval 1 year) in a patient with atypical parkinsonian syndrome (from left to right) (**c**), FDG-PET of a patient with MSA-P and lack of FDG-uptake in the putamina (**d**)

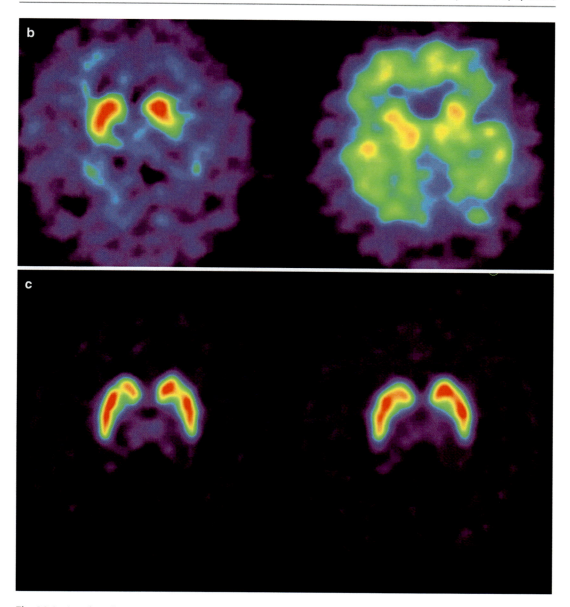

Fig. 38.3 (continued)

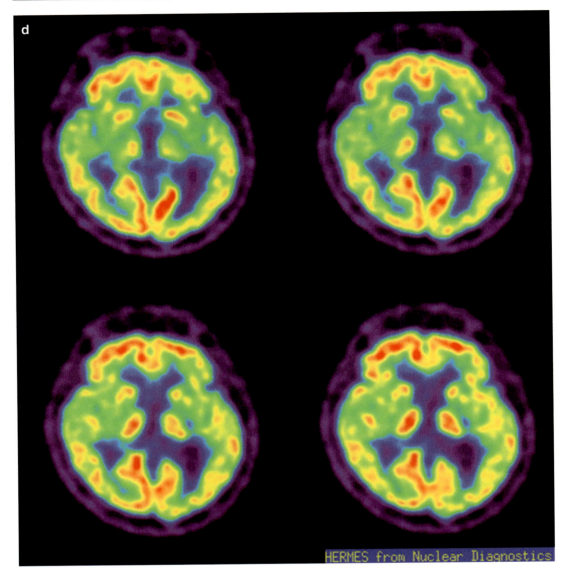

Fig. 38.3 (continued)

38.5 Neuropathology Findings

Macroscopic Features
- No obvious changes
- Substantia nigra might appear paler
- Pigment loss in locus coeruleus, motor nucleus of the vagus
- Brownish discoloration and reduction in size of the lateral-posterior putamen
- Possible atrophy of:
  - Cerebellum
  - Middle cerebellar peduncle
  - Pontine base

Microscopic Features (Figs. 38.4a–h and 38.5a–d)
- Neuronal loss in
  - Striatum

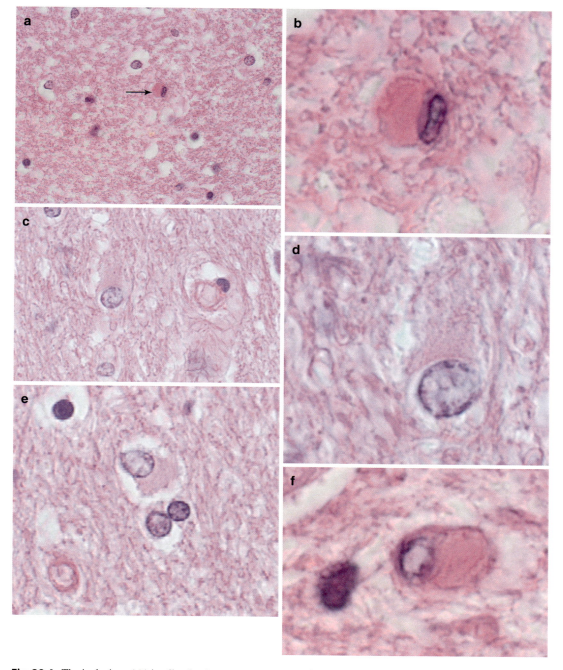

Fig. 38.4 The inclusions (➜) in oligodendrocytes appear on routine H&E stained sections eosinophilic (**a–h**)

38.5 Neuropathology Findings

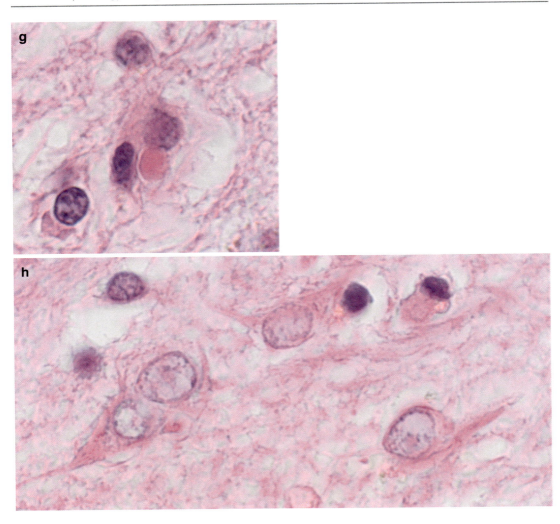

Fig. 38.4 (continued)

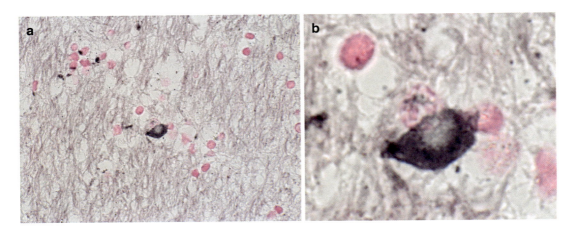

Fig. 38.5 Inclusions as seen on Gallyas stain (**a–d**)

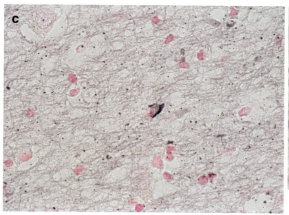
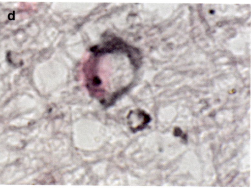

Fig. 38.5 (continued)

- Substantia nigra
- Locus coeruleus
- Inferior olives
- Purkinje cell layer of the cerebellum
- Basis pontis
- Motor nucleus of the vagus
- Intermediate column of the spinal cord
- Nucleus of Onufrowicz (Onuf's nucleus)
• Astrogliosis
• Glial cytoplasmic inclusion (GCI) or Papp-Lantos bodies in
  - Oligodendroglia
    ○ Mainly of the white matter
  - Flame-shaped
  - Best visualized by Gallyas silver stain
  - Present in:
    ○ Basal ganglia
    ○ Frontal cortex
    ○ Primary motor cortex
    ○ Reticular formation
    ○ Cerebellum
• Argyrophilic neuronal inclusions
• Nuclear inclusions
• Immunopositivity for:
  - Alpha-synuclein (hallmark) in GCI
  - Ubiquitin
  - p62
  - Tau-Protein
  - α- and ß-Tubulin

• Striato-Nigral Degeneration (SND).
  - Neuronal loss in the striatum
  - Demyelination
  - Gliosis in putamen and substantia nigra
  - Hemosiderin deposits in the posterior-lateral putamen
• Autonomic dysregulation (Shy–Drager syndrome)
  - Neuronal loss and gliosis in:
    • Striatum
    • Substantia nigra
    • Cerebellum
    • Pons
    • Nucleus olivary inferior
    • Intermediolateral cell column of the spinal cord
    • Nucleus of Onufrowicz

One abundant α-synuclein positive GCI alone is sufficient for the diagnosis of MSA in the absence of a clinical history of MSA!!!!!

Immunophenotype (Figs. 38.6, 38.7, 38.8, and 38.9)
• Alpha-synuclein (hallmark) in GCI
• Ubiquitin
• p62
• Tau-Protein
• α- and ß-Tubulin

38.5 Neuropathology Findings

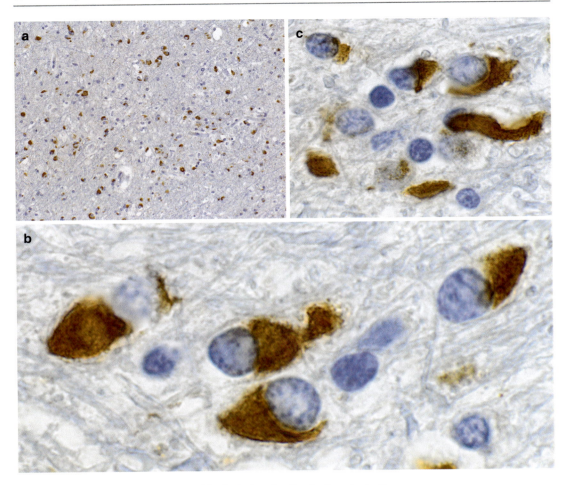

Fig. 38.6 Examples of α-synuclein-positive inclusions in oligodendrocytes (**a–f**)

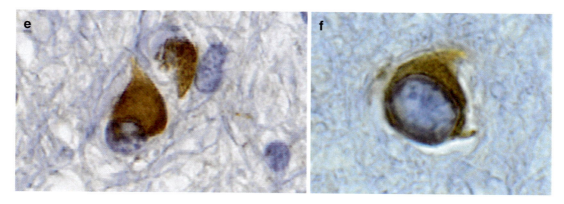

Fig. 38.6 (continued)

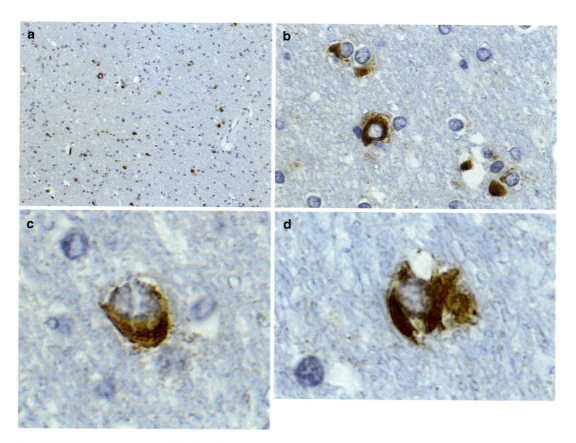

Fig. 38.7 The inclusions are positive for p62 (**a–d**)

38.5 Neuropathology Findings

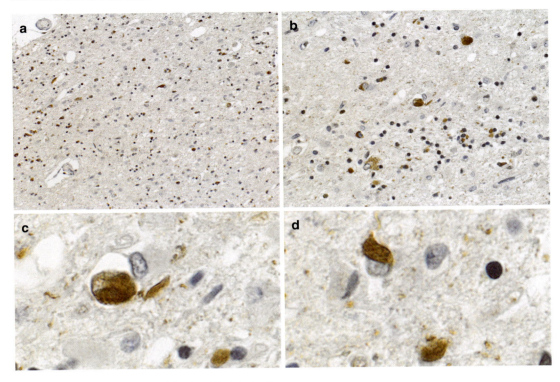

Fig. 38.8 The inclusions are positive for ubiquitin (**a–d**)

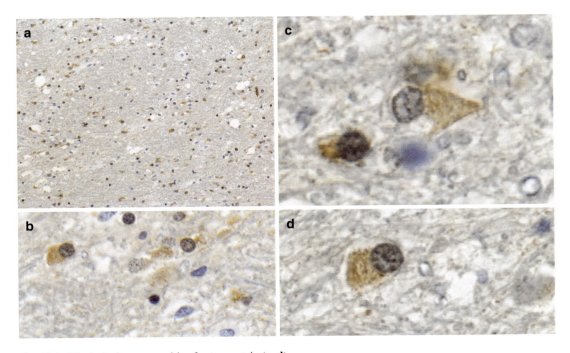

Fig. 38.9 The inclusions are positive for tau-protein (**a–d**)

38.6 Molecular Neuropathology

- Complex
- Not well understood
- Permissive templating "prion-like" propagation of misfolded α-synuclein
- Environmental factors
- Genetic or epigenetic factors
- Functionally relevant mutations in the *COQ2* gene leading to reduced 4-hydroxybenzoate polyprenyltransferase activity
- Mitochondrial dysfunction
- Relocation of phosphoprotein-25α (p25α) from the myelin sheath to the cytoplasm followed by cytoplasmic accumulation in oligodendrocytes

Differential Diagnosis
- Differences between MSA-P (predominantly parkinsonism subtype) and MSA-C (predominantly cerebellar subtype) are given in Table 38.1).

38.7 Treatment and Prognosis

Treatment
- Parkinsonism
  – Similar to Parkinson's disease, i.e., levodopa
- Dysautonomia:
  – Similar to Parkinson's disease
- Ataxia:
  – No effective treatment

Table 38.1 Differential diagnoses by etiology and MSA phenotype, modified after Krismer and Wenning (2017) reproduced with kind permission by Springer Nature

	MSA-P	MSA-C
Sporadic, degenerative	• Dementia with Lewy bodies • Neurofilament inclusion body disease • Parkinson disease • Primary lateral sclerosis • Progressive supranuclear palsy	• Prion disease (sporadic variant) • Sporadic adult-onset ataxia of unknown etiology • Idiopathic late-onset cerebellar ataxia
Genetic	• *SNCA* G51D mutation • Hereditary spastic paraplegias • Huntington disease (late-onset) • Mitochondrial encephalomyopathy, lactic acidosis and stroke-like episodes (MELAS) 3243A>G mutation in the mitochondrial *MT-TL1* gene • Perry syndrome • *SNCA* multiplications (duplication or triplications)	• *C9orf72* mutations • Cerebrotendinous xanthomatosis (*CYP27A1* mutation) • Fragile X tremor/ataxia syndrome (FXTAS) • Friedreich ataxia (late-onset) • *POLG* mutations • Prion disease (genetic variant) • Spinocerebellar ataxia type 3 (Machado–Joseph disease) • Spinocerebellar ataxia type 6 • X-linked adrenoleukodystrophy (*ABCD1* mutation)
Metabolic/inflammatory/other	• Drug-induced parkinsonism • Multiple sclerosis (primary progressive) • Vascular	• Alcoholic cerebellar degeneration • Anti-GAD ataxia • Drug-induced cerebellar degeneration • Gluten ataxia. • Hashimoto encephalopathy • Multiple sclerosis (primary progressive) • Paraneoplastic cerebellar degeneration • Vascular

- Urogenital symptoms
  - Anticholinergics
- Palliative therapies
- Physical and occupational therapy
- Clinical trials with
  - Rasagiline
  - Rifampicin
  - Lithium
  - Mesenchymal stem cells
  - Minocycline
  - Riluzole
  - Growth hormone

Biologic Behavior–Prognosis–Prognostic Factors
- More aggressive course than Parkinson's disease
- Median survival: 6–9 years
- Prognostic factors:
  - Older age of onset
  - Female sex
  - Early-onset autonomic failure

Selected References

Ahmed Z, Asi YT, Sailer A, Lees AJ, Houlden H, Revesz T, Holton JL (2012) The neuropathology, pathophysiology and genetics of multiple system atrophy. Neuropathol Appl Neurobiol 38(1):4–24. https://doi.org/10.1111/j.1365-2990.2011.01234.x

Fanciulli A, Wenning GK (2015) Multiple-system atrophy. N Engl J Med 372(3):249–263. https://doi.org/10.1056/NEJMra1311488

Federoff M, Schottlaender LV, Houlden H, Singleton A (2015) Multiple system atrophy: the application of genetics in understanding etiology. Clin Auton Res 25(1):19–36. https://doi.org/10.1007/s10286-014-0267-5

Gilman S, Wenning GK, Low PA, Brooks DJ, Mathias CJ, Trojanowski JQ, Wood NW, Colosimo C, Durr A, Fowler CJ, Kaufmann H, Klockgether T, Lees A, Poewe W, Quinn N, Revesz T, Robertson D, Sandroni P, Seppi K, Vidailhet M (2008) Second consensus statement on the diagnosis of multiple system atrophy. Neurology 71(9):670–676. https://doi.org/10.1212/01.wnl.0000324625.00404.15

Ito M, Watanabe H, Kawai Y, Atsuta N, Tanaka F, Naganawa S, Fukatsu H, Sobue G (2007) Usefulness of combined fractional anisotropy and apparent diffusion coefficient values for detection of involvement in multiple system atrophy. J Neurol Neurosurg Psychiatry 78(7):722–728. https://doi.org/10.1136/jnnp.2006.104075

Ito S, Shirai W, Hattori T (2009) Putaminal hyperintensity on T1-weighted MR imaging in patients with the Parkinson variant of multiple system atrophy. AJNR Am J Neuroradiol 30(4):689–692. https://doi.org/10.3174/ajnr.A1443

Jellinger KA (2014) Neuropathology of multiple system atrophy: new thoughts about pathogenesis. Mov Disord 29(14):1720–1741. https://doi.org/10.1002/mds.26052

Krismer F, Wenning GK (2017) Multiple system atrophy: insights into a rare and debilitating movement disorder. Nat Rev Neurol 13(4):232–243. https://doi.org/10.1038/nrneurol.2017.26

Massano J, Costa F, Nadais G (2008) Teaching neuroImage: MRI in multiple system atrophy: "hot cross bun" sign and hyperintense rim bordering the putamina. Neurology 71(15):e38. https://doi.org/10.1212/01.wnl.0000327520.99034.28

Matsusue E, Fujii S, Kanasaki Y, Sugihara S, Miyata H, Ohama E, Ogawa T (2008) Putaminal lesion in multiple system atrophy: postmortem MR-pathological correlations. Neuroradiology 50(7):559–567. https://doi.org/10.1007/s00234-008-0381-y

Matsusue E, Fujii S, Kanasaki Y, Kaminou T, Ohama E, Ogawa T (2009) Cerebellar lesions in multiple system atrophy: postmortem MR imaging-pathologic correlations. AJNR Am J Neuroradiol 30(9):1725–1730. https://doi.org/10.3174/ajnr.A1662

Peerally T (2014) Multiple system atrophy. Semin Neurol 34(2):174–181. https://doi.org/10.1055/s-0034-1381737

Ramirez EP, Vonsattel JP (2014) Neuropathologic changes of multiple system atrophy and diffuse Lewy body disease. Semin Neurol 34(2):210–216. https://doi.org/10.1055/s-0034-1381732

Seppi K, Schocke MF, Wenning GK, Poewe W (2005) How to diagnose MSA early: the role of magnetic resonance imaging. J Neural Transm (Vienna) 112(12):1625–1634. https://doi.org/10.1007/s00702-005-0332-2

Stefanova N, Bucke P, Duerr S, Wenning GK (2009) Multiple system atrophy: an update. Lancet Neurol 8(12):1172–1178. https://doi.org/10.1016/s1474-4422(09)70288-1

Watanabe H, Fukatsu H, Katsuno M, Sugiura M, Hamada K, Okada Y, Hirayama M, Ishigaki T, Sobue G (2004) Multiple regional 1H-MR spectroscopy in multiple system atrophy: NAA/Cr reduction in pontine base as a valuable diagnostic marker. J Neurol Neurosurg Psychiatry 75(1):103–109

Wenning GK, Krismer F (2013) Multiple system atrophy. Handb Clin Neurol 117:229–241. https://doi.org/10.1016/b978-0-444-53491-0.00019-5

Wenning GK, Stefanova N, Jellinger KA, Poewe W, Schlossmacher MG (2008) Multiple system atrophy: a primary oligodendrogliopathy. Ann Neurol 64(3):239–246. https://doi.org/10.1002/ana.21465

Neurodegenerative Diseases: Motor Neuron Diseases

39.1 Introduction

Motor neuron diseases are a spectrum of diseases characterized by degeneration of the:

- Upper motor neuron (UMN) and/or
- Lower motor neuron (LMN)

The following motor neuron diseases are distinguished:

- Amyotrophic lateral sclerosis (ALS)
- Primary lateral sclerosis
- Bulbar atrophy
- Progressive muscular atrophy
- Progressive bulbar palsy
- Familial myotrophic lateral sclerosis

39.2 Clinical Signs and Symptoms

- Clinical variability is high (Table 39.1):
  - Bulbar versus limb predominance
  - UMN versus LMN predominance
  - Rapid versus slow progression
  - Extent of cognitive involvement
- Clinical manifestations include:
  - Muscle cramps
  - Spasticity
  - Muscle weakness
  - Muscle atrophy
  - Dysarthria
  - Dysphagia
  - Dyspnea
  - Respiratory insufficiency
  - Cognitive impairment
  - Behavioral impairment

39.3 Diagnostic Criteria

The El Escorial World Federation of Neurology Diagnostic Criteria are given as follows (Brooks 1994):

- The presence of:
  - Evidence of lower motor neuron degeneration by clinical, electrophysiological, or neuropathological examination
  - Evidence of upper motor neuron degeneration by clinical examination
  - Progression of the motor syndrome within a region or to other regions, as determined by history or examination
- The absence of:
  - Electrophysiological and pathological evidence of other disease processes that might explain the signs of lower or upper motor neuron degeneration
  - Neuroimaging evidence of other disease processes that might explain the observed clinical and electrophysiological signs

Table 39.1 The clinical characteristics of motor neuron diseases

Disease		
Amyotrophic lateral sclerosis	Pathology	• Upper motor neuron (UMN) • Lower motor neuron (LMN)
	Signs/symptoms	• Weakness • Atrophy • Spasticity • Dysarthria • Dyspnea • Dysphagia
	Genetics	• Sporadic
	Disease course	• High variability • Depends on degree of supportive care
Primary lateral sclerosis	Pathology	• UMN
	Signs/symptoms	• Spasticity • Rigidity
	Genetics	• Familial patterns possible
	Disease course	• Often prolonged • >10 years
Bulbar atrophy	Pathology	• UMN and/or • LMN
	Signs/symptoms	• Dysarthria • Dysphagia • Dyspnea • Sialorrhea • Weakness • Atrophy • Spasticity
	Genetics	• Some familial forms
	Disease course	• Usually aggressive • Depends on degree of supportive care
Progressive muscular atrophy	Pathology	• LMN
	Signs/symptoms	• Weakness • Atrophy
	Genetics	• Familial forms = spinal muscular atrophy
	Disease course	• High variability
Progressive bulbar palsy	Pathology	• UMN > LMN
	Signs/symptoms	• Dysarthria • Dysphagia • Dyspnea • Sialorrhea
	Genetics	• Sporadic
	Disease course	• Similar to bulbar ALS

Table 39.1 (continued)

Disease		
Familial amyotrophic lateral sclerosis	Pathology	• UMN and/or • LMN
	Signs/symptoms	• High variability • Weakness • Atrophy • Spasticity • Dysarthria • Dyspnea • Dysphagia
	Genetics	• >50 mutations
	Disease course	• High variability

- **Definite ALS**
  - Upper motor signs in the bulbar region AND
  - Lower motor signs in the bulbar region AND
  - At least two regions along the neuraxis (cervical, thoracic, lumbosacral)
  - Alternatively
    o UMN AND LMN in three regions sparing bulbar areas at the time of diagnosis
- **Probable ALS**
  - UMN signs AND
  - LMN signs
  - In at least two spinal regions
  - At least one UMN sign should be present rostral to at least one LMN sign
- **Probable Laboratory Supported ALS**
  - UMN AND LMN signs in only one region
  - Electrophysiological evidence of denervation in at least two regions where other etiologies have been excluded
- **Possible ALS**
  - UMN findings AND
  - LMN findings in only one region
  - OR UMN findings in at least two regions
  - OR LMN signs rostral to UMN signs

39.4 Epidemiology

Incidence
- 1.5–2.5 per 100,000 per year
- Highest rates in Finland (2.4 per 100,000 person-years)
- Lowest rates in Italy (0.6 per 100,000 person-years)

Age Incidence
- Seventh decade (maximum)
- Disease begin in the fourth decade

Sex Incidence
- Male:Female ratio: 2:1

Localization
- Spinal cord, anterior horn, motor neurons
- Muscle

39.5 Neuroimaging Findings

General Imaging Features
- Bilateral signal abnormalities along the corticospinal tract

CT non-contrast-enhanced
- Progressive brain atrophy

CT contrast-enhanced
- No pathological enhancement

MRI-T2
- Bilateral hyperintensities along corticospinal tract
- Hypointensity in precentral gyrus due to iron deposition possible

MRI-FLAIR (Fig. 39.1a–d)
- Bilateral hyperintensities along corticospinal tract

MRI-T1
- Internal capsule most commonly isointense, sometimes hypo- or mild hyperintense signal

MRI-T1 Contrast-Enhanced
- No pathological enhancement

MRI-T2*/SWI
- Decreased signal intensity of the motor cortex due to iron accumulation possible

MR-Diffusion Tensor Imaging
- Decreased fractional anisotropy in corticospinal tract

MR-Spectroscopy
- Decreased NAA/Cr-Ratio
- Decreased NAA/Cho-Ratio

Nuclear Medicine Imaging Findings (Fig. 39.2a, b)
- FDG-PET studies with statistical parametric mapping reveal a highly significant increase in glucose metabolism in the amygdala, midbrain, pons, and cerebellum in ALS patients, possibly due to the local activation of astrocytes and microglia.
- Some radiotracers with ^{18}F are under investigation to study neuroinflammation (i.e., microglial activation). However, there is no tracer commercially available or used in daily clinical routine.
- For studies, ^{11}C (i.e., 11C-PK11195) tracers are used.
- Hypometabolism in FDG-PET with statistical parametric mapping studies was found in the frontal cortex, anterior cingulate, precuneus, and inferior parietal lobe in patients with bulbar onset in contrast to patients with spinal onset. Corresponding to degeneration of motor neurons, hypometabolism in the precentral gyrus is reported.
- Flumazenil-PET studies showed a reduction of the neuronal density in frontal, parietal, and

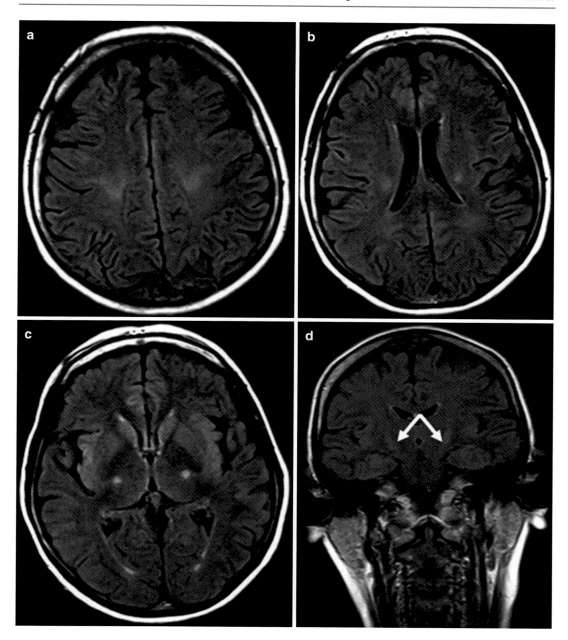

Fig. 39.1 Bilateral hyperintensities along corticospinal tract; FLAIR axial (**a–c**) and coronar (→) (**d**)

39.5 Neuroimaging Findings

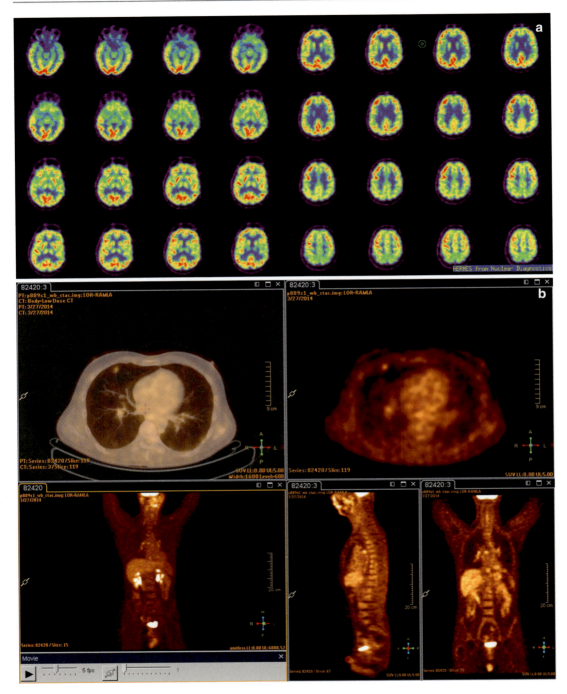

Fig. 39.2 FDG-PET of a 40-year-old patient with ALS—hypometabolism parietal, central cortex, temporal (**a**). FDG-PET of the torso of the same patient. Pulmonary and mediastinal inflammation due to aspiration (**b**)

visual association areas. These reductions were also found in the premotor and motor cortices.
- In addition, radionuclide swallow studies can show a significant retention and delayed clearance of radioactivity from the mouth.

39.6 Neuropathology Findings

Macroscopic Features (Fig. 39.3a–h)
- Muscle (limb, tongue, intercostal)
  - Atrophy
  - Wasting
- Spinal cord
  - Atrophy
  - Especially the cervical and lumbar segments
- Anterior roots
  - Discoloration
  - Atrophy
- Cerebral cortex
  - Possible atrophy
  - Rarely atrophy of the precentral gyrus

Microscopic Features (Fig. 39.4a–j)
- Muscle
  - Fascicular atrophy
  - Fiber type grouping
- Spinal cord
  - Loss of upper and lower motor neurons
  - Astrogliosis
  - Microgliosis
  - Bunina bodies
  - Abnormal inclusions
  - Myelin pallor of the antero-lateral columns
  - Central chromatolysis
  - Axonal swellings of the anterior horn

Inclusions
- Skein-like inclusions
  - Faint staining on H&E sections
  - Ubiquitin-positive intracytoplasmic filamentous structures
  - P62-positive
  - TDP-43 positive
  - FUS/TLS positive
- Round inclusions
  - Pale, eosinophilic inclusions (H&E stain)
  - Ubiquitin-positive
  - Phosphorylated neurofilament positive
- Small granules and single threads
- Bunina bodies
  - Specific hallmark of ALS
  - Small (2–5 μm) eosinophilic round inclusions
  - Purple on PTAH stain
  - Light blue on Klüver–Barrera stain
  - Red on Masson stain
  - Immunoreactive for cystatin C and transferrin
- Lewy body-like hyaline inclusions
  - Found in fALS with SOD1 mutations
  - Immunoreactive for SOD1
- Basophilic inclusions
  - Immunoreactive for ubiquitin, p62, FUS/TLS

Motor Neuron Disease with Dementia (FTD/ALS)
- Moderate atrophy of the frontal and temporal lobes
- Moderate neuronal loss
- Spongiform changes in cortical layers I–III
- Astrocytic gliosis in cortical layers I–III
- Loss of motor neurons in the spine and rarely in the medulla oblongata
- Ubiquitin-positive inclusions in:
  - Motor neurons
  - Neurons in cortical layer II of the frontal and temporal lobes
  - Dentate gyrus of the hippocampus
- Absence of Tau-positivity
- Absence of glial inclusions

Ultrastructural Features
- Skein-like inclusions
  - Bundles of fibrils with granules
  - Free fibrils with granules
- Round inclusions
  - Abnormal filaments (15–20 nm) without granules or with fuzzy granules
  - Neurofilaments

39.6 Neuropathology Findings

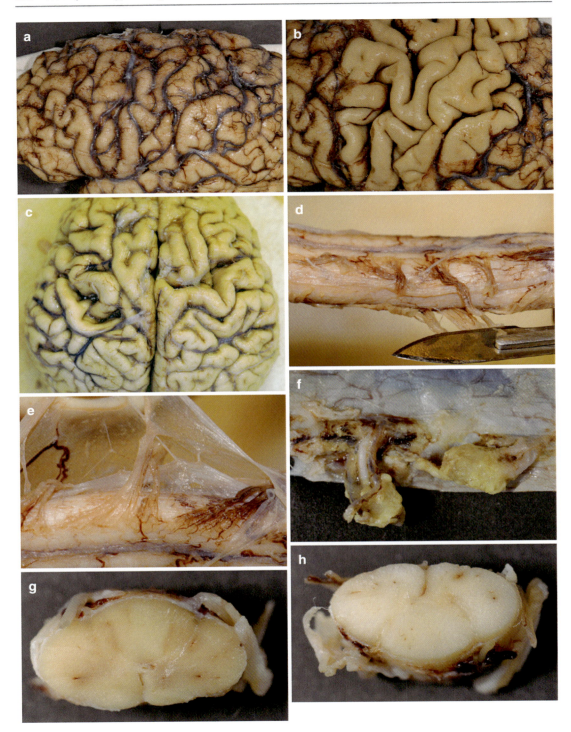

Fig. 39.3 Atrophy of the precentral gyrus (**a–c**), thinning of the nerve roots (**d–f**), no obvious changes in the gray matter of the spinal cord (**g, h**)

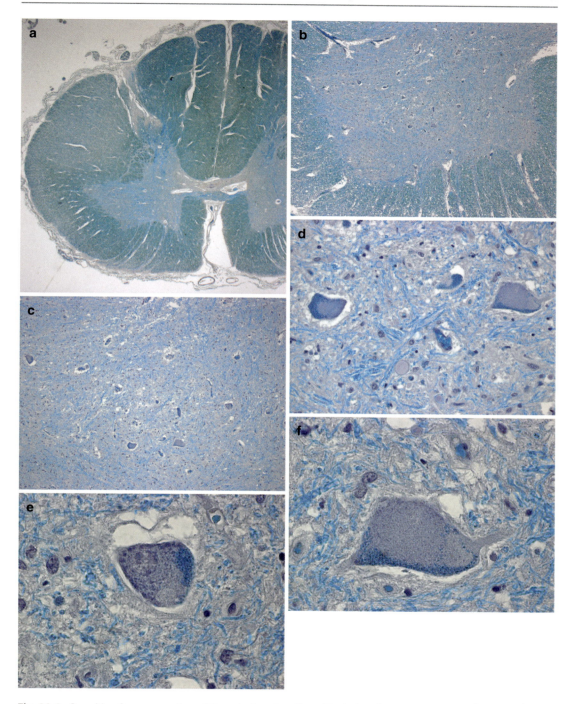

Fig. 39.4 One side of a cross-section of the spinal cord showing the butterfly-like structure of gray matter (**a**), the anterior horn (**b**), loss of neurons in the anterior horn (**c**, **d**), and inclusions in motor neurons (**e**, **f**) (→) (**a–f**: stain: LFB). Anterior horn with loss of neurons (**g–j**, stain: HE)

39.7 Molecular Neuropathology

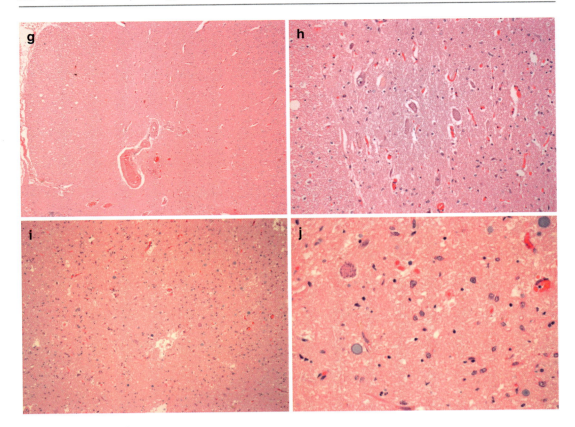

Fig. 39.4 (continued)

- Bunina bodies
  - Amorphous electron-dense material
  - Surrounded by tubular and vesicular structures

Immunophenotype (Fig. 39.5a–t)
- Ubiquitin-positive cytoplasmic inclusions
  - In neurons and glial cells
- p62-positive cytoplasmic inclusions
  - In neurons and glial cells
- TDP-43 major protein
- FUS

Differential Diagnosis
- Multifocal motor neuropathy
- Kennedy disease

39.7 Molecular Neuropathology

39.7.1 Pathogenetic Mechanisms

Possible pathogenic mechanisms include (Table 39.2):

- Excitotoxicity
- Oxidative stress
- Reactive oxygenating species toxicity
- Mitochondrial dysfunction
- Impairment of axonal transport
- Cytoskeletal derangement
- Protein aggregation
- Endoplasmic reticulum stress

- Abnormal RNA processing
- Neuroinflammation
- Role of glial cells
- Excitability of peripheral axons
- Role of targets muscles and neuromuscular junction
- mtSOD1-mediated neurotoxicity
- Protein misfolding
- Proteasome impairment
- Axonopathy

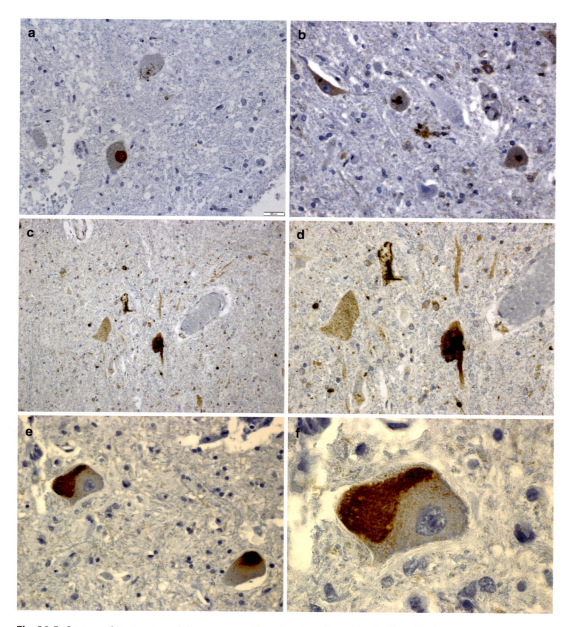

Fig. 39.5 Immunophenotype: surviving neurons with p62-positive inclusions (**a–j**) which also stain positive for ubiquitin (**k, l**), TDP-43 (**m–p**), and FUS (**q–t**)

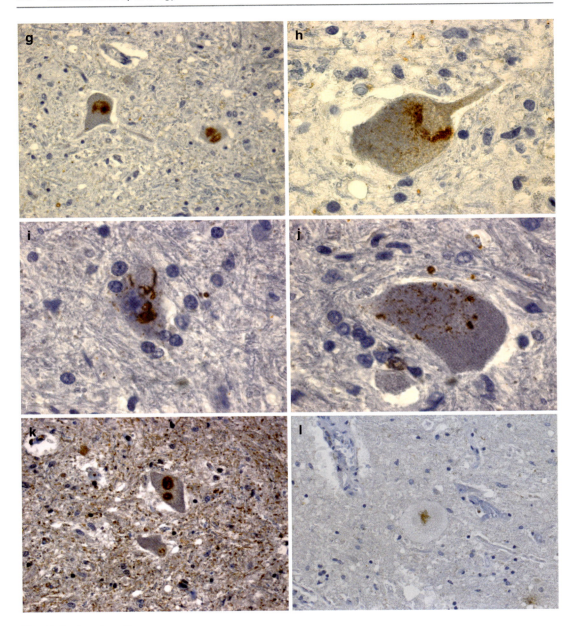

Fig. 39.5 (continued)

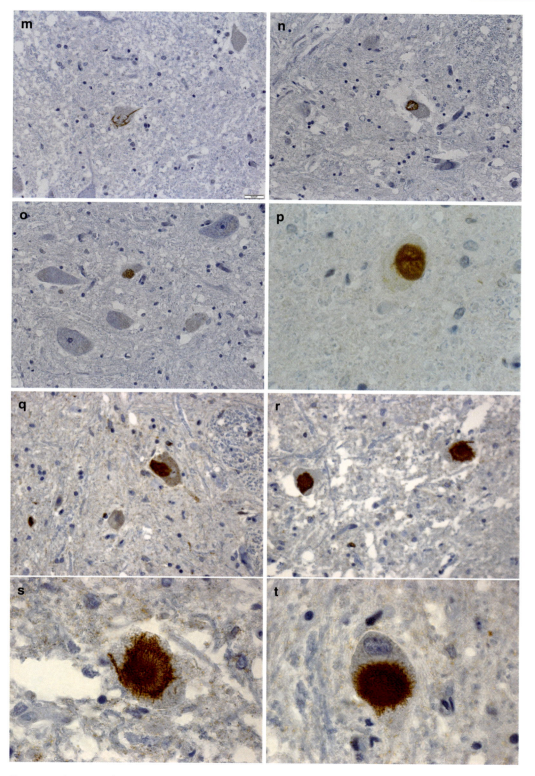

Fig. 39.5 (continued)

39.7 Molecular Neuropathology

Table 39.2 Implications of mutated genes in pathophysiological aspects, modified after Hardiman et al. (2017) reproduced with kind permission by Springer Nature

Pathophysiological component	Mutated genes
Hyperexcitability	• *SOD1*—Cu/Zn superoxide dismutase 1
Impaired protein homeostasis	• *SIGMAR1*—Sigma non-opioid intracellular receptor 1 • *CHMP2B*—Charged multivesicular body protein 2B/Chromatin-modifying protein 2B • *C9orf72*—Guanine nucleotide exchange C9orf72 • *SQSTM1*—P62/Sequestosome-1 • *UBQLN2*—Ubiquilin-2 • *SOD1*—Cu/Zn superoxide dismutase 1 • *ALS2*—Alsin • *VAPB*—VAMP (vesicle-associated membrane protein B) • *OPTN*—Optineurin • *VCP*—Valosin-containing protein • *TBK1*—Serine/threonine-protein kinase TBK1 (TANK-binding kinase)
Oxidative stress	• *SOD1*—Cu/Zn superoxide dismutase 1 • *ALS2*—Alsin • *TARDBP*—TAR DNA-binding protein 43 (TDP-43)
Mitochondrial dysfunction	• *SOD1*—Cu/Zn superoxide dismutase 1 • *CHCHd10*—coiled-coil-helix-coiled-coil-helix domain containing 10 • *TARDBP*—TAR DNA-binding protein 43 (TDP-43)
Nuclear export	• *C9orf72*—Guanine nucleotide exchange C9orf72
Impaired DNA repair	• *NEK1*—*never in mitosis gene a-related kinase 1* • *C21orf2*—*chromosome 21 open reading frame 2* • *SPG11*—Spatacsin • *FUS*—Fused in sarcoma
Aberrant TNA metabolism	• *SETX*—senataxin • *FUS*—Fused in sarcoma • *ANG*—angiogenin • *TARDBP*—TAR DNA-binding protein 43 (TDP-43) • *ELP3*—elongator acetyltransferase complex subunit 3 • *TAF15*—TATA-box binding protein associated factor 15 • *EWSR1*—Ewing sarcoma breakpoint region 1 • *ATXN2*—ataxin 2 • *HNRNPA1*—heterogeneous nuclear ribonucleoprotein A1 • *C9orf72*—Guanine nucleotide exchange C9orf72 • *HNRNPA2B1*—heterogeneous nuclear ribonucleoprotein A2/B1 • *MATR3*—matrin 3
Dysregulated vesicle transport	• *SOD1*—Cu/Zn superoxide dismutase 1 • *ALS2*—Alsin • *FIG4*—FIG4 phosphoinositide 5-phosphatase • *VAPB*—VAMP (vesicle-associated membrane protein B) • *OPTN*—Optineurin • *UNC13A*—unc-13 homolog A • *CHMP2B*—Charged multivesicular body protein 2B/Chromatin-modifying protein 2B
Axonopathy	• *SOD1—Cu/Zn superoxide dismutase 1* • *SPG11*—Spatacsin • *TUBA4A*—tubulin alpha 4a • *PFN1*—profilin 1 • *DCTN*—dynactin • *NEFH*—neurofilament, heavy polypeptide
Glial dysfunction	• *SOD1*—Cu/Zn superoxide dismutase 1 • *C9orf72*—Guanine nucleotide exchange C9orf72

Table 39.3 Genes likely causing ALS (in alphabetical order), modified after Su et al. (2014) and Mancuso and Navarro (2015) reproduced with kind permission by Elsevier and Wiley

Gene		Function	Clinical phenotype	Epidemiology
ALS2	Alsin	Cellular transport	j-ALS, j-PLS, HSP	<1% FALS
ANG	Angiogenin	RNA metabolism	ALS, PD	<1% ALS overall
C9ORF72	Chromosome 9 open reading frame 72	RNA metabolism	ALS, FTD	40% FALS, 5–6% SALS
CHMP2B		Cellular transport	ALS, FTD	Unknown
DAO		Glutamatergic signaling	ALS	<1% FALS
FUS	Fused in sarcoma/translated in liposarcoma	DNA/RNA metabolism	ALS, j-ALS, FTD	5% FALS, <1% SALS
hnRNPA1		RNA metabolism	ALS, FTD, IBMPFD	Unknown
hnRNPA2B1		RNA metabolism	ALS, FTD, IBMPFD	Unknown
OPTN	Optineurin	Protein metabolism	ALS	<1% FALS
PFN1	Profilin	Axonal outgrowth	ALS	<1% FALS
SETX	Senataxin	DNA/RNA metabolism	j-ALS	<1% FALS
SOD1	CU/Zn superoxide dismutase	Prevent oxidative damage	ALS, FTD, PMA	20% FALS, 3% SALS
SPG11	Spatacsin	Neuronal maturation	j-ALS, HSP	Unknown
SQSTM1		Protein metabolism	ALS, FTD	<2% ALS overall
TAF15		RNA metabolism	ALS	Unknown
TARDBP2	TAR DANN-binding protein 43	DNA/RNA metabolism	ALS, FTD	3% FALS, 2% SALS
UBQLN2	Ubiquilin-2	Protein metabolism	ALS, FTD	<2% FALS
VAPB	Vesicle-associated membrane protein B	Cellular transport	ALS, PMA	<1% FALS
VCP	Valosin-containing protein	Protein metabolism	ALS, FTD, IBMPFD	1–2% FALS

- Transcription factors for genes involved in resistance to oxidative stress and repair of oxidative damage

39.7.2 Genes

- Genes likely to cause ALS are given in Table 39.3, while major genes playing a role at the center of the ALS/FTD disease spectrum are listed in Table 39.4.

Genes involved in familial ALS are manifold and listed in Table 39.5. Different subtypes of familial ALS and their genotype–phenotype correlations are illustrated in Table 39.6.

Table 39.4 Major genes at the center of the ALS/FTD disease spectrum, modified after Thomas et al. (2013) reproduced with kind permission by Oxford University Press

Disease subgroup	Genes	Mode of inheritance	Protein species found in inclusions
ALS-SOD1	• SOD1	• Sporadic	• SOD1 • p62 • Ubiquitin • Ubiquilin2
ALS-TDP-43	• TARDBP • C9ORF72 • OPTN • UBQLN2	• Sporadic	• TDP-43 • p62 • Ubiquitin • Ubiquilin • Ubiquillin2 • Optineurin
ALS-FUS	• FUS • UBQLN2	• Sporadic	• FUS • p62 • Ubiquitin • Ubiquilin 2 • Optineurin

39.7 Molecular Neuropathology

Table 39.5 Genetic findings in familial ALS, modified after Zufiria et al. (2016) reproduced with kind permission by Elsevier

Name	Onset	Inheritance	Linkage	Gene	Clinical phenotype	Protein	Pathogenetic mechanism
ALS-1	Adult	AD, AR, De novo	21q22.1	*SOD1*	ALS FTD PMA	Cu/Zn superoxide dismutase 1 (SOD1)	• Oxidative stress • Ubiquitin-proteasome system • Autophagy • Protein aggregation • Possible gains of redox function • Impaired axonal transport • Metabolic alterations/ • Cytoplasmic inclusions of SOD1, ubiquitin, and p62 but not TDP-43 aggregates
ALS-2	Juvenile	AR	2q33–35	*ALS2*	jALS jPLS HSP	Alsin	• Endosomal trafficking • Oxidative stress • Membrane trafficking
ALS-3	Adult	AD	18q21	Unknown	ALS		• Unknown
ALS-4	Juvenile	AD	9q34	*SETX*	jALS	Senataxin	• DNA processing • RNA processing
ALS-5	Juvenile	AR	15q21.1	*SPG11*	jALS HSP	Spatacsin	• Intracellular cargo transport • Axonal growth
ALS-6	Adult	AD, AR	16q12	*FUS*	ALS jALS FTD	Fused in sarcoma	• RNA processing • Stress granule formation • Formation of inclusion bodies/FUS but not TDP-43 aggregates
ALS-7	Adult	AD	20q	Unknown	ALS		• Unknown
ALS-8	Adult	AD	20q13.33	*VAPB*	ALS PMA	VAMP (vesicle-associated membrane protein B)	• Endoplasmic reticulum stress • Unfolded protein response • Intracellular membrane trafficking • Vesicle trafficking/TDP43 aggregates
ALS-9	Adult	AD	14q11	*ANG*	ALS PD	Angiogenin	• RNA processing • rRNA transcription • Stress granule formation/TDP-43 aggregates
ALS-10	Adult	AD, AR	1q36	*TARDBP*	ALS FTD	TAR DNA-binding protein 43 (TDP-43)	• RNA processing • RNA splicing • Formation of protein inclusion bodies • Metabolic alterations • Mitochondrial integrity/Ubiquitin, p62, and TDP-43 positive aggregates

(continued)

Table 39.5 (continued)

Name	Onset	Inheritance	Linkage	Gene	Clinical phenotype	Protein	Pathogenetic mechanism
ALS-11	Adult	AD	6q21	FIG4		Polyphosphoinositide phosphatase	• Endosomal trafficking • Overexpression of SAC3 • Multivesicular body formation
ALS-12	Adult	AD, AR	10p13	OPTN	ALS	Optineurin	• Autophagy • Golgi maintenance • membrane trafficking and exocytosis • Formation of inclusion bodies • Interaction with huntingtin, transcription factor IIIA and RAB8/Ubiquitin, p62, optineurin and TDP-43 positive aggregates
ALS-13	Adult	AD	12q24	ATXN2		Ataxin-2	• RNA processing • Toxic to neuronal cells • ATXN2 and TDP-43 associate in a complex that depends on RNA • ATXN2 is abnormally localized in spinal cord neurons of ALS patients/ubiquitin and p62 positive aggregates
ALS-14	Adult	AD	9q13	VCP	ALS FTD IBMPFD	Valosin-containing protein	• Autophagy • Proteasomal degradation • Endosomal trafficking • Vesicle sorting/TDP-43 aggregates
ALS-15	Adult	X-LD	Xp11.21	UBQLN2	ALS FTD	Ubiquilin-2	• Ubiquitin-proteasome system • Autophagy • Proteasomal protein degradation • Inclusion body formation/Ubiquilin-2 aggregates, positive for ubiquitin, p62, TDP-43, and FUS inclusions
ALS-16	Juvenile	AD; AR	9p13.3	SIGMAR1		Sigma non-opioid intracellular receptor 1	• Autophagy • Unfolded protein response • Endoplasmic reticulum stress • Proteasome function • Modulation of potassium channels activity (Kv1.4)
ALS-17	Adult	AD	3p12.1	CHMP2B	ALS FTD	Charged multivesicular body protein 2B/Chromatin-modifying protein 2B	• Endosomal trafficking • Autophagy • Multivesicular bodies (MVBs) formation and sorting of endosomal cargo proteins/Intraneuronal inclusions immunopositive for ubiquitin

39.7 Molecular Neuropathology

Name	Onset	Inheritance	Linkage	Gene	Clinical phenotype	Protein	Pathogenetic mechanism
ALS-18	Adult	AD	17p13.2	*PFN1*	ALS	Profilin	• Cytoskeleton • Axonal growth • Disruption of cytoskeletal pathways
ALS-19	Adult	AD	2q33.3–q34	*ERBB4*		Receptor tyrosine-protein kinase erbB4	• Neuronal development • Tyrosin-kinase receptor for neuregulins that suppress induction of long-term potentiation in the hippocampal CA1 region without affecting basal synaptic transmission; glucose uptake
ALS-20	Adult	AD	12q13.1	*hnRNPA1*	ALS FTD IBMPFD	Heterogeneous nuclear ribonucleoprotein A1	• RNA processing • Pathogenic mutations strengthen a "steric zipper" motif in the PrLD, which accelerates formation of self-seeding fibrils that cross-seed polymerization of WT hnRNP
ALS-21	Adult	AD	5q31.3	*MATR3*		Matrin 3	• RNA processing • Appears in the nuclei of motor neurons interacting with TDP-43 and regulating transcription
ALS-22	Adult	AD	2q35	*TUBA4A*		Tubulin alpha 4 protein	• Cytoskeleton
ALS/FTD1	Adult	AD	9q21–22	*C9ORF72*	ALS FTD	Guanine nucleotide exchange C9orf72	• RNA processing • Endosomal trafficking • Autophagy • Endosomal trafficking and autophagy • Altered C9ORF72 RNA splicing • Formation of nuclear RNA foci/TDP-43 positive aggregates and TDP-43 negative aggregates localized in hippocampus and cerebellum positive for ubiquitin and p62
ALS/FTD2	Adult	AD	22q11.23	*CHCHD10*		Coiled-coil-helix-coiled-coil-helix domain containing 10	• Mitochondrial function
ALS/FTD3	Adult	AD	5q35.3	*SQSTM1*	ALS FTD	P62/Sequestosome-1	• Protein degradation • Autophagy • Association with the NF-kappaB pathway • Regulation of glucose metabolism
ALS/FTD4	Adult	AD	12q14.2	*TBK1*		Serine/threonine-protein kinase TBK1 (TANK-binding kinase)	• Autophagy • Neuroinflammation • Regulates inflammatory responses to foreign agents • TBK1 phosphorylates OPTN and SQSTM1 to enhance autophagy

Abbreviations used: *ALS* amyotrophic lateral sclerosis, *FALS* familial ALS, *FTD* fronto-temporal dementia, *HSP* hereditary spastic paraplegia, *IBMPFD* inclusion body myopathy, Paget disease and fronto-temporal dementia, *J* juvenile, *PD* Parkinson disease, *PLS* primary lateral sclerosis, *PMA* progressive muscular atrophy, *SALS* sporadic ALS

Table 39.6 Different subtypes of *familial ALS* and their genotype–phenotype correlations, modified after Li and Wu (2016) reproduced with kind permission by Biomed Central, open access

ALS type	ALS features	FTD	Other features
ALS-1 (21q22.1)	• AAO: adult > juvenile • Onset: LL > UL > bulbar • Progression: rapid > slow • UMN + LMN > LMN dominant	Rare	• Progressive muscular atrophy (PMA) • Progressive bulbar palsy (PBP) • Benign focal amyotrophy (BFA) • Cerebellar ataxia • Autonomic dysfunction
ALS-2 (2q33.2)	• AAO: juvenile • Onset: LL, UL • Progression: slow • UMN dominant > UMN + LMN	None	• Primary lateral sclerosis (PLS) • Infantile-onset ascending hereditary spastic paralysis (IAHSP)
ALS-3 (18q21)	• N/A	N/A	• N/A.
ALS-4 (9q34)	• AAO: juvenile > adult • Onset: LL > UL • Progression: slow • UMN + LMN > LMN dominant	None	• Ataxia and oculomotor apraxia type 2 (AOA2) • Cerebellar ataxia • Motor neuropathy
ALS-5 (15q21.1)	• AAO: juvenile > adult • Onset: bulbar, limb • Progression: slow • UMN dominant > UMN + LMN	Rare	• Hereditary spastic paraplegia (HSP) • Autonomic dysfunction • Mental retardation
ALS-6 (16q11.2)	• AAO: adult > juvenile • Onset: UL, bulbar > LL De novo • Progression: rapid > slow • UMN + LMN > LMN dominant	Rare	• Progressive muscular atrophy (PMA) • Parkinsonism • Essential tremor • Mental retardation
ALS-7 (20p13)	• N/A	N/A	• N/A
ALS-8 (20q13.3)	• AAO: adult > juvenile • Onset: limb • Progression: slow • LMN dominant	None	• SMA • Motor neuropathy • Autonomic dysfunction
ALS-9 (14q11.2)	• AAO: adult > juvenile • Onset: limb, bulbar • Progression: N/A • UMN + LMN	Yes	• Progressive bulbar palsy (PBP) • Parkinson disease (PD)
ALS-10 (1p36.22)	• AAO: adult • Onset: limb, bulbar • Progression: variable • UMN + LMN	Yes	• Progressive supranuclear palsy (PSP) • FTD with Parkinsonism • Parkinson disease (PD) • Chorea
ALS-11 (6q21)	• AAO: adult • Onset: bulbar > limb • Progression: variable • UMN + LMN > UMN dominant	None	• Charcot–Marie–Tooth disease (CMT4J) • Hereditary spastic paraplegia (HSP) • Primary lateral sclerosis (PLS) • Yunis–Varon syndrome • Epilepsy with polymicrogyria
ALS-12 (10p13)	• AAO: adult • Onset: bulbar, limb • Progression: slow • UMN + LMN	Yes	• Primary open angle glaucoma (POAG) • Parkinsonism • Aphasia
ALS-13 (12q24)	• AAO: adult > juvenile • Onset: UL, LL • Progression: variable • UMN + LMN	None	• Spinocerebellar ataxia 2 (SCA2) • Parkinsonism
ALS-14 (9p13)	• AAO: adult > juvenile • Onset: limb > bulbar • Progression: variable • UMN + LMN	Yes	• Inclusion body myopathy with Paget disease and fronto-temporal dementia (IBMPFD)

39.8 Treatment and Prognosis

Table 39.6 (continued)

ALS type	ALS features	FTD	Other features
ALS-15 (Xp11.21)	• AAO: adult > juvenile • Onset: limb, bulbar • Progression: variable • UMN + LMN > UMN dominant	Yes	• Primary lateral sclerosis (PLS)
ALS-16 (9p13.3)	• AAO: juvenile • Onset: LL > UL • Progression: N/A • UMN + LMN	Rare	• Motor neuropathy
ALS-17 (3p12.1)	• AAO: adult • Onset: bulbar, limb • Progression: N/A • UMN + LMN > LMN dominant	Yes	• Progressive muscular atrophy (PMA) • Parkinsonism
ALS-18 (17p13.2)	• AAO: adult • Onset: limb • Progression: N/A • UMN + LMN	None	• N/A
ALS-19 (2q33.3–q34)	• AAO: adult • Onset: UL, bulbar • Progression: slow • UMN + LMN	None	• N/A
ALS-20 (12q13.1)	• AAO: adult • Onset: N/A • Progression: N/A • UMN + LMN > LMN dominant	Yes	• Multi-system proteinopathy
ALS-21 (5q31.3)	• AAO: adult • Onset: bulbar, limb • Progression: slow • UMN + LMN > LMN dominant	Yes	• Distal myopathy
ALS-FTD (9p21.2)	• AAO: adult • Onset: bulbar, limb • Progression: rapid > slow • UMN + LMN	Yes	• Parkinsonism • Cerebellar ataxia

Abbreviations: *AAO* age at onset, *LL* lower limb, *LMN* lower motor neuron, *UL* upper limb, *UMN* upper motor neuron, *UN* unknown

39.8 Treatment and Prognosis

Treatment
- Drugs
  - Riluzole (2-amino-6-[trifluoromethoxy] benzothiazole)
- Nutritional support
- Respiratory support
- Symptomatic management

Biologic Behavior–Prognosis–Prognostic Factors
- Progressive disorder
- Median life expectancy:
  - 2.5–3.5 years
  - 2 years for patients with bulbar onset
  - 4 years for patients with onset of limb weakness
- Favorable prognostic factors
  - Early age of onset
  - Progressive muscular atrophy
  - Primary lateral sclerosis
- Poor prognostic factors
  - Bulbar onset
  - Older age
  - Female sex
- Staging of disease (Table 39.7)
- Genes modifying progression (Table 39.8)

Table 39.7 Staging of disease, modified after Hardiman et al. (2017) reproduced with kind permission by Springer Nature

Staging	King's clinical staging	MITOS functional staging
0	Presymptomatic	Functional involvement (disease onset)
1	Involvement of one clinical region (disease onset)	Loss of independence in one functional domain
2	Involvement of two clinical regions	Loss of independence in two functional domains
3	Involvement of three clinical regions	Loss of independence in three functional domains
4	Substantial respiratory or nutritional failure	Loss of independence in four functional domains
5	Death	Death

Table 39.8 Genes modifying ALS risk or progression, modified after Su et al. (2014) reproduced with kind permission by Wiley

Gene	Gene Locus	Protein product	Molecular function
ATXN2	12q24	Ataxin-2	• RNA metabolism • RNA translation • Endocytosis
CHGB		Chromogranin B	• Protein metabolism
CREST		nBAF component SS18L1	• DNA regulation
ELP3	8p21.1	Elongator protein 3	• Axonal outgrowth • Axonal guidance • RNA metabolism
EPHA4	2q36.1	Ephrin A4	• Axonal outgrowth
FIG4		Polyphosphoinositide phosphatise	• Lipid metabolism
GRN		Progranulin	• Growth factor
HFE	6p22.2	Human hemochromatosis protein	• Iron metabolism
KIFAP3	1q24.2	Kinesin-associated protein 3	• Cellular transport • Axonal transport.
NEFH		Neurofilament heavy subunit	• Cytoskeleton
PON1, 2, 3	7q21.3		• Detoxifying enzyme
SMN1	5q13.2		• Survival factor
SPAST	2q22.3		• Cytoskeleton
SS18L1	20q12.33		• Chromatin regulation
TMEM106B	7p21.3		• Endolysosomal pathway
UNC13A	19p13.11	UNC13A protein	• Neurotransmission • Neurotransmitter release
VEGF	6p21.1	Vascular endothelial growth factor	• Angiogenesis
ZNF512B	20q13.33		• Positive regulator of TGF-ß signaling

Selected References

Al-Chalabi A, Hardiman O, Kiernan MC, Chio A, Rix-Brooks B, van den Berg LH (2016) Amyotrophic lateral sclerosis: moving towards a new classification system. Lancet Neurol 15(11):1182–1194. https://doi.org/10.1016/s1474-4422(16)30199-5

Brooks BR (1994) El Escorial World Federation of Neurology criteria for the diagnosis of amyotrophic lateral sclerosis. Subcommittee on Motor Neuron Diseases/Amyotrophic Lateral Sclerosis of the World Federation of Neurology Research Group on Neuromuscular Diseases and the El Escorial "Clinical limits of amyotrophic lateral sclerosis" workshop contributors. J Neurol Sci 124(Suppl):96–107

Foerster BR, Welsh RC, Feldman EL (2013) 25 years of neuroimaging in amyotrophic lateral sclerosis. Nat Rev Neurol 9(9):513–524. https://doi.org/10.1038/nrneurol.2013.153

Hardiman O, Al-Chalabi A, Chio A, Corr EM, Logroscino G, Robberecht W, Shaw PJ, Simmons Z, van den Berg LH (2017) Amyotrophic lateral sclerosis. Nat Rev Dis Primers 3:17085. https://doi.org/10.1038/nrdp.2017.85

Khader SM, Greiner FG (1999) Neuroradiology case of the day. Amyotrophic lateral sclerosis. Radiographics 19(6):1696–1698. https://doi.org/10.1148/radiographics.19.6.g99no151696

Kwan JY, Jeong SY, Van Gelderen P, Deng HX, Quezado MM, Danielian LE, Butman JA, Chen L, Bayat E, Russell J, Siddique T, Duyn JH, Rouault TA,

Selected References

Floeter MK (2012a) Iron accumulation in deep cortical layers accounts for MRI signal abnormalities in ALS: correlating 7 tesla MRI and pathology. PLoS One 7(4):e35241. https://doi.org/10.1371/journal.pone.0035241

Kwan JY, Meoded A, Danielian LE, Wu T, Floeter MK (2012b) Structural imaging differences and longitudinal changes in primary lateral sclerosis and amyotrophic lateral sclerosis. Neuroimage Clin 2:151–160. https://doi.org/10.1016/j.nicl.2012.12.003

Li HF, Wu ZY (2016) Genotype-phenotype correlations of amyotrophic lateral sclerosis. Transl Neurodegener 5:3. https://doi.org/10.1186/s40035-016-0050-8

Mancuso R, Navarro X (2015) Amyotrophic lateral sclerosis: current perspectives from basic research to the clinic. Prog Neurobiol 133:1–26. https://doi.org/10.1016/j.pneurobio.2015.07.004

Riva N, Agosta F, Lunetta C, Filippi M, Quattrini A (2016) Recent advances in amyotrophic lateral sclerosis. J Neurol 263(6):1241–1254. https://doi.org/10.1007/s00415-016-8091-6

Shang Y, Huang EJ (2016) Mechanisms of FUS mutations in familial amyotrophic lateral sclerosis. Brain Res 1647:65–78. https://doi.org/10.1016/j.brainres.2016.03.036

Su XW, Broach JR, Connor JR, Gerhard GS, Simmons Z (2014) Genetic heterogeneity of amyotrophic lateral sclerosis: implications for clinical practice and research. Muscle Nerve 49(6):786–803. https://doi.org/10.1002/mus.24198

Thomas M, Alegre-Abarrategui J, Wade-Martins R (2013) RNA dysfunction and aggrephagy at the centre of an amyotrophic lateral sclerosis/frontotemporal dementia disease continuum. Brain 136(Pt 5):1345–1360. https://doi.org/10.1093/brain/awt030

Wang S, Melhem ER, Poptani H, Woo JH (2011) Neuroimaging in amyotrophic lateral sclerosis. Neurotherapeutics 8(1):63–71. https://doi.org/10.1007/s13311-010-0011-3

Weishaupt JH, Hyman T, Dikic I (2016) Common molecular pathways in amyotrophic lateral sclerosis and frontotemporal dementia. Trends Mol Med 22(9):769–783. https://doi.org/10.1016/j.molmed.2016.07.005

Yasuda K, Mili S (2016) Dysregulated axonal RNA translation in amyotrophic lateral sclerosis. Wiley Interdiscip Rev RNA 7(5):589–603. https://doi.org/10.1002/wrna.1352

Zufiria M, Gil-Bea FJ, Fernandez-Torron R, Poza JJ, Munoz-Blanco JL, Rojas-Garcia R, Riancho J, de Munain AL (2016) ALS: a bucket of genes, environment, metabolism and unknown ingredients. Prog Neurobiol 142:104–129. https://doi.org/10.1016/j.pneurobio.2016.05.004

Neurodegenerative Diseases: Huntington Disease

40.1 Introduction

Huntington disease (HD) is an autosomal dominant disorder with full penetrance and rare de novo mutations. Sporadic cases are extremely rare.

40.2 Clinical Signs and Symptoms

- Early changes include:
  - Mild motor decline with clumsiness and slowed gait
  - Irritability, anxiety, or agitation
  - Apathy or depression
  - Subtle eye movement abnormalities
  - Delusions and hallucinations
- Progressive changes include:
  - Dystonia and chorea
  - Parkinsonian symptoms
  - Slow and stiff gait
  - Dysphagia
  - Tremor
  - Depression and suicidal ideation
- Late changes include:
  - Rigidity, severe bradykinesia
  - Dysphagia, inability to swallow
  - Seizures
  - Unable to walk or speak

40.3 Epidemiology

Prevalence
- 5–10: 100,000

Age at Onset
- Late childhood to eighth decade
- Mean age: 35–40 years

Sex Incidence
- Male:female ratio: 1:1

40.4 Neuroimaging Findings

General Imaging Findings
- Atrophy of striatum (especially caudate nucleus), cortical gray matter, globus pallidus and thalamus

CT non-contrast-enhanced
- Earliest changes: Atrophy of caudate nucleus with consecutive widening of frontal horns of lateral ventricles

CT contrast-enhanced
- No pathological enhancement

MRI-T2 (Fig. 40.1a, b)
- Atrophy of basal ganglia
- Juvenile Huntington disease: hyperintensity of putamen and caudate nucleus

MRI-FLAIR (Fig. 40.1c)
- Atrophy of basal ganglia

MRI-T1 (Fig. 40.1d, e)
- Decreased volume of basal ganglia

MRI-T1 Contrast-Enhanced
- No pathological enhancement

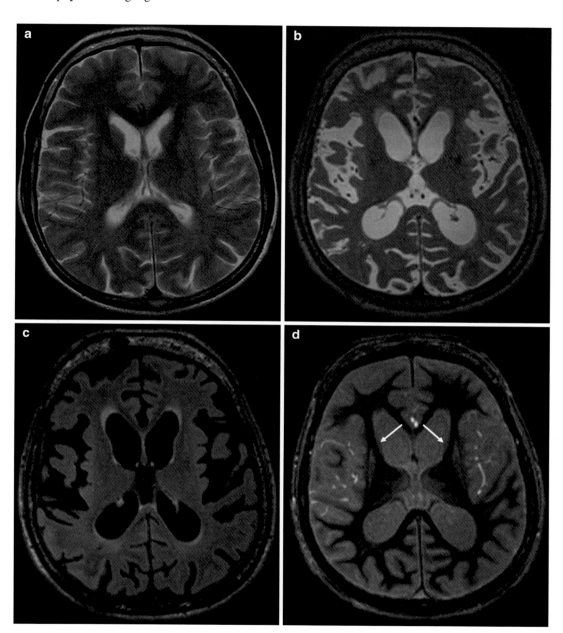

Fig. 40.1 Female patient with Huntington disease—initial MRI shows normal volume of the caudate nucleus: T2 (**a**); follow-up scan 10 years later shows general brain atrophy and atrophy of caudate nucleus with widening of frontal horns of the lateral ventricles: T2 (**b**), FLAIR (**c**), FGATIR (Fast Gray Matter Acquisition T1 Inversion Recovery) axial (**d**), coronal (**e**)

40.4 Neuroimaging Findings

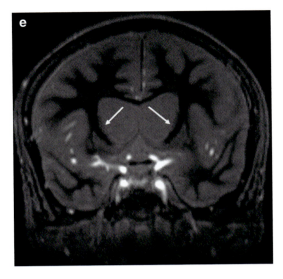

Fig. 40.1 (continued)

MR-Spectroscopy
- Decreased NAA/creatine ratio in basal ganglia

Nuclear Medicine Imaging Findings (Figs. 40.2a, b and 40.3a, b)
- FDG-PET studies demonstrate a reduction of striatal glucose consumption in patients with Huntington disease.
- FDG uptake reduction is accentuated in the caudate but also clearly visible in the putamen.
- Striatal hypometabolism can precede the onset of symptoms and morphological changes.
- In patients with genetic diagnosed Huntington disease, a normal FDG uptake is a prognostic marker that the onset of symptoms may be delayed by some years.

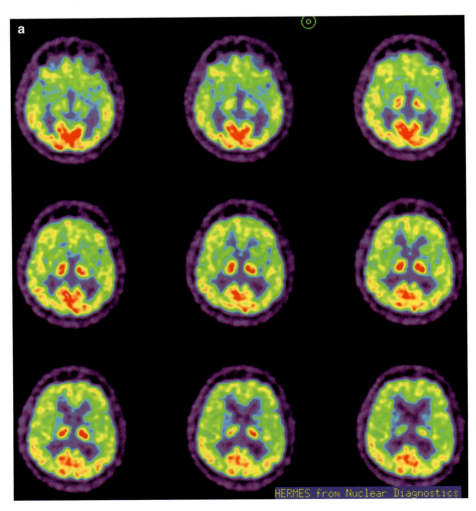

Fig. 40.2 FDG-PET of a patient with Huntington disease demonstrates loss of metabolism in the striatum (**a, b**)

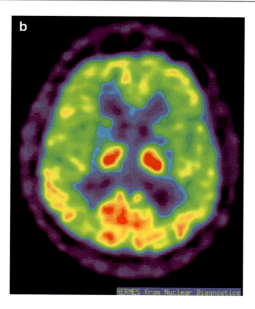

Fig. 40.2 (continued)

- Striatal hypometabolism can be so pronounced that nearly no uptake can be seen in the later course of the disease.
- Cortical glucose metabolism is reduced in Huntington disease patients too, mainly in the frontal and temporal lobe, although these reductions are little in contrast to striatal loss and mainly seen in statistical analysis.
- CBF studies reveal a similar pattern like FDG-PET but have an inferior resolution and uptake measurement and statistical analysis is more complicated.
- Striatal glucose hypometabolism can also occur in patients with hereditary chorea and Lesch–Nyhan syndrome.
- D2 receptor binding studies with SPECT and PET tracers like IBZM, epidepride, raclopride, or fallypride reveal a reduced D2 receptor binding in patients with Huntington disease.

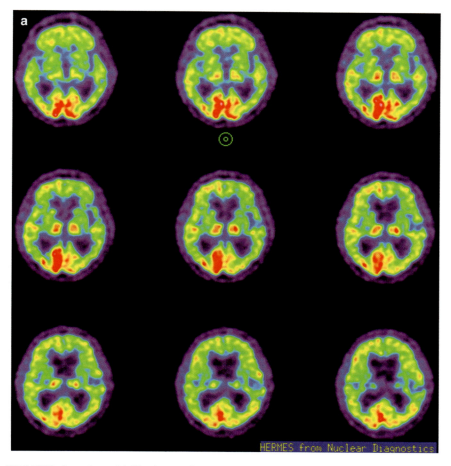

Fig. 40.3 FDG-PET of a patient with Huntington disease and dementia shows loss of metabolism not only in the striatum but also in the cerebral cortex (**a**, **b**)

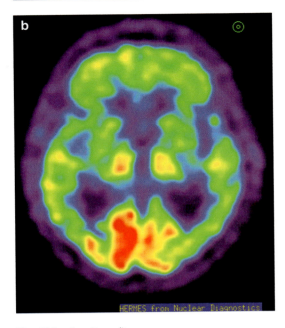

Fig. 40.3 (continued)

40.5 Neuropathology Findings

Macroscopic Findings (Fig. 40.4a–c)
- Brain weight might be reduced (1100 g)
- Cortical atrophy present in some cases
- Frontal sections: severely atrophic caudate nucleus which might have a rounded appearance and concave
- The putamen appears smaller
- Lateral ventricles are severely enlarged especially the anterior parts
- Substantia nigra appears darker due to an atrophy of the pars reticulata

Microscopic Findings (Fig. 40.5a–h)
- Loss of medium-sized spiny neurons in the caudate nucleus
  - Neurons are GABA-substance P or GABA-enkephalin positive
  - Project to the globus pallidus and pars reticulata of the substantia nigra

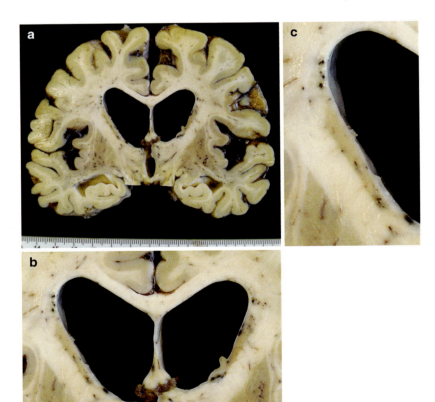

Fig. 40.4 Severe atrophy of the caudate nucleus is seen at the gross-anatomical level (**a–c**)

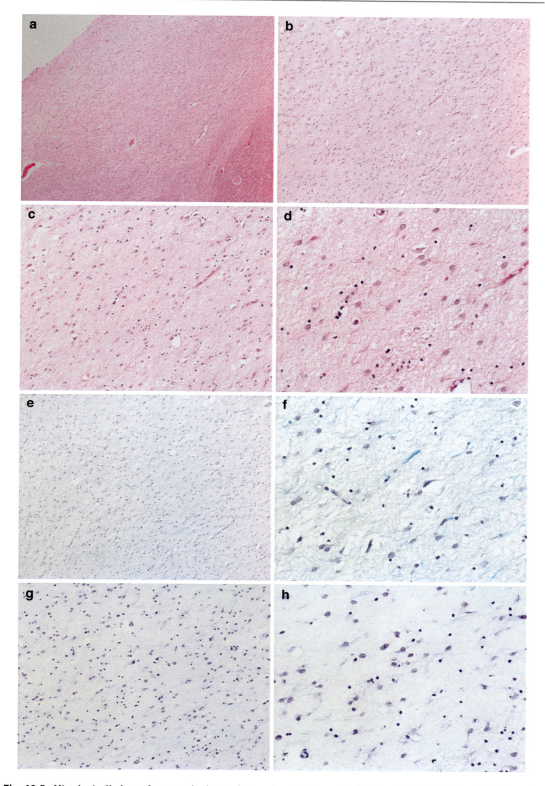

Fig. 40.5 Histologically loss of neurons in the caudate nucleus is discernible (**a–d**: stain: H&E) (**e, f**: stain: LFB; **g, h**: stain: Cresyl violet)

- Small spiny interneurons are not involved
  - They are neuropeptide Y, somatostatin and NADPH-Diaphorase positive
- Large non-spiny cholinergic interneurons not involved
- Other regions involved
  - Globus pallidus
  - Ventrolateral thalamus
  - Subthalamic nuclei
- Peculiar pattern of neuronal loss in the caudate nucleus and putamen
  - Medial to dorsal
  - Dorsal to ventral
  - From tail to head through body
- Vacuolization of the neuropil
- Strong reactive astrogliosis
- Cerebral cortex:
  - No obvious microscopic changes
  - Slight loss of pyramidal neurons in layers III, V, and VI of the frontal lobe, CA1 region of the hippocampus
  - Concomittant reactive astrogliosis
- In elderly patients:
  - ß-Amyloid deposits in variable amounts in the cerebral cortex and hippocampus
  - Absence of neuritic plaques
  - Sparse amount of neurofibrillary tangles in the cerebral cortex, hippocampus, and amygdala

The five grades of disease severity in the postmortem brain have been described by Vonsattel as follows (Vonsattel and DiFiglia 1998; Vonsattel et al. 1985, 2008, 2011):

- Grade 0
  - No indentifiable gross changes
  - Diagnosis based on clinical history, family history, and DNA test results
- Grade 1
  - No or minimal atrophy at the CAP level
  - Atrophy of the tail and body of caudate nucleus
- Grade 2
  - Atrophy of the neostriatum at the CAP level
  - Head of caudate nucleus with mildly bulging border with the anterior horn of the lateral ventricle
- Grade 3
  - Marked atrophy in the dorsal regions of the neostriatum
  - Straight caudate/ventricle border
- Grade 4
  - Slightly concave, wrinkled caudate/ventricle border
  - Atrophy of caudate nucleus, putamen, and internal capsule
- Peculiar pattern of neuronal loss in the caudate nucleus and putamen
  - Medial to dorsal
  - Dorsal to ventral
  - From tail to head through body

Immunohistochemical Staining (Fig. 40.6a–f)
- Ubiquitin-positive inclusions
- 1C2 positive inclusions

40.6 Molecular Neuropathology

- Huntington disease (HD) is an autosomal dominant monogenic disorder with full penetrance and rare de novo mutations
- Sporadic cases are extremely rare
- Expansion of CAG repeat in exon 1 in the huntingtin gene (HTT) mapped to short arm of chromosome 4q16.3
  - Encodes the protein huntingtin
  - Located at the 5′ end of the gene
- Number of repeats can increase from one generation to the next one
  - Normal alleles: 26 or fewer repeats
  - Intermediate alleles: 27–35 repeats
    - Individual nor at risk to develop the disease
    - Risk of having an affected child
  - HD-causing alleles: 36 or more repeats
    - Reduced penetrance: 36–39 repeats
    - Full penetrance: 40 or more repeats
- Inverse correlation between number of repeats and age of disease onset

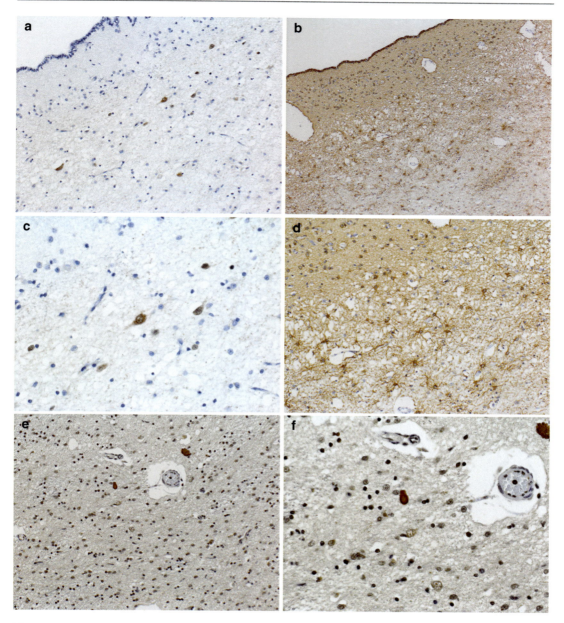

Fig. 40.6 Immunophenotype: the few surviving neurons can be identified with NeuN stain (**a**, **b**); moderate reactive astrogliosis (**c**, **d**: stain GFAP); a few neurons contain ubiquitin-positive inclusions (**e**, **f**)

- Environmental factors, genetic modifiers, and other factors determine the development of the disease over time
- Maternal or paternal transmission
  - Paternal transmission associated with higher number of repeats
- Huntingtin:
  - Wild-type (wt) HTT also appears to play several roles in regulating the dynamics of autophagy
  - Expressed in innate immune cells
  - For wild-type huntingtin in the intracellular transport of vesicles and organelles

40.6.1 Genetics

The affected gene in HD patients is *HTT* which contains 67 exons and maps to the short arm of chromosome 4p16.3 where it covers a region of ~180 kb. It encodes huntingtin (HTT), a large protein of over 3000 amino acids. Although the physiological functions of HTT are not fully established yet, it has become clear that it plays a pivotal role in cell survival and integrity, e.g., by participating in transcriptional control, intracellular vesicular trafficking, and in regulating the dynamics of autophagy.

A prominent feature of HTT is a repetitive stretch of glutamine residues (polyQ) in the N-terminal region of the protein, encoded by consecutive CAG triplets in exon1 of the *HTT* gene. In normal alleles, about 26 or fewer repeats are observed. Expanded repeats (27–35; intermediate alleles) correlate with risk of developing HD or having an affected child. HD-causing alleles exhibit even higher numbers; those with 36–39 repeats show low penetrance for the disease. Full penetrance occurs with alleles containing 40 or more CAG copies.

It should be noted that normal alleles are genetically stable, whereas expanded CAG repeats have a tendency to increase from one generation to the next. Paternal transmission appears to be associated with higher repeat numbers. Moreover, an inverse correlation between number of repeats and age of disease onset is documented. However, other factors such as environmental influences or genetic modifiers (for instance, proteins of the DNA repair machinery, DNA methylation) also affect the development of the disease over time.

40.6.2 Epigenetics

Studies with transgenic HD mouse models as well as human samples revealed altered DNA methylation patterns in HD tissues as compared to controls. Differences were found in gene regulatory sequences, i.e., promoter and CpG islands, presumably contributing to changes in transcriptional activity. However, both hyper- and hypomethylated regions have been detected in HD, a confusing finding which makes it difficult to comprehend the epigenetic processes underlying the disease. More detailed investigations studying DNA methylation changes in HD have been targeted at specific genes (e.g., *HES4, ADORA2A*) which were selected for their possible involvement in HD pathogenesis (reviewed in Thomas (2016)).

40.7   Treatment and Prognosis

Treatment
- Rigidity: baclofen and diltiazem
- Chorea: haloperidol or atypical antipsychotics
- Myoclonus: valproate

Biologic Behavior-Prognosis-Prognostic Factors
- Progressive disorder
- Mean duration of disease: 17 years (2–45 years)

Selected References

Adam OR, Jankovic J (2008) Symptomatic treatment of Huntington disease. Neurotherapeutics 5(2):181–197. https://doi.org/10.1016/j.nurt.2008.01.008

Anglada-Huguet M, Vidal-Sancho L (2017) Pathogenesis of Huntington's disease: how to fight excitotoxicity and transcriptional dysregulation. In: Tunalı NE (ed) Huntington's disease – molecular pathogenesis and current models. InTech, Rijeka, pp 37–73. https://doi.org/10.5772/66734

Apolinario TA, Paiva CL, Agostinho LA (2017) REVIEW-ARTICLE Intermediate alleles of Huntington's disease HTT gene in different populations worldwide: a systematic review. Genet Mol Res 16(2). https://doi.org/10.4238/gmr16029648

Arning L (2016) The search for modifier genes in Huntington disease – multifactorial aspects of a monogenic disorder. Mol Cell Probes. https://doi.org/10.1016/j.mcp.2016.06.006

Dayalu P, Albin RL (2015) Huntington disease: pathogenesis and treatment. Neurol Clin 33(1):101–114. https://doi.org/10.1016/j.ncl.2014.09.003

Ho VB, Chuang HS, Rovira MJ, Koo B (1995) Juvenile Huntington disease: CT and MR features. AJNR Am J Neuroradiol 16(7):1405–1412

Martin DD, Ladha S, Ehrnhoefer DE, Hayden MR (2015) Autophagy in Huntington disease and huntingtin in autophagy. Trends Neurosci 38(1):26–35. https://doi.org/10.1016/j.tins.2014.09.003

Montoya A, Price BH, Menear M, Lepage M (2006) Brain imaging and cognitive dysfunctions in Huntington's disease. J Psychiatry Neurosci 31(1):21–29

Ross CA, Aylward EH, Wild EJ, Langbehn DR, Long JD, Warner JH, Scahill RI, Leavitt BR, Stout JC, Paulsen JS, Reilmann R, Unschuld PG, Wexler A, Margolis RL, Tabrizi SJ (2014) Huntington disease: natural history, biomarkers and prospects for therapeutics. Nat Rev Neurol 10(4):204–216. https://doi.org/10.1038/nrneurol.2014.24

Rub U, Vonsattel JP, Heinsen H, Korf HW (2015) The neuropathology of Huntington's disease: classical findings, recent developments and correlation to functional neuroanatomy. Adv Anat Embryol Cell Biol 217:1–146

Sturrock A, Leavitt BR (2010) The clinical and genetic features of Huntington disease. J Geriatr Psychiatry Neurol 23(4):243–259. https://doi.org/10.1177/0891988710383573

Sturrock A, Laule C, Decolongon J, Dar Santos R, Coleman AJ, Creighton S, Bechtel N, Reilmann R, Hayden MR, Tabrizi SJ, Mackay AL, Leavitt BR (2010) Magnetic resonance spectroscopy biomarkers in premanifest and early Huntington disease. Neurology 75(19):1702–1710. https://doi.org/10.1212/WNL.0b013e3181fc27e4

Thomas EA (2016) DNA methylation in Huntington's disease: implications for transgenerational effects. Neurosci Lett 625:34–39. https://doi.org/10.1016/j.neulet.2015.10.060. Epub 2015 Nov 11

Tomé S, Dandelot E (2017) Genetic modifiers of CAG.CTG repeat instability in Huntington's disease mouse models. In: Tunalı NE (ed) Huntington's disease – molecular pathogenesis and current models. InTech, Rijeka, pp 1–20. https://doi.org/10.5772/66438

Vonsattel JP, DiFiglia M (1998) Huntington disease. J Neuropathol Exp Neurol 57(5):369–384

Vonsattel JP, Myers RH, Stevens TJ, Ferrante RJ, Bird ED, Richardson EP Jr (1985) Neuropathological classification of Huntington's disease. J Neuropathol Exp Neurol 44(6):559–577

Vonsattel JP, Keller C, Del Pilar Amaya M (2008) Neuropathology of Huntington's disease. Handb Clin Neurol 89:599–618. https://doi.org/10.1016/s0072-9752(07)01256-0

Vonsattel JP, Keller C, Cortes Ramirez EP (2011) Huntington's disease – neuropathology. Handb Clin Neurol 100:83–100. https://doi.org/10.1016/b978-0-444-52014-2.00004-5

Warby SC, Graham RK, Hayden MR (1993) Huntington disease. In: Pagon RA, Adam MP, Ardinger HH et al (eds) GeneReviews(R). University of Washington, Seattle, WA

Zheng Z, Diamond MI (2012) Huntington disease and the huntingtin protein. Prog Mol Biol Transl Sci 107:189–214. https://doi.org/10.1016/b978-0-12-385883-2.00010-2

Part VII
The Brain Diseases: Myelin Disorders

Demyelinating Diseases: Multiple Sclerosis

41.1 Introduction

Demyelination is characterized by:

- Destruction of normal myelin
- Relative preservation of axons

Demyelinating diseases include (Table 41.1):

- Multiple sclerosis (MS)
- Neuromyelitis optica (Dévic disease)
- Acute disseminated encephalomyelitis (ADEM)
- Acute hemorrhagic leukoencephalopathy (AHL)

Dysmyelination is characterized by:

- Failure to form myelin normally

Loss of myelin can be due to an inherited defect of metabolism.

41.2 Clinical Signs and Symptoms

- Clinical symptoms of MS are multiple, variable, and unspecific (Table 41.2).

The following types of MS exist:

- Classical—Charcot type
- Acute—Marburg type
- Concentric type Balo

The classical MS Charcot type is clinically characterized by:

- Relapsing remitting (RRMS)
  - Multiple acute attacks followed by clinical improvement
- Secondary progressive (SPMS)
  - After years of RRMS, stage of no recovery between acute attacks
- Primary progressive (PPMS)
  - Progressive disease without periods of recovery
- Relapsing progressive (PRMS)
  - Acute attacks are superimposed on progressive disease without episodes of recovery

More Common Symptoms of Multiple Sclerosis (MS) (Ghasemi et al. 2017)
- Primary symptoms
  - More common symptoms
    - Sensory disturbances (numbness, tingling, itching, burning)

Table 41.1 Diseases related to myelin pathology

Group	Disease
Acquired, inflammatory, or infectious	• Multiple sclerosis classic type Charcot • Multiple sclerosis variants 　– Acute multiple sclerosis—Marburg type 　– Diffuse sclerosis—Schilder type 　– Concentric sclerosis—Balò type 　– Tumefactive MS • Neuromyelitis optica—Dévic type • Optic neuritis • Clinically isolated syndrome • Acute disseminated encephalitis 　– Post-infectious encephalomyelitis 　– Post-vaccination encephalomyelitis 　– Post-immunization encephalomyelitis • Acute hemorrhagic leukoencephalopathy • Progressive multifocal leukoencephalopathy • Tabes dorsalis • Transverse myelitis
Hereditary metabolic	• Metachromatic leukodystrophy • Krabbe disease • Adrenoleukodystrophy • Pelizaeus-Merzbacher disease 　– Type I—classic 　– Type II—Seitelberger, connatal, or congenital 　– Type III—transitional 　– Type IV—adult type 　– Type V 　– Type VI • Canavan disease • Alexander disease • Alper syndrome • CAMFAK syndrome
Acquired toxic-metabolic	• Central pontine myelinolysis • Marchiafava–Bignami disease • Vitamin B12 deficiency
Traumatic	• Compression due to extrinsic factors • Tumor compression

Table 41.2 Symptoms of MS are multiple, variable, unspecific, modified after Compston and Coles (2008) reproduced with kind permission by Elsevier

Site affected	Symptoms
Cerebrum	• Cognitive impairment • Hemisensory and motor • Affective (mainly depression) • Epilepsy (rare) • Focal cortical defects (rare)
Optic nerve	• Unilateral painful loss of vision
Cerebellum	• Tremor • Clumsiness and poor balance
Brainstem	• Diplopia, oscillopsia • Vertigo • Impaired swallowing • Impaired speech and emotional lability • Paroxysmal symptoms
Spinal cord	• Weakness • Stiffness and painful spasms • Bladder dysfunction • Erectile impotence • Constipation
Other	• Pain • Fatigue • Temperature sensitivity and exercise intolerance

  o Intestinal and urinary system dysfunction (constipation and bladder dysfunction)
  o Cognitive and emotional impairment (inability to learn and depression)
  o Dizziness and vertigo
  o Sexual problems
• Less common symptoms
  o Swallowing problems (dysphagia)
  o Speech problems (dysarthria)
  o Breathing problems
  o Hearing loss
  o Seizures
  o Headache
• Secondary symptoms
  – Urinary tract infections
  – Inactivity
  – Immobility
• Tertiary symptoms
  – Social complications
  – Vocational complications
  – Psychological complications
  – Depression
  o Walking difficulties (due to fatigue, weakness, spasticity, loss of balance, and tremor)
  o Vision problems (diplopia, blurred, and pain on eye movement)

41.3 Epidemiology

Incidence
- Geographical variation of prevalence:
- >30 per 100,000 in Europe, Israel, Canada, northern USA
- 5–30 per 100,000 in southern USA, southern Mediterranean, South Africa, Latin America

Age Incidence
- <20 years: 20%
- 20–50 years: 50–60%
- >50 years: 20–30%

Sex Incidence
- Male:Female ratio: 1:1.4–3.1

Localization
- White matter
- Predominantly periventricular

41.4 Neuroimaging Findings

General Imaging Findings
- Multiple white matter lesions with dissemination in time and space

CT non-contrast-enhanced
- Iso- or hypodense lesions
- Variable brain atrophy in chronic MS

CT contrast-enhanced
- Enhancement of acute plaques

MRI-T2 (Figs. 41.1a and 41.3a)
- Hyperintense white matter lesions

MRI-FLAIR (Figs. 41.1b, c, 41.2a, and 41.3b)
- FLAIR more sensitive than T2
- Asymmetric bilateral hyperintensities, common in periventricular location, callososeptal or juxtacortical
- Supra- and/or infratentorial location
- Perpendicular arrangement to lateral ventricles following deep medullary veins—"Dawson fingers"
- As disease proceeds plaques show confluence
- Balo type: variant of MS with ring-shaped large lesions (alternating demyelinated and regular myelinated white matter)

MRI-T1 (Figs. 41.1d, 41.2b, and 41.3c)
- Iso- or hypointense ("black holes")

MRI-T1 Contrast-Enhanced (Figs. 41.1e, 41.2c, and 41.3d)
- Nodular or solid enhancement, ring or incomplete ring enhancement

MRI-T2*/SWI
- Deep medullary veins located in the center of the plaques

MR-Diffusion Imaging (Figs. 41.1f, g, 41.2d, e, and 41.3e, f)
- Diffusion restriction in acute plaques possible

MRI-Perfusion
- Decreased rCBV

MR-Diffusion Tensor Imaging
- Anisotropy very low in plaques, but also low in regular-appearing white matter

MR-Spectroscopy
- NAA low
- Choline high

The 2016 MAGNIMS consensus guidelines of MRI criteria for dissemination in time and space are shown in Table 41.3.

Nuclear Medicine Imaging Findings (Fig. 41.4)
- Some studies, mainly performed in rats, describe a focal FDG uptake in demyelinating lesions and focal uptake of novel tracers for the detection of microglial activation like 11C-PK11195.

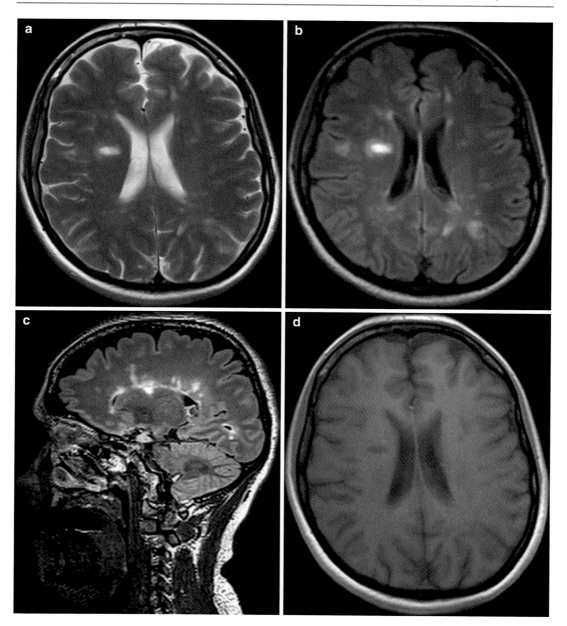

Fig. 41.1 Multiple sclerosis with bilateral periventricular and juxtacortical T2-hyperintensities, acute gadolinium-enhancing plaque in right corona radiata, T2 (**a**), FLAIR (**b**), typical "Dawson fingers" on sagittal FLAIR (**c**), T1 (**d**), T1 contrast (**e**), DWI (**f**), ADC (**g**)

41.4 Neuroimaging Findings

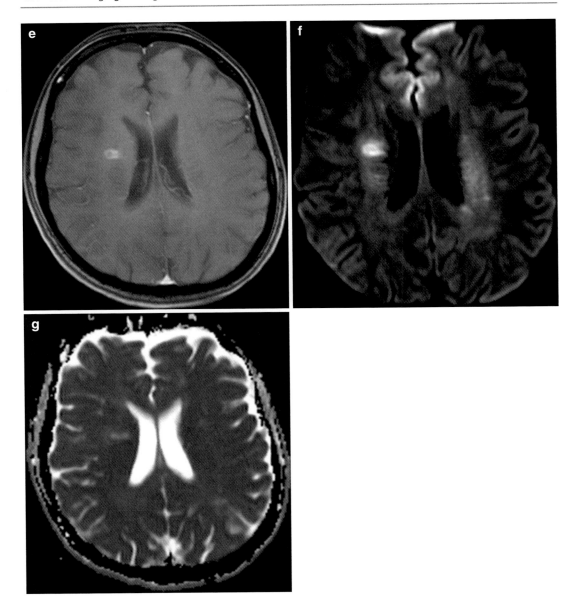

Fig. 41.1 (continued)

- 18F-FSPG-PET studies are investigating the cystine/glutamate antiporter system in MS mouse models.
- Cerebral dysfunction can be seen on FDG-PET of the brain in patients with involvement of verbal and/or long-term memory.
- In recent time, FET is considered to be a valuable diagnostic tool for the visualization of the inflammatory process, which can be seen in MRI-negative white matter. After initializing therapy response of these lesions can be seen.

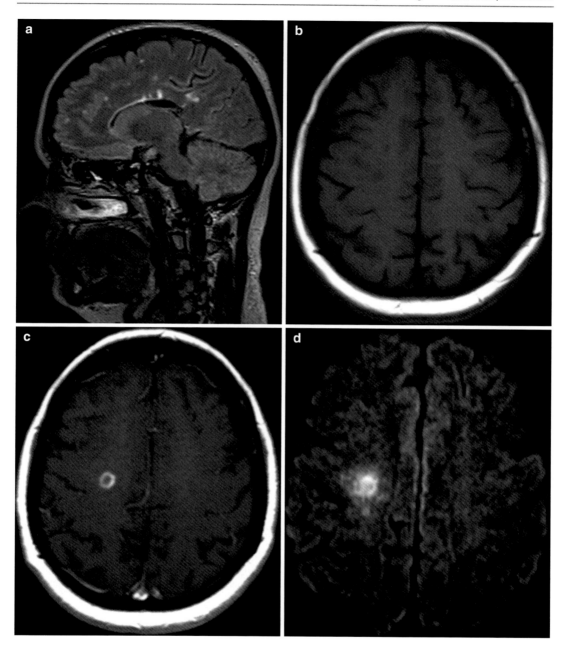

Fig. 41.2 Acute, ring-enhancing MS-plaque in right semioval center with restricted diffusion on plaque rim, sagittal FLAIR (**a**), T1 (**b**), T1 contrast (**c**), DWI (**d**), ADC (**e**)

41.5 Neuropathology Findings

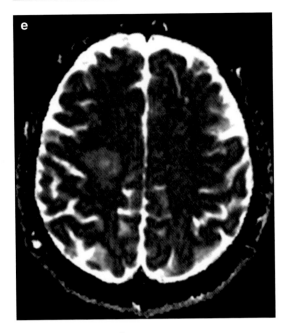

Fig. 41.2 (continued)

Table 41.3 MRI criteria for dissemination in time and space (MAGNIMS consensus guidelines 2016 (Hyun et al. 2017))

Dissemination in space	Dissemination in time
Involvement of at least two of the following five CNS regions:	New T2-hyperintense lesion and/or enhancing plaque compared to a previous MRI
• ≥3 periventricular lesions	OR
• ≥1 juxtacortical or cortical lesion	
• ≥1 infratentorial lesion	Appearance of asymptomatic enhancing lesions AND non-enhancing lesions at any time
• ≥1 spinal cord lesion	
• ≥1 optic nerve lesion	

41.5 Neuropathology Findings

Macroscopic Features (Fig. 41.5a–n)
- Plaque:
  - Well-demarcated regions of gray discoloration
  - Variable in size, shape, number, and distribution
  - Adjacent to the lateral borders of the ventricular system
  - Anywhere in the brain
    ○ Deep gray nuclei
    ○ Cerebellar white matter
    ○ Floor of the fourth ventricle
    ○ Brainstem
    ○ Spinal cord

Microscopic Features (Figs. 41.6, 41.7, 41.8, and 41.9)
Variation in appearance of plaques due to:
- Age of lesion
- Disease activity
- Presence or absence of remyelination
- Location, i.e., white matter versus gray matter

Area of demyelination is characterized by:
- Destructed myelin
- Perivascular inflammation with
  - Lymphocytes
  - Macrophages
- Disrupted blood–brain barrier
  - Immunohistochemical demonstration of interstitial accumulation of serum proteins (e.g., transthyretin)

The following types of plaques are distinguished:
- Active plaque
- Inactive plaque
- Shadow plaque

Active plaque:
- Hypercellular lesion
- Perivascular and parenchymal infiltrate of lymphocytes and macrophages
  - Greatest towards the edge of the lesion
  - Mostly T-lymphocytes
  - CD4-Helper cells predominate in active demyelinating areas
  - CD8-Suppressor/cytotoxic cells in less active areas
- Scattered reactive astrocytes
- MHC class II positive macrophages/microglia
- Preservation of axons
  - Shown by silver impregnation of immunohistochemistry for neurofilaments
- Signs of axonal damage shown by accumulation of ß-amyloid precursor protein (APP)

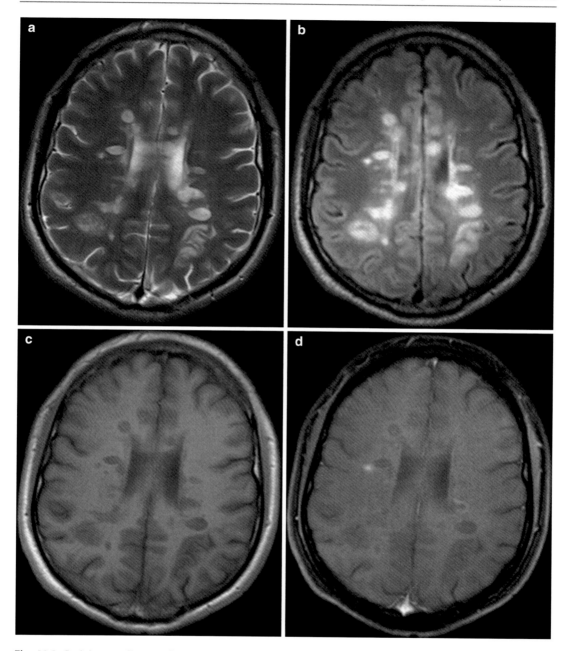

Fig. 41.3 Incipient confluence of periventricular plaques, T2 (**a**), FLAIR (**b**); multiple "black holes" in T1 (**c**), two plaques show mild enhancement on T1 contrast (**d**), DWI (**e**), ADC (**f**)

41.5 Neuropathology Findings

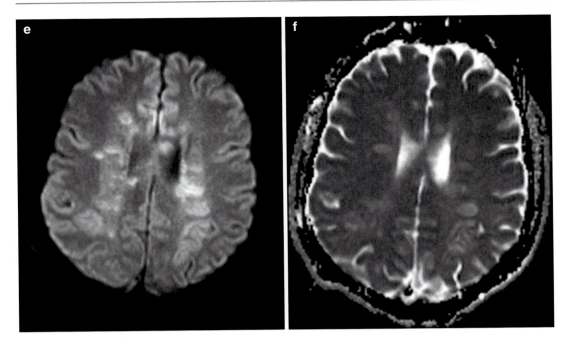

Fig. 41.3 (continued)

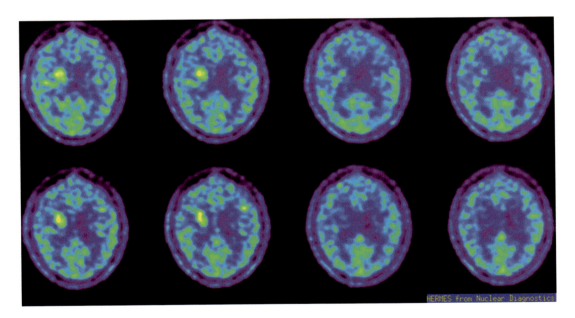

Fig. 41.4 FET-PET showing uptake within the focus of demyelination

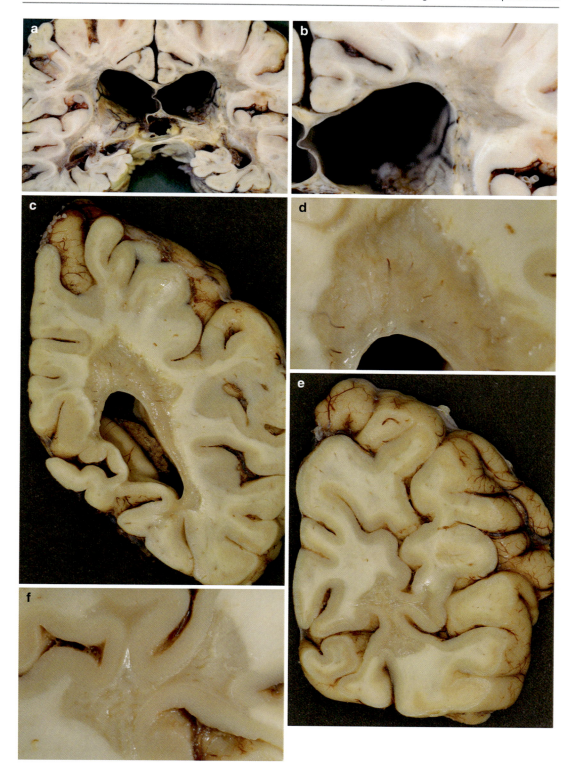

Fig. 41.5 Macroscopic appearances of demyelinating plaques: periventricular lesions in the parietal and temporal lobes (**a**, **b**); glassy appearance of a periventricular plaque in the occipital lobe (**c**, **d**); moth-eaten appearance of a lesion in the occipital lobe (**e**, **f**); frontal lobe (**g**); temporal lobe (**h–j**); corpus callosum (**k**, **l**) (→); pons (**m**, **n**) (→)

41.5 Neuropathology Findings

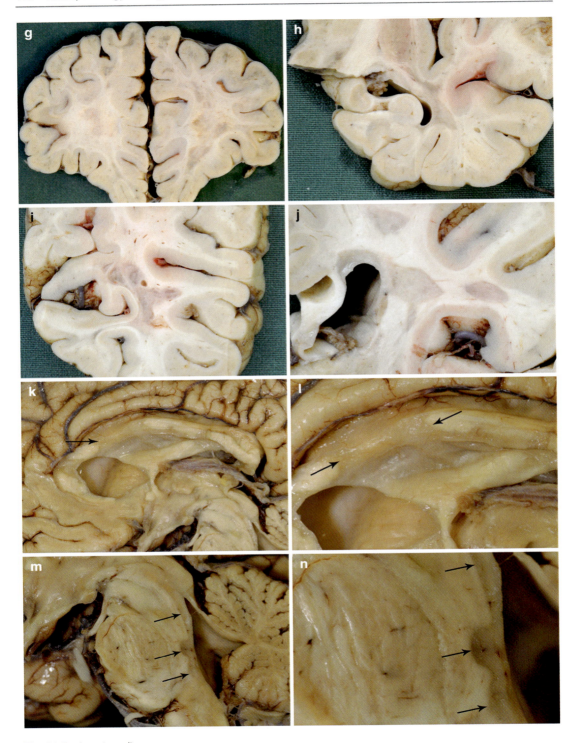

Fig. 41.5 (continued)

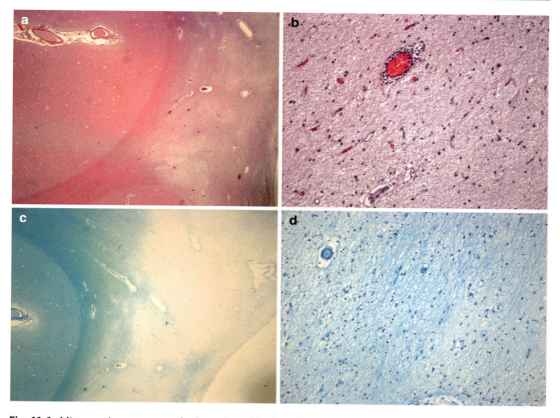

Fig. 41.6 Microscopic appearance of a demyelinated brain region (**a, b**: H&E, **c, d**: LFB). Note the paucicellular area with some perivascularly located lymphocytes

Inactive plaque:
- Hypocellular lesion
- Densely gliotic
- Marked loss of oligodendrocytes
- Groups of axons in direct apposition (cross-talk)
- Sharply defined plaque margins as seen on myelin stain
- Reduction in caliber and amount of axons
- Cavitation possible

Shadow plaque:
- Plaque with reduced but not absent myelin
- Contain remyelinated axons with thin myelin sheaths

Remyelination:
- Occurs spontaneously
- Is often structurally and functionally incomplete
- Mediated by oligodendrocyte precursor cells (OPC)
  - OPC in the white matter
  - Activation of OPC
  - Migration of OPC to the lesion
  - Differentiation into myelin-generating cells
- Remyelinated fibers
  - Thinner myelin sheaths encountered at the border of the lesion

Demyelination and remyelination can occur in the same plaque.

Classification criteria of MS based on the presence of neuropathologic changes are provided in Table 41.4. A comparison of various classification systems for MS as proposed so far is given in Table 41.5.

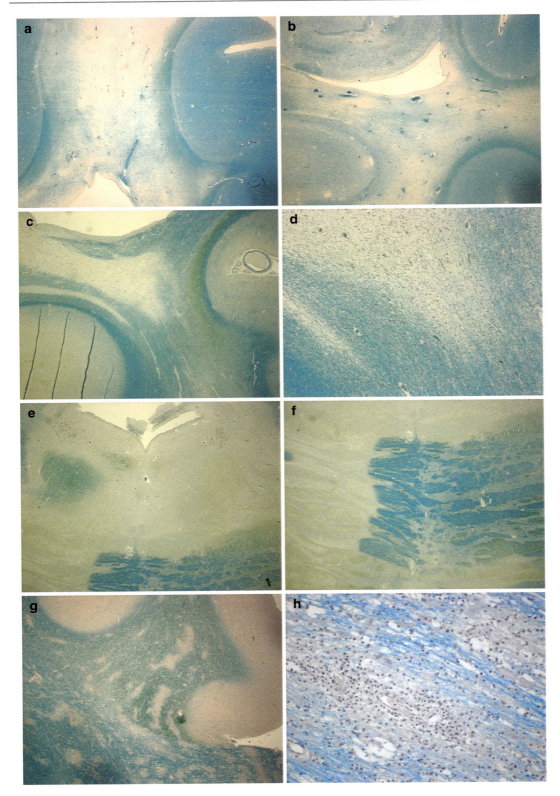

Fig. 41.7 Various appearances of demyelinated areas as seen on Luxol Fast Blue (LFB)-stained sections (**a–d**: cortical white matter; **e, f**: pons; **g, h**: moth-eaten appearance (**g**) with higher cellularity in the lesion (**h**))

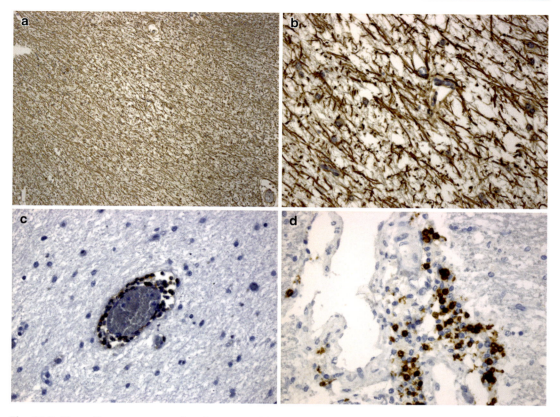

Fig. 41.8 Nerve fibers are preserved as demonstrated by immunohistochemistry for NF (neuronal filament) (**a**, **b**). Perivascularly located CD3-positive T-cells (**c**, **d**)

Recently, Kuhlmann et al. (2017) proposed a simple classification system of MS as follows:
- Active
  - Active and early demyelinating
  - Active and late demyelinating
  - Active and post-demyelinating
- Mixed active/inactive
  - Mixed active/inactive and demyelinating
  - Mixed active/inactive and postdemyelinating
- Inactive

Cortical Lesions

Cortical lesions in multiple sclerosis affect:
- Cerebral cortex
- Cerebellar cortex
- Hippocampus

Cortical lesions include:
- Primary demyelinating lesions with
  - Complete loss of myelin
  - Axonal preservation like preserved phosphorylated neurofilament-reactive profiles
  - Ramified microglia
  - Rarely macrophages
  - Sparse lymphocytes
- Degeneration of cortical
  - Neurons
  - Axons
  - Synapses

Cortical lesions best demonstrated by immunohistochemistry for:
- Myelin basic protein (MBP)
- Proteolipid protein (PLP)

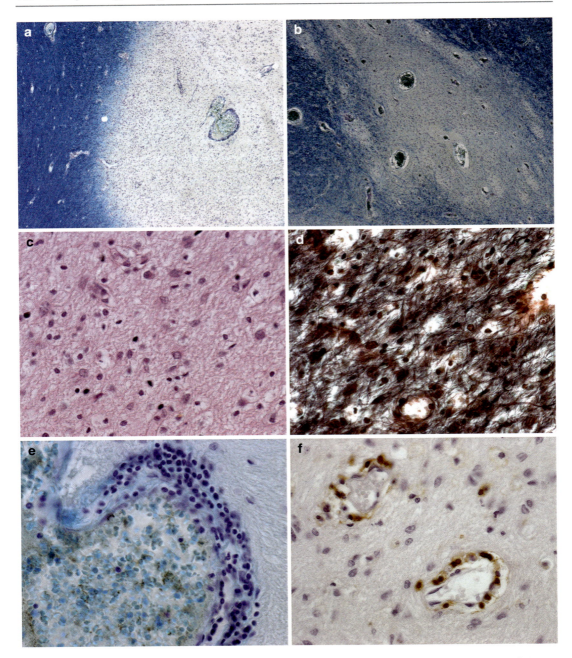

Fig. 41.9 Case of an acute demyelination resulting from acute amphetamine abuse. Demyelinated area (**a**, **b**: LFB), reactive astrogliosis (**c**: HE), preserved axons (**d**: stain: Bodian), perivascular lymphocytic cuffing (**e**, **f**: immunostain CD3), reactive microgliosis (**g**, **h**: HLA-DRII)

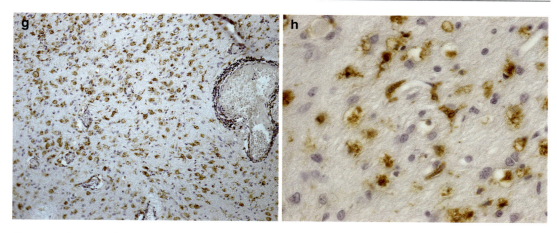

Fig. 41.9 (continued)

Table 41.4 Classification criteria of MS (Lucchinetti et al. 2000) reproduced with kind permission by Wiley

		Pattern I	Pattern II	Pattern III	Pattern IV
Inflammation	CD3 T-cells	Present	Present	Present	Present
	Plasma cells	Occasional	Moderate	Occasional	Occasional
	Macrophages	Numerous	Numerous	Numerous	Very numerous
	Activated complement (C9neo)	Absent	Present	Absent	Absent
Demyelination	Perivenous	Yes	Yes	No	Rarely
	Plaque edge	Sharp	Sharp	Ill-defined	Sharp
	Concentric	No	No	In some cases	No
Oligodendrocytes	Density in inactive center of plaque	Preserved	Preserved	Depleted	Depleted
	DNA fragmentation	Occasional	Occasional	Extensive	Extensive
	Apoptosis	No	No	Yes	No
	Loss of myelin proteins	All equally	All equally	Loss of MAG	All equally
Remyelination	Shadow plaques	Prominent	Prominent	Absent	Absent

Classification of cortical lesions as:
- Leukocortical (Type I after Peterson et al. (2001))
- Intracortical (Type II after Peterson et al. (2001))
- Subpial (Type III after Peterson et al. (2001))
- Transcortical

Cortical lesion classification after Calabrese et al. (2010)
- Type I
  - Lesion extends into the deeper cortical laminae and the subcortical white matter (cortical–juxtacortical lesions)
  - Lesion extends through both white matter and gray matter (cortical–juxtacortical lesions)
- Type II
  - Lesion extends through all cortical layers
  - Lesion within the cerebral cortex and does not extend to the surface of the brain or to the subcortical white matter
- Type III
  - Cortical lesion located in the superficial cortical layers
  - Long ribbons of subpial lesion that often affect several adjacent gyri
- Type IV
  - Lesion affecting the subcortical U-fibers (strictly subcortical)

Table 41.5 Comparison of various classification systems for MS (van der Valk and De Groot 2000; Bo et al. 1994; Bruck et al. 1994, 1995; Lassmann et al. 1998; Trapp et al. 1998)

Bö/Trapp	Van der Valk/deGroot	Lassmann/Brück	Vienna consensus
Active	• Preactive • Active + demyelination	• Early active	• 6 Inf −, Demyel − • 1 Inf +, Demyel + • 3 InfRim +, Demyel +
Chronic active	• Active − no demyelination • Chronic active	• Late active • Inactive	• 2 Inf +, Demyel − • 4 InfRim +, Demyel −
Chronic inactive	• Chronic inactive	• Inactive	• 6 Inf −, Demyel − • 5 Inf −, Demyel +

  – Lesion extends throughout the full width of the cerebral cortex, but does not reach the subcortical white matter
- Type V
  – Lesion affects all of the cortical laminae and the subcortical white matter (cortical–juxtacortical lesion)
- Type VI
  – Small, round, or ovoid lesions occurring in any part of the cortical ribbon
- Type VII
  – A large lesion affecting both banks of a gyrus, or more than one gyrus

Ultrastructural Features
- Active plaque
  – Macrophages contain myelin debris in contact with axons undergoing demyelination
- Inactive plaque
  – Loss of axons associated with concomitant increase of extracellular space

Immunohistochemical Staining Characteristics
(Figs. 41.8a–d and 41.10a–f) (Table 41.6)
- Lymphocyte population
  – CD3 T-lymphocytes
  – CD4-helper T-lymphocytes
  – CD8-suppressor/cytotoxic T-lymphocytes
- Macrophages/microglia
  – MHC class II
  – CD68
- Amyloid precursor protein (APP)
- Myelin proteins
  – Myelin basic protein (MBP)
  – Proteolipid protein (PLP)
  – 2′,3′-Cyclic nucleotide 3′-phosphodiesterase (CNP)
  – Myelin-associated glycoprotein (MAG)
  – Myelin oligodendrocyte glycoprotein (MOG)
- Blood–brain barrier leakage
  – Serum proteins, e.g., transthyretin

Differential Diagnosis
- Dysmyelinating disorder
- Other demyelinating diseases
- Vacuolar myelopathy
- Leukodystrophies (Adrenoleukodystrophy, Adrenomyeloneuropathy)
- Marchiafava–Bignami
- Vasculitis

41.6 Molecular Neuropathology

- Autoimmune hypothesis
- Inflammation
  – Innate immunity
  – Microglia and macrophages
  – Adaptive immunity
  – T-cells, regulatory T-cells
  – B-cells
  – Interleukin 1ß
- Infective hypothesis
  – Viruses—Molecular mimicry
    ○ Measles
    ○ Rubella
    ○ Epstein-Barr
    ○ Varicella-zoster
    ○ Herpes
    ○ Endogenous retroviruses
- Other hypotheses
- Environmental factors

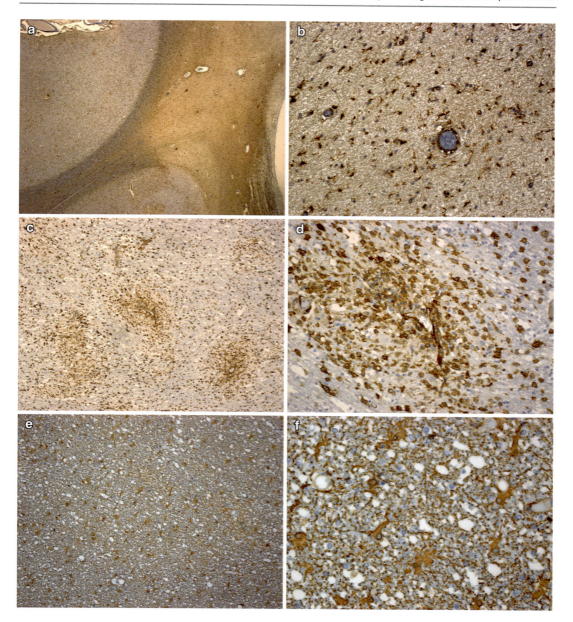

Fig. 41.10 Reaction patterns of microglia (**a–d**) partly diffuse (**a, b**), focally moderate to strong (**c, d**) as well as astrocytes (**e, f**)

- Gene expression patterns in cortical lesions include (Fischer et al. 2013):
  - Category 1: genes associated with inflammation
    - Antigen recognition of class I and II restricted T-cells
    - Regulation of TH1 and Th17 T-cell responses
    - Microglia and macrophage function
    - Chemokine/cytokine signaling and leukocyte recruitment

41.6 Molecular Neuropathology

Table 41.6 Histological and immunoprofile of active, mixed active/inactive, and inactive MS lesions, modified after Kuhlmann et al. (2017) reproduced with kind permission by Springer Nature

	Macrophages/ microglia throughout lesion	Macrophages/ microglia at the border of the lesion	Macrophages/ microglia containing degradation products of LFB, MBP, PLP	Macrophages/ microglia containing degradation products of CNP, MAG, MOG
Active	+	−	±	±
Active and early demyelinating	+	−	+	+
Active and late demyelinating	+	−	+	−
Active and post-demyelinating	+	−	−	−
Mixed active/inactive	−	+	±	±
Mixed active/inactive and demyelinating	−	+	+	±
Mixed active/inactive and post-demyelinating	−	+	−	−
Inactive	−	−	−	−

- Category 2: genes associated with cell death, DNA damage, and DNA repair
  - Apoptosis
  - DNA damage
  - P53 function
  - DNA repair
- Category 3: reaction to tissue injury and association with tissue repair
  - RNA metabolism
  - Regulation of transcription or translation
- MS risk variants determined as changed single nucleotide polymorphisms (SNP) of genes involved in human methylation pathways (Table 41.7)

Candidate **miRNA biomarkers** in MS have been described with findings in blood and proposed involved pathways and/or targets (Harris et al. 2017). Abbreviations used: *AHSCT* autologous hematopoietic stem cell transplantation, *CIS* clinically isolated syndrome, *CSF* cerebrospinal fluid, *MS* multiple sclerosis, *PBMC* peripheral blood mononuclear cell, *RRMS* relapsing-remitting MS, *SPMS* secondary progressive MS:

- *let-7a*
  - SPMS: Serum increase, RRMS: plasma increase
  - IL-12. TGFß, TLR
- *let-7c*
  - RRMS: Serum increase, after natalizumab: whole blood decrease
  - LIN28B, SMAD2, ZCCHC11, DICER1, EIF2C2
- *let-7d*
  - RRMS: Serum increase, MS: PBMC increase
  - IL-1ß, SMARCAD1, FAM178A, LIN28B, LRIG3, GATM, IGDCC3
- *let-7g*
  - MS: PBMC decrease
  - HTATIP2, LRRK1, TLR4
- *miR-16*
  - MS: PBMC increase, after AHSCT: normalized
  - FOXP3, PDCD1
- *miR-16-2-3p*
  - CIS/RRMS: Whole blood increase
  - CUL2, RAB6A, PLCXD3, INTU, SGIP1, FAM126B, CLTC
- *miR-18a*
  - After natalizumab: Whole blood increase
  - MAPK, NF-κB, NEDD9, BBX, ZBTB47, PHF19, RORA, INADL
- *miR-18b*
  - MS: PBMC increase, RRMS: increase
  - PERQ1, GAB1, SIM2, GLRB, REXO2, BTG3, HSF2, MDGA1, UBTD2, TSHZ3, C7orf42, HMBOX1, CLIP3, UBE2Z

Table 41.7 MS risk variants involved in human methylation pathways, modified after Webb and Guerau-de-Arellano (2017) reproduced with kind permission by Elsevier

SNP	Gene	Sequence change	Mutation type (amino acid)	Risk allele	Biological effect of risk allele
rs1801131	MTHFR	c.1298A>C	Missense (E/A)	A(protective)	Reduced DNA methylation and protection from MS
rs1801133	MTHFR	c.677C>T	Missense (A/V)	T	Reduced MTHFR enzymatic activity/stability
rs1051266	SLC19A1	c.80G>A	Missense (H/R)	A(protective)	Lower plasma folate levels and later age of MS onset
rs72058776	CBS	c.844_855ins68bp	Intronic		Higher expression and earlier MS disease onset
rs2726518	TET2	c.7577A>C	Intronic	C	Unknown
rs4925166	SHMT1	c.530G>T	Intronic/eQTL?	T	Increased DNA methylation at SNP locus impacting on expression
rs4410871	MYC	n.8049A>G	Non-coding	G	Unknown
rs34286592	MAZ	c.418C>T	Intronic	T	Unknown
rs2836425	ERG	c.21281C>T	Intronic	T	Unknown
rs4364506	L3MBTL3	c.374G>A	Intronic	A	Unknown

- *miR-20a-5p*
  - CIS/RRMS: Whole blood decrease
  - CDKN1A
- *miR-20b*
  - After natalizumab: Whole blood increase, MS: PBMC decrease
  - MAPK, NF-κB, ZNFX1, PTPN4, PDCD1LG2, ADARB1, PKD2, ZNF800
- *miR-22*
  - MS: Plasma increase, RRMS: increase
  - BTG-1, ESR-α
- *miR-26a*
  - RRMS relapse: PBMC increase
  - TGFß, SMAD1, SMAD4, p300, and c-Myc
- *miR-26a-5p*
  - PPMS and SPMS: Serum increase, MS and in IFNß responders: PBMC increase
  - HOMER1, GRIN3A, SLC1A1, SLC38A1, DLG4
- *miR-142-3p*
  - MS: PBMC increase, after AHSCT: normalized, MS: increase, RRMS: increase, after glatiramer acetate: reduced
  - FOXO1, FAM208B, WASL, HECTD1, CLDN12, RLF, MTUS1
- *mir-145*
  - RRMS: Serum increase, MS: increase, MS: plasma increase, MS: PBMC increase, MS: increase, MS: CSF increase
  - IFNγ, ABCE1, MPZL2, DAB2, KCNA4, ABHD17C
- *miR-146a*
  - RRMS: PBMC increase, after glatiramer acetate: reduced
  - NOVA1, SRSF6, BCORL1, SEC23IP, ZBTB2, EIF4G2
- *miR-146b*
  - MS: PBMC increase, RRMS SRSF: increase
  - SRSF6, NOVA1, SEC23IP, BCORL1, EIF4G2, ZBTB2
- *mir-150*
  - MS after natalizumab: Serum increase, after fingolimod: decrease, MS: PBMC decrease, RRMS: CSF increase, CIS-RRMS converters: increase, after natalizumab: reduced

- SOCS1, SPI1, EPHB2
- miR-155
  - MS: PBMC increase, after AHSCT: normalized, MS: increase, RRMS: increase
  - FOXP3, IRF2BP2
- miR-181c
  - Serum increase vs. CSF, MS: PBMC decrease, MS: CSF increase, CIS-RRMS: increase
  - MeCP2, XIAP, HMGA1, GDNF, VEGF
- miR-210
  - RRMS: Serum increase, MS: PBMC increase
  - FGFFRL1, ISCU, RRP1B, DENND6A, IGF2
- miR-223
  - PPMS: Serum decrease, MS: PBMC increase
  - FBXW7, RRAS2, CRIM1, HSP90B1, INPP4A
- miR-326
  - After natalizumab: Whole blood decrease, MS: PBMC increase, RRMS relapse: increase, RRMS: increase
  - MAPK, NF-κB, ETS1, CEP85, GGT7, PALM, PRR14L, SAMD4B
- miR-422a
  - MS: Plasma increase, MS: PBMC increase
  - CYP7A1, NR2C2, KIAA1522, TMEM245, SLC7A6
- miR-572
  - PPMS: Serum decrease, SPMS and RRMS relapse: increase, MS: plasma increase
  - NCAM1, SEPT8, TAOK2, QRICH2
- miR-599
  - MS: PBMC increase, RRMS relapse: increase
  - LRRC4C, ZSWIM6, NFIA, ROCK1, TGFß2, ATMIN
- miR-648a
  - MS: Plasma increase, RRMS remission: decrease
  - ONECUT, HBP1, LRRC16A, IMPDH1, MLLT4, KIF13A, MBD5
- miR-922
  - CIS-RRMS conversion: Serum increase, MS: CSF decrease, CIS-RRMS: increase
  - UCHL1, APH1A, CLIC5, STX17, RNF2, HIF1AN

Proposed Mechanisms Leading to Progressive Multiple Sclerosis

Immune effector mechanisms
- Clonal expansion of B-cells
  - Antibody production, antigen presentation, ectopic formation of follicle-like structures (FLS)
  - Induction of compartmentalized population driving CNS injury, independent of peripheral immune activity
  - Secretion of IL-6, TNFα, IL-10, and IL-35: complement activation and T-cell functions
- Ectopic formation of follicle-like structures (FLS)
  - Secretion of CXCL13: recruitment, maturation, and antigenic selection of B-cells
  - Secretion of cytotoxic factors
- EBV-infected B-cells
  - Induce CD8-mediated immune responses against brain tissue
- CD8+ cytotoxic T-lymphocytes
  - Release of TNFα: neuronal cell death via p55 receptor; IFN-γ: increased glutamate neurotoxicity and Ca^{2+} influx; secretion of perforin and granzyme: cellular membrane damage, associated to Na^+ and Ca^{2+} influx
- Microglia activation
  - Decreased expression of immune-suppressive factors: fractalkine-CX3CR1, and CD200-CD200R
  - Secretion of pro-inflammatory cytokines: IL-1, IL-6, TNFα, IFN-γ
  - Ag presentation of CD4+ T-cells via MHC Class II
  - Oxidative burst: production of ROS and RNS
  - Acquisition of aging phenotype: expression of advanced glycation end products (AGE) and AGE receptor (RAGE)
- Astrocyte activation
  - Secretion of pro-inflammatory cytokines: IL-1, IL-6, TNFα
  - Secretion of chemokines: CCL2, CCL5, IP10, CXCL12, IL-8
  - BBB breakthrough: action on endothelial cells and tight junctions
  - Production of B-cell-activating factor (BAFF): driving B-cell autoimmunity

- Activation of microglia: secretion of CXCL-10/CXXR3, granulocyte-macrophage colony stimulating factor (GM-CSF), macrophage-colony stimulating factor (M-CSF), and TGF-ß
- Production of LacCer: induces secretion of CCL2 and GM-CSF causing activation of microglia and monocytes infiltration
- Production of ROS, RNS, nitric oxide (NO), and ONOO

Mechanisms of Neurodegeneration and Axonal Dysfunction
- Mitochondrial injury
  - Impaired activity of respiratory chain complexes (I, III, and IV)
  - Alterations in mitochondrial molecular motors
  - Mitochondrial DNA (mtDNA) deletions
  - Energy deficiency: failure of Na^+/K^+ ATPase, reverse activity of sodium calcium exchanger (NCX), and excess of intra-axonal Ca^{2+}
  - Amplify oxidative stress
  - Histotoxic hypoxia, which amplifies energy deficiency
- Release of Fe^{3+} from damaged oligodendrocytes
  - Amplifies oxidative injury
- Anomalous distribution of ion channels
  - Redistribution of Na^+ channels (Na, 1.2, 1.6, and 1.8) along the denuded axon: increased energy demand
  - Activation of voltage-gated Ca^{2+} channel (VGCC), acid-sensing ion channel (ASIC1), and transient potential receptor melastatin 4 (TRPM4) contributes to excess of intra-axonal Ca^{2+}
- Astrocyte activation
  - Production of peroxynitrite (ONOO)-limited glutamate transporters, increasing glutamate excitotoxicity
  - Reactive astrogliosis: inhibition of remyelination and axonal regeneration by oversecretion of fibroblast growth factor 2 (FGF-2), chondroitin sulfate proteoglycans (CSPGs), and ephrins (EPH)
- Upregulation of purinergic receptors: increased responsiveness to ATP, formation of membrane pores, and increased Ca^{2+} influx
- Cellular senescence: low level of chronic inflammation, altered Ca^{2+} homeostasis
- Glutamate excitotoxicity
  - Massive influx of Ca^{2+} into neurons
- Excess of intra-axonal Ca^{2+}
  - Stimulates catabolic enzyme systems: proteases, calpain, and phospholipases, leading to proteolytic degradation of cytoskeletal proteins
- Loss of myelin-derived trophic support
  - Alteration of a single myelin protein (proteolipid protein (PLP), myelin-associated glycoprotein (MAG), or 2′,3′-cyclic nucleotide 3′-phosphodiesterase (CNP)) can cause axonal dysfunction
- Deficit in axonal transport
  - Reduced expression of kinesins (anterograde transport)
  - Reduced expression of dyneins (retrograde transport)

Experimental animal models used to study demyelination include:

- Experimental autoimmune encephalomyelitis
- Experimental autoimmune neuritis
- Canine distemper encephalomyelitis
- Visna
- Coonhound paralysis
- Marek disease
- Mouse hepatitis virus encephalomyelitis
- Theiler's virus encephalomyelitis
- Diphtheritic neuropathy

41.7 Treatment and Prognosis

Treatment
- Relapsing-remitting MS
  - Moderate to severe relapse
    - Methylprednisolone 1000 mg in 100 ml 5% dextrose, infused intravenously over 30–60 min for 3 days or
    - 500 mg daily for 5 days

- Long-term treatment
  - First line
    - Interferon beta-1b
    - Glatiramer acetate
    - Azathioprine
  - Second line
    - Oral agents: fingolimod, fumarate
  - Third line
    - Natalizumab
    - Alemtuzumab
- Primary or secondary progressive MS
  - High-dose methylprednisolone
  - Mitoxantrone
- Symptomatic relief of
  - Spasticity, bladder dysfunction, bowel dysfunction, sexual dysfunction, bulbar dysfunction, visual dysfunction, cognitive dysfunction and depression, tremor and ataxia, fatigue, impaired mobility, and pain
- Autologous hematopoietic stem cell transplantation
- Neural stem cell based approaches

Biologic Behavior–Prognosis–Prognostic Factors

- Classical MS Charcot type is clinically characterized by:
  - Relapsing remitting (RRMS)
    - Multiple acute attacks followed by clinical improvement
- Secondary progressive (SPMS)
    - After years of RRMS, stage of no recovery between acute attacks
- Primary progressive (PPMS)
    - Progressive disease without periods of recovery
- Relapsing progressive (PRMS)
    - Acute attacks are superimposed on progressive disease without episodes of recovery
- Acute Marburg type
  - Rapidly progressive monophasic course
  - Fatal within a few months and always within 1 year of onset
- JC virus infection under natalizumab
  - Development of progressive multifocal leukoencephalopathy (PML)

Selected References

Baranzini SE, Oksenberg JR (2017) The genetics of multiple sclerosis: from 0 to 200 in 50 years. Trends Genet. https://doi.org/10.1016/j.tig.2017.09.004

Bo L, Mork S, Kong PA, Nyland H, Pardo CA, Trapp BD (1994) Detection of MHC class II-antigens on macrophages and microglia, but not on astrocytes and endothelia in active multiple sclerosis lesions. J Neuroimmunol 51(2):135–146

Bou Fakhredin R, Saade C, Kerek R, El-Jamal L, Khoury SJ, El-Merhi F (2016) Imaging in multiple sclerosis: a new spin on lesions. J Med Imaging Radiat Oncol 60(5):577–586. https://doi.org/10.1111/1754-9485.12498

Bove RM (2017) Remyelinating pharmacotherapies in multiple sclerosis. Neural Regen Res. https://doi.org/10.1007/s13311-017-0577-0

Brandstadter R, Katz Sand I (2017) The use of natalizumab for multiple sclerosis. Neuropsychiatr Dis Treat 13:1691–1702. https://doi.org/10.2147/ndt.s114636

Bruck W, Schmied M, Suchanek G, Bruck Y, Breitschopf H, Poser S, Piddlesden S, Lassmann H (1994) Oligodendrocytes in the early course of multiple sclerosis. Ann Neurol 35(1):65–73. https://doi.org/10.1002/ana.410350111

Bruck W, Porada P, Poser S, Rieckmann P, Hanefeld F, Kretzschmar HA, Lassmann H (1995) Monocyte/macrophage differentiation in early multiple sclerosis lesions. Ann Neurol 38(5):788–796. https://doi.org/10.1002/ana.410380514

Calabrese M, Castellaro M (2017) Cortical gray matter MR imaging in multiple sclerosis. Neuroimaging Clin N Am 27(2):301–312. https://doi.org/10.1016/j.nic.2016.12.009

Calabrese M, Filippi M, Gallo P (2010) Cortical lesions in multiple sclerosis. Nat Rev Neurol 6(8):438–444. https://doi.org/10.1038/nrneurol.2010.93

Clerico M, Artusi CA, Liberto AD, Rolla S, Bardina V, Barbero P, Mercanti SF, Durelli L (2017) Natalizumab in multiple sclerosis: long-term management. Int J Mol Sci 18(5). https://doi.org/10.3390/ijms18050940

Compston A, Coles A (2008) Multiple sclerosis. Lancet 372(9648):1502–1517. https://doi.org/10.1016/s0140-6736(08)61620-7

Correale J, Gaitan MI, Ysrraelit MC, Fiol MP (2017) Progressive multiple sclerosis: from pathogenic mechanisms to treatment. Brain 140(3):527–546. https://doi.org/10.1093/brain/aww258

Dargahi N, Katsara M, Tselios T, Androutsou ME, de Courten M, Matsoukas J, Apostolopoulos V (2017) Multiple sclerosis: immunopathology and treatment update. Brain Sci 7(7). https://doi.org/10.3390/brainsci7070078

van den Berg R, Hoogenraad CC, Hintzen RQ (2017) Axonal transport deficits in multiple sclerosis: spiraling into the abyss. Acta Neuropathol 134(1):1–14. https://doi.org/10.1007/s00401-017-1697-7

van der Valk P, De Groot CJ (2000) Staging of multiple sclerosis (MS) lesions: pathology of the time frame of MS. Neuropathol Appl Neurobiol 26(1):2–10

Dulamea AO (2017) Role of oligodendrocyte dysfunction in demyelination, remyelination and neurodegeneration in multiple sclerosis. Adv Exp Med Biol 958:91–127. https://doi.org/10.1007/978-3-319-47861-6_7

Filippi M, Rocca MA, Ciccarelli O, De Stefano N, Evangelou N, Kappos L, Rovira A, Sastre-Garriga J, Tintore M, Frederiksen JL, Gasperini C, Palace J, Reich DS, Banwell B, Montalban X, Barkhof F (2016) MRI criteria for the diagnosis of multiple sclerosis: MAGNIMS consensus guidelines. Lancet Neurol 15(3):292–303. https://doi.org/10.1016/s1474-4422(15)00393-2

Filippi M, Preziosa P, Rocca MA (2017) Microstructural MR imaging techniques in multiple sclerosis. Neuroimaging Clin N Am 27(2):313–333. https://doi.org/10.1016/j.nic.2016.12.004

Fischer MT, Wimmer I, Hoftberger R, Gerlach S, Haider L, Zrzavy T, Hametner S, Mahad D, Binder CJ, Krumbholz M, Bauer J, Bradl M, Lassmann H (2013) Disease-specific molecular events in cortical multiple sclerosis lesions. Brain 136. (Pt 6:1799–1815. https://doi.org/10.1093/brain/awt110

Geginat J, Paroni M, Pagani M, Galimberti D, De Francesco R, Scarpini E, Abrignani S (2017) The enigmatic role of viruses in multiple sclerosis: molecular mimicry or disturbed immune surveillance? Trends Immunol. https://doi.org/10.1016/j.it.2017.04.006

Ghasemi N, Razavi S, Nikzad E (2017) Multiple sclerosis: pathogenesis, symptoms, diagnoses and cell-based therapy. Cell J 19(1):1–10. https://doi.org/10.1016/j.jneuroim.2017.02.002

Green AJ, Filippi M, Preziosa P, Rocca MA (2017) Brain mapping in multiple sclerosis: lessons learned about the human brain. Neurotherapeutics. https://doi.org/10.1016/j.neuroimage.2017.09.021

Harris VK, Tuddenham JF, Sadiq SA (2017) Biomarkers of multiple sclerosis: current findings. Degener Neurol Neuromuscul Dis 7:19–29

Heidker RM, Emerson MR, LeVine SM (2017) Metabolic pathways as possible therapeutic targets for progressive multiple sclerosis. Neural Regen Res 12(8):1262–1267. https://doi.org/10.4103/1673-5374.213542

Hojati Z (2017) Molecular genetic and epigenetic basis of multiple sclerosis. Adv Exp Med Biol 958:65–90. https://doi.org/10.1007/978-3-319-47861-6_6

Hyun JW, Huh SY, Kim W, Park MS, Ahn SW, Cho JY, Kim BJ, Lee SH, Kim SH, Kim HJ (2017) Evaluation of 2016 MAGNIMS MRI criteria for dissemination in space in patients with a clinically isolated syndrome. Mult Scler 24(6):758–766. https://doi.org/10.1177/1352458517706744

Kacperska MJ, Walenczak J, Tomasik B (2016) Plasmatic microRNA as potential biomarkers of multiple sclerosis: literature review. Adv Clin Exp Med 25(4):775–779. https://doi.org/10.17219/acem/60098

Kaunzner UW, Gauthier SA (2017) MRI in the assessment and monitoring of multiple sclerosis: an update on best practice. Ther Adv Neurol Disord 10(6):247–261. https://doi.org/10.1177/1756285617708911

Kawachi I, Lassmann H (2017) Neurodegeneration in multiple sclerosis and neuromyelitis optica. J Neurol Neurosurg Psychiatry 88(2):137–145. https://doi.org/10.1136/jnnp-2016-313300

Klawiter EC (2013) Current and new directions in MRI in multiple sclerosis. Continuum (Minneap Minn) 19. (4 Multiple Sclerosis:1058–1073. https://doi.org/10.1212/01.con.0000433283.00221.37

Kuhlmann T, Ludwin S, Prat A, Antel J, Bruck W, Lassmann H (2017) An updated histological classification system for multiple sclerosis lesions. Acta Neuropathol 133(1):13–24. https://doi.org/10.1007/s00401-016-1653-y

Lassmann H, Raine CS, Antel J, Prineas JW (1998) Immunopathology of multiple sclerosis: report on an international meeting held at the Institute of Neurology of the University of Vienna. J Neuroimmunol 86(2):213–217

Levite M (2017) Glutamate, T cells and multiple sclerosis. J Neural Transm (Vienna) 124(7):775–798. https://doi.org/10.1007/s00702-016-1661-z

Lucchinetti C, Bruck W (2004) The pathology of primary progressive multiple sclerosis. Mult Scler 10(Suppl 1):S23–S30

Lucchinetti C, Bruck W, Parisi J, Scheithauer B, Rodriguez M, Lassmann H (2000) Heterogeneity of multiple sclerosis lesions: implications for the pathogenesis of demyelination. Ann Neurol 47(6):707–717

Lucchinetti C, Bruck W, Noseworthy J (2001) Multiple sclerosis: recent developments in neuropathology, pathogenesis, magnetic resonance imaging studies and treatment. Curr Opin Neurol 14(3):259–269

Lucchinetti CF, Parisi J, Bruck W (2005) The pathology of multiple sclerosis. Neurol Clin 23(1):77–105., vi. https://doi.org/10.1016/j.ncl.2004.09.002

Luo C, Jian C, Liao Y, Huang Q, Wu Y, Liu X, Zou D, Wu Y (2017) The role of microglia in multiple sclerosis. Neuropsychiatr Dis Treat 13:1661–1667. https://doi.org/10.2147/ndt.s140634

Martin R, Sospedra M, Rosito M, Engelhardt B (2016) Current multiple sclerosis treatments have improved our understanding of MS autoimmune pathogenesis. Eur J Immunol 46(9):2078–2090. https://doi.org/10.1002/eji.201646485

Moccia M, Ciccarelli O (2017) Molecular and metabolic imaging in multiple sclerosis. Neuroimaging Clin N Am 27(2):343–356. https://doi.org/10.1016/j.nic.2016.12.005

Peterson JW, Bo L, Mork S, Chang A, Trapp BD (2001) Transected neurites, apoptotic neurons, and reduced inflammation in cortical multiple sclerosis lesions. Ann Neurol 50(3):389–400

Polman CH, Reingold SC, Banwell B, Clanet M, Cohen JA, Filippi M, Fujihara K, Havrdova E, Hutchinson M, Kappos L, Lublin FD, Montalban X, O'Connor P, Sandberg-Wollheim M, Thompson AJ, Waubant E, Weinshenker B, Wolinsky JS (2011) Diagnostic criteria for multiple sclerosis: 2010 revisions to the

McDonald criteria. Ann Neurol 69(2):292–302. https://doi.org/10.1002/ana.22366

Rajda C, Pukoli D, Bende Z, Majlath Z, Vecsei L (2017) Excitotoxins, mitochondrial and redox disturbances in multiple sclerosis. Int J Mol Sci 18(2). https://doi.org/10.3390/ijms18020353

Selmaj I, Mycko MP, Raine CS, Selmaj KW (2017) The role of exosomes in CNS inflammation and their involvement in multiple sclerosis. J Neuroimmunol 306:1–10. https://doi.org/10.1016/j.jneuroim.2017.02.002

Spencer JI, Bell JS, DeLuca GC (2017) Vascular pathology in multiple sclerosis: reframing pathogenesis around the blood-brain barrier. J Neurol Neurosurg Psychiatry. https://doi.org/10.1136/jnnp-2017-316011

Stampanoni Bassi M, Mori F, Buttari F, Marfia GA, Sancesario A, Centonze D, Iezzi E (2017) Neurophysiology of synaptic functioning in multiple sclerosis. Clin Neurophysiol 128(7):1148–1157. https://doi.org/10.1016/j.clinph.2017.04.006

Tommasin S, Gianni C, De Giglio L, Pantano P (2017) Neuroimaging techniques to assess inflammation in multiple sclerosis. Neuroscience. https://doi.org/10.1016/j.neuroscience.2017.07.055

Trapp BD, Peterson J, Ransohoff RM, Rudick R, Mork S, Bo L (1998) Axonal transection in the lesions of multiple sclerosis. N Engl J Med 338(5):278–285. https://doi.org/10.1056/nejm199801293380502

Vagberg M, Axelsson M, Birgander R, Burman J, Cananau C, Forslin Y, Granberg T, Gunnarsson M, von Heijne A, Jonsson L, Karrenbauer VD, Larsson EM, Lindqvist T, Lycke J, Lonn L, Mentesidou E, Muller S, Nilsson P, Piehl F, Svenningsson A, Vrethem M, Wikstrom J (2017) Guidelines for the use of magnetic resonance imaging in diagnosing and monitoring the treatment of multiple sclerosis: recommendations of the Swedish Multiple Sclerosis Association and the Swedish Neuroradiological Society. Acta Neurol Scand 135(1):17–24. https://doi.org/10.1111/ane.12667

Vidal-Jordana A, Montalban X (2017) Multiple sclerosis: epidemiologic, clinical, and therapeutic aspects. Neuroimaging Clin N Am 27(2):195–204. https://doi.org/10.1016/j.nic.2016.12.001

Webb LM, Guerau-de-Arellano M (2017) Emerging role for methylation in multiple sclerosis: beyond DNA. Trends Mol Med 23(6):546–562. https://doi.org/10.1016/j.molmed.2017.04.004

Xiao J, Yang R, Biswas S, Zhu Y, Qin X, Zhang M, Zhai L, Luo Y, He X, Mao C, Deng W (2017) Neural stem cell-based regenerative approaches for the treatment of multiple sclerosis. Mol Neurobiol. https://doi.org/10.1007/s12035-017-0566-7

Demyelinating Diseases: Neuromyelitis Optica Spectrum Disorder

42.1 Clinical Signs and Symptoms

Neuromyelitis optica (NMO) or Devic disease is characterized by:

- Optic neuritis (ON)
- Transverse myelitis

Optic Neuritis (ON)
- Visual function more severely affected than in MS or single isolated idiopathic ON
- Recurrence of attack
- May not respond to corticosteroid treatment
- Visual acuity is worser and recovery is poorer than in MS

Myelitis
- Severe paraparesis or tetraparesis
- Sensory-level and/or sphincter disturbances
- Longitudinal extensive transverse myelitis (LETM) (>3 vertebral segments)
- Painful tonic spasms

Associated with Serum Antibodies Against Aquaporin 4 (AQP4)
- 10–50% of patients with NMO might be sero-negative
- 5% of patients with single isolated idiopathic ON are sero-positive
- 5–20% of patients with isolated recurring ON are seropositive
- Patients with MS are negative

Recently published **international diagnostic consensus criteria of neuromyelitis optica spectrum disorder (NMOSD)** for adult patients are given as follows (Wingerchuk et al. 2015):

- Diagnostic criteria for NMOSD with AQP4-IgG
  - At least one core clinical characteristic
  - Positive test for AQP4-IgG using best available detection method (cell-based assay strongly recommended)
  - Exclusion of alternative diagnoses
- Diagnostic criteria for NMOSD without AQP4-IgG or NMOSD with unknown AQP4-IgG status
  - At least two core clinical characteristics occurring as a result of one or more clinical attacks and meeting all of the following requirements:
    - At least one core clinical characteristic must be optic neuritis, acute myelitis with LETM, or area postrema syndrome
    - Dissemination in space (two or more different core clinical characteristics)
    - Fulfillment of additional MRI requirements, as applicable

- Negative tests for AQP4-IgG using best available detection method, or testing unavailable
- Exclusion of alternative diagnoses
• Core clinical characteristics
  - Optic neuritis
  - Acute myelitis
  - Area postrema syndrome: episode of otherwise unexplained hiccups or nausea and vomiting
  - Acute brainstem syndrome
  - Symptomatic narcolepsy or acute diencephalic clinical syndrome with NMOSD-typical diencephalic MRI lesions
  - Symptomatic cerebral syndrome with NMOSD-typical brain lesions
• Additional MRI requirements for NMOSD without AQP4-IgG and NMOSD with unknown AQP4-IgG status
  - Acute optic neuritis: requires brain MRI showing (a) normal findings or only non-specific white matter lesions, OR (b) optic nerve MRI with T2-hyperintense lesion or T1-weighted gadolinium enhancing lesion extending over 0.1/2 optic nerve length or involving optic chiasm
  - Acute myelitis: requires associated intramedullary MRI lesion extending over ≥3 contiguous segments (LETM) OR ≥3 contiguous segments of focal spinal cord atrophy in patients with history compatible with acute myelitis
  - Area postrema syndrome: requires associated dorsal medulla/area postrema lesions
  - Acute brainstem syndrome: requires associated periependymal brainstem lesions

42.2 Epidemiology

Incidence
• 0.5–4.4 per 100,000

Age Incidence
• Fourth decade of life
• May occur in childhood as well as in elderly patients

Sex Incidence
• Male:Female ratio: 1:3

Localization
• Optic nerve
• Spinal cord

42.3 Neuroimaging Findings

General Imaging Findings
• Optic neuritis and myelitis (long segmental over more than 3 vertebral segments)

CT non-contrast-enhanced
• MRI best imaging tool

CT contrast-enhanced
• MRI best imaging tool

MRI-T2 (Fig. 42.1a,c)
• Hyperintensity and enlargement of optic nerves
• Hyperintense cord signal over more than three vertebral segments (involves central part of the cord)

MRI-FLAIR (Fig. 42.2d)
• Parenchymal lesions different from typical MS-plaques
• Typical locations of NMO lesions:
  - Dorsal medulla (area postrema)
  - Periependymal surface of ventricles
  - Subcortical/deep white matter
  - Corticospinal tract
• If corpus callosum is affected, lesions appear more heterogeneous and edematous than MS-plaques

MRI-T1 (Fig. 42.2a)
• Iso- or hypointense

MRI-T1 contrast-enhanced (Figs. 42.1d and 42.2b, c, e)
• Enhancement of optic nerves uni- or bilateral, frequently involving posterior part of optic nerves
• Enhancement of periependymal lesions possible

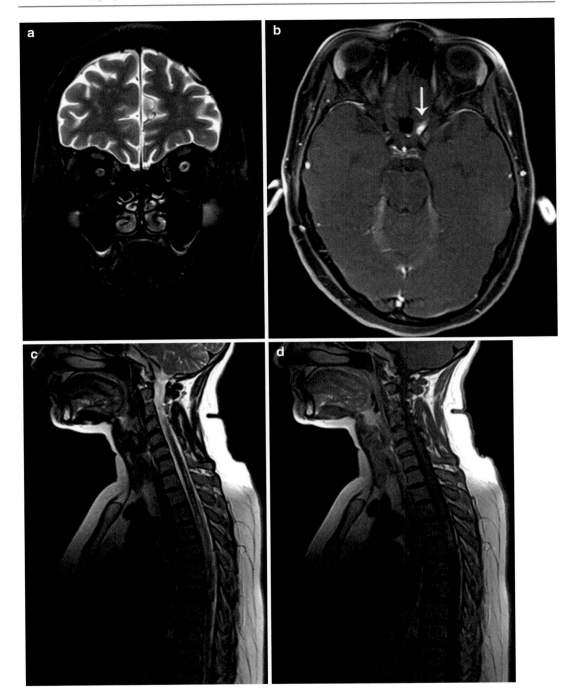

Fig. 42.1 Unilateral enhancement and mild enlargement of intraorbital and prechiasmatic left optic nerve →, coronar T2 (**a**), T1 contrast (**b**); same patient with long segmental, enhancing spinal cord lesion, sagittal T2 (**c**), sagittal T1 contrast (**d**)

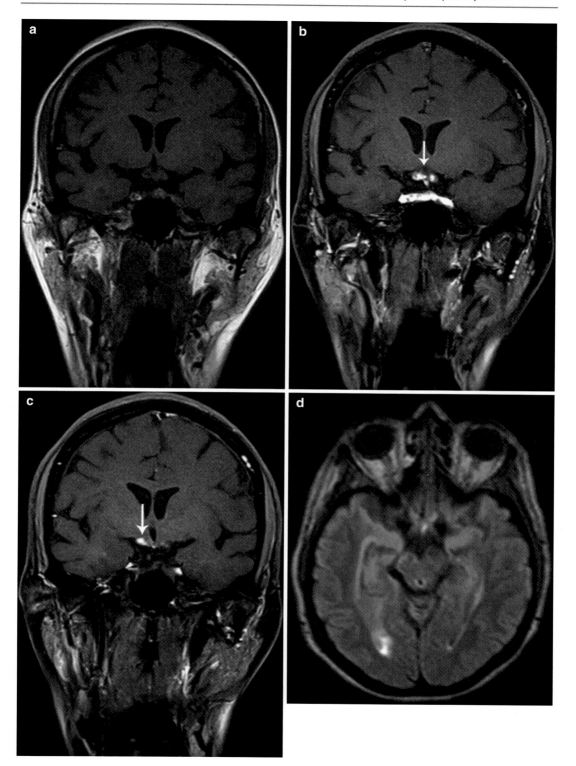

Fig. 42.2 Bilateral optic nerve enhancement extending posterior to optic chiasm and right optic tract →, coronar T1 (**a**), coronar T1 contrast (**b, c**); periependymal enhancing lesion next to right posterior horn of lateral ventricle, FLAIR (**d**), T1 contrast (**e**)

42.5 Molecular Neuropathology

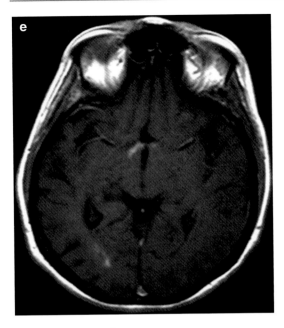

Fig. 42.2 (continued)

MR-Diffusion Tensor Imaging
- Decreased FA and increased diffusivity in corticospinal tract and optic radiation

MR-Spectroscopy
- Normal metabolites in unaffected white and gray matter (in contrast to MS)

Nuclear Medicine Imaging Findings
- Few cases have been described so far
- Some cases show focal FDG uptake in the lesions of the spinal cord, one with uptake throughout the whole spinal cord with regression after therapy

42.4 Neuropathology Findings

Macroscopic Features
- Congested optic nerves and spinal cord
- Necrosis of the spinal cord possible
- In long-survivor:
  - Thinned and gray-brown optic nerves
  - Atrophic spinal cord

Microscopic Features (Fig. 42.3a–d)
- Extensive demyelination
- Inflammatory infiltrates
  - Perivascular neutrophils and eosinophils
  - Few T-lymphocytes
  - Macrophages, lymphocytes, and plasma cells
  - Perivascular deposition of immunoglobulins (IgM) and activated complement (C9neo)
- Hyaline fibrosis of the small vessels
- Cavitation or necrosis of the spinal cord

Immunophenotype (Figs. 42.4a, b and 42.5)
- Loss of aquaporin 4 immunoreactivity
  - Auto-antigen AQP4 is expressed on the astrocytic foot processes suggesting a role for astrocytes
- Loss of excitatory amino acid transporter 2 (EEAT2)
- Deposition of activated complement C9neo in macrophages or along myelin sheaths

Differential Diagnosis
- Demyelinating plaques in multiple sclerosis

42.5 Molecular Neuropathology

- Autoantibodies against AQP4
- Aquaporin 4 regulates the transport of
  - Water
  - Glutamate
  - Potassium
- Aquaporin is expressed in:
  - Astrocytic endfeet of the blood–brain barrier
  - Nodes of Ranvier
  - Neuronal synapses

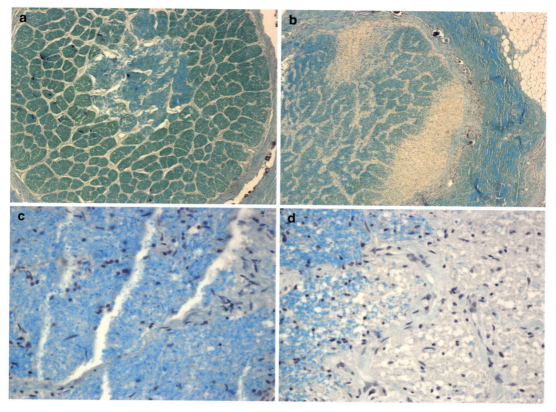

Fig. 42.3 Unaffected optic nerve (**a**), affected optic nerve with large areas of demyelination (**b**), unaffected optic nerve (**c**), affected optic nerve with large area of depigmentation (**d**). Note at the bottom normal appearing myelin. (Stain: LFB)

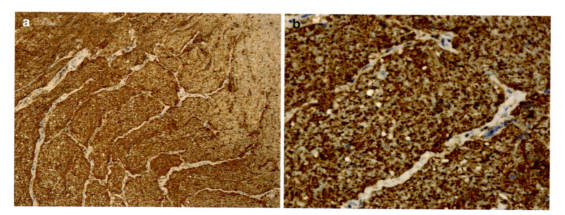

Fig. 42.4 Strong reactive microgliosis at low magnification (**a**) and high magnification (**b**)

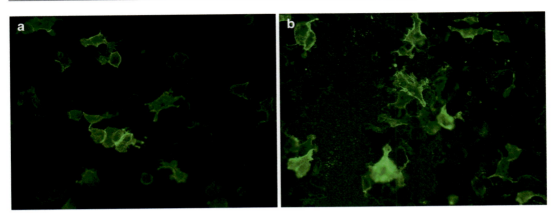

Fig. 42.5 Examples for the demonstration of anti-aquaporin 4 antibodies in the serum from affected patients (**a**, **b**)

- Association with non-organ-specific autoimmune diseases
  - Systemic lupus erythematosus (SLE)
  - Sjögren's syndrome (SS)
  - Rheumatoid arthritis (RA)
  - Undifferentiated connective tissue disease (UCTD)
  - Organ-specific autoimmune diseases (e.g., thyroid diseases, myasthenia gravis)

42.6 Treatment and Prognosis

Treatment

- Oral corticosteroids
- Plasmapheresis
- Immunosuppressant drugs (azathioprine, mycophenolate mofetil, mitoxantrone)
- Monoclonal antibodies (rituximab)
- New approaches include:
  - Targeting complement proteins, the IL-6 receptor, neutrophils, eosinophils and CD19-AQP4-blocking antibodies and AQP4-IgG enzymatic inactivation
  - Reduction of AQP4 expression, disruption of AQP4 orthogonal arrays, enhancement of complement inhibitor expression, restoration of the blood–brain barrier, and induction of immune tolerance

Biologic Behavior–Prognosis–Prognostic Factors

- Developments are needed for:
  - Better and earlier recognition of patients with relapsing-remitting disease
  - Identification of prognostic factors of treatment response
  - Development of a biomarker of disease activity

Selected References

Aboul-Enein F, Krssak M, Hoftberger R, Prayer D, Kristoferitsch W (2010) Diffuse white matter damage is absent in neuromyelitis optica. AJNR Am J Neuroradiol 31(1):76–79. https://doi.org/10.3174/ajnr.A1791

Barnett Y, Sutton IJ, Ghadiri M, Masters L, Zivadinov R, Barnett MH (2014) Conventional and advanced imaging in neuromyelitis optica. AJNR Am J Neuroradiol 35(8):1458–1466. https://doi.org/10.3174/ajnr.A3592

Filippi M, Rocca MA (2004) MR imaging of Devic's neuromyelitis optica. Neurol Sci 25(Suppl 4):S371–S373

Higashiyama A, Komori T, Inada Y, Nishizawa M, Nakajima H, Narumi Y (2017) Diffuse (18)F-FDG uptake throughout the spinal cord in the acute phase of neuromyelitis optica spectrum disorder. Eur J Nucl Med Mol Imaging 44(9):1609–1610. https://doi.org/10.1007/s00259-017-3735-z

Jarius S, Wildemann B (2013) Aquaporin-4 antibodies (NMO-IgG) as a serological marker of neuromyelitis optica: a critical review of the literature. Brain Pathol 23(6):661–683. https://doi.org/10.1111/bpa.12084

Oyama H, Miwa S, Noda T, Sobajima A, Kito A, Maki H, Hattori K, Wada K (2012) Neuromyelitis optica spectrum disorder: 2-deoxy-2-[18F]fluoro-D-glucose positron emission tomography findings—case report. Neurol Med Chir 52(10):769–773

Sato DK, Lana-Peixoto MA, Fujihara K, de Seze J (2013) Clinical spectrum and treatment of neuromyelitis optica spectrum disorders: evolution and current status. Brain Pathol 23(6):647–660. https://doi.org/10.1111/bpa.12087

Verkman AS, Phuan PW, Asavapanumas N, Tradtrantip L (2013) Biology of AQP4 and anti-AQP4 antibody: therapeutic implications for NMO. Brain Pathol 23(6):684–695. https://doi.org/10.1111/bpa.12085

Wingerchuk DM, Banwell B, Bennett JL, Cabre P, Carroll W, Chitnis T, de Seze J, Fujihara K, Greenberg B, Jacob A, Jarius S, Lana-Peixoto M, Levy M, Simon JH, Tenembaum S, Traboulsee AL, Waters P, Wellik KE, Weinshenker BG (2015) International consensus diagnostic criteria for neuromyelitis optica spectrum disorders. Neurology 85(2):177–189. https://doi.org/10.1212/wnl.0000000000001729

Demyelinating Diseases: Acute Demyelinating Encephalomyelitis (ADEM)

43.1 Introduction

Synonyms used for acute demyelinating encephalomyelitis (ADEM):

- Postinfectious encephalomyelitis
- Perivenous encephalomyelitis

Acute hemorrhagic leukoencephalopathy (AHL) considered as:

- Hyperacute form of ADEM

43.2 Clinical Signs and Symptoms

Acute demyelinating encephalomyelitis (ADEM)
- Fever
- Headache
- Impaired conscious level
- Meningism
- Seizures
- Progressive neurological signs
  - Hemiparesis, paraparesis
  - Sensory defects
  - Ataxia
  - Optic neuritis
  - Raised intracranial pressure

Acute hemorrhagic leukoencephalopathy (AHL)
- Headache
- Pyrexia
- Vomiting
- Drowsiness
- Generalized weakness
- Seizures

43.3 Epidemiology

Incidence
- Uncommon
- Most frequent after non-specific upper respiratory tract infections

Age Incidence
- 20–40 years

Sex Incidence
- Male:Female ratio: 1:1

Localization
- White matter

43.4 Neuroimaging Findings

General Imaging Findings
- Bilateral asymmetric, usually enhancing white matter lesions of same age following recent infection or vaccination, gray matter (especially basal ganglia) almost always affected.

CT non-contrast-enhanced (Fig. 43.2a)
- Often normal
- Lesions hypodense, asymmetric

CT contrast-enhanced
- Lesions may show enhancement

MRI-T2 (Figs. 43.1a and 43.2b)
- Variable, multifocal hyperintense lesions
- FLAIR more sensitive

MRI-FLAIR (Figs. 43.1b and 43.2c)
- Multifocal, asymmetric, hyperintense lesions of variable size (punctuate to expansive, tumor-like)
- Usually affecting white matter, but gray matter especially thalamus and basal ganglia often involved (rarely seen in multiple sclerosis)
- Usually callososeptal interface excluded

MRI-T1 (Figs. 43.1c and 43.2d)
- Plaques hypointense

MRI-T1 Contrast-Enhanced (Figs. 43.1d, e and 43.2e)
- Lesions usually show enhancement
- No enhancement does not exclude ADEM
- Enhancement of cranial nerves possible

MR-Diffusion Imaging (Figs. 43.1f, g and 43.2f, g)
- Variable diffusion restriction (ADC ↑ or ↓)

MRI-Perfusion (Fig. 43.2h)
- rCBV ↓ or ↑

MR-Diffusion Tensor Imaging (Fig. 43.2i)
- In contrast to MS, normal diffusivity within regular appearing white matter

MR-Spectroscopy
- Decreased NAA in T2-hyperintensities

Nuclear Medicine Imaging Findings
- CBF-SPECT can show increased uptake in white matter regions due to disrupted blood–brain barrier, presence of inflammatory cells and hyperemia
- CBF and FDG-uptake reduction correlate with neuropsychological impairment

43.5 Neuropathology Findings

Macroscopic Features (Fig. 43.3a–d)
- Acute demyelinating encephalomyelitis (ADEM)
- Congestion and swelling of the brain and spinal cord
- Foci of yellowish to gray discoloration

Acute hemorrhagic leukoencephalopathy (AHL)
- Soft and swollen brain
- Numerous foci of hemorrhage
  - In the cerebral and cerebellar white matter and pons

Microscopic Features (Figs. 43.4a–f and 43.5a–d)
- Acute demyelinating encephalomyelitis (ADEM)
- Infiltrates of lymphocytes, macrophages, and plasma cells
- Around veins and venules, in the leptomeninges
- Associated with area of demyelination
- Perivascular hemorrhages
- Loss of myelin
- Some degree of axonal damage

Acute hemorrhagic leukoencephalopathy (AHL)
- Fibrinoid necrosis of small blood vessels
- Perivascular necrosis with nuclear débris
- Zones of hemorrhage
  - Ring- and ball-shaped perivascular hemorrhages
- Inflammatory infiltrate of neutrophils and mononuclear cells around other vessels
- Fibrin exudate
- Demyelinated fibers
- Axonal fragmentation

43.5 Neuroimaging Findings

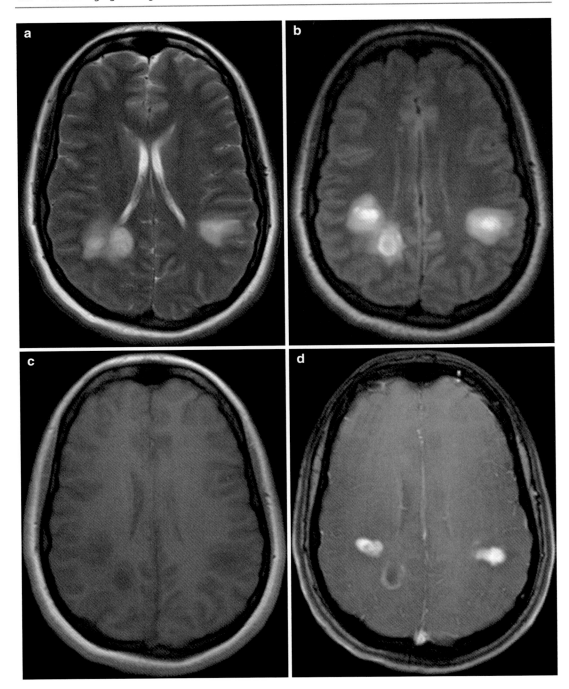

Fig. 43.1 Numerous gadolinium-enhancing white matter lesions supratentorial of variable size and restricted diffusion, enhancement of all lesions indicates monophasic course of disease; T2 (**a**), FLAIR (**b**), T1 (**c**), T1 contrast (**d**, **e**), DWI (**f**), ADC (**g**)

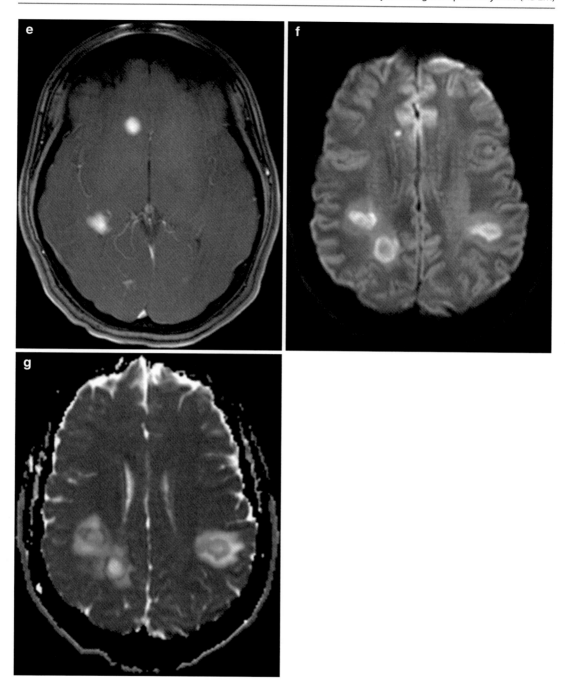

Fig. 43.1 (continued)

43.5 Neuroimaging Findings

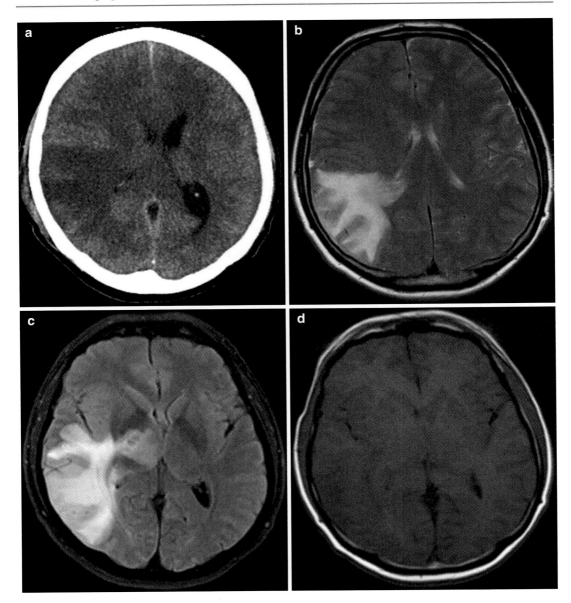

Fig. 43.2 Large, tumor-like lesion right temporo-parietal extending to deep gray matter of right thalamus, ring-shaped thalamic enhancement—histologically verified ADEM; CT non contrast-enhanced (**a**), T2 (**b**), FLAIR (**c**), T1 (**d**), T1 contrast (**e**), DWI (**f**), ADC (**g**), rCBV (**h**), DTI (**i**)

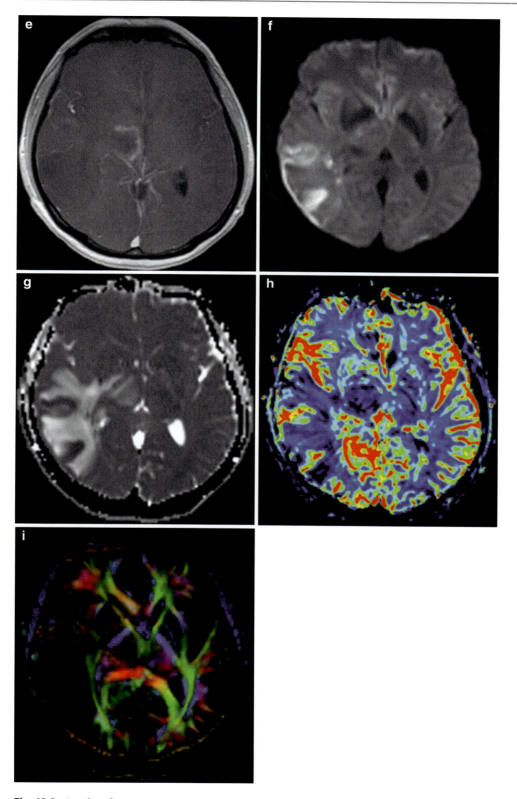

Fig. 43.2 (continued)

43.5 Neuroimaging Findings

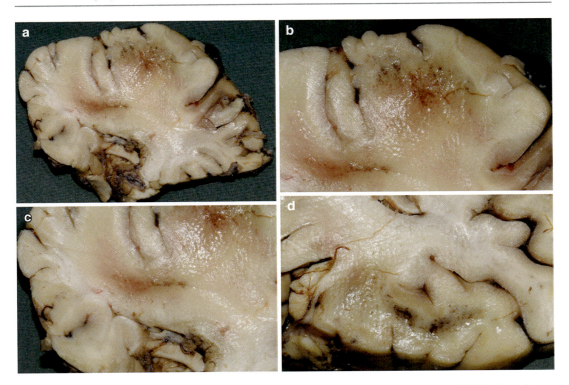

Fig. 43.3 Areas of tissue softening (**a**, **b**), perivascular exudates (reddish color) (**b**, **c**), and petechial bleedings (brown color) (**d**)

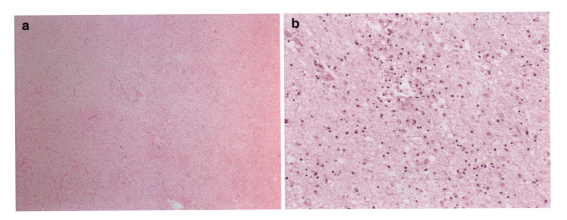

Fig. 43.4 Large areas of tissue softening (**a**), lymphocytic infiltrates in the parenchyma (**b**) and around vessels (**c**), reactive astrogliosis (**d**), petechial hemorrhages (**e**, **f**)

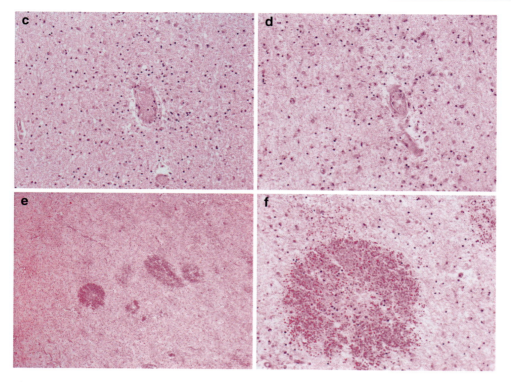

Fig. 43.4 (continued)

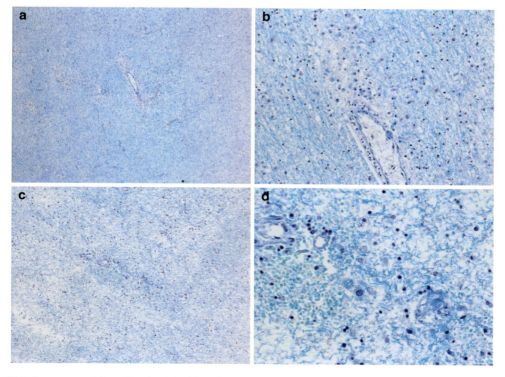

Fig. 43.5 Large area of demyelination (**a**) with perivascular lymphocytic infiltrates (**b–d**) (stain: LFB)

Immunophenotype (Figs. 43.6, 43.7, 43.8, and 43.9)
- Lymphocyte population
  - CD3 T-lymphocytes
  - CD4-helper T-lymphocytes
  - CD8-suppressor/cytotoxic T-lymphocytes
- Macrophages/microglia
  - MHC class II
  - CD68
- APP amyloid precursor protein
- Blood–brain barrier leakage
  - Serum proteins, e.g., transthyretin

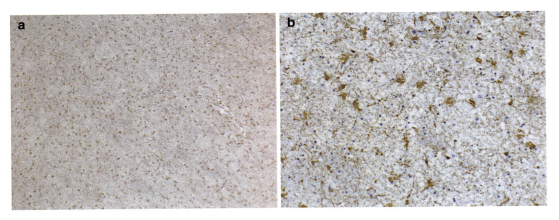

Fig. 43.6 Reactive astrogliosis (stain: GFAP) (**a**, **b**)

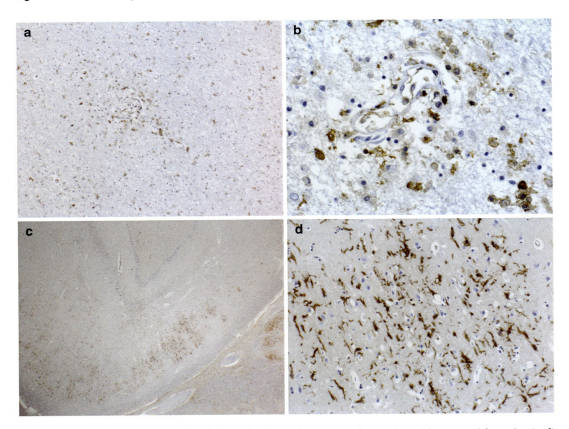

Fig. 43.7 Reactive microgliosis (stain: HLA-DRII) in the white matter (**a**, **b**), and in the hippocampal formation (**c**, **d**)

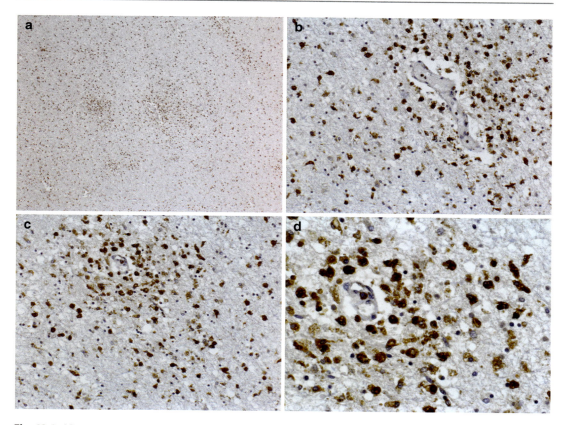

Fig. 43.8 Numerous macrophages (stain: CD68) are diffusely scattered throughout the parenchyma (**a–d**)

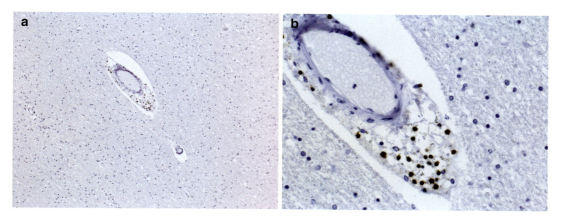

Fig. 43.9 Perivascular T-lymphocytes (stain: CD3) (**a, b**)

Differential Diagnosis

- Acute demyelinating encephalomyelitis (ADEM)
  - Multiple sclerosis
  - Inflammatory process
- Acute hemorrhagic leukoencephalopathy (AHL)
  - Fat embolism
  - Thrombotic thrombocytopenic purpura
  - Disseminated intravascular coagulation

Biologic Behavior–Prognosis–Prognostic Factors

- Acute demyelinating encephalomyelitis (ADEM)
  - Good recovery in the majority of patients
- Acute hemorrhagic leukoencephalopathy (AHL)
  - Fatal within days
- Disability
- Death

43.6 Molecular Neuropathology

Acute demyelinating encephalomyelitis (ADEM)
- Preceding infections
  - Viral: measles, mumps, chickenpox (varicella), German measles, influenza
  - *Mycoplasma pneumonia*, *Campylobacter jejuni*, Group A streptococcal infections
- Preceding vaccinations
  - Smallpox vaccination
- Iatrogenic
  - Sicca-cell preparation, gold, levamisole

Acute hemorrhagic leukoencephalopathy (AHL)
- Systemic viral infection
  - Measles
- Systemic respiratory infection
  - Atypical pneumonia (M. Pneumonia)

43.7 Treatment and Prognosis

Treatment
- Corticosteroids
- Plasmapheresis

Selected References

Bernarding J, Braun J, Koennecke HC (2002) Diffusion- and perfusion-weighted MR imaging in a patient with acute demyelinating encephalomyelitis (ADEM). J Magn Reson Imaging 15(1):96–100

Bester M, Petracca M, Inglese M (2014) Neuroimaging of multiple sclerosis, acute disseminated encephalomyelitis, and other demyelinating diseases. Semin Roentgenol 49(1):76–85. https://doi.org/10.1053/j.ro.2013.09.002

Bizzi A, Ulug AM, Crawford TO, Passe T, Bugiani M, Bryan RN, Barker PB (2001) Quantitative proton MR spectroscopic imaging in acute disseminated encephalomyelitis. AJNR Am J Neuroradiol 22(6):1125–1130

Esposito S, Di Pietro GM, Madini B, Mastrolia MV, Rigante D (2015) A spectrum of inflammation and demyelination in acute disseminated encephalomyelitis (ADEM) of children. Autoimmun Rev 14(10):923–929. https://doi.org/10.1016/j.autrev.2015.06.002

Garg RK (2003) Acute disseminated encephalomyelitis. Postgrad Med J 79(927):11–17

Inglese M, Salvi F, Iannucci G, Mancardi GL, Mascalchi M, Filippi M (2002) Magnetization transfer and diffusion tensor MR imaging of acute disseminated encephalomyelitis. AJNR Am J Neuroradiol 23(2):267–272

Javed A, Khan O (2014) Acute disseminated encephalomyelitis. Handb Clin Neurol 123:705–717. https://doi.org/10.1016/b978-0-444-53488-0.00035-3

Wender M (2011) Acute disseminated encephalomyelitis (ADEM). J Neuroimmunol 231(1–2):92–99. https://doi.org/10.1016/j.jneuroim.2010.09.019

Part VIII

The Brain Diseases: The Epilepsies

Epilepsies: General Aspects

44.1 Introduction

"Epilepsy" is not a single disease entity. Epilepsies are many syndromes and diseases that have a multitude of different manifestations and causes (Panayiotopoulos 2007). For detailed descriptions of the field of the epilepsies, the reader is referred to specialized literature.

44.2 Definitions

The International League Against Epilepsy (ILAE) commissioned a task force to develop a practical (operational) definition of epilepsy, designed for use by doctors and patients (Fisher et al. 2014).

Epileptic seizure: A transient occurrence of signs and/or symptoms due to abnormal excessive or synchronous neuronal activity in the brain (Fisher et al. 2014).

Epilepsy: A disorder of the brain characterized by an enduring predisposition to generate epileptic seizures and by neurobiological, cognitive, psychological and social consequences of this condition. The definition of epilepsy requires the occurrence of at least one epileptic seizure (Fisher et al. 2014).

The task force proposed that epilepsy be considered to be a disease of the brain defined by any of the following conditions and that a person is considered to have epilepsy if they meet any of the following conditions (Fisher et al. 2014):

- At least two unprovoked (or reflex) seizures occurring greater than 24 h apart.
- One unprovoked (or reflex) seizure and a probability of further seizures similar to the general recurrence risk (at least 60%) after two unprovoked seizures, occurring over the next 10 years.
- Diagnosis of an epilepsy syndrome.

Epilepsy is considered to be resolved for individuals who had an age-dependent epilepsy syndrome but are now past the applicable age or those who have remained seizure-free for the last 10 years, with no seizure medicines for the last 5 years (Fisher et al. 2014).

Epileptic: A class of signs and symptoms, such as epileptic seizures (Engel 2013).

Ictus and ictal event: Refers to the epileptic seizure itself, as identified clinically or electrophysiologically (Engel 2013).

Postictal period: Time during which postictal symptoms persist (usually seconds to days) (Engel 2013).

Postictal phenomena: Transient clinical or electrophysiological abnormalities in brain function that result from the ictus and appear after the ictal event has ended (Engel 2013).

Interictal period: Time between the resolution of postictal abnormalities and the beginning of the next ictal event (Engel 2013).

Seizure focus: It is the site in the brain from which the seizure originated and is most likely equivalent to the epileptogenic zone, defined as the area of cerebral cortex indispensable for the generation of clinical seizures. The seizure focus is usually defined as the site in the brain from which the seizure originated or, in the case of focal seizure discharge, the totality of the tissue involved (Nadler and Spencer 2014).

Epileptogenesis: Development and extension of tissue capable of generating spontaneous behavioral or electrographic seizures (Pitkanen 2010). It includes both the development of an epileptic condition and progression after the condition is established.

Epileptogenicity: Capacity to generate epileptic seizures (Engel 2013).

Epileptic spike focus: Brain area that appears to be the major source of interictal epileptiform EEG discharges.

EEG epileptic discharges:
- Focal: single epileptic spike focus
- Bilateral and independent: epileptic spike foci in two hemispheres
- Multifocal: three or more epileptic spike foci
- Diffuse: no apparent epileptic focus

Epileptogenic lesion: Structural abnormality responsible for the generation of epileptic seizures.

Epileptogenic zone or region: Area of brain necessary and sufficient for generation of spontaneous seizures. In 1993, Luders et al. (1993) defined the *epileptogenic zone* as the "area of cortex that is necessary and sufficient for initiating seizures and whose removal (or disconnection) is necessary for complete abolition of seizures." In 2006, Luders et al. (2006) proposed the following, simplified definition of the epileptogenic zone as "the minimum amount of cortex that must be resected (inactivated or completely disconnected) to produce seizure freedom."

During the presurgical evaluation, the following five areas are measured using different diagnostic techniques (Martinkovic et al. 2014; Carreno and Lüders 2001):

- **Irritative zone:**
  - Area of cortex which generates interictal spikes
  - Area is measured by EEG (invasive and non-invasive), magnetoencephalography (MEG), and functional magnetic resonance imaging (fMRI)
- **Seizure-onset zone:**
  - Area of cortex that initiates clinical seizures
  - Area is determined primarily by EEG (invasive and non-invasive), but can also be defined by ictal SPECT and to a lesser degree by fMRI and MEG
- **Symptomatogenic zone:**
  - Area of cortex which, when activated, produces the initial ictal symptoms or signs
  - Area is determined by analyzing the initial seizure symptomatology
- **Epileptogenic lesion:**
  - Macroscopic lesion which is causative of the epileptic seizures because the lesion itself is epileptogenic (*e.g.,* cortical dysplasia) or by secondary hyperexcitability of adjacent cortex
  - Area of cortex which is currently defined by anatomical imaging such as high resolution MRI. Further advances in imaging techniques will undoubtedly result in more accurate definition of the epileptogenic lesion and its cellular/molecular components: histo-molecular imaging
- **Functional deficit zone:**
  - Area of cortex that is not functioning normally in the interictal period
  - Area of cortex defined by a number of tests including neurological examination, neuropsychological examination, and functional imaging (interictal SPECT and PET)

44.3 Classification of the Epilepsies

44.3.1 International League Against Epilepsy (ILEA) Classification-1981

The International League Against Epilepsy (ILAE) classification of *epileptic seizures* lists the following entities (Commission on Classification and Terminology of the International League Against Epilepsy 1981):

- Partial (focal) seizures
  - Simple partial seizures (consciousness not impaired)
    - With motor signs (including Jacksonian, versive, and postural)
    - With sensory symptoms (including visual, somatosensory, auditory, olfactory, gustatory, and vertiginous)
    - With psychic symptoms (including dysphasia, dysmnestic, hallucinatory, and affective changes)
    - With autonomic symptoms (including epigastric sensation, pallor, flushing, papillary changes)
  - Complex partial seizures (consciousness impaired)
    - Simple partial onset followed by impaired consciousness
    - With impairment of consciousness at onset
    - With automatisms
  - Partial seizures evolving to secondarily generalized seizures
    - simple partial seizures evolving to generalized seizures
    - complex partial seizures evolving to generalized seizures
    - simple partial seizure evolving to complex partial seizures evolving to generalized seizures
- Generalized seizures of non-focal origin (convulsive or non-convulsive)
  - Absence seizures
    - With impaired consciousness only
    - With one or more of the following:
      - Atonic components
      - Tonic components
      - Automatisms
      - Autonomic components
  - Myoclonic seizures
    - Myoclonic jerks
  - Tonic-clonic seizures
  - Tonic seizures
  - Atonic seizures
- Unclassified epilepsies

44.3.2 International League Against Epilepsy (ILEA) Classification-1989

The International League Against Epilepsy (ILAE) classification of *epileptic seizures* lists the following entities (Commission on Classification and Terminology of the International League Against Epilepsy 1989):

- Localization-related (focal, local, partial) epilepsies and syndromes
  - Idiopathic (with age-related onset)
    - Benign childhood epilepsy with centrotemporal spikes
    - Childhood epilepsy with occipital paroxysms
    - Primary reading epilepsy
  - Symptomatic
    - Chronic progressive epilepsia partialis continua of childhood
  - Cryptogenic
    - Seizure types
    - Anatomical locations
- Generalized epilepsies and syndromes
  - Idiopathic (with age-related onset)
  - Cryptogenic or symptomatic (in order of age)
  - Symptomatic
    - Nonspecific etiology
    - Specific syndromes

- Epilepsies and syndromes undetermined as to whether they are focal or generalized
  - With both generalized and focal seizures
  - Without unequivocal generalized or focal features
- Specific syndromes
  - Situation-related seizures
    ○ Febrile convulsions
    ○ Isolated seizures or isolated status epilepticus
    ○ Seizures occurring only when there is an acute metabolic or tonic event

44.3.3 International League Against Epilepsy (ILEA) Classification-2010

The outline of the 2010 ILAE classification of focal seizures is given in Table 44.1.

44.3.4 International League Against Epilepsy (ILAE) Classification-2017

The International League Against Epilepsy (ILAE) (Fisher et al. 2017a; b) presented a revised operational classification of seizure types based upon the 1981 Classification, extended in 2010 aiming at:

- Recognizing that some seizure types can have either a focal or generalized onset
- Allowing classification when the onset is unobserved
- Including some missing seizure types
- Adopting more transparent names

The new classification does not represent a fundamental change, but allows greater flexibility and transparency in naming seizure types:

- The ILAE has constructed a revised classification of seizure types.
- The classification is operational and not based on fundamental mechanisms.

Table 44.1 Outline of the 2010 ILAE classification of focal seizures is given as follows, adapted from Berg et al. (2010) reproduced with kind permission by Wiley

Generalized seizures	• Tonic-clonic (in any combination) (tonic contraction followed by clonus usually lasting 1–2 min)	
	• Absence	• Typical • Atypical • Absence with special features – Myoclonic absence – Eyelid myoclonia
	• Myoclonic	• Myoclonic • Myoclonic atonic • Myoclonic tonic
	• Clonic	
	• Tonic	
	• Atonic	
Focal seizures (according to severity)	• Without impairment of consciousness	
	• With observable motor and/or autonomic components • With objective motor and/or autonomic symptoms (simple partial seizures)	• Involving subjective sensory or psychic phenomena only • With only subjective sensory or psychic phenomena (aura)
	• With impairment of consciousness • With impaired consciousness (complex partial seizures)	
	• With generalization to tonic, clonic, or tonic-clonic seizures • Becoming secondarily generalized	
Unknown	• Epileptic spasms	

44.3 Classification of the Epilepsies

- Reasons for revision include:
  - Clarity of nomenclature
  - Ability to classify some seizure types as either focal or generalized
  - Classification when onset is unknown
- Seizures are divided into:
  - Focal
  - Generalized
  - Onset unknown
  - With subcategories of
    - Motor
    - Non-motor
    - With retained awareness
    - Impaired awareness
    - Unknown awareness
- Glossaries of new seizure terms, of common descriptive terms for behaviors during seizures and mapping tables of old to new terms are provided, along with examples (Table 44.2).

44.3.5 International Classification of Diseases Classification (ICD)-2012

The International Classification of Diseases (ICD-10) lists epilepsy and recurrent seizures as follows (http://www.cdc.gov./nchs/icd/icd10cm.htm):

- Localization-related (focal) (partial) idiopathic epilepsy and epileptic syndromes with seizures of localized onset
- Localization-related (focal) (partial) idiopathic epilepsy and epileptic syndromes with simple partial seizures
- Localization-related (focal) (partial) idiopathic epilepsy and epileptic syndromes with complex partial seizures
- Generalized idiopathic epilepsy and epileptic syndromes
- Absence epileptic seizures
- Epileptic seizures related to external causes
- Grand mal seizures unspecified (with or without petit mal)
- Petit mal unspecified (without grand mal seizures)

Table 44.2 Glossaries of new seizure terms, of common descriptive terms for behaviors during seizures and mapping tables of old to new terms are provided, along with examples

Focal	• Motor	• Tonic • Atonic • Myoclonic • Clonic • Myoclonic • Epileptic spams • Hypermotor
	• Non-motor	• Sensory • Cognitive • Emotional • Autonomic
	• Awareness	• Aware • Impaired awareness • Unknown awareness
Generalized	• Motor	• Tonic-clonic • Tonic • Atonic • Myoclonic • Myoclonic atonic • Clonic • Clonic-tonic-clonic • Epileptic spasms
	• Absence	• Typical • Atypical • Myoclonic • Eyelid myoclonia
Unknown onset	• Motor	• Tonic-clonic • Tonic • Atonic • Epileptic spasms
	• Awareness	• Aware • Impaired awareness • Unknown awareness
	• Unclassifiable	

- Other epilepsy and recurrent seizures
- Epilepsy unspecified

44.3.6 Electroclinical Syndromes

Electroclinical syndromes and other epilepsies are given in Table 44.3.

Table 44.3 Electroclinical syndromes and other epilepsies, modified after Engel (2013) and Berg et al. (2010) reproduced with kind permission by Wiley

Electroclinical syndromes arranged by age at onset	
Neonatal period	• Benign familial neonatal epilepsy (BFNE) • Early myoclonic encephalopathy (EME) • Ohtahara syndrome
Infancy	• Epilepsy of infancy with migrating focal seizures • West syndrome • Myoclonic epilepsy in infancy (MEI) • Benign infantile epilepsy • Benign familial infantile epilepsy • Dravet syndrome • Myoclonic encephalopathy in non-progressive disorders
Childhood	• Febrile seizures plus (FS+) (can start in infancy) • Panayiotopoulos syndrome • Epilepsy with myoclonic atonic (previously astatic) seizures • Benign epilepsy with centrotemporal spikes (BECTS) • Autosomal dominant nocturnal frontal lobe epilepsy (ADNFLE) • Late onset childhood occipital epilepsy (Gastaut type) • Epilepsy with myoclonic absences • Lennox–Gastaut syndrome • Epileptic encephalopathy with continuous spike-and-wave during sleep (CSWS) • Landau–Kleffner syndrome (LKS) • Childhood absence epilepsy (CAE)
Adolescence—Adult	• Juvenile absence epilepsy (JAE) • Juvenile myoclonic epilepsy (JME) • Epilepsy with generalized tonic-clonic seizures alone • Progressive myoclonus epilepsies (PME) • Autosomal dominant epilepsy with auditory features (ADEAF) • Other familial temporal lobe epilepsies
Less specific age relationship	• Familial focal epilepsy with variable foci (childhood to adult) • Reflex epilepsies
Distinctive constellations	

(continued)

Table 44.3 (continued)

	• Mesial temporal lobe epilepsy with hippocampal sclerosis (MTLE with HS) • Rasmussen syndrome • Gelastic seizures with hypothalamic hamartoma • Hemiconvulsion–hemiplegia–epilepsy • Head nodding syndrome • Epilepsies that do not fit into any of these diagnostic categories can be distinguished first on the basis of the presence or absence of a known structural or metabolic condition (presumed cause) and then on the basis of the primary mode of seizure onset (generalized vs. focal)
Epilepsies attributed to and organized by structural-metabolic causes	
	• Malformations of cortical development (hemimegalencephaly, heterotopias, etc.) • Neurocutaneous syndromes (tuberous sclerosis complex, Sturge-Weber, etc.) • Tumor • Infection • Trauma • Angioma • Perinatal insults • Stroke • Etc.
Epilepsies of unknown cause	
Not diagnosed as forms of epilepsy per se	
	• Benign neonatal seizures • Febrile seizures • Reactive seizures • Neonatal seizures due to structural and metabolic disorders

44.4 Neuroimaging Findings

44.4.1 Transient Seizure Related Imaging Features

General Imaging Findings
- Reversible swelling and T2-hyperintensity of involved brain area

44.4 Neuroimaging Findings

CT non-contrast-enhanced
- Increased volume of affected brain area with blurred gray/white matter junction
- Hypodense

CT contrast-enhanced
- Variable enhancement

MRI-T2/FLAIR (Fig. 44.1a, b)
- Hyperintense edema of affected gray and white matter

MRI-T1 (Fig. 44.1c)
- Hypointensity and swelling of involved gray and white matter

MRI-T1 contrast-enhanced (Fig. 44.1d)
- Variable enhancement, often leptomeningeal or gyriform

MRI-T2*/SWI
- No hemorrhage

MR-Diffusion Imaging (Fig. 44.1e, f)
- Restricted diffusion

MRI-Perfusion (Fig. 44.1g, h)
- Increased rCBF and rCBV (hyperemia)

MR-Spectroscopy
- Patients with temporal lobe epilepsy may show lipid/lactate peaks within 24 h after seizure

Nuclear Medicine: General Aspects (Fig. 44.2)
- Brain perfusion SPECT with HMPAO and ECD is most commonly used for the assessment of focal epilepsy (in primary generalized epilepsy, nuclear medicine plays no role because there is no indication for surgery).
- ECD has some advantages over HMPAO (faster clearing rate of the blood, longer stabilization) but is at the moment commercially available with limitations.
- For ictal SPECT acquisition, the time of injection is crucial. The tracer should be injected as early in the course of the seizure as possible to identify the source of the seizure.
- Later injected doses show a larger area with hyperperfusion (corresponding to the propagation pathways) and are of limited usefulness for the accurate localization of the onset. The time from the injection to the brain has to be considered (30 s).
- Postictal hypoperfusion of the epileptogenic focus has been reported after 1–2 min postictal, the propagation pathways show hyperperfusion at this time. Hypoperfusion can be seen in other brain regions during the seizure and can persist after the seizure too. Thus, hypoperfusion shortly after a seizure cannot be used for a distinct diagnostic tool for localization of the focus. Some studies reported that the overall hypoperfused hemisphere can be used postictal for the assessment of the hemisphere of the seizure onset.
- It has to be understood that the seizure process is a dynamic one and thereby the time of injection plays a major role because the acquired image is a snapshot of the perfusion when the tracer reaches the brain. To guarantee best results, video-EEG monitoring and a trained staff is crucial to perform injection immediately after seizure onset. Automated injection systems are available to allow the injection from the neighboring room.
- Interictal: There is an inhomogeneous hypoperfusion in the epileptogenic focus with a difference in perfusion on 10–40%. It has to be mentioned that ictal hypoperfusion, postictal and interictal hyperperfusion has been reported (interictal SPECT should be performed after a seizure-free interval of at least 24 h to guarantee best results).
- Studies proved that even in MRI negative patients nuclear medicine diagnostics can be useful in the detection of the epileptogenic zone.

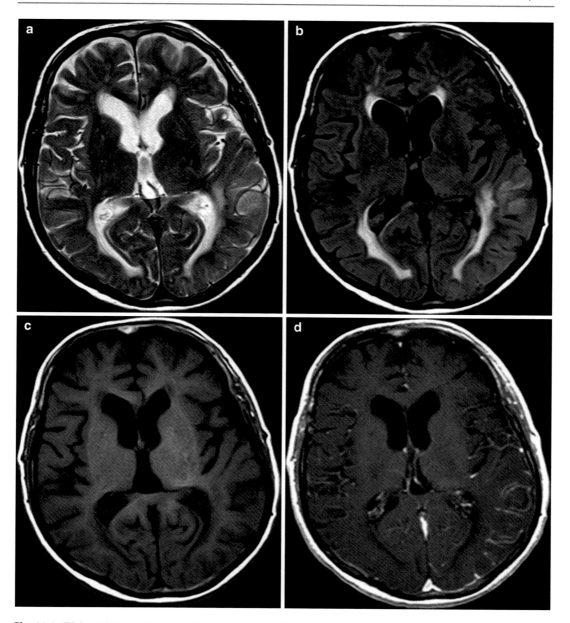

Fig. 44.1 T2-hyperintense edema in left temporo-occipital lobe with leptomeningeal enhancement, restricted diffusion and hyperperfusion after seizure; T2 (**a**), FLAIR (**b**), T1 (**c**), T1 contrast (**d**), DWI (**e**), ADC (**f**), CBV (**g**), CBF (**h**)

- In comparison to FDG-PET, ictal SPECT has the advantage to be rapidly incorporated in the brain tissue and thereby presenting a real snapshot of the seizure activity. FDG uptake is a prolonged process for about 30–40 min. Thereby in the ictal situation SPECT is the best modality to reflect seizure activity. In the interictal situation, FDG-PET has the advantage of a much better spatial resolution than interictal SPECT.
- Hypometabolism is seen in the epileptogenic focus in FDG-PET scans. Often there is at

44.4 Neuroimaging Findings

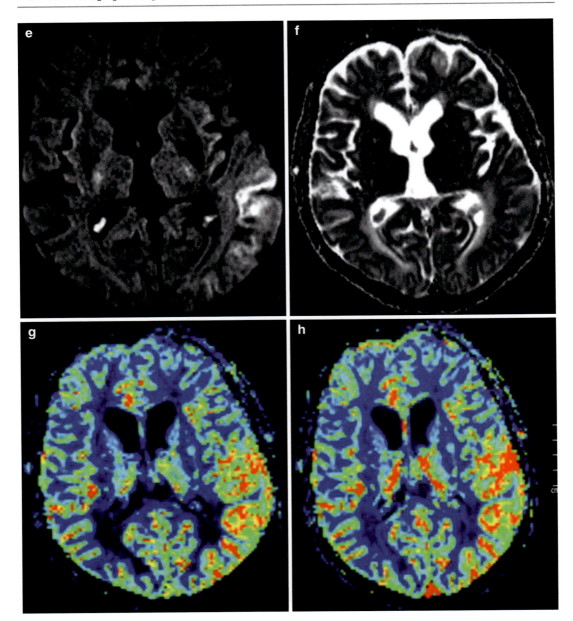

Fig. 44.1 (continued)

least the possibility of lateralization. A pitfall can be the seizure onset after FDG-injection in an interictal study. FDG-PET can be analyzed visually, semi-quantitatively or quantitatively with automated methods like SPM. FDG findings can be correlated to the contralateral side, the whole brain or cerebellum. It has to be taken into account that hypometabolism in FDG-PET is not specific for an epileptogenic focus and study results have to be carefully analyzed. FDG-PET is most helpful in temporal lobe epilepsy.

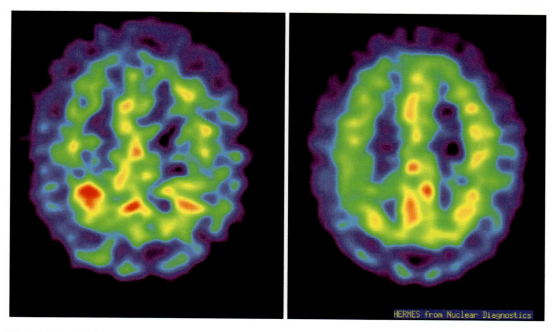

Fig. 44.2 Ictal (left) and interictal (right) perfusion SPECT of a patient with an epileptogenic focus parietal right with hyperperfusion in the ictal and hypoperfusion in the interictal state

In addition, receptor-PET studies can be performed but are in most cases limited for research.

- Flumazenil (nowadays as ^{18}F-flumazenil) is a benzodiazepine receptor binding tracer.
  - It has been reported that flumazenil is more sensitive than FDG in localizing the epileptogenic focus.
  - Flumazenil demonstrates the neuronal loss in patients with epilepsy.
  - Similar to FDG, reduced binding should help to identify the epileptogenic focus.
- Opiate receptor studies with ^{11}C and ^{18}F labeled tracers show increased µ-receptor density in the epileptogenic focus.
- PET studies with $5HT_{1A}$ receptors show a reduction in temporal lobe epilepsy ipsilateral to the focus. For these patients it has to be taken into account that depression is associated with changes in $5HT_{1A}$ receptor density.

In general, it has been shown that

- Nuclear medicine diagnostic has a better sensitivity in temporal lobe epilepsy than in extratemporal lobe epilepsy, especially in patients with normal MRI scans.
- In these patients, nuclear medicine can be useful in lateralization of the seizure-onset zone and thereby giving the opportunity to place the intracranial EEG.
- It has been discussed that in extratemporal lobe epilepsy the propagation is quicker and the postictal changes occur earlier than in temporal lobe epilepsy.
- In contrast to sensitivity in extratemporal lobe epilepsy, specificity is higher than in temporal lobe epilepsy.

Interpretation of the scans can be done as follows:

- Visually by comparing the SPECT or PET study with MRI and the regions with the contralateral side.
- Automated methods are available,
  - One of them is SISCOM (subtraction ictal SPECT coregistered to MRI). This means that the normalized interictal SPECT images are subtracted from the normalized ictal ones, thereby mainly eliminating the background activity and by coregistration to MRI allowing a topographic orientation.
  - Another automated method is SPM (statistical parametric mapping) where individual ictal SPECT images are compared to a database of normal scans or interictal scans from patients with epilepsy.
- These automated systems have some technical limitations too and it has to be kept in mind that minor changes in the analysis criteria can cause substantial different outcomes or even show multiple foci; thus, these findings have to be verified by the physician. SPM has the limitation of a complex statistical modeling due to the created database.

44.5 Etiological Classification of Epilepsies

Etiological causes of the epilepsies are manifold (Table 44.4):

- Single gene disorder
- Complex inheritance
- Disorders of chromosome function
- Encephalopathies
- Progressive myoclonic epilepsies
- Neurocutaneous syndromes
- Developmental anomalies of cerebral structure
- Hippocampal sclerosis
- Perinatal and infantile causes
- Cerebral trauma
- Cerebral tumor
- Cerebral infection
- Cerebrovascular disorders
- Cerebral immunological disorders
- Degenerative and other neurological conditions

44.6 Neuropathological Lesions Associated with the Epilepsies

Neuropathological lesions which are associated with the epilepsies in *adulthood* are classified as follows:

- Tumors
  - Astrocytomas
    - Pilocytic astrocytoma
    - Pleomorphic xanthoastrocytoma
    - Subependymal giant cell astrocytoma (SEGA)
  - Ganglioglioma and gangliocytoma
  - Dysembryoplastic neuroepithelial tumor (DNT)
- Trauma
- Vascular disorders
  - Arteriovenous malformations
  - Cavernous hemangiomas
  - Vein of Galen aneurysm
  - Sturge-Weber Syndrome
- Inflammatory and infectious disorders
- Degenerative and genetic disorders
- Neuronal migration disorders
  - Gray matter heterotopia
  - Periventricular/subependymal nodular heterotopia
  - Diffuse laminar/band heterotopia (double cortex syndrome)
  - Cerebral microdysgenesis
- Focal cortical dysplasia
- Hamartomas and hamartias
- Changes secondary to epilepsy
- Sudden unexpected death in epilepsy (SUDEP)
- Aging
- Hippocampal sclerosis and double pathology

Table 44.4 The etiological classification of the epilepsies, modified after Shorvon (2011)

Main category	Subcategory	Examples
Idiopathic epilepsy	Pure epilepsies due to single gene disorders	• Benign familial neonatal convulsions • Autosomal dominant nocturnal frontal lobe epilepsy • Generalized epilepsy with febrile seizures plus • Severe myoclonic epilepsy of childhood • Benign adult familial myoclonic epilepsy
	Pure epilepsies with complex inheritance	• Idiopathic generalized epilepsy (and its subtypes) • Benign partial epilepsies of childhood
Symptomatic epilepsy Predominately genetic or developmental causation	Childhood epilepsy syndromes	• West syndrome • Lennox–Gastaut syndrome
	Progressive myoclonic epilepsies	• Unverricht–Lundborg disease • Dentato-rubro-pallido-luysian atrophy • Lafora body disease • Mitochondrial cytopathy • Sialidosis • Neuronal ceroid lipofuscinosis • Myoclonus renal failure syndrome
	Neurocutaneous syndromes	• Tuberous sclerosis • Neurofibromatosis • Sturge-Weber syndrome
	Other neurologic single gene disorders	• Angelman syndrome • Lysosomal disorders • Neuroacanthocytosis • Organic acidurias and peroxisomal disorders • Porphyria • Pyridoxine dependent epilepsy • Rett syndrome • Urea cycle disorders • Wilson disease • Disorders of cobalamin and folate metabolism
	Disorders of chromosome function	• Down syndrome • Fragile X syndrome • 4p-syndrome • Isodicentric chromosome 15 • Ring chromosome 20
	Developmental anomalies of cerebral structure	• Hemimegalencephaly • Focal cortical dysplasia • Agyria-pachygyria-band spectrum • Agenesis of corpus callosum • Polymicrogyria • Schizencephaly • Periventricular nodular heterotopias • Microcephaly • Arachnoid cyst

(continued)

44.6 Neuropathological Lesions Associated with the Epilepsies

Table 44.4 (continued)

Main category	Subcategory	Examples
Symptomatic epilepsy Predominately acquired causation	Hippocampal sclerosis	• Hippocampal sclerosis
	Perinatal and infantile causes	• Neonatal seizures • Postneonatal seizures • Cerebral palsy • Vaccination and immunization
	Cerebral trauma	• Open head injury • Closed head injury • Neurosurgery • Epilepsy after epilepsy surgery • Nonaccidental head injury in infants
	Cerebral tumor	• Glioma • Ganglioglioma and hamartoma • DNT • Hypothalamic hamartoma • Meningioma • Secondary tumors
	Cerebral infection	• Viral meningitis and encephalitis • Bacterial meningitis and abscess • Malaria • Neurocysticercosis • Tuberculosis • HIV
	Cerebrovascular disorders	• Cerebral hemorrhage • Cerebral infarction • Degenerative vascular disease • Arteriovenous malformation • Cavernous hemangioma
	Cerebral immunologic disorders	• Rasmussen encephalitis • SLE and collagen vascular disorders • Inflammatory and immunologic disorders
	Degenerative and other neurologic conditions	• Alzheimer disease and other dementing disorders • Multiple sclerosis and demyelinating disorders • Hydrocephalus and porencephaly
Provoked epilepsy	Provoking factors	• Fever • Menstrual cycle and catamenial epilepsy • Sleep-wake cycle • Metabolic and endocrine-induced seizures • Drug-induced seizures • Alcohol and toxin-induced seizures
	Reflex epilepsies	• Photosensitive epilepsies • Startle-induced epilepsies • Reading epilepsy • Auditory-induced epilepsy • Eating epilepsy • Hot-water epilepsy
Cryptogenic epilepsies		

Neuronal and glial malformations associated with the epilepsies in *children* are classified as follows:

- Cortical malformations
  - Lissencephaly
    - Type I
      - Miller Dieker
      - Isolated Lissencephaly sequence
      - X-linked Lissencephaly
    - Type II
      - Walker Warburg
      - Cerebro-ocular muscular syndromes
    - Type III
    - Type IV
  - Regional cortical dysplasias
    - Schizencephaly
    - Focal cortical dysplasia
    - Perisylvian dysplasia
    - Hippocampal dysplasia
- Heterotopias
  - Periventricular, nodular, diffuse
  - Subcortical, band, laminar, double cortex, diffuse
  - Subarachnoid, diffuse
  - Subcortical and subependymal, focal
- Hemimegalencephaly
- Microdysgenesis

Changes secondary to epilepsy include:

- Nerve cell loss
- Cerebellar atrophy
- Cerebral hemiatrophy
- Contralateral cerebellar atrophy
- Changes in status epilepticus

Neuropathological lesions as diagnosed after epilepsy surgery are given in Table 44.5, while tumor entities diagnosed after epilepsy surgery are listed in Table 44.6.

Age OP: age of patients at surgery (in years)
Onset: age at onset of spontaneous seizure activity (in years)
Duration: duration of seizure disorder before surgical treatment (in years)

The frequencies (in %) of occurrence of lesions differ for the whole group, between adults and children (Blumcke et al. 2017).

Disease category	All patients	Adults	Children
Number of cases	9523	6900	2623
Hippocampal sclerosis	36.4	44.5	15.0
Tumor	23.6	22.2	27.2
Cortical malformations	19.8	12.4	39.3
No lesion	7.7	8.4	6.1
Vascular malformations	6.1	7.2	3.2
Glial scar	4.9	4.5	5.8
Encephalitis	1.5	0.9	3.3

44.7 Molecular Neuropathology

The proposed pathogenetic mechanisms are abundant.

- Any neuron, or aggregate of neurons, may be made to discharge abnormally electric stimulation, by alterations in basic metabolic environment, or excitatory drugs (strychnine, pentylenetetrazol) as well as neurotransmitter substances.
- Seizures originate from an abnormal structural focus producing excessive discharge of the gray matter of the brain.
- Convulsion results from sudden, excessive, and temporary, but not necessarily "disorderly," nervous discharges.
- Some material of the cells which make up the discharging lesion has, by morbid nutrition, become a very high tension and unstable equilibrium, briefly of high instability, and occasionally discharging excessively.
- The various pathologic disorders that produce recurrent seizures, or epilepsy, operate on:
  - basic predisposition
  - specific abnormal processes
  - precipitating or triggering disturbances
- The different kinds of seizures are determined by the functions of the part of the brain involved.
- Seizure sensitive brain regions
  - The vascularity of these structures is vulnerable to compression, and the tissues themselves are sensitive to biochemical disturbances produced by hypoxia, metabolic agents, viruses, and genetic states,

44.7 Molecular Neuropathology

Table 44.5 Neuropathological lesions as diagnosed after epilepsy surgery. Data are based on the European Epilepsy Brain Bank (Blumcke et al. 2014) reproduced with kind permission by Springer Nature

Category	Numbers	%	Onset of seizures (in years)	Age at operation (in years)	Duration of disease (in years)
Hippocampal sclerosis (HS)	1908	32.7	11.3 ± 7.7	33.9 ± 10.4	22.7 ± 10.0
Dual pathology	294	5.0	9.5 ± 7.8	25.5 ± 12.8	15.9 ± 9.9
Long-term epilepsy-associated tumors (LEAT)	1551	26.5	16.5 ± 10.1	27.9 ± 12.3	11.8 ± 8.8
Malformations of cortical development (MCD)	930	15.9	5.9 ± 5.7	18.2 ± 12.0	12.3 ± 9.1
Vascular	328	5.6	23.4 ± 11.4	36.1 ± 12.3	12.7 ± 9.0
Glial scars	284	4.9	10.3 ± 8.0	25.6 ± 12.4	14.7 ± 8.6
Encephalitis	96	1.6	13.3 ± 9.4	20.4 ± 12.6	8.2 ± 7.1
No lesion	451	7.7	12.6 ± 7.7	29.2 ± 10.8	16.1 ± 8.0
Total	5842		12.4 ± 8.9	28.6 ± 12.5	16.5 ± 10.1

Table 44.6 The various tumor entities as diagnosed after epilepsy surgery. Data are based on the European Epilepsy Brain Bank (Blumcke et al. 2014) reproduced with kind permission by Springer Nature

Tumor entity	Numbers	%	Onset of seizures (in years)	Age at operation (in years)	Duration of disease (in years)
Ganglioglioma GG I°	673	43.3	12.8	24.9	12.7
Ganglioglioma GG II°/III°	77	5.0	14.2	26.9	11.0
Dysembryoplastic neuroepithelial tumor WHO I	256	16.5	14.7	25.2	10.7
Pleomorphic xanthoastrocytoma (PXA)	38	2.5	18.8	29.3	12.2
INET	29	1.9	14.4	27.9	17.7
Subependymal giant cell astrocytoma (SEGA)	16	1.0	12.3	20.1	9.0
ANET	5	0.3	2.0	19.7	13.0
Astrocytoma WHO II/III	110	7.1	29.5	36.2	6.7
Oligodendroglioma WHO II/III	97	6.3	24.5	38.6	12.5
Pilocytic astrocytoma WHO I	81	5.2	14.8	25.1	12.1
Cysts	31	2.0	21.7	32.4	11.6
Meningioma	26	1.7	38.9	46.5	8.4
Not Otherwise Specified (NOS)	62	3.2	16.1	29.2	13.3
Other	50	4.0	25.0	31.5	11.3
Total	1551		16.5	27.9	11.7

i.e., having a low threshold and high susceptibility
- motor cortex
- limbic structures
- regions involved in autonomic function
- temporal lobe
- amygdala
- hippocampus
  - abnormal dentate gyrus network circuitry
  - mossy fiber sprouting in the dentate gyrus

- Intrinsic membrane instabilities related to
  - intracellular metabolic disturbances
  - extracellular metabolic disturbances
- Excessive and prolonged depolarization
- Defect in recovery following excitation
- No synchronous activity
- Mutation of a specific family of ion (potassium) channels
- Deficiency of glucose transporter Glut-1
- Aberrant formation of local neuronal circuits
- Synaptic reorganization
- Synaptic proteins

- Gliosis
  - might form a barrier, progressively isolating neuronal ensembles from presynaptic influx producing an epileptogenic state
- Neuronal plasticity
  - possibly underlies the long-term potentiation of synaptic efficacy that could be related to epileptogenesis
- Dendritic spines
  - volume changes could profoundly affect synaptic potentials
- Glutamate receptors
  - in hippocampal foci, an increased density has been found
- Immediate Early Genes (IGE)
  - Neuronal excitation by experimentally induced seizures elicits the rapid induction of a set of immediate early genes IGE.
  - IEG encoded proteins act as third messengers in an intracellular signal transduction cascade between neural cell surface receptors, cytoplasmic second messenger systems, and specific target genes in the nucleus → stimulus transcription coupling.
  - IGE encoded transcription factors are thought to up- or down-regulate effector genes with preferential expression in the central nervous system, including genes for neurotransmitters, growth factors, synaptic and axonal proteins.
  - May help explain synaptic efficacy, kindling, and sprouting.
- The neuronal disturbances probably involve intrinsic membrane instabilities related to intracellular and extracellular metabolic disturbances.
- The instabilities produce excessive and prolonged depolarization, implying a defect in recovery following excitation.
- Neuronal excitability
  - Voltage-gated Na⁺ channels
  - Ligand-gated channels
- Ion channels
- Channelopathies
  - Sodium channel defects
  - Potassium channel defects
  - T-type Ca^{2+} and hyperpolarization-activated cyclic nucleotide-gated (HCN) ion channel defects and thalamocortical loops
  - Voltage-gated calcium channels
  - Other Ca^{2+} channel defects
  - Phasic $GABA_A$-mediated inhibition
  - Tonic $GABA_A$ receptor-mediated signaling
  - Glutamate receptors
  - Nicotinic acetylcholine receptors
- Neuronal synchronization and thalamocortical rhythms
- Limbic network synchronization
- Reticulocortical synchronization
- Dendritic excitability
- Neurogenesis
- Epilepsy genes
  - Sodium channel mutations
  - Potassium channelopathies
  - Voltage-gated calcium channel
  - $GABA_A$ receptors
  - Nicotinic acetylcholine receptor
  - Haploinsufficiency of *STXBP1*
  - Gene interactions and modifiers
- Mechanisms of epileptogenesis
  - Immediate initiating processes
    - Cell death
    - Inflammation/blood–brain barrier breakdown
    - Denervation
    - Loss of developmental guidance factors
    - Metabolic changes
    - Changes in gene expression
  - Subsequent delayed changes
    - Altered cell properties
    - Loss of inhibitory constraints
    - Altered synaptic and network organization
    - Altered glial function
    - Changes of the extracellular space
    - Reversion of cellular/synaptic properties to an immature state
    - Subclinical electrical activity/oscillatory activity
- non-coding RNAs
- and many more

44.8 Malformations Due to Genetic Changes

Genetic changes lead to the following varieties of malformations:

- Abnormal proliferation of neurons and glia
  - Tuberous sclerosis
    - Autosomal dominant disorder
    - *TSC1*, located on chromosome 9q34, encoded protein: hamartin
    - *TSC2*, located on chromosome 16p13.3
- Abnormal neuronal migration
  - Bilateral periventricular nodular heterotopia Filamin-A gene (orthogonal branching of actin filaments)
  - Lissencephaly and subcortical band heterotopia
    - Lissencephaly (*LIS1*) gene
    - Doublecortin (*DCX*) (*XLIS*) gene
  - Autosomal recessive lissencephaly with cerebellar hypoplasia
    - Reelin (*RELN*) gene
- Abnormal cortical organization
  - Schizencephaly
    - EMX2
  - Polymicrogyria
    - Xq28
    - 22q11.2 deletion
    - 16q12.2-21

Further genetic changes include:

- Genes leading to epilepsy syndromes in a single gene mode of inheritance (Table 44.7)
- Major linkage loci
- Copy number variants (CNVs)
- Gene variants associated with epilepsy derived from whole-exome sequencing

Major linkage loci have been reported for the epilepsies (Chen et al. 2017) and include:

- 2q24: Benign familial infantile convulsions; *SCN3A;* Generalized epilepsy with febrile seizures plus (GEFS+); *SCN1A;* Generalized epilepsy with febrile seizures plus (GEFS+); *SCN2A;* Generalized epilepsy with febrile seizures plus (GEFS+); *SCN9A*
- 2q34: Genetic generalized epilepsy (GGE)
- 3q26: A benign form of mesial temporal lobe epilepsy (TLE)
- 5q34: A broad spectrum of familial genetic generalized epilepsy (GGE) syndromes
- 5q14-q15: Febrile seizures and epilepsy
- 6p12: Juvenile myoclonic epilepsy (JME)
- 6p21.3: Juvenile myoclonic epilepsy (JME); *TAP-1*
- Juvenile myoclonic epilepsy (JME); *BRD2*
- 6q24: Lafora progressive myoclonus epilepsy; *EPM2A*
- 7p12.1-7q11.22: Progressive myoclonic epilepsy (PME); *KCTD7*
- 7q32: Myoclonic seizures-related photosensitivity
- 8q24: Idiopathic generalized epilepsy (IGE); *KCNQ3*
- Childhood absence epilepsy (CAE); *KCNK9*
- 10q24: Partial epilepsy, autosomal dominant partial epilepsy with auditory features
- 10q22-24: Autosomal dominant partial epilepsy with auditory features (ADPEAF); *LGI1*
- 10q25-q26: Generalized tonic-clonic seizure
- 13q31.3: Genetic generalized epilepsy (GGE)
- 15q14: Rolandic epilepsy (RE)
- 16p13: Familial autodominant recessive infantile myoclonic epilepsy (IME) of infancy; *TBC1D24*
- 19q13: Generalized epilepsy with febrile seizures plus (GEFS+); *SCN1B*
- 22q11-12: Familial partial epilepsy with variable foci; *DEPDC5*
- 22q13.11: Recessive genetic epilepsy with febrile seizures plus; *TBC1D22A*

Copy number variants (CNVs) identified for epilepsy were described and include (Chen et al. 2017).

Table 44.7 Epilepsy syndromes having a single gene mode of inheritance, modified after Guerrini et al. (2011)

Epilepsy syndrome	Type of seizures	Gene	Protein	Locus
Generalized epilepsy with febrile seizures plus (GEFS+)	• Febrile • Afebrile • Complex partial • Generalized tonic-clonic • Abscence • Myoclonic	SCN1A	Sodium channel, neuronal type 1, α-subunit	2q24.3
		SCN1B	Sodium channel, neuronal type 1, β-subunit	19q13.1
		GABRG2	Gamma-aminobutyric acid receptor, γ-2	5q31.1-q33.1
Severe myodonic epilepsy of infancy (SMEI) or Dravet syndrome	• Febrile • Partial • Absences • Myoclonic • Generalized • Unilateral clonic • Generalized tonic-clonic	SCN1A	Sodium channel, neuronal type 1, α-subunit	2q24.3
Benign familial neonatal seizures (BFNS)	• Multifocal neonatal convulsions • Generalized tonic-clonic	KCNQ2	Potassium channel, voltage-gated, KQT-like subfamily, member 2	20q13.3
		KCNQ3	Potassium channel, voltage-gated, KQT-like subfamily, member 3	8q24
Benign familial neonatal/infantile seizures (BFNIS)	• Multifocal neonatal convulsions • Generalized tonic-clonic	SCN2A	Sodium channel, voltage-gated, type 2, α-subunit	2q23-q24.3
Benign familial infantile seizures (BFIS) with familial hemiplegic migraine	• Multifocal neonatal convulsions • Generalized tonic-clonic • Hemiplegic migraine	ATP1A2	ATPase, Na +/K+ transporting, α-2 polypeptide	1q21-q23
Autosomal dominant nocturnal frontal lobe epilepsy (ADNFLE)	• Partial nocturnal motor seizures with hyperkinetic manifestations	CHRNA4	Cholinergic receptor, neuronal nicotinic, α polypeptide 4	20q13.2-q13.3
		CHRNB2	Cholinergic receptor, neuronal nicotinic, β polypeptide 2	1q21
		CHRNA2	Cholinergic receptor, neuronal nicotinic, α polypeptide 2	8q21
Autosomal dominant temporal lobe epilepsy (ADTLE)	• Partial seizures with auditory or visual GLH hallucinations	LGI1	Leucine-rich, glioma-inactivated 1	10q24
Childhood absence epilepsy (CAE)	• Absences • Tonic-clonic	GABRG2	Gamma-aminobutyric acid receptor, γ-2	5q31.1-q33.1
		CLCN2	Chloride channel 2	3q26
Absence epilepsy and paroxysmal dyskinesia	• Absences • Paroxysmal dyskinesia	KCNMA1	Calcium-sensitive potassium (BK) channel	10q22
Juvenile myoclonic epilepsy (JME)	• Myoclonic • Tonic-clonic • Absence	GABRA1	Gamma-aminobutyric acid receptor, α-1	5q34-q35
		EFHC1	Protein with an EF-hand motif	6q12-p11
Infantile spasms, West Syndrome	• Infantile spasms • Hypsarrhythmia	ARX	Gene homeobox Aristaless-related	Xq22.13

(continued)

44.8 Malformations Due to Genetic Changes

Table 44.7 (continued)

Epilepsy syndrome	Type of seizures	Gene	Protein	Locus
Early infantile epileptic encephalopathy, infantile spasms	• Myoclonic • Infantile spasms	CDKL5	Cyclin-dependent kinase 5	Xp22X
Epilepsy and mental retardation restricted to females	• Febrile • Partial • Absences • Myoclonic • Generalized tonic-clonic	PCDH19	Protocadherin 19	Xq22
Early epileptic encephalopathy with suppression burst (Ohtahara syndrome)	• Tonic • Infantile spasms	SIXBP1	Syntaxin binding protein 1	9q34.1

- *NRXN1*—2p16.3; exon-disrupting deletions
- *SCN1A*—2q24.2-q24.3; duplication/deletion
- *SCN2A*—2q24.2-q24.3; duplication/deletion
- *BMP5*—6p12.1; Microduplication
- *AUTS2*—7q11.22; deletion
- *PODXL*—7q32.3; microdeletion
- *CNTNAP2*—7q35; deletion, hemizygous deletions
- *NIPA2*—15q11.2; microdeletion
- *CYFIP1*—15q11.2; microdeletion
- *CHRNA7*—15q13.3; microdeletion
- *NDE1*—16p13.11; deletion
- *GRIN2A*—16p13.2; microdeletion
- *PRRT2*—16p13.2; microdeletion

Variants of genes (and their locus) associated with epilepsy derived from whole-exome sequencing were published (Chen et al. 2017) and include:

- *INHA*—Inhibin, alpha, 2q35
  - Epilepsy with generalized tonic-clonic seizures on awakening (EGTCA)
- *PRICKLE2*—Homolog 2 on chromosome 3, 3p14.1
  - Progressive myoclonus epilepsy (PME)
- *SCARB2*—Scavenger receptor class B, member 2, 4q21.1
  - Progressive myoclonus epilepsy (PME)
- *SYNGAP1*—Synaptic RasGTPase activating protein 1, 6p21.3
  - Epilepsy with myoclonic absences (EMA)
- *PRICKLE*—Prickle homolog 1 on chromosome 12, 12q12
  - Progressive myoclonus epilepsy (PME)
- *CARS2*—Cysteinyl-tRNA synthetase 2, mitochondrial (putative), 13q34
  - Progressive myoclonus epilepsy (PME)
- *CLN6*—Ceroid lipofuscinosis, neuronal 6, 15q23
  - Teenage-onset progressive myoclonus epilepsy (TOPME)
- *GOSR2*—Golgi SNAP receptor complex member 2, 17q21.34
  - Progressive myoclonus epilepsy (PME)
- *PRRT2*—Proline-rich transmembrane protein 2, 16p11.2
  - BFNIS
- *RBFOX1*—RNA-binding protein, fox-1 homolog (*Caenorhabditis elegans*) 1, 16p13.3
  - Idiopathic generalized epilepsy/Rolandic epilepsy (IGE/RE)
- *RBFOX3*—RNA-binding protein, fox-1 homolog (*C. elegans*) 3, 17q25.3
  - Rolandic epilepsy (RE)
- *COL6A2*—Collagen type VI alpha 2—21q22.3
  - Progressive myoclonus epilepsy (PME)
- *DEPDC5*—Disheveled, Egl-10 and Pleckstrin domain-containing protein 5, 22q12
  - Autosomal dominant focal epilepsy (ADFE)

44.9 Treatment

The definition of the type of epilepsy offers the best guide to both management and prognosis. The short- and long-term management of epilepsies is syndrome-related and differs markedly between the various syndromes (Panayiotopoulos, 2007).

- Pharmacological treatment with various agents (see below)
  - Standard older drugs
  - Newer drugs
  - Special and rarely used drugs
- Non-pharmacological therapies
  - Surgical resection
    - Hippocampus, amygdala, parts of the temporal lobe (see Chap. 45)
    - Malformations of cortical development (see Chaps. 46 and 47)
    - Other pathologies, i.e., brain tumors, vascular malformations
  - Vagus nerve stimulation
  - Hormone therapy
  - Immune therapy
  - MRI-guided laser interstitial thermal therapy

Antiepileptic drugs are classified based on the category of their mode of action, their target molecules (Hanada 2014). Typical antiepileptic drugs include:

- Ion-channel modulators (reduce neuronal excitability)
  - Calcium ion channel
    - Ethosuximide
    - Gabapentin
    - Pregabalin
  - Potassium ion channel
    - Retigabine (ezogabine)
  - Sodium ion channel
    - Carbamazepine
    - Eslicarbazepine
    - Lacosamide
    - Lamotrigine
    - Oxcarbazepine
    - Phenytoin
    - Rufinamide
- Enhancers of GABA-ergic transmission (enhance inhibitory neurotransmission)
  - $GABA_A$
    - Clobazam
    - Clonazepam
    - Diazepam
    - Phenobarbital
  - GABA transporter
    - Tiagabine
  - GABA transaminase
    - Vigabatrin
- Modulators of presynaptic machinery
  - SV2A
    - Levetiracetam
- Selective postsynaptic inhibitors of excitatory neurotransmission (reduce excitatory neurotransmission)
  - AMPA receptor
    - Perampanel
- Multiple modes of action
  - Sodium ion channel
  - GABAA receptors
  - NMDA receptors
    - Felbamate
  - Sodium ion channel
  - AMPA/kainate receptors
  - GABAA receptors
    - Topiramate
  - Sodium ion channel
  - GABA turnover
  - NMDA receptors
    - Valproate

Control: Frequency or severity of epileptic seizures is reduced treatment to some acceptable level for some period (Engel 2013).

Complete control: Patient is seizure-free, i.e., epileptic seizures no longer exist.

Cure: Seizure-free patient without treatment.

Drug resistance: Failure of two appropriate drug trials because of inefficacy but not intolerance (Kwan et al. 2010). Epilepsy is considered as drug-resistant if seizures persist despite adequate medication with two, tolerated antiepileptic drugs (single drugs or in combination).

Pharmacosensitive: Patients whose seizures can be controlled by antiseizure medications (Engel 2013).

Pharmacoresistant: Patients whose seizures continue despite adequate treatment (Engel 2013).

Several major theories trying to explain drug resistance in epilepsy include (Tang et al. 2017):

- Pharmacokinetic hypothesis
- Neural network hypothesis
- Intrinsic severity hypothesis
- Gene variant hypothesis
- Target hypothesis
- Transporter hypothesis

Epilepsy surgery outcome scales are widely used to classify outcome after surgical treatment for medically refractory outcome.

Engel Outcome Scale (Engel et al. 1993)

- Class I: Free of disabling seizures
    - IA: Completely seizure-free since surgery
    - IB: Nondisabling simple partial seizures only since surgery
    - IC: Some disabling seizures after surgery, but free of disabling seizures for at least 2 years
    - ID: Generalized convulsions with antiepileptic drug withdrawal only
- Class II: Rare disabling seizures ("almost seizure-free")
    - IIA: Initially free of disabling seizures but has rare seizures now
    - IIB: Rare disabling seizures since surgery
    - IIC: More than rare disabling seizures after surgery, but rare seizures for at least 2 years
    - IID: Nocturnal seizures only
- Class III: Worthwhile improvement
    - IIIA: Worthwhile seizure reduction
    - IIIB: Prolonged seizure-free intervals amounting to greater than half the follow-up period, but not less than 2 years
- Class IV: No worthwhile improvement
    - IVA: Significant seizure reduction
    - IVB: No appreciable change
    - IVC: Seizures worse

ILAE Outcome Scale (Wieser et al. 2001)

- Class 1: Completely seizure free; no auras
- Class 2: Only auras; no other seizures
- Class 3: 1–3 seizure days per year; ± auras
- Class 4: 4 seizure days per year to 50% reduction of baseline seizure days; ± auras
- Class 5: Less than 50% reduction of baseline seizure days; ± auras
- Class 6: More than 100% increase of baseline seizure days; ± auras

Selected References

Abdul Rahim MI, Thomas RH (2017) Gamification of medication adherence in epilepsy. J Neurol 52:11–14. https://doi.org/10.1016/j.seizure.2017.09.008

Bauer S, van Alphen N, Becker A, Chiocchetti A, Deichmann R, Deller T, Freiman T, Freitag CM, Gehrig J, Hermsen AM, Jedlicka P, Kell C, Klein KM, Knake S, Kullmann DM, Liebner S, Norwood BA, Omigie D, Plate K, Reif A, Reif PS, Reiss Y, Roeper J, Ronellenfitsch MW, Schorge S, Schratt G, Schwarzacher SW, Steinbach JP, Strzelczyk A, Triesch J, Wagner M, Walker MC, von Wegner F, Rosenow F (2017) Personalized translational epilepsy research—novel approaches and future perspectives: part II: experimental and translational approaches. Epilepsy Behav 76:7–12. https://doi.org/10.1016/j.yebeh.2017.06.040

Berg AT, Berkovic SF, Brodie MJ, Buchhalter J, Cross JH, van Emde Boas W, Engel J, French J, Glauser TA, Mathern GW, Moshe SL, Nordli D, Plouin P, Scheffer IE (2010) Revised terminology and concepts for organization of seizures and epilepsies: report of the ILAE Commission on Classification and Terminology, 2005–2009. Epilepsia 51(4):676–685. https://doi.org/10.1111/j.1528-1167.2010.02522.x

Blumcke I, Aronica E, Urbach H, Alexopoulos A, Gonzalez-Martinez JA (2014) A neuropathology-based approach to epilepsy surgery in brain tumors and proposal for a new terminology use for long-term epilepsy-associated brain tumors. Acta Neuropathol 128(1):39–54. https://doi.org/10.1007/s00401-014-1288-9

Blumcke I, Spreafico R, Haaker G, Coras R, Kobow K, Bien CG, Pfafflin M, Elger C, Widman G, Schramm J, Becker A, Braun KP, Leijten F, Baayen JC, Aronica E, Chassoux F, Hamer H, Stefan H, Rossler K, Thom M, Walker MC, Sisodiya SM, Duncan JS, McEvoy AW, Pieper T, Holthausen H, Kudernatsch M, Meencke HJ, Kahane P, Schulze-Bonhage A, Zentner J, Heiland DH, Urbach H, Steinhoff BJ, Bast T, Tassi L, Lo Russo G, Ozkara C, Oz B, Krsek P, Vogelgesang S, Runge U, Lerche H, Weber Y, Honavar M, Pimentel J, Arzimanoglou A, Ulate-Campos A, Noachtar S, Hartl E, Schijns O, Guerrini R, Barba C, Jacques

TS, Cross JH, Feucht M, Muhlebner A, Grunwald T, Trinka E, Winkler PA, Gil-Nagel A, Toledano Delgado R, Mayer T, Lutz M, Zountsas B, Garganis K, Rosenow F, Hermsen A, von Oertzen TJ, Diepgen TL, Avanzini G (2017) Histopathological findings in brain tissue obtained during epilepsy surgery. N Engl J Med 377(17):1648–1656. https://doi.org/10.1056/NEJMoa1703784

Caplan R (2017) Epilepsy, language, and social skills. Brain Lang. https://doi.org/10.1016/j.bandl.2017.08.007

Carreno M, Lüders HO (2001) General principles of presurgical evaluation. In: Lüder HO, Comair YG (eds) Epilepsy surgery, 2nd edn. Lippincott Williams & Wilkins, Philadelphia, pp 185–200

Chen T, Giri M, Xia Z, Subedi YN, Li Y (2017) Genetic and epigenetic mechanisms of epilepsy: a review. Neuropsychiatr Dis Treat 13:1841–1859. https://doi.org/10.2147/ndt.s142032

Commission on Classification and Terminology of the International League Against Epilepsy (1981) Proposal for revised clinical and electroencephalographic classification of epileptic seizures. Epilepsia 22(4):489–501

Commission on Classification and Terminology of the International League Against Epilepsy (1989) Proposal for revised classification of epilepsies and epileptic syndromes. Epilepsia 30(4):389–399

Cukiert A, Lehtimaki K (2017) Deep brain stimulation targeting in refractory epilepsy. Epilepsia 58 suppl 1:80–84. https://doi.org/10.1111/epi.13686

Engel J Jr (2013) Seizures and epilepsies. Oxford University Press, Oxford

Engel JJ, Van Ness PC, Rasmussen TB (1993) Outcome with respect to epileptic seizures. In: Engel JJ (ed) Surgical treatment of the epilepsies, 2nd edn. Raven Press, New York, pp 609–621

Falco-Walter J, Owen C, Sharma M, Reggi C, Yu M, Stoub TR, Stein MA (2017) Magnetoencephalography and new imaging modalities in epilepsy. Neurotherapeutics 14(1):4–10. https://doi.org/10.1007/s13311-016-0506-7

Fisher RS (2017) The new classification of seizures by the International League Against Epilepsy 2017. Curr Neurol Neurosci Rep 17(6):48. https://doi.org/10.1007/s11910-017-0758-6

Fisher RS, Acevedo C, Arzimanoglou A, Bogacz A, Cross JH, Elger CE, Engel Jr J, Forsgren L, French JA, Glynn M, Hesdorffer DC, Lee BI, Mathern GW, Moshe SL, Perucca E, Scheffer IE, Tomson T, Watanabe M, Wiebe S (2014) ILAE official report: a practical clinical definition of epilepsy. Epilepsia 55(4):475–482. https://doi.org/10.1111/epi.12550

Fisher RS, Cross JH, D'Souza C, French JA, Haut SR, Higurashi N, Hirsch E, Jansen FE, Lagae L, Moshe SL, Peltola J, Roulet Perez E, Scheffer IE, Schulze-Bonhage A, Somerville E, Sperling M, Yacubian EM, Zuberi SM (2017a) Instruction manual for the ILAE 2017 operational classification of seizure types. Epilepsia 58(4):531–542. https://doi.org/10.1111/epi.13671

Fisher RS, Cross JH, French JA, Higurashi N, Hirsch E, Jansen FE, Lagae L, Moshe SL, Peltola J, Roulet Perez E, Scheffer IE, Zuberi SM (2017b) Operational classification of seizure types by the International League Against Epilepsy: position paper of the ILAE Commission for Classification and Terminology. Epilepsia 58(4):522–530. https://doi.org/10.1111/epi.13670

Fukata Y, Fukata M (2017) Epilepsy and synaptic proteins. Curr Opin Neurobiol 45:1–8. https://doi.org/10.1016/j.conb.2017.02.001

Guerrini R, Shorvon SD, Andermann F, Andermann E (2011) Introduction to the concept of genetic epilepsy. In: Shorvon SD, Andermann F, Guerrini R (eds) The causes of epilepsy. Cambridge University Press, Cambridge, pp 43–61

Hanada T (2014) The AMPA receptor as a therapeutic target in epilepsy: preclinical and clinical evidence. J Receptor Ligand Channel Res 7:39–50

Hu Q, Zhang F, Teng W, Hao F, Zhang J, Yin M, Wang N (2018) Efficacy and safety of antiepileptic drugs for refractory partial-onset epilepsy: a network meta-analysis. J Neurol 265(1):1–11. https://doi.org/10.1007/s00415-017-8621-x

Kim JA, Chung JI, Yoon PH, Kim DI, Chung TS, Kim EJ, Jeong EK (2001) Transient MR signal changes in patients with generalized tonicoclonic seizure or status epilepticus: periictal diffusion-weighted imaging. AJNR Am J Neuroradiol 22(6):1149–1160

Kwan P, Arzimanoglou A, Berg AT, Brodie MJ, Allen Hauser W, Mathern G, Moshé SL, Perucca E, Wiebe S, French J (2010) Definition of drug resistant epilepsy: consensus proposal by the ad hoc Task Force of the ILAE Commission on Therapeutic Strategies. Epilepsia. 51(6):1069-77. https://doi.org/10.1111/j.1528-1167.2009.02397.x

Luders HO, Burgess R, Noachtar S (1993) Expanding the international classification of seizures to provide localization information. Neurology 43(9):1650–1655

Luders HO, Najm I, Nair D, Widdess-Walsh P, Bingman W (2006) The epileptogenic zone: general principles. Epileptic Disord 8(Suppl 2):S1–S9

Martinkovic L, Hecimovic H, Sulc V, Marecek R, Marusic P (2014) Modern techniques of epileptic focus localization. Int Rev Neurobiol 114:245–278. https://doi.org/10.1016/b978-0-12-418693-4.00010-8

Middlebrooks EH, Ver Hoef L, Szaflarski JP (2017) Neuroimaging in epilepsy. Curr Neurol Neurosci Rep 17(4):32. https://doi.org/10.1007/s11910-017-0746-x

Nadler JV, Spencer DD (2014) What is a seizure focus. Adv Exp Med Biol 813:55–62. https://doi.org/10.1007/978-94-017-8914-1_4

North RY, Raskin JS, Curry DJ (2017) MRI-guided laser interstitial thermal therapy for epilepsy. Neurosurg Clin N Am 28(4):545–557. https://doi.org/10.1016/j.nec.2017.06.001

Orsini A, Zara F, Striano P (2018) Recent advances in epilepsy genetics. Neurosci Lett 667:4–9. https://doi.org/10.1016/j.neulet.2017.05.014

Panayiotopoulos CP (2007) A clinical guide to epileptic syndromes and their treatment, 2nd edn. Springer Verlag, Berlin

Pitkanen A (2010) Therapeutic approaches to epileptogenesis—hope on the horizon. Epilepsia 51(suppl 3):2–17. https://doi.org/10.1111/j.1528-1167.2010.02602.x

Rosenow F, van Alphen N, Becker A, Chiocchetti A, Deichmann R, Deller T, Freiman T, Freitag CM, Gehrig J, Hermsen AM, Jedlicka P, Kell C, Klein KM, Knake S, Kullmann DM, Liebner S, Norwood BA, Omigie D, Plate K, Reif A, Reif PS, Reiss Y, Roeper J, Ronellenfitsch MW, Schorge S, Schratt G, Schwarzacher SW, Steinbach JP, Strzelczyk A, Triesch J, Wagner M, Walker MC, von Wegner F, Bauer S (2017) Personalized translational epilepsy research—novel approaches and future perspectives: Part I: clinical and network analysis approaches. Epilepsy Behav 76:13–18. https://doi.org/10.1016/j.yebeh.2017.06.041

Seneviratne U, Cook MJ, D'Souza WJ (2017) Electroencephalography in the diagnosis of genetic generalized epilepsy syndromes. Front Neurol 8:499. https://doi.org/10.3389/fneur.2017.00499

Shao Y, Chen Y (2017) Pathophysiology and clinical utility of non-coding RNAs in epilepsy. Front Mol Neurosci 10:249. https://doi.org/10.3389/fnmol.2017.00249

Shorvon SD (2011) The etiological classification of epilepsy. In: Shorvon SD, Andermann F, Guerrini R (eds) The causes of epilepsy. Cambridge University Press, Cambridge, pp 21–23

Sprengers M, Vonck K, Carrette E, Marson AG, Boon P (2017) Deep brain and cortical stimulation for epilepsy. Cochrane Database Syst Rev (7):CD008497. https://doi.org/10.1002/14651858.CD008497.pub3

Tang F, Hartz AMS, Bauer B (2017) Drug-resistant epilepsy: multiple hypotheses, few answers. Front Neurol 8:301. https://doi.org/10.3389/fneur.2017.00301

Wieser HG, Blume WT, Fish D, Goldensohn E, Hufnagel A, King D, Sperling MR, Luders H, Pedley TA (2001) ILAE Commission Report. Proposal for a new classification of outcome with respect to epileptic seizures following epilepsy surgery. Epilepsia 42(2):282–286

Epilepsies: Temporal Lobe Epilepsy

45.1 Introduction

Temporal lobe epilepsy (also called mesial temporal lobe epilepsy) is the most frequent form of partial epilepsy in adults.

45.2 Clinical Signs

- Alterations in consciousness
- Combined by various functional manifestations including
  - Sensory
  - Motor
  - Psychic
  - Autonomic

Hippocampal sclerosis is the most commonly ncountered pathological substrate of mesial temporal lobe epilepsy in adults with drug-resistant TLE.

Formerly used names to describe hippocampal sclerosis include:

- Ammon's Horn Sclerosis (Bouchet and Cazauvieilh 1825; Sommer 1880)
- Incisural Sclerosis (Earle et al. 1953)
- Pararhinal Sclerosis (Gastaut 1959)
- Mesial Temporal Sclerosis (Falconer et al. 1964)
- End Folium Sclerosis (Margerison and Corsellis 1966)
- Total Ammon's Horn Sclerosis (Bruton 1988)

45.3 Neuroimaging Findings

General Imaging Findings

Most frequently caused by mesial temporal sclerosis—atrophy and T2-hyperinensity of hippocampus.

CT non-contrast-enhanced
- Usually normal, enlargement of temporal horn of lateral ventricle in severe cases of hippocampal atrophy

CT contrast-enhanced
- No pathological enhancement

MRI-T2 (Figs. 45.1a, b and 45.2a)
- Hyperintensity and atrophy of hippocampus
- Most commonly unilateral, in some cases bilateral atrophy
- Atrophy of fornix and/or mammillary body possible

MRI-FLAIR (Fig. 45.2b)
- Hyperintensity of hippocampus

MRI-T1 (Fig. 45.1c)
- Loss of hippocampal gray-white differentiation

MRI-T1 Contrast-Enhanced
- No pathological enhancement

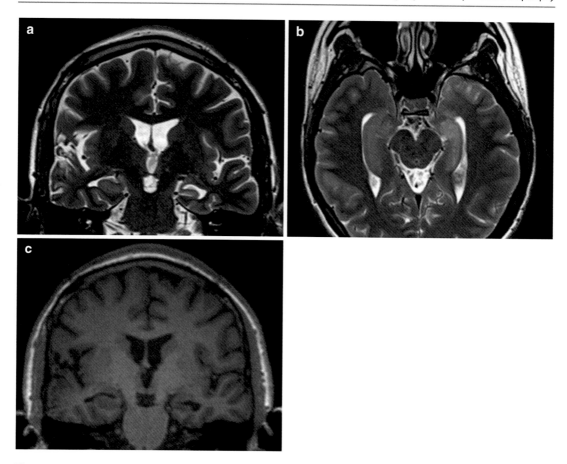

Fig. 45.1 Atrophy and T2-hyperintensity of the left hippocampus; T2 axial and coronal (**a** and **b**), T1 (**c**)

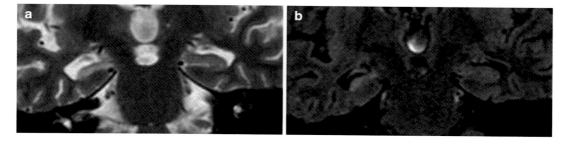

Fig. 45.2 Atrophy and T2-hyperintensity of the right hippocampus; T2 coronal (**a**), FLAIR (**b**)

MR-Diffusion Imaging
- High signal on ADC
- Restricted diffusion after seizure

MRI-Perfusion
- Increased peri-ictal, decreased interictal

MR-Spectroscopy
- Low NAA values in hippocampus/temporal lobe, decreased NAA/Cho and NAA/Cr ratios

Nuclear Medicine Imaging Findings (Figs. 45.3 and 45.4)
- FDG-PET (Chassoux et al. 2016)

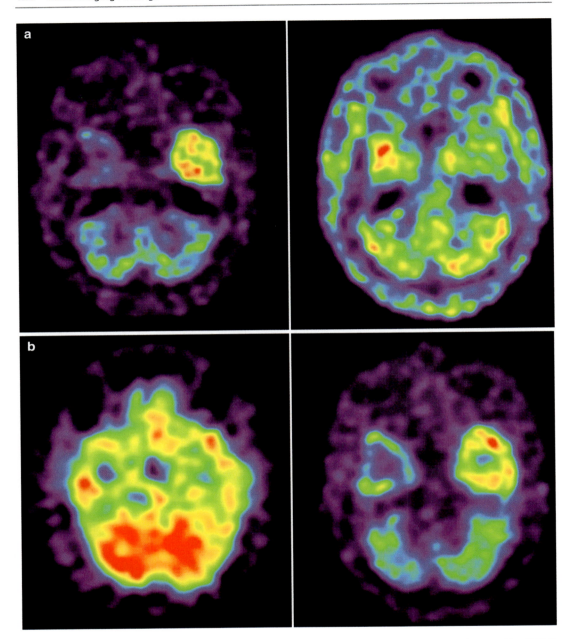

Fig. 45.3 Patient with epileptogenic focus right temporal: FMZ-PET (left) demonstrating neuronal loss and ictal FDG-PET (right) with hypermetabolism (**a**). The same patient with ictal perfusion scan (left) and FMZ-PET (right) (**b**)

- has assisted in localizing the seizure-onset zone, especially in TLE
- is a confirmatory test if adequate MRI shows no structural correlate in patients with MTLE, especially if it is in agreement with ictal electroencephalography (EEG) findings

- The characteristic interictal finding in TLE is a
  ○ diffuse regional hypometabolism of both mesial and lateral temporal structures.
  ○ Ipsilateral hypometabolism involves temporal (mesial structures, pole, and

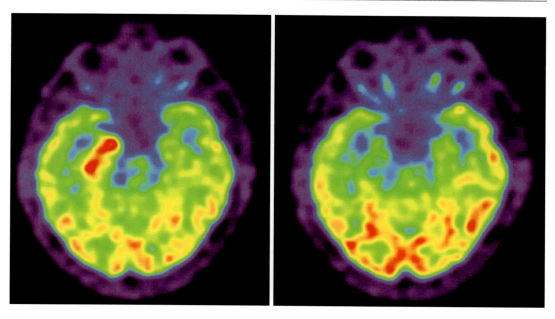

Fig. 45.4 Patient with epileptogenic focus right temporal: FDG-PET (ictal right) and (interictal left)

lateral cortex) and extratemporal areas including the insula, frontal lobe, perisylvian regions, and thalamus, more extensively in right HS (RHS).
- The exact reasons for the interictal hypometabolism are
  - not clear.
  - hypometabolism results from HS in the temporolimbic region, not necessarily affecting other parts of the temporal lobe.
  - may reflect the preferential networks involved by ictal discharges and spread pathways (Chassoux et al. 2004).
- Ipsilateral PET hypometabolism had
  - a predictive value of 86% for good outcome
  - The predictive value was 80% in patients with normal MRI.
  - It is not possible to distinguish between localizing and lateralizing findings.
- A relative increase of metabolism (hypermetabolism) is found in the nonepileptic temporal lobe and in posterior areas bilaterally.
- The topography of hypometabolism correlates strongly with the extent of epileptic networks (mesial, anterior-mesiolateral, widespread mesiolateral, and bitemporal according to the ictal spread), which were larger in RHS. Widespread perisylvian and bitemporal hypometabolism is found only in RHS.
- Mirror hypermetabolism is grossly proportional to the hypometabolic areas, coinciding partly with the default mode network.
- Gender-related effect is significant mainly in the contralateral frontal lobe, in which metabolism is higher in female patients.
- Epilepsy duration correlated with the contralateral temporal metabolism, positively in LHS and negatively in RHS.
- Opposite results are found with age at onset.
- High seizure frequency correlates negatively with the contralateral metabolism in LHS.
- FMZ-PET
  - Flumazenil (FMZ) is a specific antagonist of central benzodiazepine receptors (cBZR)

45.4 Neuropathology Findings

and is a marker of the complex of GABAA/cBZR using PET scanning.
- In MTLE with HS, cBZRs numbers in the hippocampus are reduced.
- Moreover, reduced FMZ binding is most prominent in the hippocampal subfields with the most pronounced neuronal loss.
- [18F]FP BP (Werhahn et al. 2006)
  - Significant decrease in the epileptogenic temporal lobe in all patients.
  - Reduction is evident in areas surrounding the seizure-onset zone at the pole and lateral aspects of the temporal lobe.
  - No significant decrease of [18F]FP BP the hippocampus.
  - No correlation between the reduction of [18F]FP BP and hippocampal atrophy.
- Focal hypometabolism on 18F-fluorodeoxyglucose-positron emission tomography (FDG-PET) ipsilateral to the symptomatic temporal lobe predicts a good surgical outcome; the added value of (11) C-Flumazenil-PET (FMZ-PET) and proton magnetic resonance spectroscopy (MRS) is less clear.
- Ictal and interictal CBF studies help in identifying the epileptogenic focus, especially when subtracting the images (SISCOM).

45.4 Neuropathology Findings

Macroscopic Features
- Shrinkage of the hippocampal formation
- Induration of the hippocampal formation

Microscopic Features
- The knowledge of the histological built-up of the hippocampus is a prerequisite for the analysis of the structure, which might be supplied by the neurosurgeons in "small pieces" (Fig. 45.5).

Recently the International League Against epilepsy (ILAE) presented a modified version of the previous classification as follows (Blumcke et al. 2014) (Fig. 45.6):

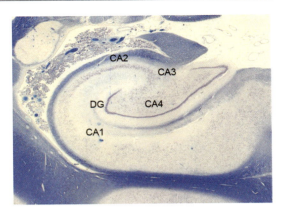

Fig. 45.5 Normal hippocampus with sectors CA1, CA2, CA3, CA4, and dentate gyrus (DG)

- Hippocampal sclerosis ILAE type 1
- Hippocampal sclerosis ILAE type 2 (CA1 predominant neuronal cell loss and gliosis)
- Hippocampal sclerosis ILAE type 3 (CA4 predominant neuronal cell loss and gliosis)
- No hippocampal sclerosis, gliosis only (no-HS)

Hippocampal Sclerosis ILAE Type 1
- The most common type of HS (approximately 60–80% of all TLE-HS cases)
- CA1 segment is most severely affected (with >80% cell loss)
- Significant neuronal cell loss in other segments, affecting
  - 30–50% of pyramidal neurons in CA2
  - 30–90% of neurons in CA3
  - 40–90% of neurons in CA4
- Dentate gyrus (DG) affected by 50–60% granule cell loss
- Cell loss is sometimes focal in the DG and accompanied by granule cell dispersion (GCD)

Hippocampal Sclerosis ILAE Type 2 (CA1 Predominant Neuronal Cell Loss and Gliosis)
(Figs. 45.7a–j and 45.8a–f)
- Predominant neuronal loss in CA1.
- Affecting almost 80% of pyramidal cells.
- Mild cell loss in all other sectors:
  - CA2 < 20%, in CA3 < 20%, and in CA4 < 25% of principal cells

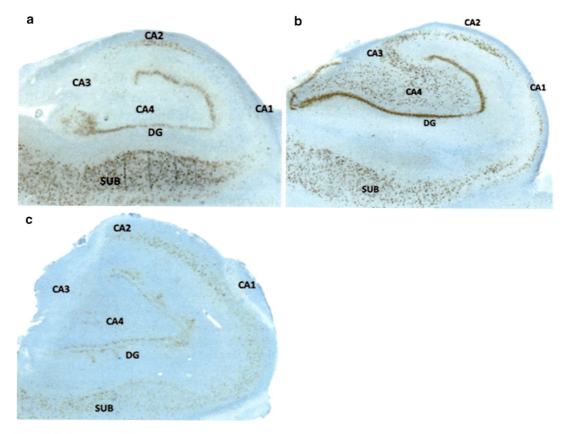

Fig. 45.6 Summary of hippocampal sclerosis: (**a**) Type 1, (**b**) Type 2, (**c**) Type 3. Modified after Blümcke, Sarnat, Coras (2015)

- This pattern is uncommon (5–10% of all TLE surgical cases).
- DG pathology patterns may include:
  - granule cell dispersion
  - absence of severe granule cell loss

Hippocampal Sclerosis ILAE Type 3 (CA4 Predominant Neuronal Cell Loss and Gliosis)
- Predominant cell loss in CA4 (approximately 50% cell loss)
- Cell loss in the dentate gyrus (35% cell loss)
- Moderate changes in CA3 (<30%), CA2 (<25%), and CA1 (<20%)
- Rare HS variant (4–7.4% of all TLE surgical cases)

Granule Cell Dispersion (GCD) (Fig. 45.9)
- Broadening of the granule cell layer above ten layers
  - ill-defined boundary with the molecular layer
  - ectopic granule cells (either isolated, clustered, or bilayered)
  - separated from the main layer by intervening neuropil
- Occurs in approximately 50% of all TLE cases.
- GCD is variably described in ILAE HS types 1, 2, and 3.
- May also occur in patients without hippocampal neuronal cell loss.
- GCD as a result of Reelin deficiency in the DG.

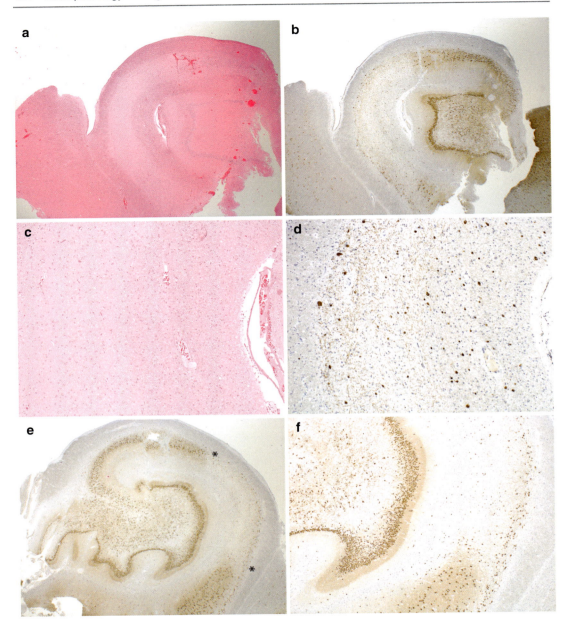

Fig. 45.7 Hippocampal sclerosis type 2: severe loss of neurons in CA1 (asterisk) and mild loss of neurons in CA2 and CA4 (H&E: **a**, **c**; IHC for NeuN: **b**, **d–f**). Neuronal loss in the dentate gyrus (H&E: **g**, **h**; IHC for NeuN: **i**, **j**)

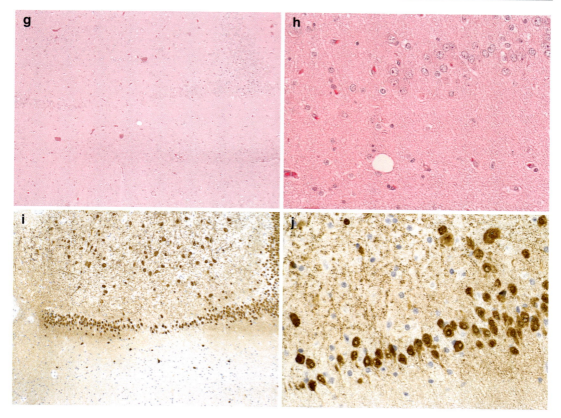

Fig. 45.7 (continued)

- The presence of GCD is associated with greater cell loss in the hilus, an older age at epilepsy surgery, and longer epilepsy duration.

No Hippocampal Sclerosis, Gliosis Only (no-HS) (Fig. 45.10)
- About 20% of TLE cases show
  - No significant neuronal cell loss
  - Only various degrees of reactive gliosis

Additional microscopic changes include:

- Outer molecular layer
  - Reduced number of Cajal–Retzius cells
- Inner molecular layer
  - Expansion of supragranular calretinin-positive axonal plexuses
  - Reduction of hilar cells
  - Increase of substance P receptor positive cells
- Granule cell layer
  - Increased complexity of chandelier cells
  - Loss of calbindin in granule cells
- Hilus
  - Reduction of calretinin-positive interneurons
  - Reduction of neuropeptide Y- and somatostatin-positive hilar cells
  - Sprouting of axons
  - Hypertrophy of calbindin-positive hilar neurons

Previously, a classification of hippocampal changes in mesial temporal lobe epilepsy was proposed and reads as follows (Blumcke et al. 2007):

- *Type 1a* (sixfold standard deviation)
  - CA1 most severe neuronal loss

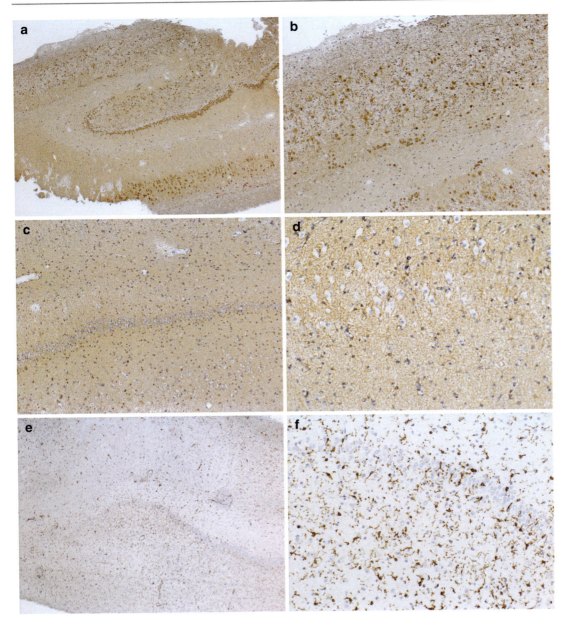

Fig. 45.8 Hippocampal sclerosis type 2: sometimes the hippocampal formation is not complete which makes the typing difficult. CA1 is grossly lacking. Moderate neuronal loss in CA2–CA4. (**a** and **b**) (IHC for NeuN). Mild reactive astrogliosis (**c** and **d**; IHC for GFAP) and moderate reactive microgliosis (**e** and **f**; IHC for HLA-DRII) are seen in the dentate gyrus

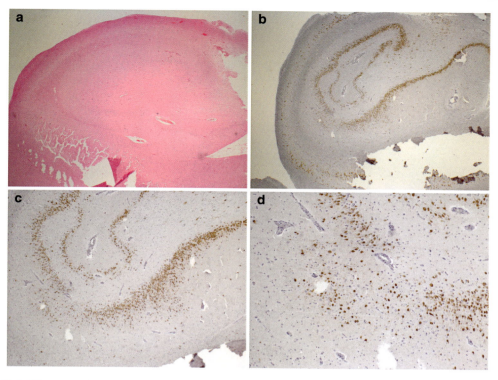

Fig. 45.9 Hippocampal sclerosis with dispersion of dentate gyrus neurons (H&E: **a**; NeuN: **b–d**)

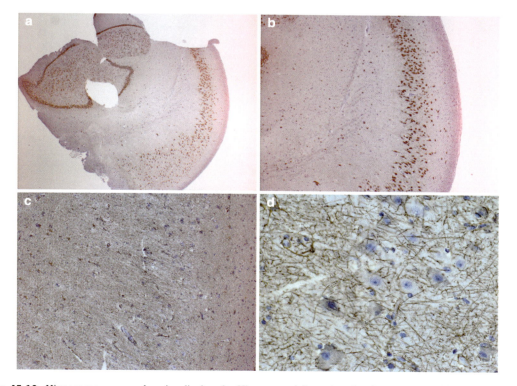

Fig. 45.10 Hippocampus—no sclerosis, gliosis only: Hippocampal formation showing no neuronal loss but moderate reactive astrogliosis (NeuN: **a**, **b**; GFAP: **c**, **d**)

Table 45.1 Neuropathological grading of hippocampal sclerosis, modified after Wyler et al. (1995), Wyler and Vossler (1997) with permission from Elsevier and Oxford University Press

Grade	Classification	Neuropathological description	MRI
Wyler I	Mild mesial temporal damage	Gliosis with slight (10%) or no hippocampal neuronal dropout involving sectors CA1, CA3, and/or CA4	Not visible
Wyler II	Moderate mesial temporal damage	Gliosis with moderate (10–50%) neuronal dropout of CA1, CA3, and/or CA4. If involvement limited to CA3 and 4 = end folium sclerosis	Loss of internal structure on high resolution T2-weighted images
Wyler III	"Classical" ammon's horn sclerosis	Gliosis with 50% neuronal dropout of CA1, CA3, and CA4, but sparing CA2	Atrophy and increased T2/FLAIR signal
Wyler IV	"Total" ammon's horn sclerosis	Gliosis with 50% neuronal dropout of all sectors	Atrophy and increased T2/FLAIR signal visible

- *Type 1b* (sixfold standard deviation)
  - Severe neuronal loss in all subfields
- *Type 2*
  - Severe loss restricted to CA1
- *Type 3* (second standard deviation)
  - Significant loss in all subfields except CA1

For historical reasons, the grading of hippocampal sclerosis after Wyler is given in Table 45.1.

45.5 Molecular Neuropathology

- Initial precipitating injury before the age of 4 years
  - Complex febrile seizures
  - Birth trauma
  - Head injury
  - Meningitis
- Not yet fully understood
- Altered inhibitory mechanisms
- Interneurons
- Mossy cells
- Impact of persisting calretinin-immunoreactive neurons with Cajal–Retzius cell morphology
- Astrocytic tenascin-C induction and redistribution as potential regulator of aberrant axonal sprouting
- Alterations of Ca^{2+}-mediated hippocampal signaling pathways
- Astrocytes
  - Causative of the generation or spread of seizure activity
  - Alterations in expression, localization, and function of astroglial inwardly rectifying K1 (Kir) channels, particularly Kir4.1, which is suspected to entail impaired K1 buffering.
  - Gap junctions in astrocytes appear to play a dual role:
    o on the one hand they counteract the generation of hyperactivity by facilitating clearance of elevated extracellular K1 levels
    o constitute a pathway for energetic substrate delivery to fuel neuronal (hyper) activity
- Changes of GABA receptors
- Changes of GABA transmission
- Enhanced excitatory mechanisms through mossy fiber sprouting
- Gene expression
  - Dentate granule cells—37 altered genes related to:
    o Structural integrity
    o Axonal outgrowth
    o Proliferation
  - Hippocampi—21 altered genes related to:
    o Gene-transcription control
    o Calcium homeostasis
    o Neuronal signaling
  - Entorhinal cortex—altered genes related to:
    o Serotonin receptor (HTR2A)
    o Neuropeptide Y receptor
    o Protein (FHL2) associated with the KCNE1 potassium channel subunit
    o Immune system-related proteins

- Subfield-specific regulation of microRNAs
- Synaptic reorganization
- Reinnervation of denervated dendrites in the hippocampus leading to laminar collateral axon sprouting.
- True hippocampal epilepsy results from early damage to the hippocampus, followed by reorganization of synaptic circuitry sufficient to generate seizures.
- Denervation of rat fascia dentata with sprouted Timm-stained mossy fiber terminals forming a monosynaptic excitatory feedback circuit.
- Aberrant feedback circuits on granule cells produce synaptically driven multiple spikes that correlate with the density of Timm-stained terminals.

45.6 Treatment and Prognosis

Treatment

- Tailored neurosurgical resection of the sclerotic hippocampus, parts of the amygdala and the temporal cortex

Biologic Behavior-Prognosis-Prognostic Factors

- 2-year postoperative seizure control: 60–80%
- Completeness of surgical resection
- Resected brain regions
- Type of hippocampal sclerosis
  - Type 1 60–80%
  - Type 2 and Type 3: fewer patients
- Class IA outcome was associated with
  - a focal anteromesial temporal hypometabolism
- Non-IA outcome correlated with
  - extratemporal metabolic changes that differed according to the lateralization:
    - ipsilateral mesial frontal and perisylvian hypometabolism in right HS
    - contralateral frontoinsular hypometabolism and posterior white matter hypermetabolism in left HS
- Suboptimal outcome presented a
  - metabolic pattern similar to the best outcome
  - but with a larger involvement of extratemporal areas, including the contralateral side in left HS.
- Failure was characterized by a
  - mild temporal involvement sparing the hippocampus
  - relatively high extratemporal hypometabolism on both sides (Chassoux et al. 2017)

Selected References

Alexander A, Maroso M, Soltesz I (2016) Organization and control of epileptic circuits in temporal lobe epilepsy. Prog Brain Res 226:127–154. https://doi.org/10.1016/bs.pbr.2016.04.007

Alonso Vanegas MA, Lew SM, Morino M, Sarmento SA (2017) Microsurgical techniques in temporal lobe epilepsy. Epilepsia 58(suppl 1):10–18. https://doi.org/10.1111/epi.13684

Andres-Mach M, Fike JR, Luszczki JJ (2011) Neurogenesis in the epileptic brain: a brief overview from temporal lobe epilepsy. Pharmacol Rep 63(6):1316–1323

Bernhardt BC, Hong S, Bernasconi A, Bernasconi N (2013) Imaging structural and functional brain networks in temporal lobe epilepsy. Front Hum Neurosci 7:624. https://doi.org/10.3389/fnhum.2013.00624

Blumcke I, Pauli E, Clusmann H, Schramm J, Becker A, Elger C, Merschhemke M, Meencke HJ, Lehmann T, von Deimling A, Scheiwe C, Zentner J, Volk B, Romstock J, Stefan H, Hildebrandt M (2007) A new clinico-pathological classification system for mesial temporal sclerosis. Acta Neuropathol 113(3):235–244. https://doi.org/10.1007/s00401-006-0187-0

Blumcke I, Aronica E, Urbach H, Alexopoulos A, Gonzalez-Martinez JA (2014) A neuropathology-based approach to epilepsy surgery in brain tumors and proposal for a new terminology use for long-term epilepsy-associated brain tumors. Acta Neuropathol 128(1):39–54. https://doi.org/10.1007/s00401-014-1288-9

Bonilha L, Keller SS (2015) Quantitative MRI in refractory temporal lobe epilepsy: relationship with surgical outcomes. Quant Imaging Med Surg 5(2):204–224. https://doi.org/10.3978/j.issn.2223-4292.2015.01.01

Burtscher J, Schwarzer C (2017) The opioid system in temporal lobe epilepsy: functional role and therapeutic potential. Front Mol Neurosci 10:245. https://doi.org/10.3389/fnmol.2017.00245

Bruton CJ (1988) The neuropathology of temporal lobe epilepsy. Oxford University Press, Oxford

Caciagli L, Bernasconi A, Wiebe S, Koepp MJ, Bernasconi N, Bernhardt BC (2017) A meta-analysis on progressive atrophy in intractable temporal lobe epilepsy: time is brain? Neurology 89(5):506–516. https://doi.org/10.1212/wnl.0000000000004176

Camacho DL, Castillo M (2007) MR imaging of temporal lobe epilepsy. Semin Ultrasound CT MR 28(6):424–436

Capizzano AA, Vermathen P, Laxer KD, Matson GB, Maudsley AA, Soher BJ, Schuff NW, Weiner MW (2002) Multisection proton MR spectroscopy for mesial temporal lobe epilepsy. AJNR Am J Neuroradiol 23(8):1359–1368

Cataldi M, Avoli M, de Villers-Sidani E (2013) Resting state networks in temporal lobe epilepsy. Epilepsia 54(12):2048–2059. https://doi.org/10.1111/epi.12400

Chassoux F, Artiges E, Semah F, Desarnaud S, Laurent A, Landre E, Gervais P, Devaux B, Helal OB (2016) Determinants of brain metabolism changes in mesial temporal lobe epilepsy. Epilepsia 57(6):907–919. https://doi.org/10.1111/epi.13377

Chassoux F, Artiges E, Semah F, Laurent A, Landre E, Turak B, Gervais P, Helal BO, Devaux B (2017) (18) F-FDG-PET patterns of surgical success and failure in mesial temporal lobe epilepsy. Neurology 88(11):1045–1053. https://doi.org/10.1212/wnl.0000000000003714

Curia G, Lucchi C, Vinet J, Gualtieri F, Marinelli C, Torsello A, Costantino L, Biagini G (2014) Pathophysiogenesis of mesial temporal lobe epilepsy: is prevention of damage antiepileptogenic? Curr Med Chem 21(6):663–688

Earle KM, Baldwin M, Penfield W (1953) Incisural sclerosis and temporal lobe seizures produced by hippocampal herniation by birth. Arch Neurol Psychiatry 69:27–42

Falconer MA, Serafetinides EA, Corsellis JA (1964) Etiology and pathogenesis of temporal lobe epilepsy. Arch Neurol 10:233–248

Gastaut H (1959) Etiology, pathology and pathogenesis of temporal lobe epilepsy. Epilepsy News, International League Against Epilepsy 15:15–24

Gross DW (2011) Diffusion tensor imaging in temporal lobe epilepsy. Epilepsia 52(suppl 4):32–34. https://doi.org/10.1111/j.1528-1167.2011.03149.x

Hamelin S, Depaulis A (2015) Revisiting hippocampal sclerosis in mesial temporal lobe epilepsy according to the "two-hit" hypothesis. Rev Neurol 171(3):227–235. https://doi.org/10.1016/j.neurol.2015.01.560

Hwang SK, Hirose S (2012) Genetics of temporal lobe epilepsy. Brain Dev 34(8):609–616. https://doi.org/10.1016/j.braindev.2011.10.008

Jan MM, Sadler M, Rahey SR (2010) Electroencephalographic features of temporal lobe epilepsy. Can J Neurol Sci 37(4):439–448

Josephson CB, Dykeman J, Fiest KM, Liu X, Sadler RM, Jette N, Wiebe S (2013) Systematic review and meta-analysis of standard vs selective temporal lobe epilepsy surgery. Neurology 80(18):1669–1676. https://doi.org/10.1212/WNL.0b013e3182904f82

Kandratavicius L, Ruggiero RN, Hallak JE, Garcia-Cairasco N, Leite JP (2012) Pathophysiology of mood disorders in temporal lobe epilepsy. Braz J Psychiatry 34(Suppl 2):S233–S245

Kawamura MJ, Ruskin DN, Masino SA (2016) Metabolic therapy for temporal lobe epilepsy in a dish: investigating mechanisms of ketogenic diet using electrophysiological recordings in hippocampal slices. Front Mol Neurosci 9:112. https://doi.org/10.3389/fnmol.2016.00112

Kim SR (2016) Control of granule cell dispersion by natural materials such as eugenol and naringin: a potential therapeutic strategy against temporal lobe epilepsy. J Med Food 19(8):730–736. https://doi.org/10.1089/jmf.2016.3712

Kim JA, Chung JI, Yoon PH, Kim DI, Chung TS, Kim EJ, Jeong EK (2001) Transient MR signal changes in patients with generalized tonicoclonic seizure or status epilepticus: periictal diffusion-weighted imaging. AJNR Am J Neuroradiol 22(6):1149–1160

Landazuri P (2014) Mesial temporal lobe epilepsy: a distinct electroclinical subtype of temporal lobe epilepsy. Neurodiagn J 54(3):274–288. https://doi.org/10.1016/j.neuroscience.2014.12.047

Leyden KM, Kucukboyaci NE, Puckett OK, Lee D, Loi RQ, Paul B, McDonald CR (2015) What does diffusion tensor imaging (DTI) tell us about cognitive networks in temporal lobe epilepsy? Quant Imaging Med Surg 5(2):247–263. https://doi.org/10.3978/j.issn.2223-4292.2015.02.01

Londono A, Castillo M, Lee YZ, Smith JK (2003) Apparent diffusion coefficient measurements in the hippocampi in patients with temporal lobe seizures. AJNR Am J Neuroradiol 24(8):1582–1586

Magerison JH, Corsellis JA (1966) Epilepsy and the temporal lobes. Brain 89:499–530

Malmgren K, Thom M (2012) Hippocampal sclerosis—origins and imaging. Epilepsia 53(suppl 4):19–33. https://doi.org/10.1111/j.1528-1167.2012.03610.x

McNamara JO, Scharfman HE (2012) Temporal lobe epilepsy and the BDNF receptor, TrkB. In: Noebels JL, Avoli M, Rogawski MA, Olsen RW, Delgado-Escueta AV (eds) Jasper's basic mechanisms of the epilepsies. National Center for Biotechnology Information, Bethesda

Muhlhofer W, Tan YL, Mueller SG, Knowlton R (2017) MRI-negative temporal lobe epilepsy-what do we know? Epilepsia 58(5):727–742. https://doi.org/10.1111/epi.13699

Muzumdar D, Patil M, Goel A, Ravat S, Sawant N, Shah U (2016) Mesial temporal lobe epilepsy—an overview of surgical techniques. Int J Surg 36(pt B):411–419. https://doi.org/10.1016/j.ijsu.2016.10.027

Palleria C, Coppola A, Citraro R, Del Gaudio L, Striano S, De Sarro G, Russo E (2015) Perspectives on treatment options for mesial temporal lobe epilepsy with hippocampal sclerosis. Expert Opin Pharmacother 16(15):2355–2371. https://doi.org/10.1517/14656566.2015.1084504

Pascual MR (2007) Temporal lobe epilepsy: clinical semiology and neurophysiological studies. Semin Ultrasound CT MR 28(6):416–423

Peter J, Houshmand S, Werner TJ, Rubello D, Alavi A (2016) Applications of global quantitative 18F-FDG-PET analysis in temporal lobe epilepsy. Nucl Med

Commun 37(3):223–230. https://doi.org/10.1097/mnm.0000000000000440

Pillai JJ, Williams HT, Faro S (2007) Functional imaging in temporal lobe epilepsy. Semin Ultrasound CT MR 28(6):437–450

Puttachary S, Sharma S (2015) Seizure-induced oxidative stress in temporal lobe epilepsy. Biomed Res Int 2015:745613. https://doi.org/10.1155/2015/745613

Rogawski MA, Delgado-Escueta AV, Noebels JL, Avoli M, Olsen RW (eds) (2012) Jasper's basic mechanisms of the epilepsies, 4th edn. National Center for Biotechnology Information, Bethesda

Rowley S, Patel M (2013) Mitochondrial involvement and oxidative stress in temporal lobe epilepsy. Free Radic Biol Med 62:121–131. https://doi.org/10.1016/j.freeradbiomed.2013.02.002

Schipper S, Aalbers MW, Rijkers K, Swijsen A, Rigo JM, Hoogland G, Vles JS (2016) Tonic GABAA receptors as potential target for the treatment of temporal lobe epilepsy. Mol Neurobiol 53(8):5252–5265. https://doi.org/10.1007/s12035-015-9423-8

Sommer W (1880) Erkrankung des Ammonshorns als ätiologischen Moment der Epilepsie. Arch Psychiat Nervenkr 10:631–675

Stark S, Steinhauser C, Grunnet M, Carmignoto G (2016) Crucial role of astrocytes in temporal lobe epilepsy. Biomed Res Int 323:157–169. https://doi.org/10.1016/j.neuroscience.2014.12.047

Steinhauser C, Seifert G, Bedner P (2012) Astrocyte dysfunction in temporal lobe epilepsy: K+ channels and gap junction coupling. Glia 60(8):1192–1202. https://doi.org/10.1002/glia.22313

Stylianou P, Hoffmann C, Blat I, Harnof S (2016a) Neuroimaging for patient selection for medial temporal lobe epilepsy surgery: part 1 structural neuroimaging. J Clin Neurosci 23:14–22. https://doi.org/10.1016/j.jocn.2015.04.019

Stylianou P, Kimchi G, Hoffmann C, Blat I, Harnof S (2016b) Neuroimaging for patient selection for medial temporal lobe epilepsy surgery: part 2 functional neuroimaging. J Clin Neurosci 23:23–33. https://doi.org/10.1016/j.jocn.2015.04.031

Tatum WO (2012) Mesial temporal lobe epilepsy. J Clin Neurophysiol 29(5):356–365. https://doi.org/10.1097/WNP.0b013e31826b3ab7

Thippeswamy T, Toth K, Magloczky Z (2014) The vulnerability of calretinin-containing hippocampal interneurons to temporal lobe epilepsy. Front Neuroanat 8:100. https://doi.org/10.3389/fnana.2014.00100

Tramoni-Negre E, Lambert I, Bartolomei F, Felician O (2017) Long-term memory deficits in temporal lobe epilepsy. Rev Neurol 173(7–8):490–497. https://doi.org/10.1016/j.neurol.2017.06.011

Werhahn KJ, Landvogt C, Klimpe S, Buchholz HG, Yakushev I, Siessmeier T, Muller-Forell W, Piel M, Rosch F, Glaser M, Schreckenberger M, Bartenstein P (2006) Decreased dopamine D2/D3-receptor binding in temporal lobe epilepsy: an [18F]fallypride PET study. Epilepsia 47(8):1392–1396. https://doi.org/10.1111/j.1528-1167.2006.00561.x

Wyler AR, Vossler DG (1997) Recent advancements in epilepsy. Surg Neurol 48(2):106–109

Wyler AR, Hermann BP, Somes G (1995) Extent of medial temporal resection on outcome from anterior temporal lobectomy: a randomized prospective study. Neurosurgery 37(5):982–990; discussion 990–981

Yilmazer-Hanke D, O'Loughlin E, McDermott K (2016) Contribution of amygdala pathology to comorbid emotional disturbances in temporal lobe epilepsy. J Neurosci Res 94(6):486–503. https://doi.org/10.1002/jnr.23689

Zhong Q, Ren BX, Tang FR (2016) Neurogenesis in the hippocampus of patients with temporal lobe epilepsy. Curr Neurol Neurosci Rep 16(2):20. https://doi.org/10.1007/s11910-015-0616-3

Epilepsies: Malformations of Cortical Development—Focal Cortical Dysplasia (FCD)

46.1 Introduction

One major cause of the epilepsies is related to malformations of cortical development which include:

- Focal cortical dysplasia (FCD)
  - FCD ILAE Type I
  - FCD ILAE Type II
  - FCD ILAE Type III
- Mild malformation of cortical development (mMCD)
- Hemimegalencephaly (HME)
- Cortical tubers in tuberous sclerosis complex (TSC)
- White matter heterotopias
- Polymicrogyria, including schizencephaly and opercular syndrome
- Generalized (non-focal) cortical dysplasias

Dysplasia

- The developmental alteration of an entire organ. *Andersen CE in: Duckett S. Pediatric Neuropathology, 1995*
- In the context of malformation, congenital dysplasia describes an abnormal organization of cells. *Robbins: Pathologic Basis of Diseases, 1994, page 438*
- To describe disorderly but non-neoplastic proliferation. It is a loss of the uniformity of the individual cell as well as a loss of their architectural orientation. It exhibits considerable pleomorphism and hyperchromatic cells. *Robbins: Pathologic Basis of Diseases, 1994, page 247*

46.2 Neuroimaging Findings

General Imaging Findings
- Imaging findings in FCD type 1 more subtle than in FCD type 2
- Cortical thickening (FCD type 2)
- Blurred white-gray matter junction
- Abnormal sulcal or gyral pattern
- Focal signal abnormality of gray and/or white matter
- Loss of regional white matter volume (FCD type 1)
- Transmantle sign (FCD type 2)

CT
- No pathological findings

MRI-T2/FLAIR (Figs. 46.1a–c and 46.2a, d)
- Focal hyperintensity of white matter
- Focal hyperintensity of the cortex
- Transmantle sign: Hyperintensity of white matter extending from the ventricle to the cortex—specific for FCD type 2

MRI-T1 (Fig. 46.2b, c)
- Hypointense signal of white matter

MRI-T1 Contrast-Enhanced
- No pathological enhancement

Nuclear Medicine Imaging Findings (Fig. 46.3a, b)
- FDG-PET: hypometabolism

46.3 Neuropathology Findings

Macroscopical Findings
- Cortex appears thicker
- Less well delineated from white matter

Microscopical Findings
- Focal cortical dysplasia is subdivided into the following three major types:
- Type I (Fig. 46.4a–l)
  - Ia: FCD with abnormal radial cortical lamination
  - Ib: FCD with abnormal tangential cortical lamination
  - Ic: FCD with abnormal radial and tangential cortical lamination
- Type II
  - IIa: FCD with dysmorphic neurons (Fig. 46.5a–l)
  - IIb: FCD with dysmorphic neurons and balloon cells (Fig. 46.6a–n)
- Type III
  - IIIa: cortical lamination abnormalities in the temporal lobe associated with hippocampal sclerosis
  - IIIb: cortical lamination abnormalities adjacent to a glial or glioneuronal tumor
  - IIIc: cortical lamination abnormalities adjacent to vascular malformation
  - IIId: cortical lamination abnormalities adjacent to another lesion acquired during early life (e.g., trauma, ischemic injury, encephalitis)

Cellular Abnormalities
- Dysmorphic neurons
  - Misshapen cells with
    - Abnormal orientation
    - Size
    - Cytoskeletal structure
    - Atypical dendritic processes
    - Nissl substance can be seen in clumps
    - Rich in cytoplasmic neurofilaments (SMI 31)
- Balloon cells
  - Abnormal large cells (20–90 μm)
  - Pale, glassy eosinophilic cytoplasm
  - Eccentric nucleus
  - Immunopositive for neuronal or glial markers
    - Vimentin (hallmark)
    - Neurofilament
    - Nestin
    - MAP 1b
    - NeuN
    - GFAP
- Giant neurons
  - Neurons of increased size
  - Central nuclei
  - With pyramidal morphology
  - Do not overexpress cytoplasmic neurofilaments
  - Are not dysmorphic
- Immature neurons
  - Round or oval cells
  - With large (immature) nucleus and
  - A thin rim of cytoplasm
  - Are not dysmorphic
  - Are not giant

Architectural Abnormalities
- *Isolated architectural abnormalities: dyslamination*
  - Intracortical lesions characterized by
    - Dyslamination
    - Columnar disorganization
  - Mildest end of the histopathologic spectrum of FCD
  - In the hippocampus
    - Abnormalities of the infolding of the dentate gyrus and focal dyslamination
- *Architectural abnormalities associated with giant neurons*
  - Presence of giant neurons
  - Absence of dysmorphic or balloon cells

46.3 Neuropathology Findings

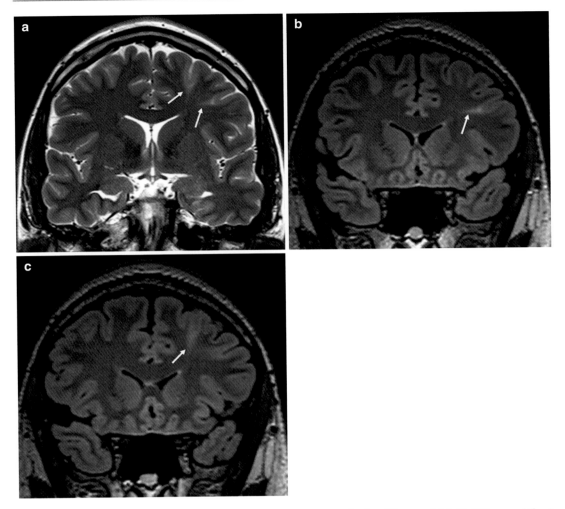

Fig. 46.1 Two areas with focal cortical dysplasia showing the transmantle sign; T2 coronal (**a**), FLAIR coronal (**b, c**)

- *Architectural abnormalities associated with dysmorphic neurons*
  - Presence of clearly dysmorphic neurons
  - More severe abnormalities from a histopathologic standpoint
- *Architectural abnormalities associated with dysmorphic neurons and balloon cells*
  - Presence of balloon cells
  - Intermixed typically with dysmorphic neurons in patients with severe architectural disorganization
  - Most severe end of the spectrum of histopathologic abnormalities of FCD

A summary of histological changes encountered in focal cortical dysplasias and the recommended markers can be given as follows (Iffland and Crino 2017):

FCD Type I
- Type Ia
  - Abnormal radial cortical lamination
  - Heterotopic neurons
  - Small immature neurons
  - Hypertrophic pyramidal cells outside layer 5
  - Markers:
    - NeuN or similar for cortical structure

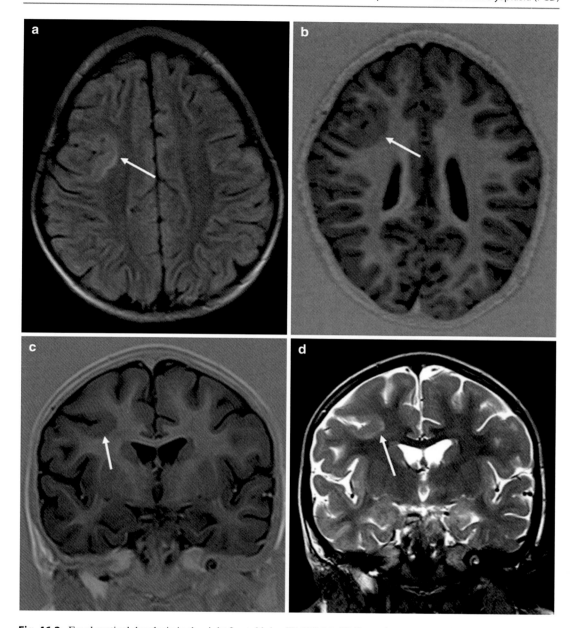

Fig. 46.2 Focal cortical dysplasia in the right frontal lobe; FLAIR (**a**), IR (Inversion recovery—T1-weighted) axial (**b**) and coronal (**c**), T2 coronal (**d**)

- ○ MAP2 for neuronal morphology
- ○ Pax6, OTX1, or similar for immature cell identification
- Type Ib
  - Loss of hexalaminar cortical structure
  - Immature small neurons
  - Hypertrophic pyramidal cells outside layer 5
  - Disoriented dendrites
  - Markers:
    - ○ NeuN or similar for cortical structure
    - ○ MAP2 for neuronal morphology
    - ○ Pax6, OTX1, or similar for immature cell identification

46.3 Neuropathology Findings

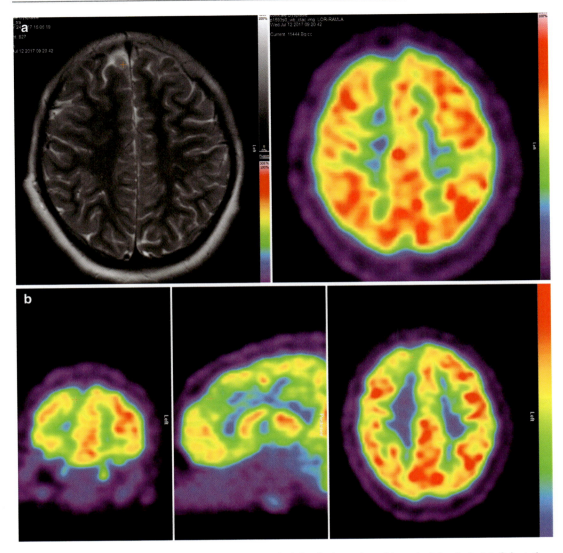

Fig. 46.3 T2 combined with FDG-PET showing metabolic defect in the region with cortical dysplasia (**a**). Orientations of the cortical dysplasia (+) in the 3D space (left: coronal, middle: sagittal, right: axial) (**b**)

- Type Ic
  - Combined features of FCD Ia and Ib
  - Abnormalities listed for types Ia and Ib
  - Markers:
    ○ NeuN or similar for cortical structure
    ○ MAP2 for neuronal morphology
    ○ Pax6, OTX1, or similar for immature cell identification

FCD Type II
- Type IIa
  - Loss of cortical lamination.
  - Blurred gray-white matter junction.
  - Dysmorphic neurons in cortex or subcortical white matter.
  - Markers:
    ○ H&E staining
    ○ Neurofilament stains (e.g., SMI32) for identification of dysmorphic neurons
- Type IIb
  - Loss of cortical lamination.
  - Blurred gray-white matter junction
  - Dysmorphic neurons as in FCD IIa plus balloon cells in cortex or subcortical white matter

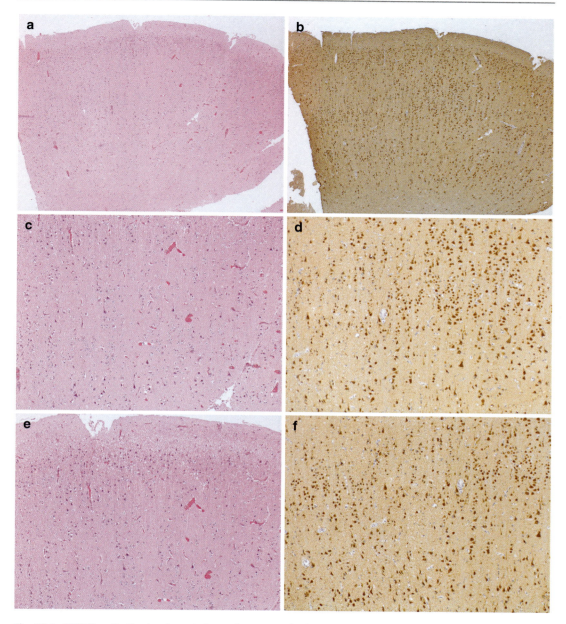

Fig. 46.4 FCD Type Ic. Section through the cortical gray matter showing a disturbed lamination, partly in the vertical as well as in the horizontal axis (H&E: **a, c, e**; NeuN: **b, d, f**) with focal neuronal loss (∗). Heterotopic neurons in the white matter (**g, h**: NeuN). Patchy reactive astrogliosis (**i, j**: GFAP). Some of the reactive astrocytes are immunopositive for vimentin (**k, l**)

- Markers:
  - Vimentin, nestin, and CD34 can be used to identify balloon cells
  - Dysmorphic neurons are identified as described for FCD IIa

FCD Type III
- Type IIIa
  - Abnormal cortical lamination
  - With mesial temporal lobe sclerosis

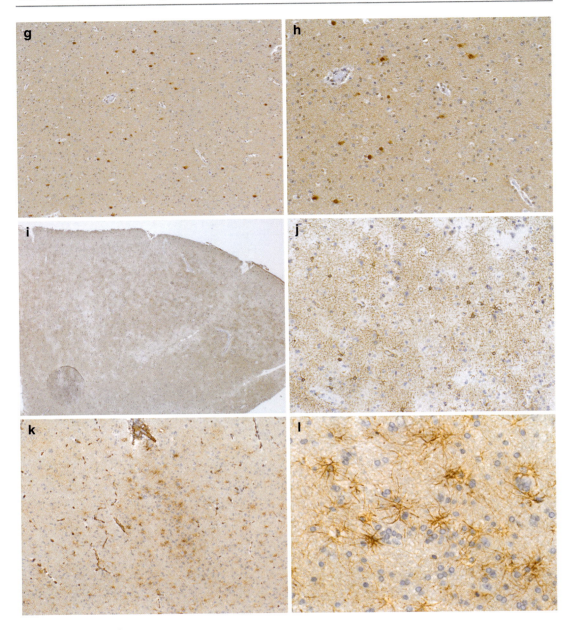

Fig. 46.4 (continued)

- Cellular and architectural abnormalities in the temporal lobe (see types I and II) with concomitant hippocampal sclerosis
- Markers:
  - MAP2 or similar to identify neurons
  - GFAP for gliosis
- Type IIIb
  - Abnormal cortical lamination adjacent to a glial or neuroglial tumor

- Cellular and architectural abnormalities (see types I and II) adjacent to tumors/neoplasms
- Markers:
  - MAP2 or similar to identify neurons
  - Appropriate tumor maker (e.g., CD34 for ganglioglioma)

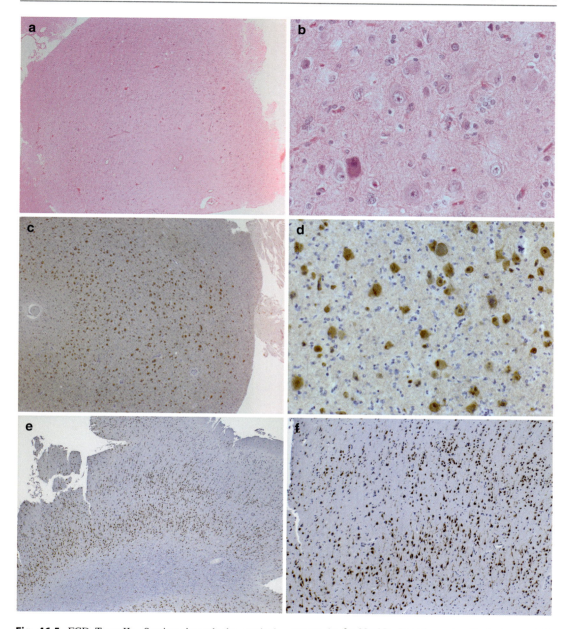

Fig. 46.5 FCD Type IIa. Section through the cortical gray matter showing dyslamination and the presence of larger dysmorphic neurons (**a**, **b**: H&E; **c–f**: NeuN) with focal neuronal loss (∗). Heterotopic neurons in the white matter (**g**, **h**: NeuN). Reactive astrogliosis is scant (**i**: GFAP). Some astrocytes are immunopositive for S-100 (**j**). Reactive astrocytes are immunopositive for vimentin (**k, l**)

- Type IIIc
  - Abnormal cortical lamination and
  - vascular malformation or glial scars
  - Cellular and architectural abnormalities (see types I and II) adjacent to vascular malformations or glial scars
  - Markers:
    - MAP2 or similar to identify neurons
    - GFAP for gliosis
- Type IIId
  - Abnormal cortical lamination located next to an acquired lesion (e.g., trauma)

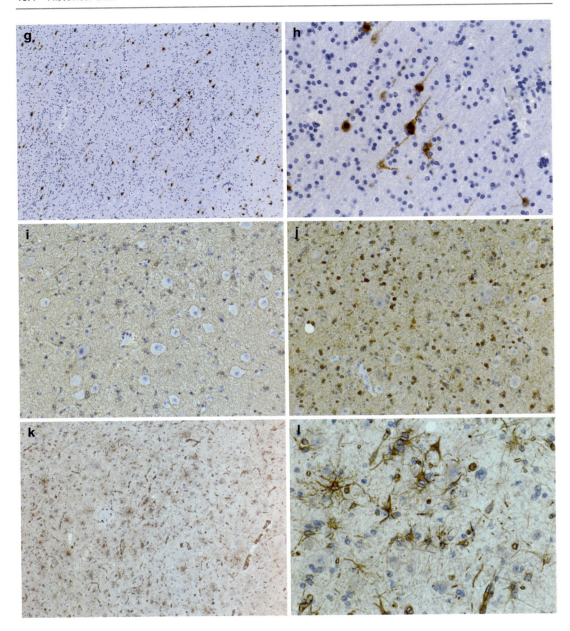

Fig. 46.5 (continued)

– Cellular and architectural abnormalities (see types I and II) adjacent to a lesion not included in type IIIa–c
– Markers:
  o MAP2 or similar to identify neurons
  o GFAP for gliosis
  o Other markers as appropriate

46.4 Historical Classification

Taylor Classification 1971 (Taylor et al. 1971)
Taylor dysplasia is determined histologically due to the presence of
- Disruption of the normal cortical lamination
- Giant neurons

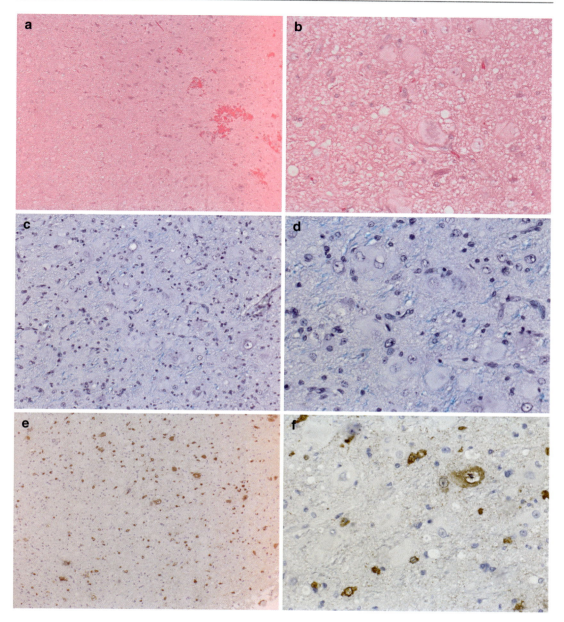

Fig. 46.6 FCD Type IIb. Cortical gray matter with severe dyslamination and presence of large balloon cells (→) (**a, b**: H&E; **c, d**: Luxol Fast Blue). A few balloon cells stain positive for NeuN (∗) while others are NeuN-negative (→) (**e, f**). A few balloon cells stain positive for MAP2abc (∗) while others are MAP2abc negative (→) (**g, h**). Faint staining of the balloon cells for GFAP (**i, j**). Intense staining of the balloon cells for vimentin (**k, l**). Note the binucleated cell (∗) (**l**). Patchy reactive astrogliosis (**m, n**: GFAP)

- Dysmorphic neurons
- Presence or absence of balloon cells (first description by Taylor)

The latter divides FCDT further into two main subtypes:

- **Taylor type I**: no balloon cells
- **Taylor type II**: balloon cells present

Palmini Classification 2004 (Palmini et al. 2004)

- Type I: no dysmorphic neurons or balloon cells

46.4 Historical Classification

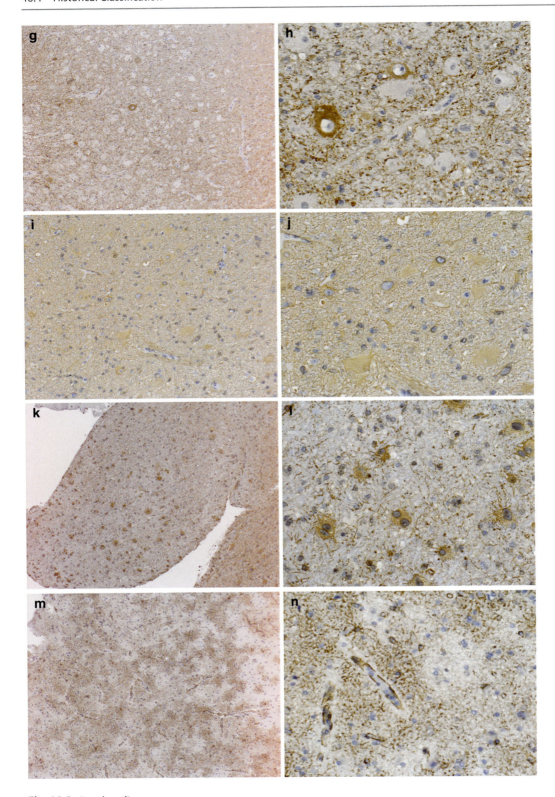

Fig. 46.6 (continued)

- Type IA: isolated architectural abnormalities (dyslamination, accompanied or not by other abnormalities of mild MCD)
- Type IB: architectural abnormalities, plus giant or immature, *but not dysmorphic* neurons
• Type II: Taylor-type FCD (dysmorphic neurons without or with balloon cells)
  - Type IIA: architectural abnormalities with dysmorphic neurons but without balloon cells
  - Type IIB: architectural abnormalities with dysmorphic neurons and balloon cells

Differential Diagnosis
• Ganglioglioma
• Tubers
• Hemimegalencephaly

46.5 Molecular Neuropathology

• Abnormal intrinsic membrane properties
• Ion channel dysfunction
• AMPA receptor expression in dysmorphic neurons
• Expression of cytoskeletal elements
  - Nestin
  - Vimentin
  - MAP 1b
  - α-Internexin
  - Peripherin
• Failure of cytoskeletal regulatory proteins to direct proper organization of the cortex at the earliest stages of brain development
• Expression of neurotransmitter subunits
  - Altered expression of neurotransmitter receptors and uptake sites
  - NMDA receptor assembly
  - Increased NMDA receptor subunit NR2B
  - GABA transmission
  - Increased immature gamma-2 $GABA_A$ receptor
• Inflammatory response
  - Enhanced expression of TNFα and NFκB
  - CD-68 positive microglia/macrophages
  - Expression of
    ○ Major histocompatibility complex class I and II
    ○ Toll-like receptors (TLR) 2 and 4
    ○ Receptor for advanced glycation end products (RAGE)
• mTOR pathway
  - Activation of mTOR signaling
  - Aberrant signaling of the cascade
  - Enhanced mTOR signaling

Mutations in mTOR regulatory genes associated with focal cortical dysplasias (FCDs) have been described as follows (Iffland and Crino 2017):

• *DEPDC5*
  - Somatic or germline mutation
  - Inactivating, enhances mTOR signaling
  - FCD Type IIa, FCD Type IIb
• *MTO*
  - Somatic mutation
  - Activating, enhances mTOR signaling
  - FCD Type IIa, FCD Type IIb
• *NPRL2*
  - Germline mutation
  - Activating, enhances mTOR signaling
  - FCD Type Ia
• *NPRL3*
  - Germline mutation
  - Inactivating, enhances mTOR signaling
  - FCD Type IIa
• *PIK3CA*
  - Somatic mutation
  - Activating, enhances mTOR signaling
  - FCD Type IIa
• *TSC1/TSC2*
  - Germline and somatic mutation
  - Inactivating, enhances mTOR signaling
  - Cortical tubers

Selected References

Abdijadid S, Mathern GW, Levine MS, Cepeda C (2015) Basic mechanisms of epileptogenesis in pediatric cortical dysplasia. CNS Neurosci Ther 21(2):92–103. https://doi.org/10.1111/cns.12345

Adler S, Lorio S, Jacques TS, Benova B, Gunny R, Cross JH, Baldeweg T, Carmichael DW (2017) Towards in vivo focal cortical dysplasia phenotyping using quantitative MRI. Neuroimage Clin 15:95–105. https://doi.org/10.1016/j.nicl.2017.04.017

Selected References

Blumcke I, Spreafico R (2011) An international consensus classification for focal cortical dysplasias. Lancet Neurol 10(1):26–27. https://doi.org/10.1016/s1474-4422(10)70225-8

Blumcke I, Thom M, Aronica E, Armstrong DD, Vinters HV, Palmini A, Jacques TS, Avanzini G, Barkovich AJ, Battaglia G, Becker A, Cepeda C, Cendes F, Colombo N, Crino P, Cross JH, Delalande O, Dubeau F, Duncan J, Guerrini R, Kahane P, Mathern G, Najm I, Ozkara C, Raybaud C, Represa A, Roper SN, Salamon N, Schulze-Bonhage A, Tassi L, Vezzani A, Spreafico R (2011) The clinicopathologic spectrum of focal cortical dysplasias: a consensus classification proposed by an ad hoc Task Force of the ILAE Diagnostic Methods Commission. Epilepsia 52(1):158–174. https://doi.org/10.1111/j.1528-1167.2010.02777.x

Colombo N, Tassi L, Deleo F, Citterio A, Bramerio M, Mai R, Sartori I, Cardinale F, Lo Russo G, Spreafico R (2012) Focal cortical dysplasia type IIa and IIb: MRI aspects in 118 cases proven by histopathology. Neuroradiology 54(10):1065–1077. https://doi.org/10.1007/s00234-012-1049-1

Gaitanis JN, Donahue J (2013) Focal cortical dysplasia. Pediatr Neurol 49(2):79–87. https://doi.org/10.1016/j.pediatrneurol.2012.12.024

Guerrini R, Duchowny M, Jayakar P, Krsek P, Kahane P, Tassi L, Melani F, Polster T, Andre VM, Cepeda C, Krueger DA, Cross JH, Spreafico R, Cosottini M, Gotman J, Chassoux F, Ryvlin P, Bartolomei F, Bernasconi A, Stefan H, Miller I, Devaux B, Najm I, Giordano F (2015) Diagnostic methods and treatment options for focal cortical dysplasia. Epilepsia 56(11):1669–1686. https://doi.org/10.1111/epi.13200

Iffland PH 2nd, Crino PB (2017) Focal cortical dysplasia: gene mutations, cell signaling, and therapeutic implications. Annu Rev Pathol 12:547–571. https://doi.org/10.1146/annurev-pathol-052016-100138

Kim DW, Kim S, Park SH, Chung CK, Lee SK (2012) Comparison of MRI features and surgical outcome among the subtypes of focal cortical dysplasia. Seizure 21(10):789–794. https://doi.org/10.1016/j.seizure.2012.09.006

Leach JL, Greiner HM, Miles L, Mangano FT (2014) Imaging spectrum of cortical dysplasia in children. Semin Roentgenol 49(1):99–111. https://doi.org/10.1053/j.ro.2013.10.007

Marin-Valencia I, Guerrini R, Gleeson JG (2014) Pathogenetic mechanisms of focal cortical dysplasia. Epilepsia 55(7):970–978. https://doi.org/10.1111/epi.12650

Mellerio C, Labeyrie MA, Chassoux F, Daumas-Duport C, Landre E, Turak B, Roux FX, Meder JF, Devaux B, Oppenheim C (2012) Optimizing MR imaging detection of type 2 focal cortical dysplasia: best criteria for clinical practice. AJNR Am J Neuroradiol 33(10):1932–1938. https://doi.org/10.3174/ajnr.A3081

Mellerio C, Labeyrie MA, Chassoux F, Roca P, Alami O, Plat M, Naggara O, Devaux B, Meder JF, Oppenheim C (2014) 3T MRI improves the detection of transmantle sign in type 2 focal cortical dysplasia. Epilepsia 55(1):117–122. https://doi.org/10.1111/epi.12464

Najm IM, Tilelli CQ, Oghlakian R (2007) Pathophysiological mechanisms of focal cortical dysplasia: a critical review of human tissue studies and animal models. Epilepsia 48(Suppl 2):21–32

Palmini A, Najm I, Avanzini G, Babb T, Guerrini R, Foldvary-Schaefer N, Jackson G, Luders HO, Prayson R, Spreafico R, Vinters HV (2004) Terminology and classification of the cortical dysplasias. Neurology 62(6 Suppl 3):S2–S8

Rickert CH (2006) Cortical dysplasia: neuropathological aspects. Childs Nerv Syst 22(8):821–826. https://doi.org/10.1007/s00381-006-0126-3

Siedlecka M, Grajkowska W, Galus R, Dembowska-Baginska B, Jozwiak J (2016) Focal cortical dysplasia: molecular disturbances and clinicopathological classification (Review). Int J Mol Med 38(5):1327–1337. https://doi.org/10.3892/ijmm.2016.2760

Taylor DC, Falconer MA, Bruton CJ, Corsellis JA (1971) Focal dysplasia of the cerebral cortex in epilepsy. J Neurol Neurosurg Psychiatry 34(4):369–387

Vonck K, Barba C, Blumcke I, Crino PB (2015) Focal cortical dysplasia. Epilepsia 35(3):201–208. https://doi.org/10.1055/s-0035-1552617

Widdess-Walsh P, Diehl B, Najm I (2006) Neuroimaging of focal cortical dysplasia. J Neuroimaging 16(3):185–196. https://doi.org/10.1111/j.1552-6569.2006.00025.x

Epilepsies: Malformations of Cortical Development—Heterotopia

47.1 Definition

Heterotopia

- Cells displaced within their organ of origin, i.e., brain

Ectopia

- Cells displaced outside their organ of origin, e.g., isolated neurons in the leptomeninges

47.2 Neuroimaging Findings

General Imaging Findings
- Tissue isointense to gray matter in wrong location
- Subependymal heterotopia—nodules of gray matter localized next to the ependymal layer of the lateral ventricles (Fig. 47.1)
- Subcortical heterotopia—gray matter located in the subcortical or deep white matter contiguous with overlying cortex and underlying ventricle (Fig. 47.2)
- Band heterotopia—subcortical band of gray matter with thinned overlying cortex ("double cortex") (Fig. 47.3)

CT Non-Contrast-Enhanced
- Isodense with gray matter

CT Contrast-Enhanced
- No enhancement

MRI-T2/FLAIR/T1 (Figs. 47.1a–c, 47.2a–e, and 47.3a–d)
- Heterotopia isointense to gray matter

MRI-T1 Contrast-Enhanced (Fig. 47.1d)
- No enhancement

MR-Spectroscopy
- Decreased NAA/Cr ratio compared to healthy subjects

47.3 Neuropathology Findings

47.3.1 White Matter Heterotopia
(Figs. 47.4 and 47.5)

Heterotopic white matter neurons
- Present in normal brains
  - Temporal lobes
  - Located near the cortex
- Increased in focal cortical dysplasia
  - Lie deeper in the subcortical white matter and near the cortex

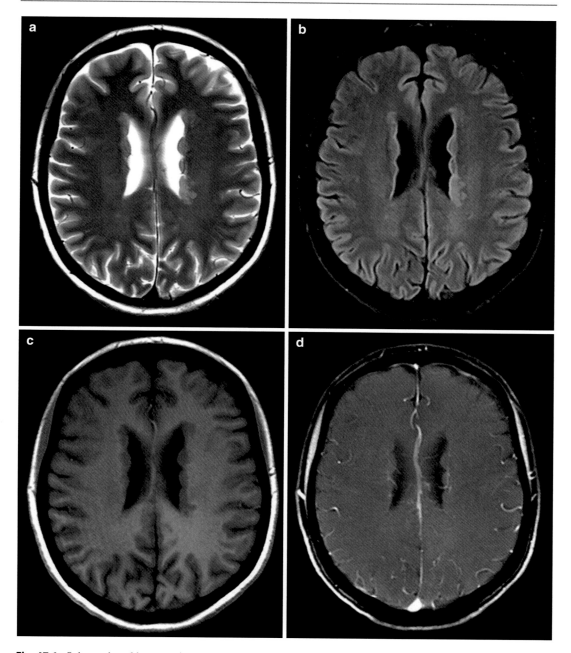

Fig. 47.1 Subependymal heterotopia; T2 (**a**), FLAIR (**b**), T1 (**c**), T1 contrast (**d**)

- Discussed as a pathogenic factor in major psychiatric diseases
- Immunoreactive for
  - Synaptophysin
    - Axons, terminal axons at their somatic membrane
    - Sign of neuronal immaturity
  - NeuN
  - SMI-32
  - MAP 2
  - Neuron-specific enolase
  - Calcium-binding markers
    - Calretinin
    - Parvalbumin
    - Identify neurons arrived by tangential migration

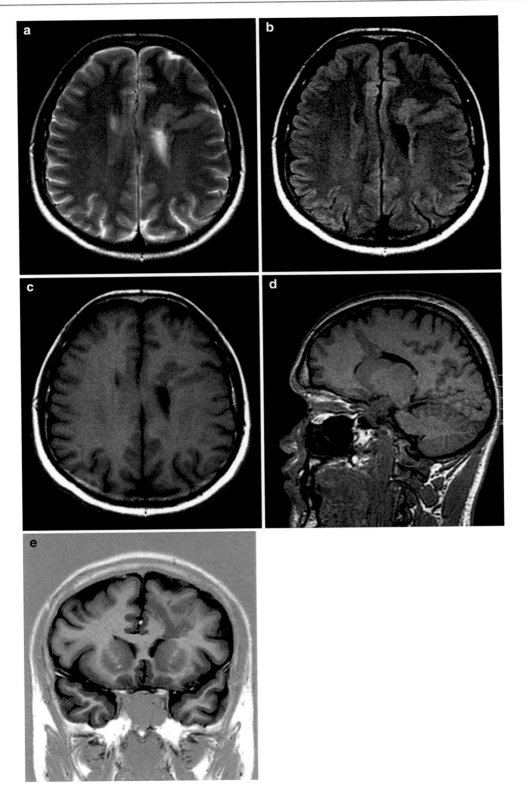

Fig. 47.2 Subcortical heterotopia; T2 (**a**), FLAIR (**b**), T1 axial (**c**) and sagittal (**d**), IR (Inversion recovery—T1-weighted) coronal (**e**)

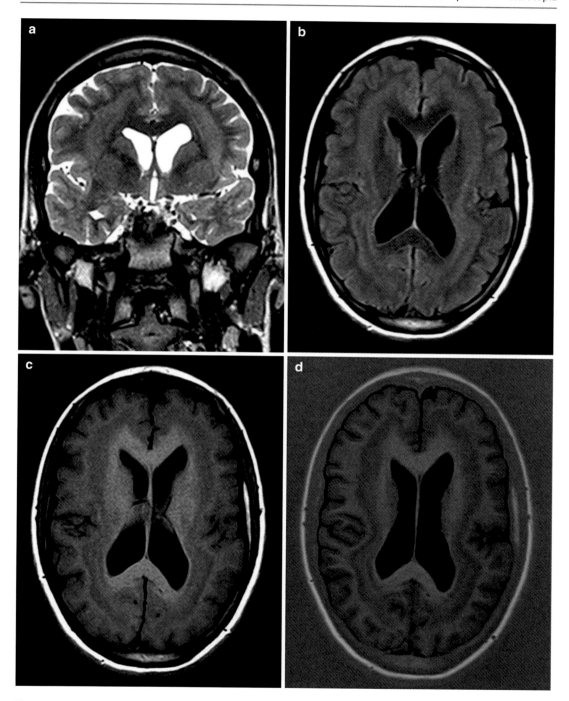

Fig. 47.3 Band heterotopia; T2 coronal (**a**), FLAIR (**b**), T1 (**c**), IR (**d**)

47.3 Neuropathology Findings

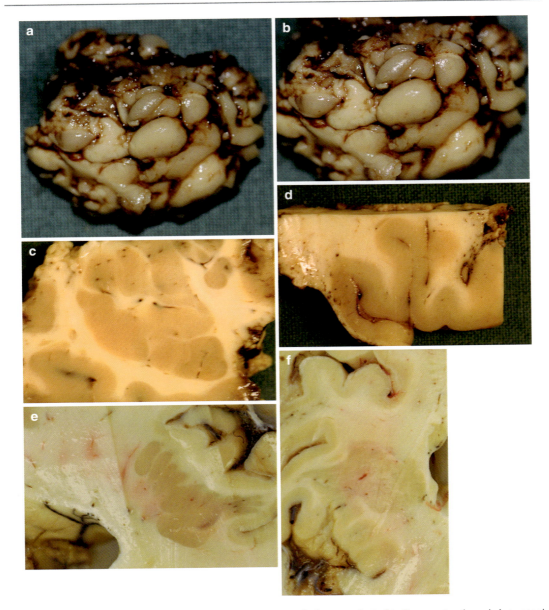

Fig. 47.4 White matter heterotopia: Cobblestone appearance of a heterotopia (**a**, **b**). Gray matter tissue is heterotopically located within the white matter (**c**, **e**, **f**). The cortical ribbon appears widened with a nodular formation (→) (**d**)

- Connect with other white matter neurons and overlaying cortex

47.3.2 Nodular Heterotopia (Fig. 47.6)

- Clustering of heterotopic neurons into aggregates
- Identified by MRI or on neuropathologic examination
- Principal sites of nodular heterotopias
  - Periventricular region
  - Centrum semiovale and other subcortical white matter
  - Dysplastic nodules within the cortical plate, e.g., molecular zone

- Classification
  - Bilateral symmetric
  - Bilateral asymmetric
  - Bilateral focal
  - Unilateral with no cortical involvement
  - Unilateral with cortical involvement

47.3.3 Periventricular Nodular Heterotopia

- Composed of
  - Mature neurons
    - Pyramidal cells
    - Subtypes of inhibitory interneurons

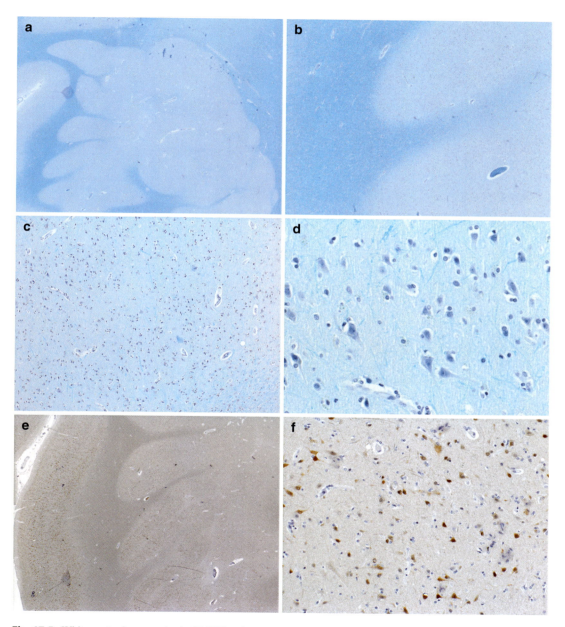

Fig. 47.5 White matter heterotopia: (**a**, **b**) LFB stain: neurons are clearly discernible (**c**, **d**) and immunostains for NeuN (**e**, **f**), synaptophysin (**g**, **h**), and MAP2 (**i**, **j**)

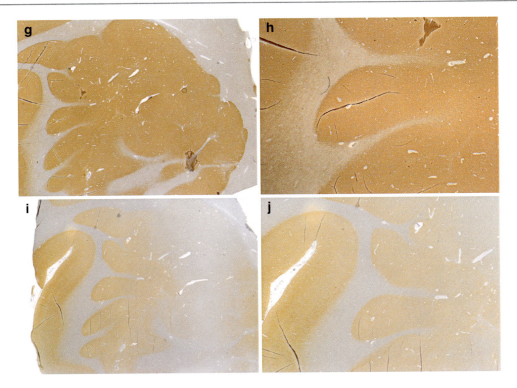

Fig. 47.5 (continued)

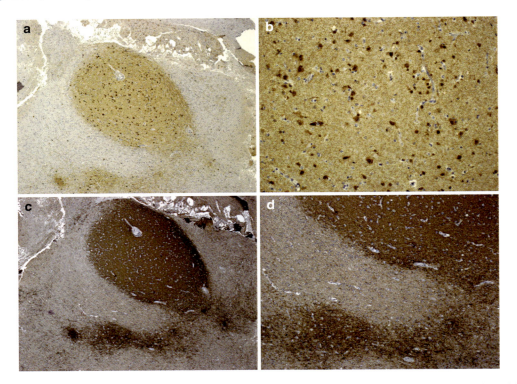

Fig. 47.6 Nodular heterotopia. Neurons within the heterotopias stain positive for NeuN (**a**, **b**); the neuropil is positive for synaptophysin (**c**, **d**)

- Small Reelin-immunoreactive neurons
- Layer VI and layer V neurons in the external border of the nodule
- Layer IV neurons in the internal region of the nodule
  - Glial cells
  - No mineralization
- Occipital horn, trigone region temporal horn, frontal horns
- Well-defined boundaries surrounded by white matter fibers
- Did not attach to radial glial fibers for migration
- Causes include
  - Mutations in various genes (Table 47.1)
  - Chromosomopathies
  - Chromosomal translocations and deletions
  - Filamin-A (FLNA) mutation
    X-linked dominant cause of bilateral periventricular nodular heterotopias
  - SCN1A gene mutation

- Associated with other brain malformations
  - Agenesis or dysgenesis of the corpus callosum
  - Cerebellar cortical dysgenesis
  - Spinal cord malformations

47.3.4 Subcortical Laminar Heterotopias

- Layer of neurons within the white matter composed of
  - Mature neurons
    - *Pyramidal cells*
    - *Subtypes of inhibitory interneurons*
    - *Small Reelin-immunoreactive neurons*
- Synonyms: band heterotopia or double cortex
- The neurons do not form a real cortex
- Mutated gene: doublecortin (DCX) (Table 47.2)
- Mutations in various genes (Table 47.2)

Table 47.1 Genes and phenotypes associated with periventricular heterotopias, modified after Watrin et al. (2015) reproduced with kind permission by Wiley

Gene (Locus)	Protein	Etiology	Phenotype
FLNA (Xq28)	Filamin-A	• In females: de novo germline mutations (missense, nonsense, and frameshift mutations) • Intragenic deletions, and duplications • In males: lethal in the majority of cases	Bilateral PNH associated with coagulopathy and cardiovascular abnormalities in some patients
ARFGEF2 (20q13.13) ADP-ribosylation factor guanine nucleotide exchange factor 2	BIG2 (brefeldin A-inhibited guanine nucleotide exchange protein 2)	• Inherited mutations (missense and frameshift) • Autosomal recessive	Bilateral PNH associated with microcephaly
C6orf70 (6q27) chromosome 6 open reading frame 70	ERMARD (ER membrane-associated RNA degradation)	• De novo deletions and missense mutation (one)	Bilateral PNH
FAT4 (4q28.1) (FAT atypical cadherin 4)	FAT atypical cadherin 4	• Inherited compound heterozygous (nonsense and missense) or homozygous (nonsense) mutations	Posterior PNH (partially penetrant)
DCHS1 (11p15.4)	Dachsous cadherin-related 1	• Inherited homozygous (nonsense and missense) mutations	Posterior PNH (partially penetrant)

Table 47.2 Genes and phenotypes associated with subcortical band heterotopias (SBH), modified after Watrin et al. (2015) reproduced with kind permission by Wiley

Gene (Locus)	Protein	Etiology	Phenotype
DCX (Xq22.3-q23) doublecortin	DCX	In females: de novo germline mutations (missense, nonsense, and frameshift mutations), deletions, and duplications	• Anteriorly predominant SBH • De novo mutations generally associated with the most severe phenotype (thick band frequently associated with frontal pachygyria, shallow sulci, and ventricular enlargement)
		In females: inherited mutations (missense, nonsense, and frameshift)	• Anteriorly predominant SBH • Inherited mutations generally associated with a milder phenotype (thin band)
		In males: de novo somatic mosaic mutations (missense, nonsense, and frameshift) and deletions	• Anteriorly predominant SBH
		In males: inherited mutations (missense mutations only)	• Anteriorly predominant SBH • Milder phenotype
LIS1 or PAFAH1B1 (17p13.3) lissencephaly-1 platelet-activating factor acetylhydrolase 1b, regulatory subunit 1	LIS1	De novo somatic mosaic heterozygous (missense and nonsense) mutations	• Posteriorly predominant SBH
KIF2A (5q12.1) kinesin heavy chain member 2A	KIF2A	De novo germline heterozygous (missense) mutation, dominant negative effect	• Frontal band heterotopia • Posterior predominant pachygyria • Severe congenital microcephaly
TUBA1A (12q13.12) tubulin, alpha 1a	α1-tubulin	De novo germline heterozygous (missense) mutation, dominant negative effect	• Laminar heterotopia • Partial agenesis of the corpus callosum • Hypoplasia of the cerebellar vermis
TUBG1 (17q21.2) tubulin, gamma 1	TUBG1 (c-Tubulin)	De novo germline heterozygous (missense) mutation, dominant negative effect	• Laminar heterotopia • Posterior pachygyria • Thick and dysmorphic corpus callosum
EML1 (14q32) echinoderm microtubule-associated protein-like 1	EML1	Inherited compound heterozygous (nonsense and missense) or homozygous (missense) mutations	• Giant bilateral periventricular and ribbon-like subcortical heterotopia with polymicrogyria and agenesis of the corpus callosum

47.4 Molecular Neuropathology

- Cajal–Retzius cells producing Reelin
  - Remain displaced in the subplate during early stages of cortical development
  - Attract migrating neurons into a heterotopic position
- Neuroepithelial cells fail to attach to radial glial fibers for migration

Selected References

Abdel Razek AA, Kandell AY, Elsorogy LG, Elmongy A, Basett AA (2009) Disorders of cortical formation: MR imaging features. AJNR Am J Neuroradiol 30(1):4–11. https://doi.org/10.3174/ajnr.A1223

Barkovich AJ (2000) Morphologic characteristics of subcortical heterotopia: MR imaging study. AJNR Am J Neuroradiol 21(2):290–295

Barkovich AJ, Raybaud CA (2004) Malformations of cortical development. Neuroimaging Clin N

Am 14(3):401–423. https://doi.org/10.1016/j.nic.2004.04.003

Barkovich AJ, Dobyns WB, Guerrini R (2015) Malformations of cortical development and epilepsy. Cold Spring Harb Perspect Med 5(5):a022392. https://doi.org/10.1101/cshperspect.a022392

Bieniek KF, Dickson DW (2015) Concurrent neurodegenerative pathologies in periventricular nodular heterotopia. Acta Neuropathol 130(6):895–897. https://doi.org/10.1007/s00401-015-1490-4

Broix L, Jagline H, LI E, Schmucker S, Drouot N, Clayton-Smith J, Pagnamenta AT, Metcalfe KA, Isidor B, Louvier UW, Poduri A, Taylor JC (2016) Mutations in the HECT domain of NEDD4L lead to AKT-mTOR pathway deregulation and cause periventricular nodular heterotopia. Nat Genet 48(11):1349–1358. https://doi.org/10.1038/ng.3676

Christodoulou JA, Walker LM, Del Tufo SN, Katzir T, Gabrieli JD, Whitfield-Gabrieli S, Chang BS (2012) Abnormal structural and functional brain connectivity in gray matter heterotopia. Epilepsia 53(6):1024–1032. https://doi.org/10.1111/j.1528-1167.2012.03466.x

Christodoulou JA, Barnard ME, Del Tufo SN, Katzir T, Whitfield-Gabrieli S, Gabrieli JD, Chang BS (2013) Integration of gray matter nodules into functional cortical circuits in periventricular heterotopia. Epilepsy Behav 29(2):400–406. https://doi.org/10.1016/j.yebeh.2013.08.028

Farquharson S, Tournier JD, Calamante F, Mandelstam S, Burgess R, Schneider ME, Berkovic SF, Scheffer IE, Jackson GD, Connelly A (2016) Periventricular nodular heterotopia: detection of abnormal microanatomic fiber structures with whole-brain diffusion MR imaging tractography. Radiology 281(3):896–906. https://doi.org/10.1148/radiol.2016150852

Feng Y, Walsh CA (2004) The many faces of filamin: a versatile molecular scaffold for cell motility and signalling. Nat Cell Biol 6(11):1034–1038. https://doi.org/10.1038/ncb1104-1034

Fox JW, Walsh CA (1999) Periventricular heterotopia and the genetics of neuronal migration in the cerebral cortex. Am J Hum Genet 65(1):19–24. https://doi.org/10.1086/302474

Gonzalez G, Vedolin L, Barry B, Poduri A, Walsh C, Barkovich AJ (2013) Location of periventricular nodular heterotopia is related to the malformation phenotype on MRI. AJNR Am J Neuroradiol 34(4):877–883. https://doi.org/10.3174/ajnr.A3312

Ito K, Nakata Y, Matsuda H, Sugai K, Watanabe M, Kamiya K, Kimura Y, Shigemoto Y, Okazaki M, Sasaki M, Sato N (2014) Evaluation of FDG-PET and ECD-SPECT in patients with subcortical band heterotopia. Brain Dev 36(7):578–584. https://doi.org/10.1016/j.braindev.2013.07.017

Jang MA, Woo HI, Kim JW, Lee J, Ki CS (2013) Identification of DCX gene mutation in lissencephaly spectrum with subcortical band heterotopia using whole exome sequencing. Pediatr Neurol 48(5):411–414. https://doi.org/10.1016/j.pediatrneurol.2012.12.033

Kato K, Miya F, Hori I, Ieda D, Ohashi K, Negishi Y, Hattori A, Okamoto N, Kato M, Tsunoda T, Yamasaki M, Kanemura Y, Kosaki K, Saitoh S (2017) A novel missense mutation in the HECT domain of NEDD4L identified in a girl with periventricular nodular heterotopia, polymicrogyria and cleft palate. J Hum Genet. https://doi.org/10.1038/jhg.2017.53

Kielar M, Tuy FP, Bizzotto S, Lebrand C, de Juan Romero C, Poirier K, Oegema R, Mancini GM, Bahi-Buisson N, Olaso R, Le Moing AG, Boutourlinsky K, Boucher D, Carpentier W, Berquin P, Deleuze JF, Belvindrah R, Borrell V, Welker E, Chelly J, Croquelois A, Francis F (2014) Mutations in Eml1 lead to ectopic progenitors and neuronal heterotopia in mouse and human. Nat Neurosci 17(7):923–933. https://doi.org/10.1038/nn.3729

Kim H, McCulloch CA (2011) Filamin A mediates interactions between cytoskeletal proteins that control cell adhesion. FEBS Lett 585(1):18–22. https://doi.org/10.1016/j.febslet.2010.11.033

Kini LG, Nasrallah IM, Coto C, Ferraro LC, Davis KA (2016) Advanced structural multimodal imaging of a patient with subcortical band heterotopia. Epilepsia Open 1(3–4):152–155. https://doi.org/10.1002/epi4.12019

Lange M, Kasper B, Bohring A, Rutsch F, Kluger G, Hoffjan S, Spranger S, Behnecke A, Ferbert A, Hahn A, Oehl-Jaschkowitz B, Graul-Neumann L, Diepold K, Schreyer I, Bernhard MK, Mueller F, Siebers-Renelt U, Beleza-Meireles A, Uyanik G, Janssens S, Boltshauser E, Winkler J, Schuierer G, Hehr U (2015) 47 patients with FLNA associated periventricular nodular heterotopia. Orphanet J Rare Dis 10:134. https://doi.org/10.1186/s13023-015-0331-9

Leite CC, Lucato LT, Sato JR, Valente KD, Otaduy MC (2007) Multivoxel proton MR spectroscopy in malformations of cortical development. AJNR Am J Neuroradiol 28(6):1071–1075; discussion 1076–1077. https://doi.org/10.3174/ajnr.A0511

Lian G, Sheen VL (2015) Cytoskeletal proteins in cortical development and disease: actin associated proteins in periventricular heterotopia. Front Cell Neurosci 9:99. https://doi.org/10.3389/fncel.2015.00099

Liu W, Yan B, An D, Xiao J, Hu F, Zhou D (2017) Sporadic periventricular nodular heterotopia: classification, phenotype and correlation with Filamin A mutations. J Hum Genet 133:33–40. https://doi.org/10.1016/j.eplepsyres.2017.03.005

Matsumoto N, Hoshiba Y, Morita K, Uda N, Hirota M, Minamikawa M, Ebisu H, Shinmyo Y, Kawasaki H (2017) Pathophysiological analyses of periventricular nodular heterotopia using gyrencephalic mammals. Hum Mol Genet 26(6):1173–1181. https://doi.org/10.1093/hmg/ddx038

Ramos RL, Siu NY, Brunken WJ, Yee KT, Gabel LA, Van Dine SE, Hoplight BJ (2014) Cellular and axonal constituents of neocortical molecular layer heterotopia. Dev Neurosci 36(6):477–489. https://doi.org/10.1159/000365100

Selected References

Robertson SP (2005) Filamin A: phenotypic diversity. Curr Opin Genet Dev 15(3):301–307. https://doi.org/10.1016/j.gde.2005.04.001

Rossini L, Tassi L, Spreafico R, Garbelli R (2012) Heterotopic reelin in human nodular heterotopia: a neuropathological study. Epileptic Disord 14(4):398–402. https://doi.org/10.1684/epd.2012.0541

Sato M, Nagano T (2005) Involvement of filamin A and filamin A-interacting protein (FILIP) in controlling the start and cell shape of radially migrating cortical neurons. Anat Sci Int 80(1):19–29. https://doi.org/10.1111/j.1447-073x.2005.00101.x

Sheen VL (2012) Periventricular heterotopia: shuttling of proteins through vesicles and actin in cortical development and disease. Scientifica 2012:480129. https://doi.org/10.6064/2012/480129

Watrin F, Manent JB, Cardoso C, Represa A (2015) Causes and consequences of gray matter heterotopia. CNS Neurosci Ther 21(2):112–122. https://doi.org/10.1111/cns.12322

Zajac-Mnich M, Kostkiewicz A, Guz W, Dziurzynska-Bialek E, Solinska A, Stopa J, Kucharska-Miasik I (2014) Clinical and morphological aspects of gray matter heterotopia type developmental malformations. Pol J Radiol 79:502–507. https://doi.org/10.12659/pjr.890549

Part IX

The Brain Diseases: Trauma and Intoxication

Trauma

48.1 Definition

Traumatic brain injury (TBI) is the result of head injury due to various causes.

48.2 Epidemiology

Incidence
- Leading cause of death in people under 45 years of age
- 200–300 patients per 100,000 population

Age Incidence
- Bimodal pattern
  - 65 years and older
  - Children under 14 years old

Sex Incidence
- Male:Female ratio: 3:1

Localization
- Brain
- Brain stem
- Spinal cord
- Cranial nerves
  - Olfactory nerve
  - Optic nerve
  - Oculomotor nerves
  - Trigeminal nerve
  - Facial and auditory nerves
  - Glossopharyngeal, vagus, spinal accessory, and hypoglossal nerves
- Traumatic arterial injuries

48.3 Clinical Signs and Symptoms

Traumatic brain injury symptoms include:
- Vomiting
- Dizziness and balance problems
- Lethargy
- Breathing problems
- Headache
- Slow pulse
- Confusion
- Difficulty swallowing
- Paralysis
- Ringing in the ears, or changes in hearing
- Cognitive difficulties
- Loss of consciousness
- Inappropriate emotional responses
- Dilated pupils
- Body numbness or tingling
- Vision changes (blurred vision or seeing double, not able to tolerate bright light, loss of eye movement, blindness)
- Cerebrospinal fluid (which may be clear or blood tinged) coming out of the ears or nose
- Slow breathing rate, with an increase in blood pressure

- Speech difficulties (slurred speech, inability to understand and/or articulate words)
- Droopy eyelid or facial weakness
- Loss of bowel control or bladder control
- Coma

48.4 Classification of TBI

Classification of TBI can be done under various aspects:

- Clinical classification
- Clinical/neuroradiological classification
- Neuropathological classification
- Mechanistic classification

The **clinical classification** is based on the *Glasgow Coma Scale (GCS)* as follows (Table 48.1) (Teasdale and Jennett 1974; Teasdale et al. 1979, 2014):

- Three clinical parameters are evaluated
  - Eye response
  - Verbal response
  - Motor response
- For each response a value between 1 and 6 is given
- The values for the three responses are added up
- A score between 3 and 15 can be summed up

A *mild brain injury* is often caused by a blunt head trauma, and/or acceleration or deceleration forces to the head, and refers to the initial impact of the injury.

The diagnosis of mild traumatic brain injury based on WHO 2004 criteria is given as follows (Mayer et al. 2017):

- Inclusion criteria
  GCS 13–15 after 30 min postinjury or later and one or more of the following:
  (1) Confusion or disorientation
  (2) LOC ≤ 30 min
  (3) Posttraumatic amnesia ≤24 h
  (4) Transient neurologic abnormalities (focal signs or seizure)
  (5) Intracranial lesion not requiring surgery
- Exclusion criteria
  (1) GCS < 13 after 30 min postinjury
  (2) Symptoms caused by other noncranial injuries
  (3) Caused by other problems (psychological or substance-related)
  (4) Caused by penetrating craniocerebral injury

Table 48.1 Glasgow Coma Scale

Points	Eye response	Verbal response	Motor response
1	Does not open eyes	Makes no sounds	Makes no movements
2	Opens eyes in response to voice	Incomprehensible sounds	Extension to painful stimuli (decerebrate response)
3	Opens eyes in response to voice	Utters inappropriate words	Abnormal flexion to painful stimuli (decorticate response)
4	Opens eyes spontaneously	Confused, disoriented	Flexion/Withdrawal to painful stimuli
5	N/A	Oriented, converses normally	Localizes painful stimuli
6	N/A	N/A	Obeys commands
Score	1–4	1–5	1–6
Grades of TBI		**GCS**	
Mild		13–15	
Moderate		9–12	
Severe		<9	

48.4 Classification of TBI

The most common causes of a *moderate or severe TBI* are

- Falls (40.5%)
- Motor vehicle accidents (14.3%)
- Assaults (10.7%)
- Being struck by or against (15.5%)

Concussion (commotion cerebri)

- Temporary, reversible neurologic deficiency
- Caused by trauma
- Results in immediate, temporary loss of consciousness
- Retrograde and posttraumatic amnesia always accompany a concussion

Contusion

- Bruise of the brain's surface
- The overlying dura mater nearly always remains intact
- Contusions formed at the site of cranial impact are coup contusions; those opposite the cranial impact contrecoup contusions

Laceration

- Mechanical tear or rent in normal tissues

The **clinical/neuroradiological classification** categorizes TBI as follows:

- Focal TBI
- Diffuse or multifocal TBI

The **neuropathological classification** is done as follows:

- Anatomical
  - Focal including
    - Scalp lacerations
    - Skull fractures
    - Contusions/lacerations
    - Intracranial hemorrhage
    - Focal lesions secondary to raised intracranial pressure
  - Diffuse including
    - Global ischemic injury
    - Traumatic axonal injury
    - Diffuse vascular injury
    - Brain swelling
- Pathophysiological
  - Primary (injuries occurring at the moment of injury)
  - Secondary (injuries occurring in a mechanically injured brain)

The **mechanistic classification** results in the following types of injury:

- Impact injury
  - Head makes contact with an object
  - Forces of impact are transmitted to the brain
  - Leads to hemorrhages and traumatic axonal injury
- Acceleration-deceleration injury
  - Unrestricted movement of the head leads to shear and compressive strains
  - Leads to traumatic axonal injury
- Penetrating injury (Figs. 48.1, 48.2, 48.3, and 48.4)
  - An object passes through the skull producing brain damage
  - Leads to focal tissue necrosis
- Blast injury
  - Shock waves produce brain damage
  - Leads to brain swelling

A blast TBI (bTBI) is a

- Unique subtype of traumatic injury
- Occurs due to direct or indirect exposure to an explosion, primarily in combat situations

A "blast wave" generated from an explosion

- Consists of a front of high pressure
- Quickly compresses the surrounding air
- Gives rise to negative pressure
- Rapidly expands and displaces an equal volume of air
- This displacement of air then generates a "blast wind"

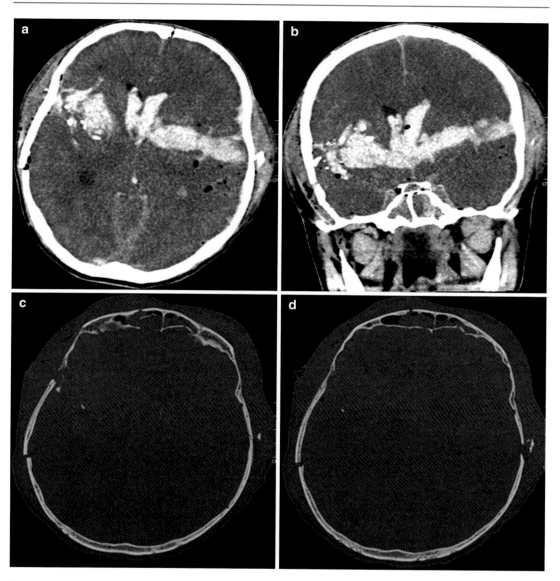

Fig. 48.1 Perforating gunshot injury—CT showing missile track (**a**, **b**), entry (**c**), and exit wound (**d**)

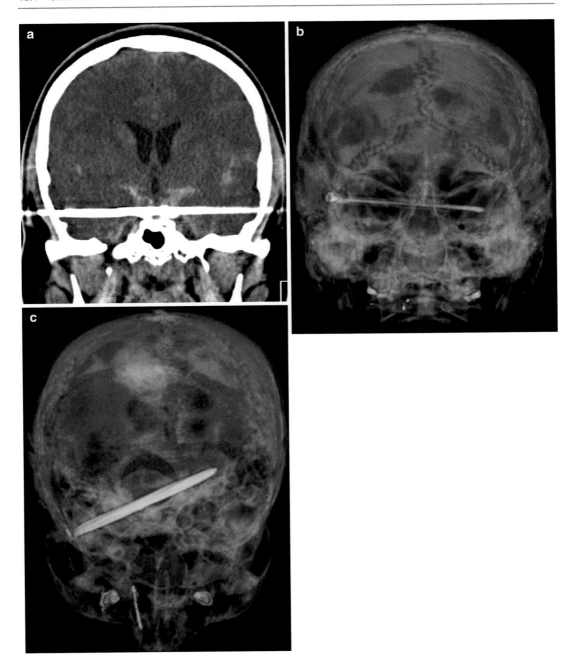

Fig. 48.2 Nail gun shot—CT non-contrast (**a**), 3D reconstruction of CT-scan (**b, c**)

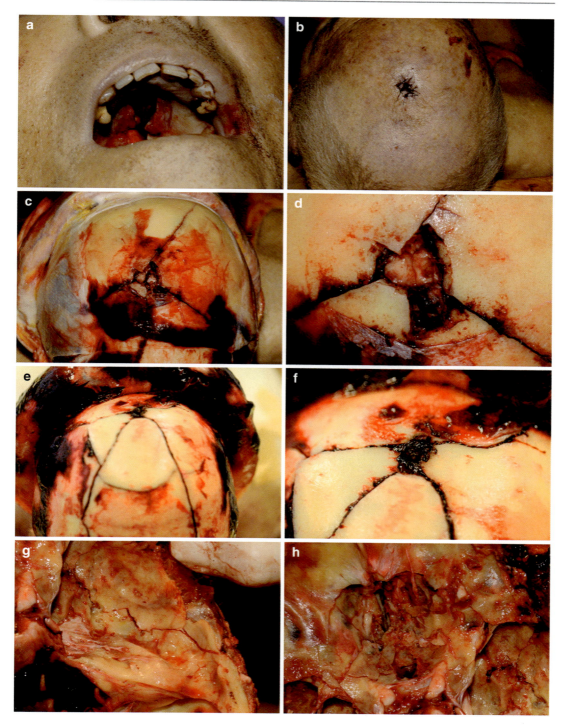

Fig. 48.3 Gunshot through the mouth (**a**) with exit at the occiput (**b**). Fractures of the skull after gunshot impact (**c–h**)

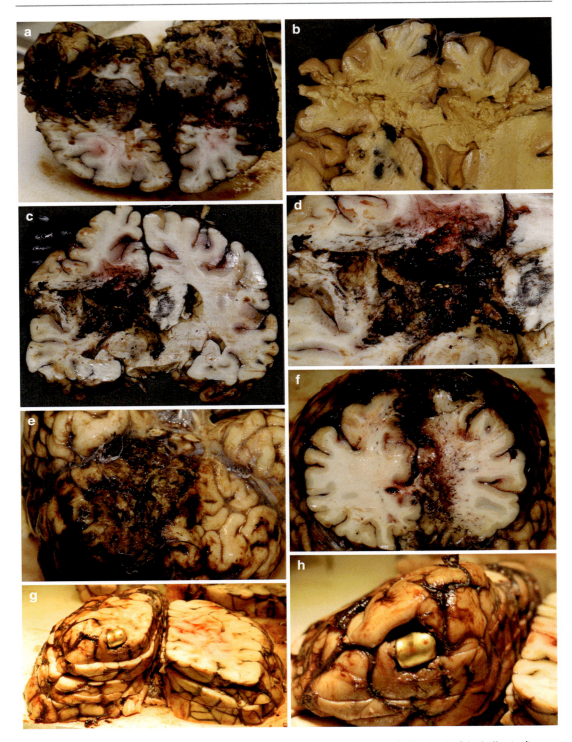

Fig. 48.4 Gunshot through the brain with tissue destruction and hemorrhages (**a–f**). Retrieval of the bullet (**g–j**)

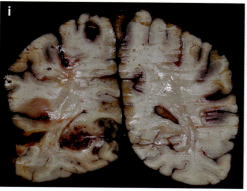
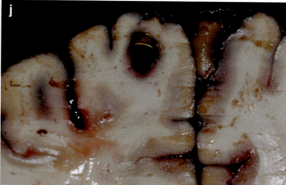

Fig. 48.4 (continued)

48.5 Neuroimaging Findings

48.5.1 Cerebral Contusions

General Imaging Features
- Hemorrhagic or non-hemorrhagic edematous lesions—typical location: anterior inferior frontal lobes and temporal poles
- Coup-contrecoup injury—brain damage located at the site of impact and the opposite side of the brain

CT Non-Contrast-Enhanced (Figs. 48.5a)
- Ill-defined hypodense lesions (edema) with hyperdense hemorrhages

MRI-T2/FLAIR
- Hyperintense edema

MRI-T1
- Hypointense edema

MRI-T2*/SWI
- Hypointense hemorrhages

MR-Diffusion Imaging
- Restricted diffusion in lesions possible

MR-Spectroscopy
- Choline elevated
- NAA decreased

48.5.2 Chronic Traumatic Brain Injury

General Imaging Features
- General brain atrophy
- Encephalomalacia: focal loss of brain parenchyma following
  - Contusions
  - Ischemia
  - Hemorrhage
  - Often with surrounding gliosis

Nuclear Medicine Imaging Findings (Fig. 48.6a–d)
- Nuclear medicine studies can be used to assess the functional damage caused by trauma.
- The imaging results can be correlated to clinical findings and help to understand the functional deficits of the patient or promise a good prognostic outcome for the patients with normal findings after trauma.
- Nuclear medicine studies have been reported to be useful in the monitoring of neurological improvements in trauma patients.
- CBF-SPECT, presynaptic and postsynaptic dopaminergic SPECT, FDG-PET, pre- and postsynaptic dopaminergic PET, perfusion PET, and flumazenil PET can be used depending on the trauma, the clinical findings, and morphological findings of the patient.
- Especially flumazenil would give the opportunity to visualize neuronal loss.

48.5 Neuroimaging Findings

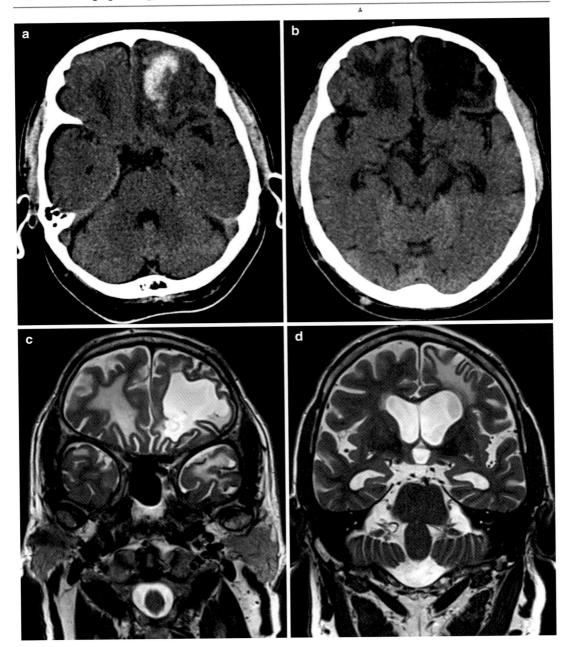

Fig. 48.5 Contusions/chronic traumatic brain injury: Partly hemorrhagic contusions in frontal and temporal lobes (not shown)—CT non-contrast (**a**); CT/MRI scans 8 years later show general brain atrophy and encephalomalacia in frontotemporal lobes—CT non-contrast (**b**), T2 coronal (**c, d**), FLAIR (**e**)

- Interestingly, for FDG it is reported that hypermetabolism in the cerebellar vermis can be used to assess traumatic brain injury and be a prognostic marker of recovery if the hypermetabolism remains over time.
- Perfusion PET studies can be used to assess the response of the brain to memory tasks.
- Interpretation of SPECT and PET studies can be done visually or with automated methods

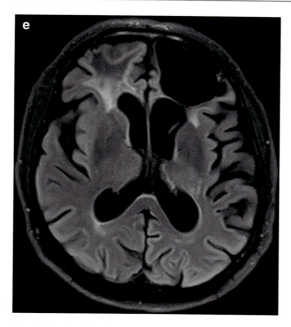

Fig. 48.5 (continued)

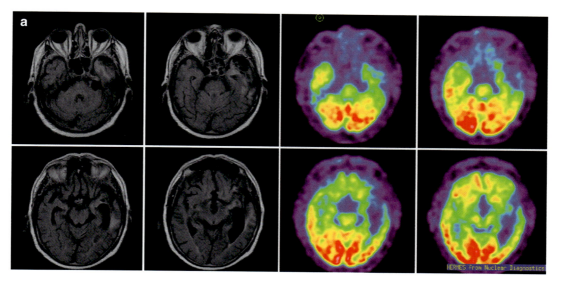

Fig. 48.6 FDG-PET with correlating MRI and FP-CIT SPECT of a patient with a history of brain trauma (**a–d**). Scars in the left temporal lobe and the right putamen cause movement disorder and changes in personality, memory, and speech

48.5 Neuroimaging Findings 1195

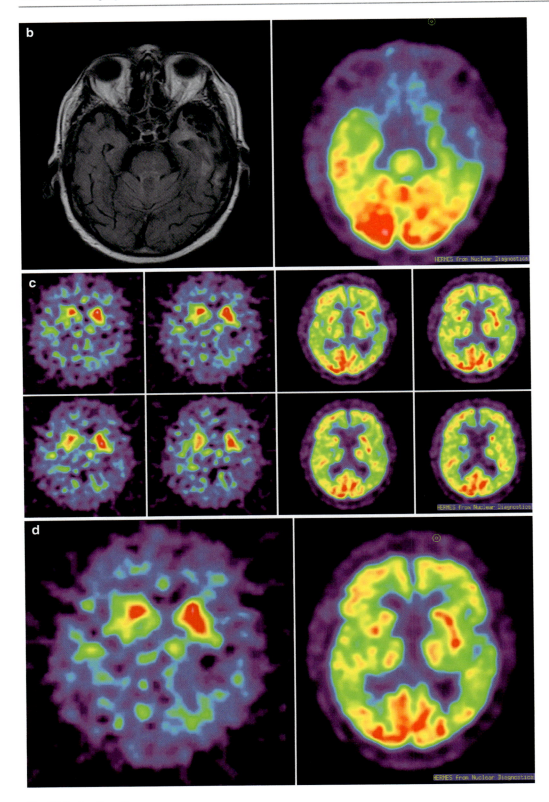

Fig. 48.6 (continued)

like SPM (statistical parametric mapping), 3D-SSP (three-dimensional stereotactic surface projections), BRASS (brain registration analysis of SPECT studies).
- The physician has to be careful in interpreting the studies because functional changes in SPECT and PET studies can be correlated to other causative diseases (like dementia, vascular changes, depression, intoxication, and Parkinson disease) as well and we have to be attentive not to over-interpret the results.
- It has been reported that diffusely decreased white matter glucose metabolism is a general phenomenon in trauma patients.

48.6 Focal Injuries

The focal injuries include:

- Scalp lesions (Fig. 48.7a–r)
- Skull lesions (fractures) (Fig. 48.8a–p)
- Contusions and lacerations (Figs. 48.9, 48.10, and 48.11)
- Intracranial hemorrhages
    - Extradural (epidural) hemorrhage
    - Subdural hemorrhage
    - Subdural hygroma
    - Subarachnoidal hemorrhage
    - Intracerebral hemorrhage
    - Intraventricular hemorrhage

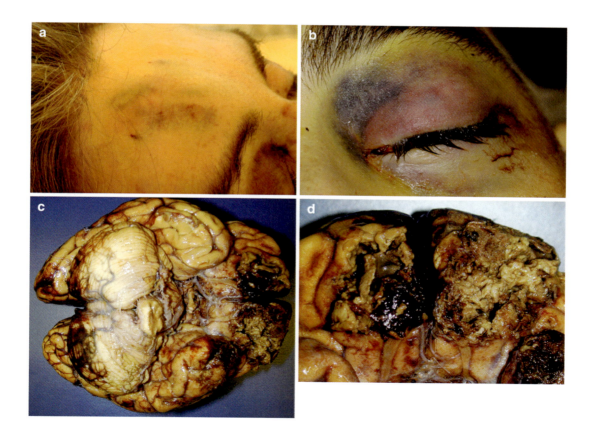

Fig. 48.7 Trauma: Bruising of the skin (**a**) and eye (**b**). Tissue destruction with hemorrhages (**c–p**), bilateral fronto-orbital cortex (**c–f**), left temporal cortex (**g**, **h**), left temporal pole (**i**, **j**), bilateral frontal poles (**k**, **l**), right temporal cortex (**m**, **n**), left straight gyrus (**o**, **p**). Retropulsion of the eyeball (**q**, **r**)

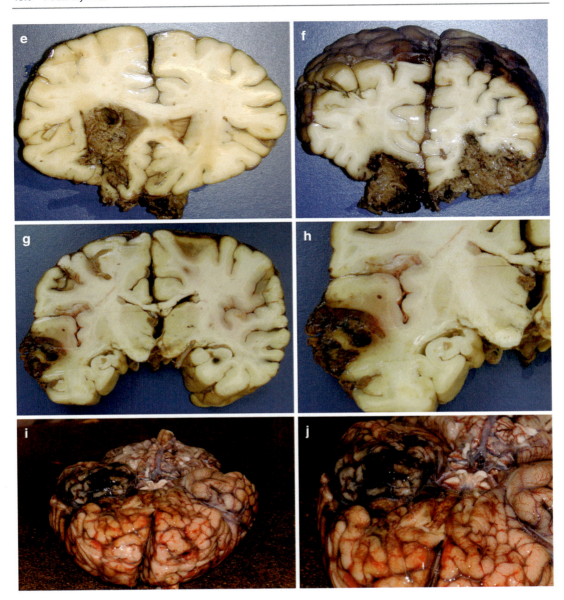

Fig. 48.7 (continued)

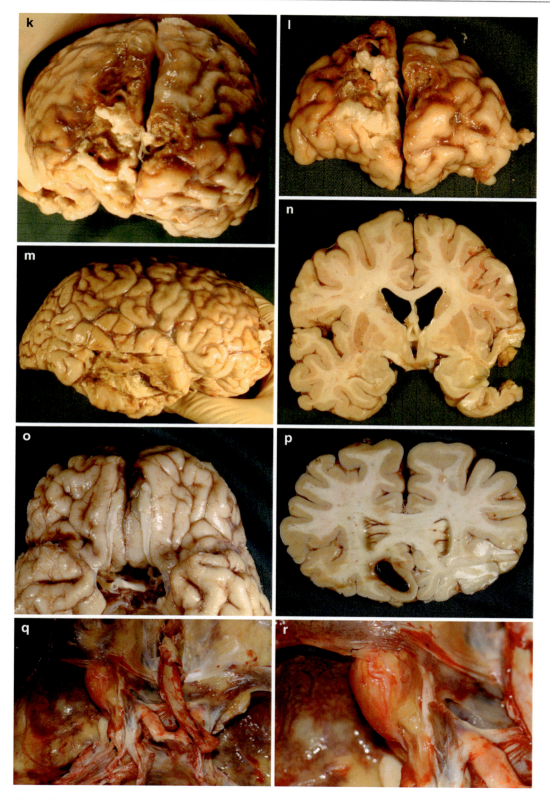

Fig. 48.7 (continued)

48.6 Focal Injuries

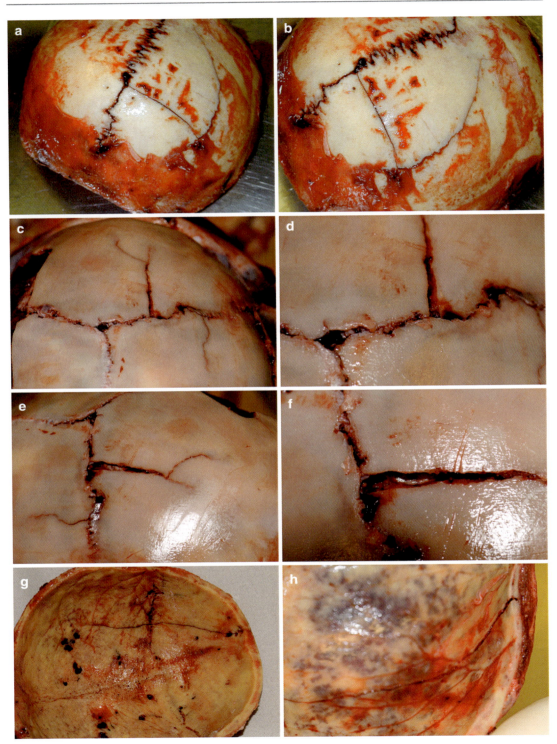

Fig. 48.8 Fracture lines affecting the outer aspects of the skull (**a–j**), the inner aspects of the skull (**g, h**), and the skull base (**i–p**)

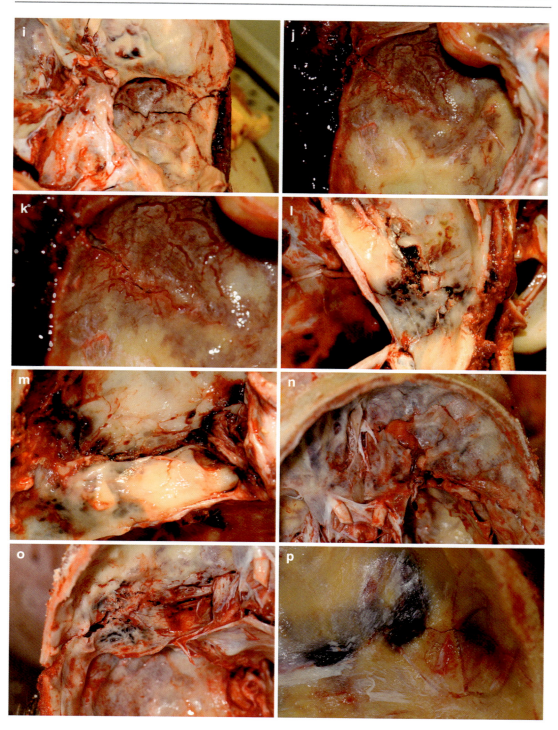

Fig. 48.8 (continued)

48.6 Focal Injuries

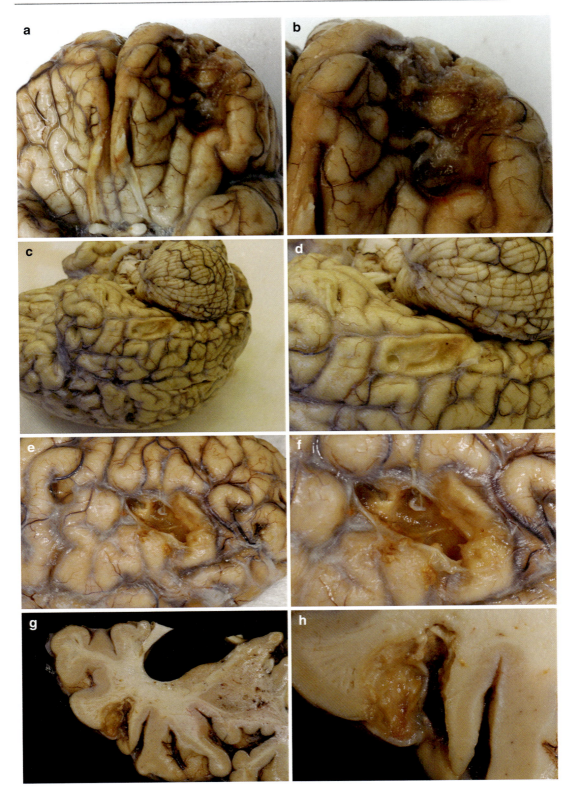

Fig. 48.9 Old traumatic contusional lesions (**a–l**) with tissue destruction and brownish coloration, left fronto-orbital cortex (**a, b**), right inferior temporal gyrus (**c, d**), surface of the right parietal lobe (**e, f**), cross-section of the parietal lobe (**g, h**), left temporal lobe (**i, j**), surface and cross-section of the left fronto-orbital cortex (**k, l**)

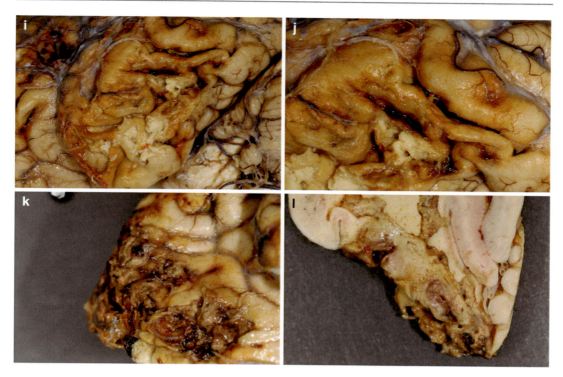

Fig. 48.9 (continued)

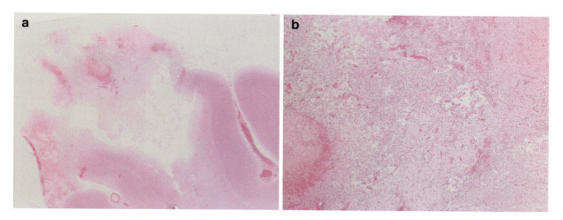

Fig. 48.10 Trauma: Tissue destruction (**a**) with large areas of necroses (**b–d**), fresh petechial hemorrhages (**e**) and hemosiderinophages (**f**). Beginning tissue destruction with softening of the tissue (**g**, **h**), hemorrhagic tissue destruction of the spinal cord (**i**, **j**). Patterns of hemorrhages (**k–r**) include large hemorrhagic areas (**k**, **l**), accumulation of monomorphonuclear cells (**m**, **n**), perivascular accumulation of erythrocytes (**o–q**), intravascular stasis and perivascular erythrocytes (**r–t**)

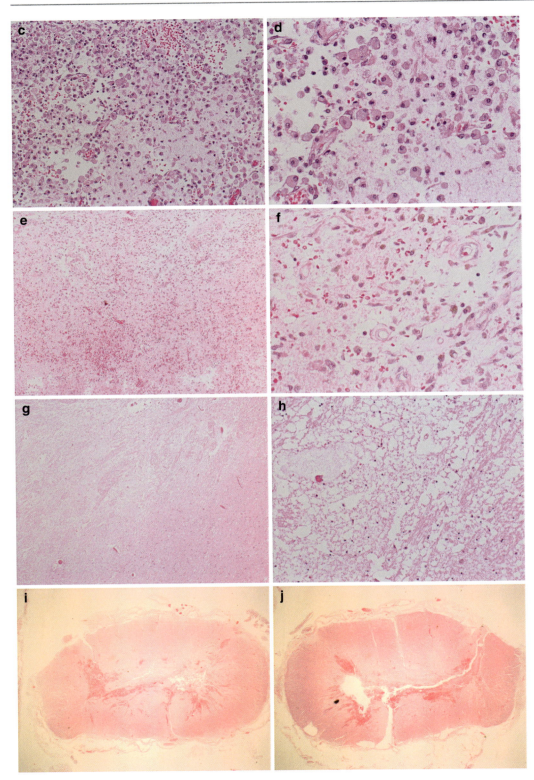

Fig. 48.10 (continued)

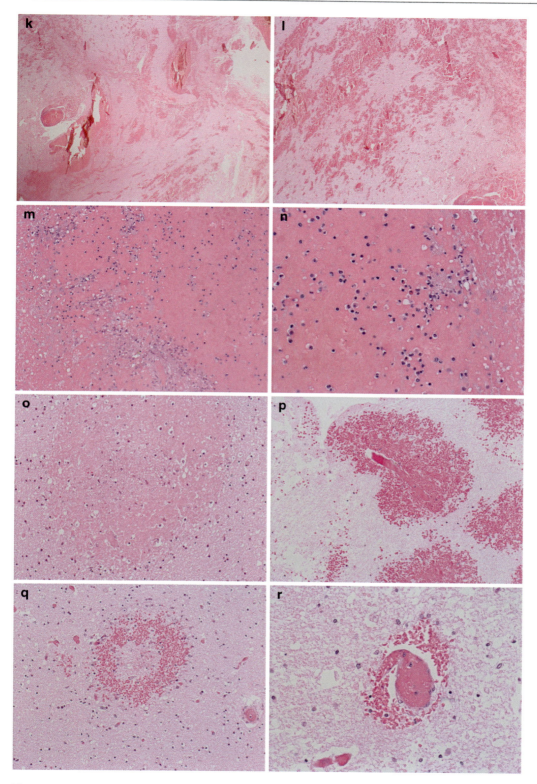

Fig. 48.10 (continued)

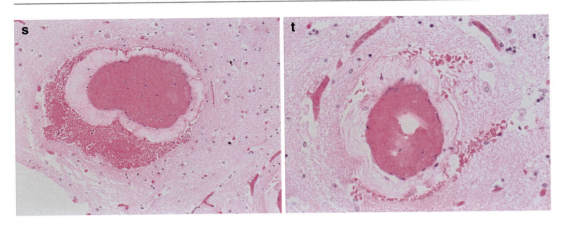

Fig. 48.10 (continued)

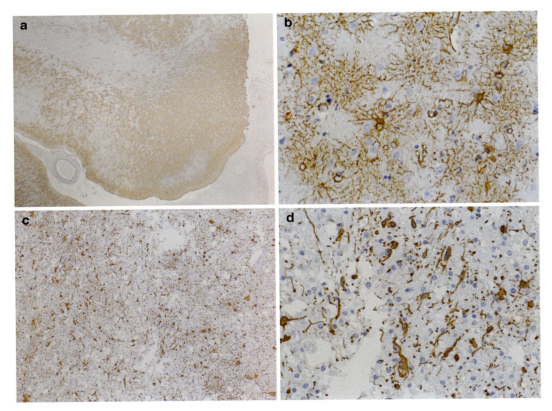

Fig. 48.11 Immunophenotype: Reactive GFAP-positive astrocytes (**a–f**) as star-like cells with strong ramifications (**a, b**), cells with reduced cytoplasmic ramifications (**c, d**) in perivascular locations (**e, f**). Reactive microgliosis (immunohistochemistry for HLA-DRII) with rod-like cells (**g, h**), round cells with macrophage morphology (**i, j**), and a mixture of both cell phenotypes at the border of necroses (**k, l**)

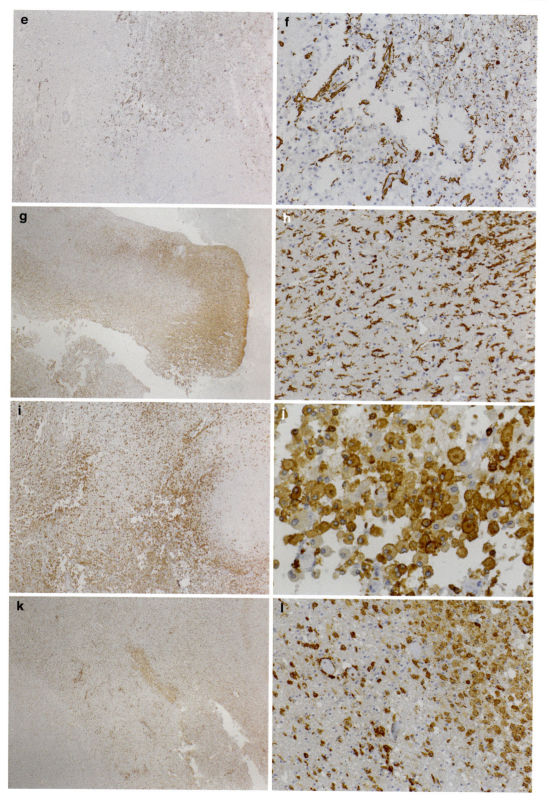

Fig. 48.11 (continued)

48.7 Diffuse Injuries

Diffuse traumatic injuries include:

- Diffuse axonal injury (DAI)
- Ischemia
- Brain swelling
- Diffuse vascular injury

Diffuse Axonal Injury (DAI)/Traumatic Axonal Injury (TAI)

General Imaging Features
- Multiple punctate, usually hemorrhagic lesions—typical location: white-gray matter junction, corpus callosum, brain stem

CT Non-Contrast-Enhanced (Fig. 48.12a, b)
- Detection of large hemorrhagic lesions and contusions, punctate lesions not detectable—MRI more sensitive

CT Contrast-Enhanced
- No enhancement

MRI-T2/FLAIR (Fig. 48.12c–e)
- Multiple punctate hyperintense lesions
- Accompanying edema hyperintense

MRI-T1 (Fig. 48.12f)
- Small lesions often not detectable
- Larger hemorrhagic lesions hypo-, iso-, or hyperintense (depending on age of hematoma)

MRI-T1 Contrast-Enhanced
- No enhancement

MRI-T2*/SWI (Fig. 48.12g, h)
- Multiple punctate, hypointense microbleeds
- Most sensitive sequences
- Including corpus callosum = grade II, with brain stem = grade III

MR-Diffusion Imaging
- Restricted diffusion in lesions possible

MR-Diffusion Tensor Imaging
- Decreased anisotropy

MR-Spectroscopy
- Choline elevated
- NAA decreased

Three grades of TAI are described:

- Grade 1:
  - Only microscopic changes are seen in the white matter of the cerebral cortex, corpus callosum, brain stem, and cerebellum
- Grade 2:
  - Macroscopic changes in the corpus callosum
- Grade 3:
  - Additional macroscopic lesions are found in the dorsolateral quadrants of the rostral brain stem

Microscopic Findings (Fig. 48.13a–l)
- H&E
  - Eosinophilic swellings as sign of damaged axons
- Silver stains
  - Allow the detection of abnormal axons only between 12 and 18 h
- Amyloid precursor protein (APP) IHC
  - Detects axonal flow disruption
- Particular vulnerability of white matter tracts:
  - Corpus callosum, internal capsule, cerebellar peduncles, descending long tracts of the brain stem
- Microglial markers
  - Formation of microglial clusters or stars around degenerating axons

Pathogenetic Mechanisms
- Primary axotomy:
  - Axonal disconnection at the time of impact leading to axonal retraction and axoplasmic pooling

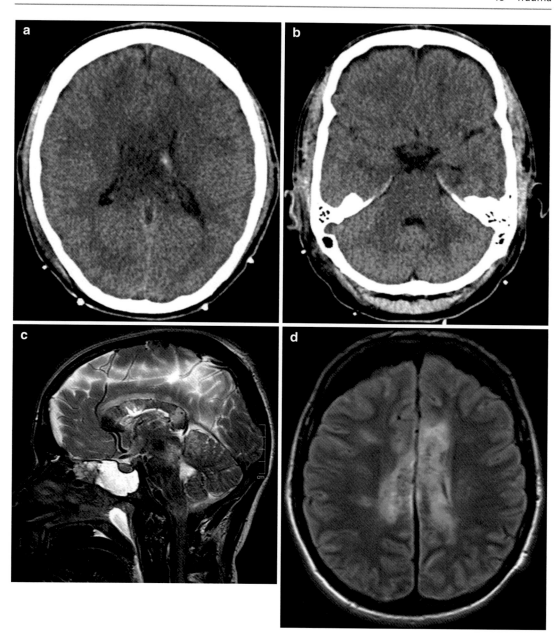

Fig. 48.12 Diffuse axonal injury grade 3 (involvement of white matter, corpus callosum, and brain stem); MRI more sensitive than CT detecting multiple microbleeds supra- and infratentorial—CT non-contrast (**a**, **b**), T2 sagittal (**c**), FLAIR (**d**, **e**), T1 (**f**), SWI (**g**, **h**)

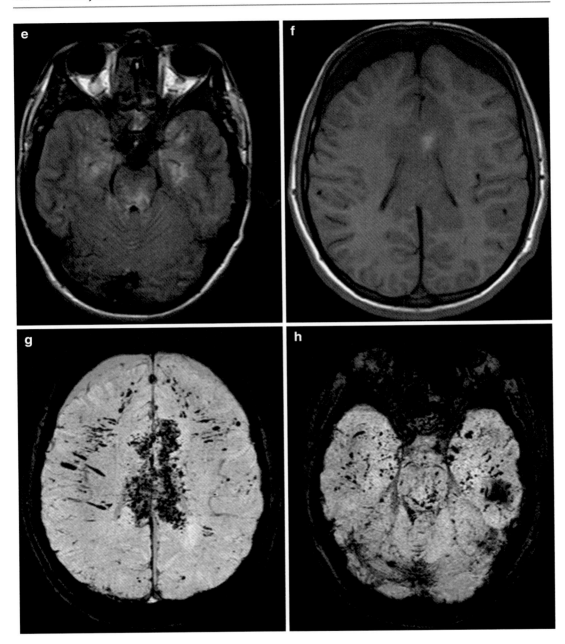

Fig. 48.12 (continued)

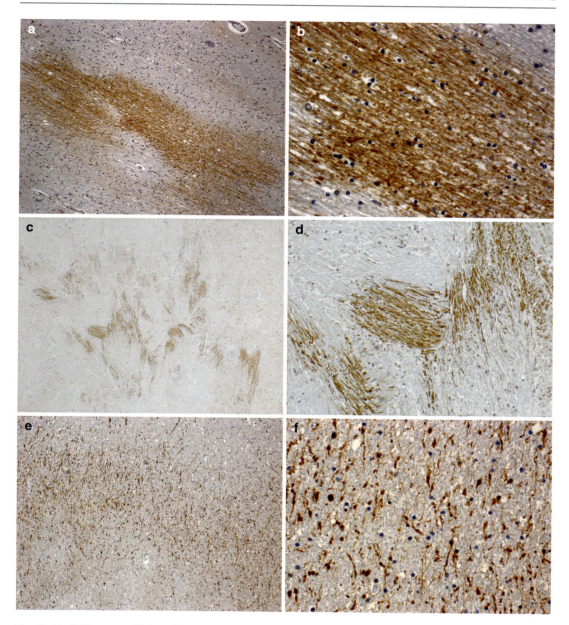

Fig. 48.13 Diffuse axonal injury (DAI) is best visualized immunohistochemically with anti-amyloid precursor protein (APP) antibodies (**a–i**). Damaged axons are present in bundles of various sizes (**a–e**), show protrusions (bulb formations) (**f–h**) or torpedos (**i, j**), or round varicosities when cut perpendicular to its length (**k, l**)

48.7 Diffuse Injuries

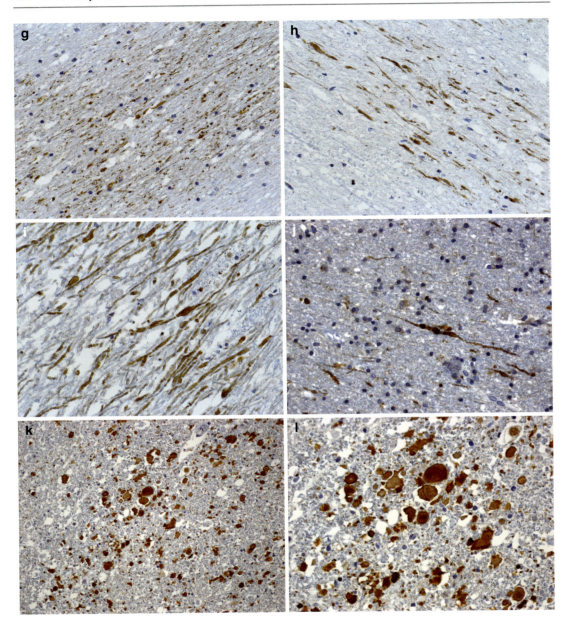

Fig. 48.13 (continued)

- Mechanoporation:
  - Focal affection of axons by applied forces resulting in mechanically induced membrane pores allowing calcium influx
  - Calcium influx leads to activation of calcium-dependent proteases and caspases
  - Modification of neurofilament subunits, i.e., phosphorylated sider arms result in microtubule compaction causing local axonal transport impairment and axonal swelling
  - Final result: rupture of the axon

48.8 Chronic Traumatic Encephalopathy

Chronic traumatic encephalopathy (CTE) is defined as progressive neurological deterioration resulting from repetitive brain trauma. It occurs in play of sports (boxing, American football, soccer, ice hockey, rugby), blast injuries, and other neurotrauma.

Clinical Signs and Symptoms
- Clinical signs include a variety of changes (Table 48.2):
- Behavioral changes
- Mood changes
- Memory loss
- Cognitive impairment
- Dementia

Neuropathology Diagnostic Criteria
- The criteria for the diagnosis of CTE are as follows (McKee et al. 2013):
- Perivascular foci of p-tau immunoreactive neurofibrillary tangles, pre-tangles, and dot-like and thread-like neurites in the neocortex (Table 48.3)
- Irregular distribution of p-tau immunoreactive neurofibrillary tangles, astrocytic tangles, and dot-like and thread-like neurites at the depths of cerebral sulci, often alongside penetrating vessels
- Neurofibrillary tangles in the crests of the cerebral cortex located preferentially in superficial layers II and III, prominent in the temporal lobes
- Clusters of subpial astrocytic tangles in the cerebral cortex, most pronounced at the sulcal depths
- Subependymal astrocytic tangles in the periventricular region of the lateral ventricles, periaqueductal gray, and lateral brain stem
- Definition of four stages based on macroscopical and microscopical features (Table 48.4)

Table 48.2 Symptoms encountered in CTE, modified after Vile and Atkinson (2017) reproduced with kind permission from Elsevier

Cognitive features	Behavioral features	Mood features	Motor features
Memory impairment	Physical violence	Depression	Ataxia
Executive dysfunction	Verbal violence	Hopelessness	Dysarthria
Impaired attention	Explosivity	Suicidality	Parkinsonism
Dysgraphia	Loss of control	Anxiety	Gait
Lack of insight	Short fuse	Fearfulness	Tremor
Preservation	Impulsivity	Irritability	Masked facies
Language difficulties	Paranoid delusions	Apathy	Rigidity
Dementia	Aggression	Loss of interest	Weakness
Alogia	Rage	Labile emotions	Spasticity
Visuospatial difficulties	Inappropriate speech	Fatigue	Clonus
Cognitive impairment	Boastfulness	Flat affect	
Reduced intelligence	Childish behavior	Insomnia	
	Socially inappropriate	Mania	
	Disinhibited behavior	Euphoria	
	Psychosis	Mood swings	
	Social isolation	Prolix	

48.8 Chronic Traumatic Encephalopathy

Table 48.3 Distinctions in hyperphosphorylated tau pathology between CTE and Alzheimer disease (McKee et al. 2013) reproduced with kind permission by Oxford University Press

Pathological features		CTE	Alzheimer disease
Tau-protein	Six isoforms	All six isoforms present	All six isoforms present
	3 or 4 repeat tau	3 repeat and 4 repeat tau present	3 repeat and 4 repeat tau present
Cell origin	Neuronal	NFTs and pre-tangles	NFTs and pre-tangles
	Astrocytic	Prominent astrocytic tangles	Not present
Neuronal domain	Cell body	Prominent	Prominent
	Dendrite	Prominent	Prominent
	Axon	Prominent	Sparse
Cell pattern	Perivascular	Prominent NFTs and astrocytic tangles	Not present
	Foci at depths of cerebral sulci	Prominent NFTs and astrocytic tangles	Not present
	Irregular, patchy cortical distribution	Prominent	Not present
	Cortical laminae	NFTs predominantly in laminae II–III	NFTs predominantly in laminae III and V
	Subpial astrocytic tangles	Prominent	Not present
	Periventricular astrocytic tangles	Present	Not present
Distribution	Mild pathology	CTE stages I–II: • NFTs in focal epicenters in cerebral cortex, usually frontal lobe	Braak stages I–III: • NFTs in entorhinal cortex, amygdala, and hippocampus
	Advanced pathology	CTE stages III–IV: • High density of NFTs in widespread cortical areas and medial temporal lobe, patchy irregular distribution • High densities of NFTs in thalamus, hypothalamus, mammillary bodies, brain stem. Moderate densities of NFTs in basal ganglia, especially nucleus accumbens • Prominent p-tau pathology in white matter tracts	Braak stages IV–VI: • High density of NFTs in widespread cortical areas and medial temporal lobe, uniform distribution • Low densities of NFTs in basal ganglia and brain stem; none in mammillary bodies • White matter tracts relatively uninvolved

Table 48.4 The following four stages of CTE are distinguished (McKee et al. 2015) reproduced with kind permission by Wiley-Blackwell

Stage	Macroscopy	Microscopy
I	• Unremarkable	• Isolated perivascular foci of p-tau NFT and neuropil neurites (discrete foci in the cerebral cortex, most commonly in the superior, dorsolateral, or lateral frontal cortices, and typically around small vessels at the depths of sulci) • Occasional p-tau immunopositive glia • Rare TDP-43 neurites • Reactive microglia in the white matter • Hemosiderin-laden macrophages around small vessels in the white matter

(continued)

Table 48.4 (continued)

Stage	Macroscopy	Microscopy
II	• Subtle changes • Mild enlargement of anterior horns of the ventricular system • Cavum septi pellucidi • Pallor of locus coeruleus and substantia nigra	• Multiple perivascular foci of p-tau NFT, pre-tangles, and neurites at the depths of the cerebral cortex (multiple epicenters at the depths of the cerebral sulci and localized spread of neurofibrillary pathology from these epicenters to the superficial layers of adjacent cortex. The medial temporal lobe is spared neurofibrillary p-tau pathology) • Occasional p-tau positive glia, astrocytic tangle • Mild TDP-43 pathology • Reactive microglia in clusters in the white matter
III	• Minor structural changes • Reduced brain weight • Mild atrophy of frontal and temporal lobes • Enlargement of lateral and third ventricles • Cavum septi pellucidi, septal perforations or fenestrations • Pallor of locus coeruleus and substantia nigra • Atrophy of mammillary bodies, thalamus, and hypothalamus • Thinning of the corpus callosum	• Confluent patches of NFT, NT, astrocytic tangles around blood vessels at the sulcal depths (widespread; the frontal, insular, temporal, and parietal cortices show neurofibrillary degeneration with greatest severity in the frontal and temporal lobe, concentrated at the depths of the sulci. The amygdala, hippocampus, and entorhinal cortex also show neurofibrillary pathology) • NFT in the cerebral cortex • TDP-43 positive neurites and inclusions • Loss of myelinated fibers, axonal dystrophy, axonal loss

48.9 Molecular Neuropathology

Axonal injury in traumatic brain injuries (Blennow et al. 2016)

- Microtubule disruption
  - Impaired axonal transport
  - Varicosity formation
  - Axonal disconnection
  - Impaired synaptic function
  - Aberrant colocalization of APP, BACE, PS1, and Aß within the varicosity
  - Intra-axonal Aß production
- Membrane leakage
  - Increased intra-axonal Ca^{2+} levels
  - Calpain and caspase activation
  - Cytoskeletal proteolysis
  - Neurofilament compaction
  - Axonal collapse
- Glutamate excitotoxicity (Munakomi and Cherian 2017)
  - Efflux of excitatory amino acid contributes to the development of neuronal damage
  - High extracellular glutamate initiates and accelerates the process of apoptosis and parthanatos
  - Extracellular glutamate level in TBI is cleared within 5 min, and the effect of glutamate receptors antagonists remains effective even after 30 min of insult
  - Theory of spreading depression due to the sodium extrusion, sequelae of calcium influx, and subsequent hyperpolarization
  - Astrocytic glutamate transporters such as GLAST and GLT-1 and splice variant are downregulated shortly following the insult precipitating glutamate-mediated excitotoxic conditions
- Lactate Storm
  - The injured brain continues to produce lactate within minutes following severe TBI
  - There is a glial–neuronal uncoupling resulting in a lactate storm in the already failing metabolic environment
  - Extracellular lactate increase is independent of brain hypoxic ischemia in severe TBI

- It is thereby a safe option to safely
  - Chelate the excess lactate
  - Buffer the pH effect
  - Inhibit glial metabolism
- Lactate, because of its role as a supplementary fuel to the brain, can be a friend only in an aerobic environment. Lactate substitution is, in fact, a foe in such a lethal and stormy metabolic milieu, and can paradoxically lead to the unsalvageable brain
- Tauopathy
  - There has been a recent upsurge in the link between lymphatic pathways in the brain and its association with tauopathies following TBI.
  - This pathway facilitates the clearance of interstitial solutes, including amyloid, from the brain.
  - Extracellular tau is cleared from the brain along these paravascular pathways mediated by Aquaporin-4 channel.
  - After TBI, glymphatic pathway function was significantly impaired for at least 1 month postinjury, thereby promoting the development of neurofibrillary pathology and neurodegeneration in the posttraumatic brain.
  - Chronic impairment of glymphatic pathway function after TBI may be a key factor that renders the posttraumatic brain vulnerable to tau aggregation and the onset of neurodegeneration thereafter.
- Immunoexcitotoxicity
  - TBI can prime microglia.
  - This leads to its activation to either of neurotrophic, neurodestructive, or intermediate states each responding to a different set of membrane signals, which can be time and cytokine dose dependent.
  - The release of chemokines like monocyte chemoattractant protein-1 also stimulates the recruitment of peripheral monocytes/macrophages to the central nervous system, especially via the circumventricular organs.
  - At the face of the excitotoxic environment, microglial cells release NO and interleukin-1b, thereby contributing to subacute neuronal degeneration.
  - Normally, the activated microglial cells go into reparative ramified mode wherein they secrete neurotrophins and the anti-inflammatory cytokines helping in the repair process.
  - Repeated trauma leads to priming of these activated microglia cells to become hyperreactive, releasing much higher concentrations of inflammatory cytokines and excitotoxins than are normally released.
  - It has been proposed that with chronic microglial neurodegeneration, this switching process to ramified form does not occur, leading to progressive and prolonged neuronal injury.
  - Gliosis and the scar associated with the neurodegeneration lead to the impairment of the paravascular clearance pathway of the amyloid and the tau-proteins.
  - Amyloid deposits are known to occur rapidly after TBI and persist in 30% of severe head trauma cases, even in children.
- Hemodynamic Alteration
  - There are specific hemodynamic alterations following the TBI
    - In the first 24 h, there is oligemia attributable to cellular edema, sympathetic adrenergic surge at the face of trauma, and the microvascular thrombi.
    - In the subsequent 3 days, there is a phase of hyperemia because of vasomotor paralysis, luxury perfusion, and the hyperglycolysis.
    - Then from the fourth day to following 2 weeks, the phase of vasospasm sets in because of the degraded blood products such as deoxyhemoglobin and bilirubin.
  - Hence, the concept of correct fluid resuscitation and replacement has a paramount importance while managing patients with TBI. Fluids should be restricted in the hyperemic phase, whereas induced hypertension, hemodilution, and hypervolemia

should be instituted during the phase of vasospasm.
- Role of opening the cisternal webs in the brain
  - The implications of opening the cisterns in TBI, though demanding, can have ripple effects in the management of TBI.
  - It immediately lax the tight brain due to egress of the CSF.
  - Furthermore, it improves the compliance of the vessels and reduces the risk of subsequent vasospasm clearing the cisternal and subarachnoid blood invariably associated with TBI.
  - Cisternal drain helps in clearing away the lactate and tau-proteins, thereby reducing the hazardous cellular milieu and also minimizing the risk of subsequent development of neurodegenerative lesions.

TBI is currently classified based on:

- Clinical observations
  - Mild
  - Moderate
  - Severe
- History
  - Duration of loss of consciousness
  - Posttraumatic amnesia

Damage to nervous tissue can be classified as:

- Primary injury, which occurs as a direct result of the experienced physical forces
- Secondary injury, which arises from pathophysiological processes following the traumatic event

The primary injury process

- Consists of the rapid acceleration-deceleration applied to the head
- Is thought to damage the brain
- Produces shear forces within nervous tissue
- Results in axonal injury and impact with the cranial wall
- These injuries can be ipsilateral or contralateral to the blow, and have been described in literature as "coup" and "contre-coup," respectively
- In more severe cases, injury can cause
  - Intracranial hemorrhage
  - Subsequent intracranial hypertension
  - This increase in pressure not only damages brain tissue by compression, but also by causing cerebral hypoperfusion and potential ischemic injury by decreasing cerebral perfusion pressure
- Following the initial trauma:
  - Axonal damage from the shear forces of primary injury affects membrane permeability and ionic balance
  - Uptake of calcium through either membrane disruption or activation of NMDA and AMPA receptors by glutamate can result in
    - Mitochondrial dysfunction
    - Overproduction of free radicals
    - Activation of apoptotic caspase signaling
- Subsequent inflammatory processes:
  - Activation of native microglia
  - Contributing to oxidative stress via oxidative burst or through secondary effects of inflammatory cytokines
  - The reactive radicals can overwhelm endogenous antioxidant systems and inflict cellular damage via lipid peroxidation and protein modifications
- The secondary products of free radical mediated lipid peroxidation
  - As reactive carbonyl species
  - Are also electrophilic
  - Further propagate oxidative damage to biomacromolecules
- The major endogenous antioxidants glutathione and ascorbic acid may remain diminished for 3 and 14 days post injury
- Lipid peroxidation byproduct
  - Elevation of F2-isoprostane
  - 4-hydroxynoneal was elevated

48.9 Molecular Neuropathology

- Involvement of oxidative stress in
  - Excitotoxicity
  - Reperfusion injury
  - Central role in secondary neuronal injury following TBI

Secondary injury in TBI:

- Occurs in the days, weeks, and months following the traumatic event
- Results from biochemical changes in nervous tissue
- Damage is frequently mediated by free radicals and reactive oxygen species (ROS)
  - Produced from ischemia reperfusion injury
  - Glutamatergic excitotoxicity
  - Neuroinflammation
- Capacity to prolong cellular injury beyond the initial traumatic event:
  - Oxidative stress
  - Excitotoxicity

Pathophysiology of Mild TBI (Dixon 2017)
- After a violent hit to the head
- The soft brain inside hits the intracranial surface of the skull
- May damage the area of the brain that comes in contact with the skull
- This damage may occur in both the forward and the reverse locations as the brain "bounces" within the skull
- Any rotational movement to the brain following the impact may stretch, and sometimes tear, axons within white matter tracts of the brain, which is known as "diffuse axonal injury"
- This type of injury may impair neuronal function
- Diffuse axonal injury may induce neuronal degeneration
- It may only induce neuronal atrophy due to axotomy of the axon initial segment
  - Two types of axonal abnormality have been observed:
    - The first is progressive swellings along the axon termed "bulbs" that eventually lead to axonal disconnection and loss of function
    - The second is a production of axonal varicosities and is thought to be due to microtubule breakage, thus slowing axonal transport to cause the varicosities
  - These abnormalities may lead to delayed secondary disconnection and/or prolonged neuronal dysfunction
- Induce other pathophysiologic responses
  - A sustained proinflammatory cytokine upregulation
  - A reduction in oligodendrocyte cell numbers
  - Glial reactivity
  - Disrupt the function of the cerebral vasculature
    - Initial reduction in cerebral blood flow (within hours of the injury), which can remain low for days, depending on injury severity
    - This reduced blood flow could be attributed to increased nitric oxide expression after injury, causing vasodilation instead of a pressure-induced increase in vasoconstriction
    - A reduction in blood vessel density in the perilesional region during the first few days after injury
    - The cerebral blood vessels may be less able to respond to dilatory stimuli

Pathophysiology of Severe TBI
- Cause the brain to hit against the intracranial portion of the skull, with or without penetration (from either skull fragments or foreign objects)
- The location and severity of the impact, as well as the depth and amount of brain penetration, likely have a significant impact on the patient's outcome
- Any penetration of the brain's fragile structure can mechanically tear apart neurons and shear their axons to disrupt neuronal circuitry as well as damage the vasculature, allowing movement of blood and leukocytes into the normally immune privileged brain

- These effects have an immediate impact on the brain by
  - Inducing necrotic cell loss
  - Inducing apoptosis of the surrounding cells
  - Local inflammatory response occurs within minutes of these changes
  - Astrocytes and microglia secrete proinflammatory cytokines, such as tumor necrosis factor, interleukin-6, and interleukin-1b, into the perilesional region
  - Proinflammatory cytokines mobilize immune and glial cells to the injury site, causing edema and further inflammation
  - This phase is associated with gliosis, demyelination, and continued apoptosis
  - Simultaneously, the cerebral vasculature is also undergoing further changes
    ○ Hypoperfusion may occur acutely after injury
    ○ Likely caused by reduced blood pressure, impaired vasodilation (vascular reactivity), and elevated intracranial pressure
  - Over the next few days, this may be followed by hyperemia, after which hypoperfusion may return and be accompanied by vasospasms
  - There may also be a reduction in the cerebral metabolic rate for oxygen suggesting impairments in energy metabolism

Pathophysiology of Blast Induced Trauma (bTBI)
- The blast wave caused by an explosion may interact with the brain in several ways:
  - The kinetic energy passes through the skull, directly inducing acceleration or rotation of the brain, which causes diffuse axonal injury and subsequent secondary injury mechanisms
  - The type of axonal injury caused by a blast is unique to bTBI
    ○ Diffusion tensor imaging of military service members following brain injury indicates the axonal damage from bTBI is more widespread and spatially variable compared with non-blast civilian TBI and includes brain regions such as the superior corona radiata of the frontal cortex, the cerebellum, and optic tracts
  - bTBI-induced axonal damage may need to be considered a separate type of diffuse axonal injury
- The secondary mechanisms of injury produced from a bTBI
  - Appear to be similar to non-blast TBI
  - A robust inflammatory response occurs that includes increased proinflammatory cytokines expression and glial reactivity
- In addition
  - Edema and vasospasms are also far more prevalent following bTBI
    ○ Due to narrowing of primary arteries
    ○ Reduced vascular integrity following a blast injury
- The blast wave may also act indirectly through two possible mechanisms
  - First, the blast may cause gas-containing compartments in the brain to compress, and subsequently expand, leading to damage of surrounding tissues
  - Second, the blast wave may also cause shock waves in the blood or cerebrospinal fluid to be delivered to the brain within seconds of the impact
    ○ This shock wave can lead to an acceleration of the elements of the tissue from their resting state to a rate dependent on the density of the medium, which may subsequently cause deformation and/or rupture of the affected brain tissue

48.10 Treatment and Prognosis

Treatment
- Emergency treatment
  - Intubation
  - Hyperventilation

48.10 Treatment and Prognosis

- Rapid intravenous administration of mannitol (i.e., 1 g/kg)
- Hypertonic saline solution
- Surgery
- Post-surgical treatment
  - Observation in the intensive care unit
  - Placement of an ICP monitor
    - Elevated ICP > 20 mmHg
    - Ventricular drainage
    - Mannitol (0.25–0.50 g/kg)
    - Hyperventilation (PCO_2 30–35 mmHg)
  - Cerebral perfusion pressure management
  - Head elevation (range 30°)

Outcome

- Outcome depends on:
  - Glasgow Outcome Scale (Table 48.5)
  - Gene polymorphisms (Table 48.6)
- Severe TBI majority of patients
  - Disability
  - Death
  - Mortality of 30%
- Mild moderate TBI
  - Physical disabilities
  - Neuropsychological disabilities
  - 10–20% coma
  - 10% severe morbidity to death

Table 48.5 Glasgow Outcome Scale (GOS) and the Extended Glasgow Outcome Scale (GOSE), modified after Gardner and Zafonte (2016) reproduced with kind permission from Elsevier

Glasgow Outcome Scale			Extended Glasgow Outcome Scale	
Score	Outcome	Definition	Score	Outcome
1	Dead	Dead	1	Dead (D)
2	Persistent vegetative state	Wakefulness without awareness	2	Vegetative state (VS)
3	Severe disability	Conscious but dependent	3	Lower severe disability (SD−)
4	Moderate disability	Independent but disabled	4	Upper severe disability (SD+)
5	Good recovery	Fully integrated into society (may have nondisabling sequelae)	5	Lower moderate disability (MD−)
			6	Upper moderate disability (MD+)
			7	Lower good recovery (GR−)
			8	Upper good recovery (GR+)

Table 48.6 Genes affecting outcome after traumatic brain injury, modified after McAllister (2015) reproduced with kind permission by Elsevier

Gene	Domain affected	Polymorphism	Functional mechanism
Response to neurotrauma			
TP53	Initiation of apoptosis	G/C (arg to pro) at codon 72	Arg allele more efficient initiator of apoptosis
BCL-2	Modulation of apoptosis	rs17759659	Unknown
PARP-1	Modulation of apoptosis	rs3219119, rs2771347	Rs3219119 is tag SNP spanning catalytic domain rs2771347 associated with activity and is tag SNP spanning promoter region
Angiotensin converting enzyme gene	Effect on vascular response to trauma	Insertion/deletion in intron 16	Alters circulating levels of ACE (higher in D/D)
Nitric oxide synthase (NOS3)	Vascular response to trauma	−786C variant	Unknown

(continued)

Table 48.6 (continued)

Gene	Domain affected	Polymorphism	Functional mechanism
Calcium channel subunit gene (CACNA1A)	Calcium influx into cell	C/T substitution at codon 218 (serine to leucine switch)	Alters configuration of Ca++ pore forming component
NGB	Resilience to hypoxia/ischemia	Tag SNP rs3783988	Unknown Ngb may facilitate oxygen transfer across BBB
Interleukin-1b (proinflammatory cytokine)	Inflammatory response	Restriction site at position +3953 exon 5	Not known—presumed effect on degree of inflammatory response
Interleukin-6 (proinflammatory cytokine)	Inflammatory response	G/C SNP in promoter region (position 174)	G allele associated with increased production of IL-6
Repair and plasticity			
Brain-derived neurotrophic factor (BDNF)	Repair and plasticity	G/A SNP in promoter region (codon 66). Results in val to met switch	Met allele associated with abnormal storage and secretion of BDNF
Apolipoprotein E	Repair	Three major alleles: e2, e3, e4 differ in amino acids at positions 112 and 158. Also several polymorphisms in the promoter region	Mechanism of allele effect for this gene is not known
Pre- and postinjury cognitive capacity and reserve			
Dopamine D2 receptor region DRD2 and ANKK1	Catecholamine receptors	Numerous polymorphisms in this region. Unclear how many are functional	Rs1800497 associated with reduced expression of D2 receptors in striatum
Dopamine transporter (DAT)	Catecholamine transporters	40 base pair variable number tandem repeat (VNTR)	Different alleles impact on expression of DAT
Catechol-O-methyl transferase (COMT)	Catecholamine metabolism	G/A SNP (val158met) resulting in Met/Val switch at position 472	Met allele less efficient in metabolizing DA
Dopamine b-hydroxylase (DBH)	Catecholamine synthesis	Functional polymorphism affects gene transcription	Not known
Monoamine oxidase-A (MAO-A)	Monoamine oxidase	VNTR	2, 3, and 5 repeats associated with lower transcriptional activity

Selected References

Algattas H, Huang JH (2013) Traumatic brain injury pathophysiology and treatments: early, intermediate, and late phases post-injury. Int J Mol Sci 15(1):309–341. https://doi.org/10.3390/ijms15010309

Armstrong RA, McKee AC, Alvarez VE, Cairns NJ (2017) Clustering of tau-immunoreactive pathology in chronic traumatic encephalopathy. J Neural Transm (Vienna) 124(2):185–192. https://doi.org/10.1007/s00702-016-1635-1

Bauer D, Tung ML, Tsao JW (2015) Mechanisms of traumatic brain injury. Semin Neurol 35(1):e14–e22. https://doi.org/10.1055/s-0035-1549095

Baugh CM, Stamm JM, Riley DO, Gavett BE, Shenton ME, Lin A, Nowinski CJ, Cantu RC, McKee AC, Stern RA (2012) Chronic traumatic encephalopathy: neurodegeneration following repetitive concussive and subconcussive brain trauma. Brain Imaging Behav 6(2):244–254. https://doi.org/10.1007/s11682-012-9164-5

Besenski N (2002) Traumatic injuries: imaging of head injuries. Eur Radiol 12(6):1237–1252. https://doi.org/10.1007/s00330-002-1355-9

Blennow K, Brody DL, Kochanek PM, Levin H, McKee A, Ribbers GM, Yaffe K, Zetterberg H (2016) Traumatic brain injuries. Nat Rev Dis Primers 2:16084. https://doi.org/10.1038/nrdp.2016.84

Braun M, Vaibhav K, Saad NM, Fatima S, Vender JR, Baban B, Hoda MN, Dhandapani KM (2017) White matter damage after traumatic brain injury: a role for damage associated molecular patterns. Biochim Biophys Acta. https://doi.org/10.1016/j.bbadis.2017.05.020

Selected References

Byrnes KR, Wilson CM, Brabazon F, von Leden R, Jurgens JS, Oakes TR, Selwyn RG (2014) FDG-PET imaging in mild traumatic brain injury: a critical review. Front Neuroenerg 5:13. https://doi.org/10.3389/fnene.2013.00013

Castellani RJ (2015) Chronic traumatic encephalopathy: a paradigm in search of evidence? Lab Invest 95(6):576–584. https://doi.org/10.1038/labinvest.2015.54

Croall I, Smith FE, Blamire AM (2015) Magnetic resonance spectroscopy for traumatic brain injury. Top Magn Reson Imaging 24(5):267–274. https://doi.org/10.1097/rmr.0000000000000063

Cruz-Haces M, Tang J, Acosta G, Fernandez J, Shi R (2017) Pathological correlations between traumatic brain injury and chronic neurodegenerative diseases. Transl Neurodegener 6:20. https://doi.org/10.1186/s40035-017-0088-2

Dixon KJ (2017) Pathophysiology of traumatic brain injury. Phys Med Rehabil Clin N Am 28(2):215–225. https://doi.org/10.1016/j.pmr.2016.12.001

Donat CK, Scott G, Gentleman SM, Sastre M (2017) Microglial activation in traumatic brain injury. Transl Neurodegener 9:208. https://doi.org/10.3389/fnagi.2017.00208

Eme R (2017) Neurobehavioral outcomes of mild traumatic brain injury: a mini review. Brain Sci 7(5). https://doi.org/10.3390/brainsci7050046

Feinberg M, Mai JC, Ecklund J (2015) Neurosurgical management in traumatic brain injury. Semin Neurol 35(1):50–56. https://doi.org/10.1055/s-0035-1544244

Gandy S, DeKosky ST (2014) [18F]-T807 tauopathy PET imaging in chronic traumatic encephalopathy. F1000Res 3:229. https://doi.org/10.12688/f1000research.5372.1

Gardner AJ, Zafonte R (2016) Neuroepidemiology of traumatic brain injury. Handb Clin Neurol 138:207–223. https://doi.org/10.1016/b978-0-12-802973-2.00012-4

Hannawi Y, Stevens RD (2016) Mapping the connectome following traumatic brain injury. Curr Neurol Neurosci Rep 16(5):44. https://doi.org/10.1007/s11910-016-0642-9

Hay J, Johnson VE, Smith DH, Stewart W (2016) Chronic traumatic encephalopathy: the neuropathological legacy of traumatic brain injury. Annu Rev Pathol 11:21–45. https://doi.org/10.1146/annurev-pathol-012615-044116

Hayes JP, Bigler ED, Verfaellie M (2016) Traumatic brain injury as a disorder of brain connectivity. Neural Regen Res 22(2):120–137. https://doi.org/10.1017/s1355617715000740

Holleran L, Kim JH, Gangolli M, Stein T, Alvarez V, McKee A, Brody DL (2017) Axonal disruption in white matter underlying cortical sulcus tau pathology in chronic traumatic encephalopathy. Acta Neuropathol 133(3):367–380. https://doi.org/10.1007/s00401-017-1686-x

Hutchinson EB, Schwerin SC, Avram AV, Juliano SL, Pierpaoli C (2017) Diffusion MRI and the detection of alterations following traumatic brain injury. J Neurosci Res. https://doi.org/10.1002/jnr.24065

Irimia A, Van Horn JD (2015) Functional neuroimaging of traumatic brain injury: advances and clinical utility. Neuropsychiatr Dis Treat 11:2355–2365. https://doi.org/10.2147/ndt.s79174

Iverson GL, Gardner AJ, McCrory P, Zafonte R, Castellani RJ (2015) A critical review of chronic traumatic encephalopathy. Neurosci Biobehav Rev 56:276–293. https://doi.org/10.1016/j.neubiorev.2015.05.008

Joseph B, Khan M, Rhee P (2017) Non-invasive diagnosis and treatment strategies for traumatic brain injury: an update. J Neurosci Res. https://doi.org/10.1002/jnr.24132

Karve IP, Taylor JM, Crack PJ (2016) The contribution of astrocytes and microglia to traumatic brain injury. Br J Pharmacol 173(4):692–702. https://doi.org/10.1111/bph.13125

Kazam JJ, Tsiouris AJ (2015) Brain magnetic resonance imaging for traumatic brain injury: why, when, and how? Top Magn Reson Imaging 24(5):225–239. https://doi.org/10.1097/rmr.0000000000000061

Khong E, Odenwald N, Hashim E, Cusimano MD (2016) Diffusion tensor imaging findings in post-concussion syndrome patients after mild traumatic brain injury: a systematic review. Front Neurol 7:156. https://doi.org/10.3389/fneur.2016.00156

Kowall NW, Ryu H, McKee AC, Willis MD, Robertson NP (2017) Chronic traumatic encephalopathy: identifying those at risk and understanding pathogenesis. Exp Mol Med 264(6):1298–1300. https://doi.org/10.1007/s00415-017-8508-x

Lenihan MW, Jordan BD (2015) The clinical presentation of chronic traumatic encephalopathy. Curr Neurol Neurosci Rep 15(5):23. https://doi.org/10.1007/s11910-015-0541-5

Ling H, Neal JW, Revesz T (2017) Evolving concepts of chronic traumatic encephalopathy as a neuropathological entity. Neuropathol Appl Neurobiol. https://doi.org/10.1111/nan.12425

Lipsky RH, Lin M (2015) Genetic predictors of outcome following traumatic brain injury. Handb Clin Neurol 127:23–41. https://doi.org/10.1016/b978-0-444-52892-6.00003-9

Liu J, Kou Z, Tian Y (2014) Diffuse axonal injury after traumatic cerebral microbleeds: an evaluation of imaging techniques. Neural Regen Res 9(12):1222–1230. https://doi.org/10.4103/1673-5374.135330

Lu C, Xia J, Bin W, Wu Y, Liu X, Zhang Y (2015) Advances in diagnosis, treatments, and molecular mechanistic studies of traumatic brain injury. Biosci Trends 9(3):138–148. https://doi.org/10.5582/bst.2015.01066

Mahar I, Alosco ML, McKee AC (2017) Psychiatric phenotypes in chronic traumatic encephalopathy. Neurosci Biobehav Rev. https://doi.org/10.1016/j.neubiorev.2017.08.023

Mayer AR, Quinn DK, Master CL (2017) The spectrum of mild traumatic brain injury: a review. Neurology 89(6):623–632. https://doi.org/10.1212/wnl.0000000000004214

McAllister TW (2015) Genetic factors in traumatic brain injury. Handb Clin Neurol 128:723–739. https://doi.org/10.1016/b978-0-444-63521-1.00045-5

McGinn MJ, Povlishock JT (2016) Pathophysiology of traumatic brain injury. Neurosurg Clin N Am 27(4):397–407. https://doi.org/10.1016/j.nec.2016.06.002

McKee AC, Daneshvar DH (2015) The neuropathology of traumatic brain injury. Handb Clin Neurol 127:45–66. https://doi.org/10.1016/b978-0-444-52892-6.00004-0

McKee AC, Stern RA, Nowinski CJ, Stein TD, Alvarez VE, Daneshvar DH, Lee HS, Wojtowicz SM, Hall G, Baugh CM, Riley DO, Kubilus CA, Cormier KA, Jacobs MA, Martin BR, Abraham CR, Ikezu T, Reichard RR, Wolozin BL, Budson AE, Goldstein LE, Kowall NW, Cantu RC (2013) The spectrum of disease in chronic traumatic encephalopathy. Brain 136(Pt 1):43–64. https://doi.org/10.1093/brain/aws307

McKee AC, Stein TD, Kiernan PT, Alvarez VE (2015) The neuropathology of chronic traumatic encephalopathy. Brain Pathol 25(3):350–364. https://doi.org/10.1111/bpa.12248

McKee AC, Alosco ML, Huber BR (2016) Repetitive head impacts and chronic traumatic encephalopathy. Neurosurg Clin N Am 27(4):529–535. https://doi.org/10.1016/j.nec.2016.05.009

Medaglia JD (2017) Functional neuroimaging in traumatic brain injury: from nodes to networks. Front Neurol 8:407. https://doi.org/10.3389/fneur.2017.00407

Mez J, Solomon TM, Daneshvar DH, Murphy L, Kiernan PT, Montenigro PH, Kriegel J, Abdolmohammadi B, Fry B, Babcock KJ, Adams JW, Bourlas AP, Papadopoulos Z, McHale L, Ardaugh BM, Martin BR, Dixon D, Nowinski CJ, Chaisson C, Alvarez VE, Tripodis Y, Stein TD, Goldstein LE, Katz DI, Kowall NW, Cantu RC, Stern RA, McKee AC (2015) Assessing clinicopathological correlation in chronic traumatic encephalopathy: rationale and methods for the UNITE study. Alzheimers Res Ther 7(1):62. https://doi.org/10.1186/s13195-015-0148-8

Mez J, Daneshvar DH, Kiernan PT, Abdolmohammadi B, Alvarez VE, Huber BR, Alosco ML, Solomon TM, Nowinski CJ, McHale L, Cormier KA, Kubilus CA, Martin BM, Murphy L, Baugh CM, Montenigro PH, Chaisson CE, Tripodis Y, Kowall NW, Weuve J, McClean MD, Cantu RC, Goldstein LE, Katz DI, Stern RA, Stein TD, McKee AC (2017) Clinicopathological evaluation of chronic traumatic encephalopathy in players of American football. JAMA 318(4):360–370. https://doi.org/10.1001/jama.2017.8334

Munakomi S, Cherian I (2017) Newer insights to pathogenesis of traumatic brain injury. Asian J Neurosurg 12(3):362–364. https://doi.org/10.4103/1793-5482.180882

Mutch CA, Talbott JF, Gean A (2016) Imaging evaluation of acute traumatic brain injury. Neurosurg Clin N Am 27(4):409–439. https://doi.org/10.1016/j.nec.2016.05.011

Posti JP, Dickens AM, Oresic M, Hyotylainen T, Tenovuo O (2017) Metabolomics profiling as a diagnostic tool in severe traumatic brain injury. Front Neurol 8:398. https://doi.org/10.3389/fneur.2017.00398

Seo JS, Lee S, Shin JY, Hwang YJ, Cho H, Yoo SK, Kim Y, Lim S, Kim YK, Hwang EM, Kim SH, Kim CH, Hyeon SJ, Yun JY, Kim J, Kim Y, Alvarez VE, Stein TD, Lee J, Kim DJ, Kim JI (2017) Transcriptome analyses of chronic traumatic encephalopathy show alterations in protein phosphatase expression associated with tauopathy. Exp Mol Med 49(5):e333. https://doi.org/10.1038/emm.2017.56

Shetty T, Raince A, Manning E, Tsiouris AJ (2016) Imaging in chronic traumatic encephalopathy and traumatic brain injury. Sports Health 8(1):26–36. https://doi.org/10.1177/1941738115588745

Shin SS, Bales JW, Edward Dixon C, Hwang M (2017) Structural imaging of mild traumatic brain injury may not be enough: overview of functional and metabolic imaging of mild traumatic brain injury. Brain Imaging Behav 11(2):591–610. https://doi.org/10.1007/s11682-017-9684-0

Teasdale G, Jennett B (1974) Assessment of coma and impaired consciousness. A practical scale. Lancet 2(7872):81–84

Teasdale G, Murray G, Parker L, Jennett B (1979) Adding up the Glasgow Coma Score. Acta Neurochir Suppl 28(1):13–16

Teasdale G, Maas A, Lecky F, Manley G, Stocchetti N, Murray G (2014) The Glasgow Coma Scale at 40 years: standing the test of time. Lancet Neurol 13(8):844–854. https://doi.org/10.1016/s1474-4422(14)70120-6

Vile AR, Atkinson L (2017) Chronic traumatic encephalopathy: the cellular sequela to repetitive brain injury. J Clin Neurosci 41:24–29. https://doi.org/10.1016/j.jocn.2017.03.035

Wintermark M, Coombs L, Druzgal TJ, Field AS, Filippi CG, Hicks R, Horton R, Lui YW, Law M, Mukherjee P, Norbash A, Riedy G, Sanelli PC, Stone JR, Sze G, Tilkin M, Whitlow CT, Wilde EA, York G, Provenzale JM (2015) Traumatic brain injury imaging research roadmap. AJNR Am J Neuroradiol 36(3):E12–E23. https://doi.org/10.3174/ajnr.A4254

Xiao H, Yang Y, Xi JH, Chen ZQ (2015) Structural and functional connectivity in traumatic brain injury. Neural Regen Res 10(12):2062–2071. https://doi.org/10.4103/1673-5374.172328

Xiong KL, Zhu YS, Zhang WG (2014) Diffusion tensor imaging and magnetic resonance spectroscopy in traumatic brain injury: a review of recent literature. Brain Imaging Behav 8(4):487–496. https://doi.org/10.1007/s11682-013-9288-2

Intoxication: Alcohol

49.1 Introduction

Alcohol abuse and dependence are serious medical and economic problems in the Western countries. The effects of alcohol on the central nervous system (CNS) are wide ranging. Direct toxicity of ethanol and its first metabolite acetaldehyde alters first basic physiological and neurochemical functions, which ultimately result in structural damage (Büttner and Weis 2008).

49.2 Ethanol: Acute and Chronic Alcoholism

49.2.1 Clinical Signs and Symptoms

- Acute and chronic alcohol abuse
- Neurologic and psychiatric complications
  - Ocular, motor, sensory, autonomic
  - Memory and cognitive defects (progressing to dementia)
  - Hallucinations
  - Stupor, coma
- Cognitive dysfunction
  - Personality and behavioral changes
  - Disinhibition
  - Social and personal neglect
  - Lack of insight
  - Lack of empathy
  - Lack of emotional control

49.2.2 Epidemiology

Incidence
- 86.4% of people aged 18 or older drank alcohol at some point in their lifetime
- 70.1% drank in the past year
- 56.0% drank in the past month
- 26.9% of people aged 18 or older engaged in binge drinking in the past month
- 7.0% engaged in heavy alcohol use in the past month
- 6.2% of people aged 18 had alcohol use disorder (AUD)
  - Men: 8.4%
  - Women: 4.2%
- Eighty eight thousand people (approximately 62,000 men and 26,000 women) die from alcohol-related causes annually, making alcohol the third leading preventable cause of death in the United States
- Alcohol-impaired driving fatalities account for 31% of overall driving fatalities

Age Incidence
- Under age 18
- All age classes
  - Men: the prevalence rate of lifetime alcohol use is highest among those aged 25–55 and lowest among the 18–24 and 55 or older age groups

Sex Incidence
- Male:Female ratio: 2:1

Localization
- Corpora mammillaria
- Cerebral cortex
  - Frontal cortex
- White matter
- Cerebellar vermis
- Corpus callosum

49.2.3 Neuroimaging Findings

General Imaging Findings
- Generalized brain atrophy, atrophy of superior vermis

CT Non-Contrast-Enhanced
- Brain atrophy, especially of superior vermis

CT Contrast-Enhanced
- No enhancement

MRI-T2/FLAIR/T1 (Fig. 49.1a–g)
- Generalized brain atrophy
- Atrophy of the superior cerebellar vermis
- Non-specific white matter lesions

MRI-T1 Contrast-Enhanced
- No enhancement

MR-Spectroscopy
- Low NAA/Cr and Cho/Cr in frontal lobes and cerebellum (reversible)

Nuclear Medicine Imaging Findings (Fig. 49.2)
- SPECT and PET studies with β-CIT, FPCIT, raclopride, and (desmethoxy) fallypride have been performed for assessing the pre- and postsynaptic dopaminergic system, revealing lower striatal tracer bindings in patients abusing alcohol.
- After withdrawal DAT binding levels are increasing (in the first few days rapidly) with a return to control levels after 4 weeks. D2 receptors are improving after withdrawal of alcohol too.
- CBF-SPECT and FDG-PET show a global reduction of perfusion as well as glucose metabolism in patients consuming alcohol at low alcohol levels and regional effects (i.e., the inferior parietal region) have been described.
- It has to be mentioned that
  - Other diseases with reduction of CBF or glucose metabolism have to be taken into account
  - Alcohol consumption can mimic changes due to other diseases

49.2.4 Neuropathology Findings

Macroscopic Findings
- Signs of atrophy which resolve after abstinence
- Reduced volume of the white matter, frontal lobes
- Reduced brain weight and volume
  - Brain atrophy is due to a reduction in the volume of the white matter
- These abnormalities may be reversed by abstinence from alcohol
- Affected regions
  - The frontal lobes are more seriously affected than other cortical regions
  - The superior frontal association cortex is mostly affected
    - Disruption of fronto-cerebellar circuitry and function
- A significant thinning of the corpus callosum was detected in older alcoholics

Microscopic Findings
- Neuronal loss
  - Especially in the frontal association cortex
  - Diencephalon (especially in patients with Wernicke–Korsakoff syndrome)
  - Cerebellum including loss of Purkinje cells and cells of the molecular layer
  - Contradictory data on neuronal loss in the hippocampus of chronic alcoholics
    - An early neuronal loss
    - No significant neuronal loss in any sub-region of the hippocampus, despite a significant reduction in hippocampal

volume which occurred exclusively in the white matter
- No significant neuronal dropout was reported for
  - The temporal cortex or motor cortex
  - The basal ganglia
  - Nucleus basalis of Meynert
- Number of serotonergic neurons
  - Reduced in the brain stem
  - Not reduced in the raphe nuclei
  - No reduction of pigmented cells in the locus coeruleus

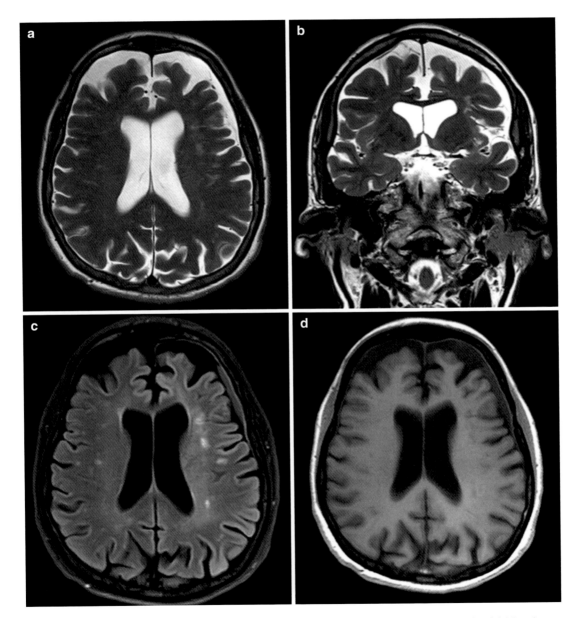

Fig. 49.1 Sixty-year-old female patient with chronic alcohol abuse; generalized brain atrophy—T2 axial (**a**) and coronal (**b**), FLAIR (**c**), T1 (**d**); atrophy of cerebellum (especially of superior vermis, →)—T2 (**e**), T1 (**f**), T1 sagittal (**g**)

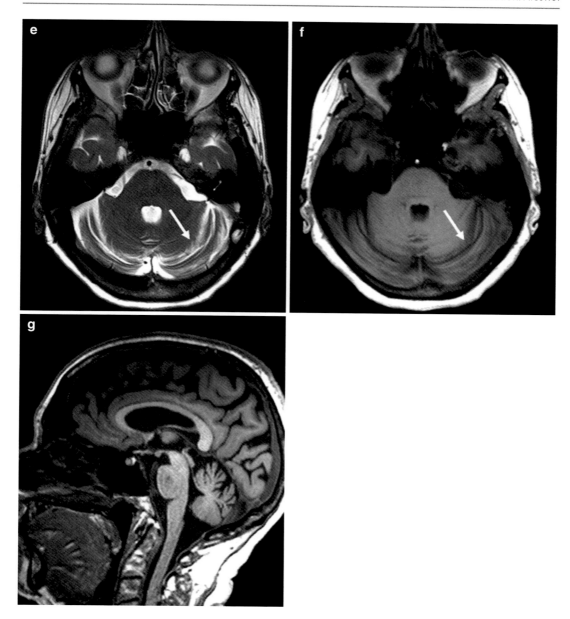

Fig. 49.1 (continued)

- Reactive astrogliosis
  - Enlargement of their cell bodies
  - Beading of the cellular processes
  - Significant loss of glial cells (astrocytes and oligodendrocytes, to a lesser degree microglial cells) was found globally in the hippocampus
  - Increased cytochrome P4502E1 and induced oxidative stress in astrocytes

- Alzheimer II astroglial (Fig. 49.3a–d)
  - A large, round, lobulated or crescent-shaped vesicular nucleus
  - Scant chromatin
  - Prominent nucleolus
  - Perikaryon is unstained with eosin
  - Immunonegative for GFAP and positive for S100

49.2 Ethanol: Acute and Chronic Alcoholism

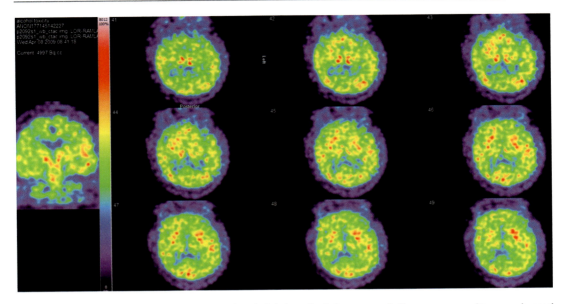

Fig. 49.2 FDG-PET showing a significantly reduced global cerebral glucose metabolism as compared to an unchanged striatal uptake

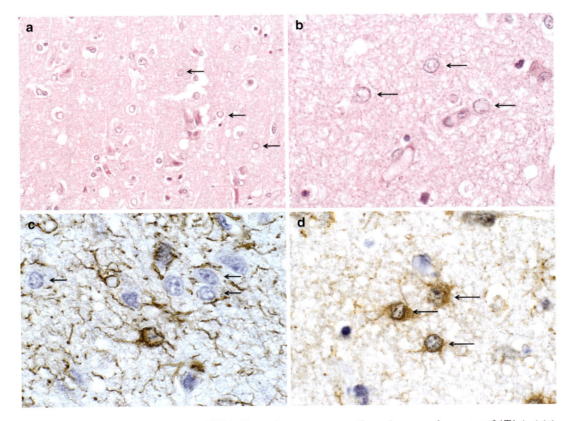

Fig. 49.3 Alzheimer Type II astrocytes (ATA): Tissue shows some spongiform changes and presence of ATA (→) (**a**), three ATA at higher magnification (**b**), GFAP-negative ATA (→) (**c**), S-100 positive ATA (→) (**d**)

- Affects microglial cell development and function
- There is also proliferation of Bergmann glia
- Dendritic alterations
- Synaptic loss in the superior layers of frontal Brodmann area 10
- An alcohol-induced degeneration of myelinated fibers in the white matter could not be demonstrated
- At the cellular level, alcohol affects the action of glutamate, gamma-aminobutyric acid (GABA), and other neurotransmitters

49.3 Wernicke–Korsakoff Encephalopathy

The Wernicke–Korsakoff syndrome (WKS) is one of the most frequently seen neurological disorders associated with long-term and heavy alcohol abuse (Victor et al. 1971).

49.3.1 Clinical Signs

- Acute or subacute onset
- Ocular alterations consist of:
  - Retinal hemorrhage
  - Pupillary changes
  - Extra-ocular muscle palsy
  - Gaze palsy
  - Nystagmus
  - The site of pathology is the tegmentum of the brainstem
- Autonomic changes include:
  - Hypo- or hypertension
  - Hypo- or hyperthermia
  - Cardiac arrhythmias
  - Respiratory failure
  - The site of pathology is the hypothalamus and the dorsal nucleus of the vagus
- Depression of consciousness
  - Reduced alertness from obtundation
  - Coma may exist
  - The site of pathology is the periaqueductal gray
- Ataxia (vestibular and/or cerebellar dysfunction)
  - The site of pathology is the vestibular region of the medulla and cerebellum

Korsakoff amnestic syndrome is characterized by:

- Impairment of recent memory including verbal and non-verbal material
- Occurs after recovery from Wernicke encephalopathy
- Sites of pathologic changes are the dorsomedial nuclei of the thalamus, mammillary bodies, and relay stations of the limbic lobe

Involved brain regions

- Walls of the third ventricle
- Mammillary bodies (atrophy in chronic cases)
- Dorsomedial nuclei of the thalami
- Periaqueductal gray matter
- Floor of the fourth ventricle

49.3.2 Neuroimaging Findings

General Imaging Findings
- Abnormal signal of mammillary bodies, medial thalamus, and periaqueductal gray

CT Non-Contrast-Enhanced
- Often normal

CT Contrast-Enhanced
- Usually no enhancement

MRI-T2/FLAIR (Fig. 49.4a, b)
- Hyperintensity of medial thalamus, mammillary bodies, and periaqueductal gray

MRI-T1
- Hypointensity of involved brain areas possible

MRI-T1 Contrast-Enhanced (Fig. 49.4d, e)
- Enhancement of mammillary bodies most common
- Enhancement of medial thalamus and periaqueductal gray possible

49.3 Wernicke–Korsakoff Encephalopathy

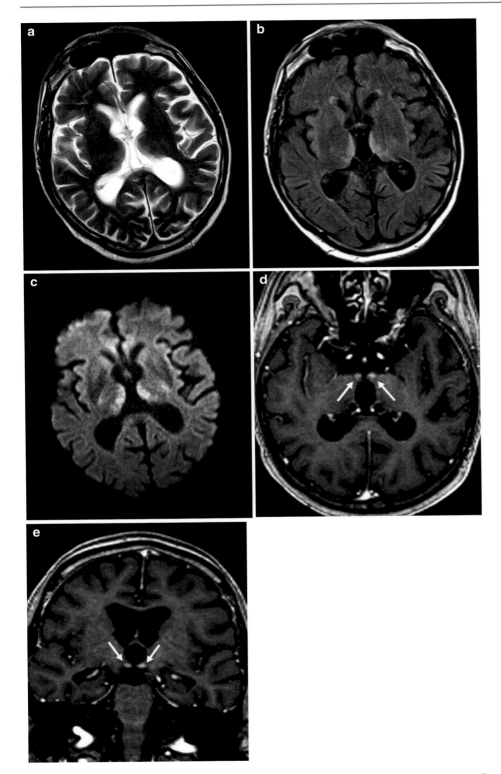

Fig. 49.4 Wernicke encephalopathy: T2-hyperintense signal in medial thalami and enhancement of mammillary bodies (white arrows); T2 (**a**), FLAIR (**b**), DWI (**c**), T1 contrast axial (**d**), and coronal (**e**)

MR-Diffusion Imaging (Fig. 49.4c)
- Restricted diffusion in involved regions possible

49.3.3 Neuropathology Findings

Acute Wernicke–Korsakoff Encephalopathy
- Macroscopic changes:
  - Soft consistency
  - Yellow to brown discoloration of the tissue
- Petechial hemorrhages
  - Around the third and fourth ventricles, medial hypothalamus, thalamus, and periaqueductal gray matter
- Microscopic changes include:
  - Edema
  - Hypertrophy of endothelial cells
  - Extravasation of erythrocytes
  - Reactive astrogliosis
  - No apparent changes in neurons

Chronic Wernicke–Korsakoff Encephalopathy
- Macroscopic changes:
  - Shrinkage and brown discoloration of the mammillary bodies
- Microscopic findings include (Fig. 49.5a–l):
  - Spongiform changes of the tissue
  - Reactive astrogliosis
  - Capillary endothelial hyperplasia
  - Presence of lipid-laden macrophages
  - Hemosiderin-laden macrophages as residues of microhemorrhages
  - Deposition of hemosiderin pigments
  - Fresh pericapillary hemorrhages
  - Endothelial hypertrophy and proliferation
  - Destruction of myelin and axons
  - Relative sparing of neurons

49.3.4 Molecular Neuropathology

- Very complex
- Multifactorial disorder
- Interaction of multiple genes and environment

- Complication of thiamine deficiency
  - Thiamine: cofactor of several enzymes implicated in the glucose metabolism
- No direct toxic effect of alcohol
- The association of vitamin B1 deficiency with intracellular and extracellular edema by glutamate (N-methyl-D-aspartate) receptor-mediated excitotoxicity seems to be an important mechanism

Genetic studies

- Controversial and non-conclusive results
- Candidate genes
  - Thiamine-dependent enzymes
  - Alcohol-metabolizing enzymes
  - GABA receptors
  - Thiamine transporters (SLC19A2 and SLC19A3)

Proteomics

- Each brain region reacts in significantly different manner to chronic alcohol ingestion
- Abnormalities in vitamin B1 (thiamine)-related biochemical pathways
- Significant differences in protein expression profiles
- Ammonia has significant additive influences on brain protein expression

49.4 Cerebellar Degeneration

49.4.1 Clinical Signs

- Cerebellar ataxia
- Slowly progressive ataxia of the trunk and lower extremities
- Broad-based irregular gait

49.4.2 Neuropathology Findings

Macroscopic Findings
- Atrophy of the superior cerebellar vermis
- Might involve the entire vermis as well as the hemisphere

49.4 Cerebellar Degeneration

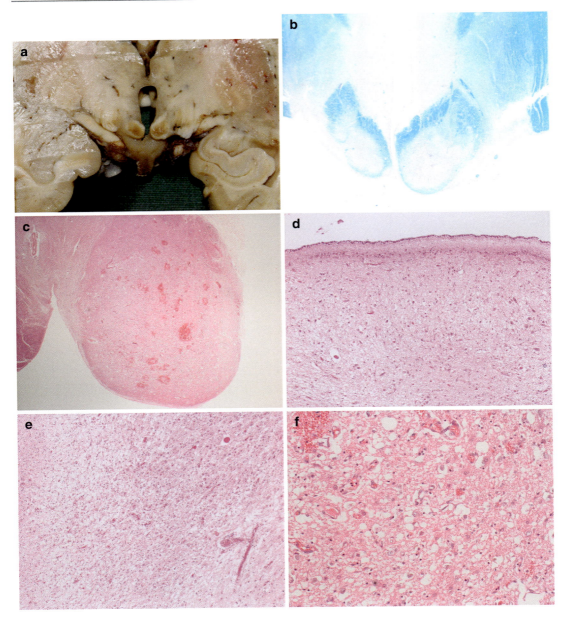

Fig. 49.5 Wernicke encephalopathy: Brown discoloration of the mammillary bodies (**a**), overview of the affected mammillary bodies (**b**) (Stain: LFB), hemorrhages and spongiform changes (**c**) (Stain: H&E), spongiform changes in the periventricular region around the third ventricle (**d**) (Stain: H&E), spongiform changes and neuronal loss (**e**) (Stain: H&E), spongiform changes and neuronal loss (**f**) (Stain: H&E), small hemorrhages (**g**) (Stain: H&E), preserved neurons (**h**) (NeuN), endothelial proliferation (**i**) (Stain. LFB), reactive astrogliosis (**j**) (Immunostain: GFAP), reactive microgliosis (**k**) (Immunostain: HLA-DRII), reactive microgliosis (**l**) (Immunostain: HLA-DRII)

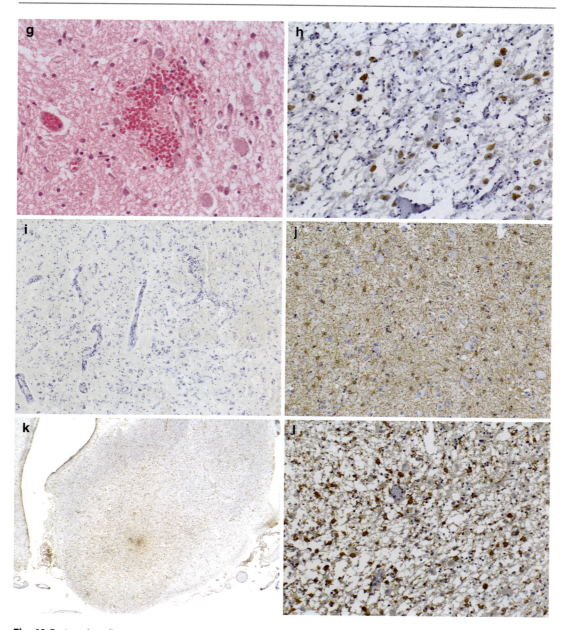

Fig. 49.5 (continued)

Microscopic Findings
- Degeneration of Purkinje cells
- Lesser involvement of the granule cells
- Atrophy of the molecular layer
- Atrophy of the myelin core of the folia
- Prominent layer of Bergmann astrocytes replacing the Purkinje cell layer
- Axonal torpedos of degenerated Purkinje cells found in the granular cell layer
- Inferior olivary nucleus:
  - Neuronal loss resulting from retrograde trans-synaptic degeneration
  - Reactive astrogliosis

49.5 Central Pontine Myelinolysis

Central pontine myelinolysis (CPM), first described by Adams et al. (1959), is a demyelinating disease of the central portion of the base of the pons often associated with demyelination of other brain areas.

49.5.1 Clinical Signs

- Acute onset
- Para-quadriparesis
- Dysarthria
- Dysphagia
- Emotional lability
- Locked-in syndrome
- Seen in:
  - In malnourished chronic alcoholics
  - Liver diseases, liver transplants
  - Severe burns
  - Hyponatremia

49.5.2 Neuroimaging Findings

General Imaging Findings
- Abnormal signal in central pons, extrapontine myelinolysis possible (basal ganglia, midbrain, white matter), often reversible

CT Non-Contrast-Enhanced
- Hypodensity of involved brain areas (central pons, basal ganglia, white matter)

CT Contrast-Enhanced
- Usually no enhancement

MRI-T2/FLAIR (Fig. 49.6a, b)
- Hyperintensity of central pons, periphery not involved
- Hyperintensity of basal ganglia, midbrain, or white matter if extrapontine myelinolysis
- Often reversible

MRI-T1 (Fig. 49.6c)
- Lesions mildly hypointense

MRI-T1 Contrast-Enhanced (Fig. 49.6d)
- Usually no enhancement, sometimes enhancement possible

MRI-T2*/SWI
- Rarely hemorrhagic

MR-Diffusion Imaging (Fig. 49.6e, f)
- Acute: Restricted diffusion ($\uparrow$DWI, $\downarrow$ADC)

49.5.3 Neuropathology Findings

Macroscopic Findings
- Oval or round or butterfly-shaped grayish softened lesion in the center of the pons
- Other regions involved (i.e., extrapontine myelinolysis, EPM) include:
  - Striatum
  - Thalamus
  - Lateral geniculate bodies
  - Cerebral white matter
  - Cerebral cortex
  - Cerebellum

Microscopic Findings (Fig. 49.7a–h)
- Demyelination of fiber tracts (transverse pontine fibers)
- Relatively preserved axons
- Lipid-laden macrophages in acute stage
- Reactive astrocytes in chronic stage
- No inflammatory changes
- Blood vessels are unaffected

49.5.4 Molecular Neuropathology

- Too rapid correction of hyponatremia
- Hyperosmotically induced demyelination process
  - Results from rapid intracellular/extracellular to intravascular water shifts producing relative glial dehydration and myelin degradation
  - Oligodendroglial apoptosis
- The etiology and pathogenesis of myelin loss is still unclear

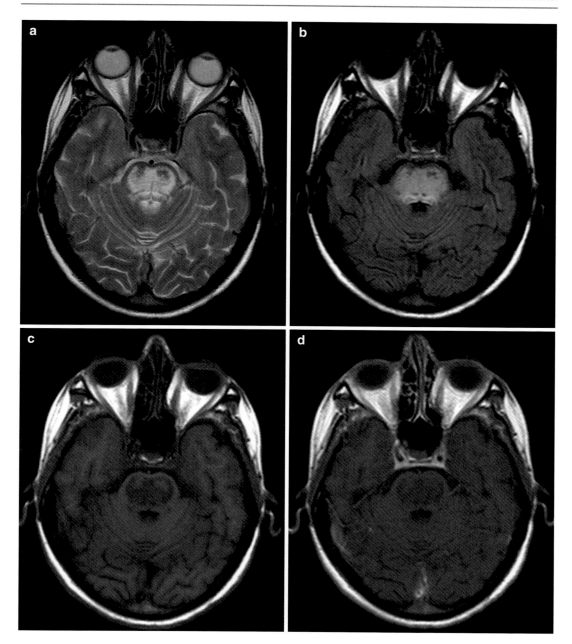

Fig. 49.6 Central pontine myelinolysis: T2 (**a**), FLAIR (**b**), T1 (**c**), T1 contrast (**d**), DWI (**e**), ADC (**f**)

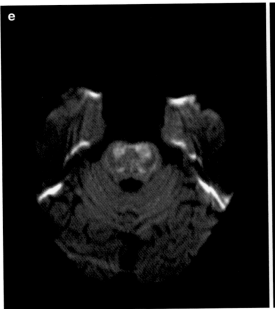 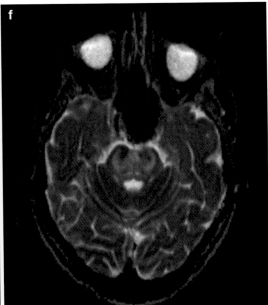

Fig. 49.6 (continued)

49.6 Marchiafava–Bignami Disease

Marchiafava–Bignami disease (MBD) is an extremely rare, severe, and usually fatal neurological disorder associated with chronic alcoholism.

49.6.1 Clinical Signs

- Interhemispheric disconnection syndrome
- Frontal lobe syndrome
- Dementia

49.6.2 Neuroimaging Findings

General Imaging Findings
- Edema of corpus callosum (acute), atrophy of corpus callosum with necrotic foci (chronic)

CT Non-Contrast-Enhanced
- Hypodense callosal lesions
- Atrophy of corpus callosum in chronic stage

CT Contrast-Enhanced
- Usually no enhancement, acute lesions may enhance

MRI-T2/FLAIR (Fig. 49.8a, b)
- Hyperintense lesions in the corpus callosum

MRI-T1 (Fig. 49.8c)
- Hypointense

MRI-T1 Contrast-Enhanced (Fig. 49.8d)
- Usually no enhancement, acute lesions may enhance

MR-Diffusion Imaging (Fig. 49.8e, f)
- Acute: restricted diffusion

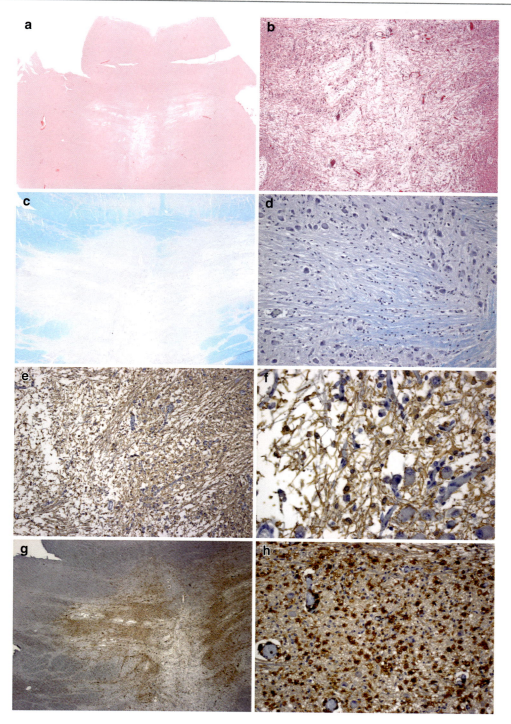

Fig. 49.7 Central pontine myelinolysis. Central softening and loss of the tissue (**a**) (Stain: H&E), central softening and loss of the tissue (**b**) (Stain: H&E, higher magnification), central softening and loss of the tissue (**c**) (Stain: LFB), central softening and loss of the tissue (**d**) (Stain: LFB, higher magnification), reactive astrogliosis (**e**) (Immunostain: GFAP), reactive astrogliosis (**f**) (Immunostain: GFPA, higher magnification), reactive microgliosis (**g**) (Immunostain: HLA-DRII), reactive microgliosis (**h**) (Immunostain: HLA-DR II, higher magnification)

49.6 Marchiafava–Bignami Disease

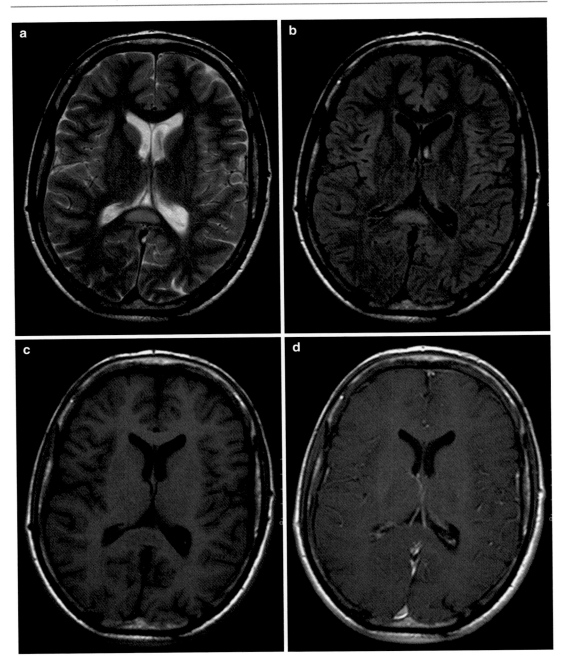

Fig. 49.8 Marchiafava–Bignami disease: Edema and restricted diffusion in the splenium of corpus callosum; T2 (**a**), FLAIR (**b**), T1 (**c**), T1 contrast (**d**), DWI (**e**), ADC (**f**)

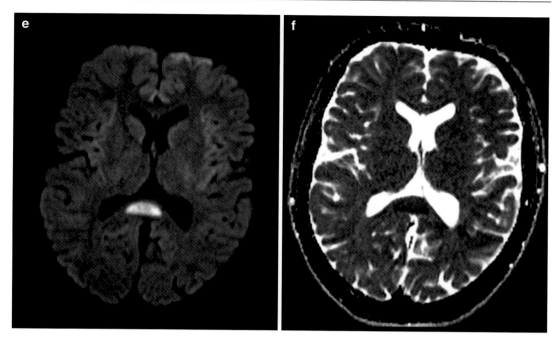

Fig. 49.8 (continued)

49.6.3 Neuropathology Findings

Macroscopic Findings
- Necrotizing, often cystic lesions of the corpus callosum

Microscopic Findings
- Prominent demyelination of the genu and body of the corpus callosum
- Demyelination might extend symmetrically into the centrum semiovale
- Further involvement of
  - Anterior commissure
  - Optic chiasm
  - Middle cerebral peduncles
- Relative sparing of the axons
- Oligodendrocytes are reduced in number
- Numerous lipid-laden macrophages
- Astrocytes with mild reactive changes, but are more prominent in and around necrotizing lesions
- Blood vessels often show proliferation and hyalinization of their walls
- The lesions also affect the corticocortical and cortico-subcortical projections due to disconnection which might cause frontal lobe syndromes and dementia

49.7 Fetal Alcohol Spectrum Disorders (FASD)

Fetal Alcohol Spectrum Disorders (FASD) includes a continuum of disorders that occur in children as a result of their mothers' consumption of alcohol during pregnancy. The most severe of these disorders is Fetal Alcohol Syndrome (FAS).

49.7.1 Clinical Signs

Many individuals with FASD have

- Abnormal facial features
  - Flat nasal bridge
  - Smooth ridge between the nose and upper lip
  - Thin upper lip
  - Extra crease in the outer ears
  - An upturned nose

- Smaller head size
- Low body weight
- Shorter than average height
- Medical issues
  - Vision problems
  - Hearing problems
  - Sleep and sucking problems as a baby
  - Heart, kidneys, or bones
- Cognitive impairments
  - General intellectual function
    ○ Decreased general intellectual functioning
    ○ IQ deficits are similar with and without dysmorphology, and persist into adulthood
  - Learning disabilities
    ○ Verbal learning and memory deficits characterized by encoding and retrieval deficits with spared retention
    ○ Deficits in non-verbal, facial, and object and spatial memory
  - Executive function
    ○ Executive dysfunction, including planning, set shifting, cognitive flexibility, mental manipulation, working memory, and reasoning deficits. Deficits exist after controlling for IQ and regardless of facial dysmorphology
    ○ Response inhibition deficits
  - Cognitive processing speed and attention
    ○ Impaired processing speed, particularly within the context of complex cognition and less apparent in automatic processing
    ○ Impaired vigilance, reaction time, organizing and maintaining attention, and information processing
    ○ Some studies report poorer visual compared to auditory attention
  - Problems following directions
  - Difficulty understanding the consequences of their actions
  - Poor memory skills
  - Hyperactive behavior
  - Inattentiveness
  - Poor reasoning skills
  - Language
    ○ Dysarthria, lisping, and articulation difficulties
    ○ Expressive and receptive language deficits
    ○ Impaired phonologic processing
  - Behavioral characteristics
    ○ Problem behaviors
      • Elevated externalizing and internalizing behaviors
      • Higher rates of delinquent behavior
      • Impaired moral decision making and more likely to lie about behavior
      • Higher rates of legal issues, substance abuse, and suicide attempts
    ○ Psychopathology
      • High rate of concomitant attention-deficit hyperactivity disorder, psychiatric diagnoses, and secondary disabilities
    ○ Social skills and communication
      • Diminished interpersonal and social skills
      • Poor ability to balance linguistic and social-cognitive demands
      • Failure to provide information in narrative communication and consider perspective
  - Academic achievement
    ○ Academic achievement impaired beyond diminished
    ○ Impaired math, reading, and spelling
    ○ High rate of learning disabilities

49.7.2 Neuropathology Findings

Morphological Changes
- Facial abnormalities
- Growth retardation
- Microencephaly
- Neural tube defects
- Cerebellar dysgenesis
- Neuroglial heterotopia

49.7.3 Molecular Neuropathology

- Cause-effect relationship cannot be determined
- Not a monotoxic disorder
- Malnutrition
- Vitamin deficiencies
  - Thiamine (vitamin B1)
- Metabolic disturbances
  - Hepatic
- Direct toxic effect of alcohol on nervous tissue
- List of gene-ethanol interactions
  - *ADH1B*
  - *ADH1C*
  - *MLLT3*
  - *SMC2*
  - *Aldh2*
  - *Fancd2*
  - *Cdon*
  - *Gli2*
  - *Shh*
  - *Nos1*
  - *hinfp*
  - *foxi1*
  - *mars*
  - *plk1*
  - *vangl2*

Selected References

Adams RD, Victor M, Mancall EL (1959) Central pontine myelinolysis: a hitherto undescribed disease occurring in alcoholic and malnourished patients. AMA Arch Neurol Psychiatry 81(2):154–172

Alfonso-Loeches S, Guerri C (2011) Molecular and behavioral aspects of the actions of alcohol on the adult and developing brain. Crit Rev Clin Lab Sci 48(1):19–47. https://doi.org/10.3109/10408363.2011.580567

Ba A (2017) Alcohol and thiamine deficiency trigger differential mitochondrial transition pore opening mediating cellular death. Apoptosis 22(6):741–752. https://doi.org/10.1007/s10495-017-1372-4

Bengochea O, Gonzalo LM (1990) Effect of chronic alcoholism on the human hippocampus. Histol Histopathol 5(3):349–357

Brown WD (2000) Osmotic demyelination disorders: central pontine and extrapontine myelinolysis. Curr Opin Neurol 13(6):691–697

Brun A, Andersson J (2001) Frontal dysfunction and frontal cortical synapse loss in alcoholism—the main cause of alcohol dementia? Dement Geriatr Cogn Disord 12(4):289–294. https://doi.org/10.1159/000051271

Büttner A, Weis S (2008) Central nervous system alterations in alcohol abuse. In: Tsokos M (ed) Forensic pathology, vol 5. Humana Press, Totowa, NJ, pp 69–89

Chastain LG, Sarkar DK (2014) Role of microglia in regulation of ethanol neurotoxic action. Int Rev Neurobiol 118:81–103. https://doi.org/10.1016/b978-0-12-801284-0.00004-x

Clarke R, Adermark L (2015) Dopaminergic regulation of striatal interneurons in reward and addiction: focus on alcohol. Neural Plast 2015:814567. https://doi.org/10.1155/2015/814567

Cullen KM, Halliday GM (1994) Chronic alcoholics have substantial glial pathology in the forebrain and diencephalon. Alcohol Alcohol Suppl 2:253–257

Del Campo M, Jones KL (2017) A review of the physical features of the fetal alcohol spectrum disorders. Eur J Med Genet 60(1):55–64. https://doi.org/10.1016/j.ejmg.2016.10.004

Dorrie N, Focker M, Freunscht I, Hebebrand J (2014) Fetal alcohol spectrum disorders. Eur Child Adolesc Psychiatry 23(10):863–875. https://doi.org/10.1007/s00787-014-0571-6

Dupuy M, Chanraud S (2016) Imaging the addicted brain: alcohol. Int Rev Neurobiol 129:1–31. https://doi.org/10.1016/bs.irn.2016.04.003

Eberhart JK, Parnell SE (2016) The genetics of fetal alcohol spectrum disorders. Alcohol Clin Exp Res 40(6):1154–1165. https://doi.org/10.1111/acer.13066

Erdozain AM, Callado LF (2014) Neurobiological alterations in alcohol addiction: a review. Adicciones 26(4):360–370

Geibprasert S, Gallucci M, Krings T (2010a) Addictive illegal drugs: structural neuroimaging. AJNR Am J Neuroradiol 31:803–808

Geibprasert S, Gallucci M, Krings T (2010b) Alcohol-induced changes in the brain as assessed by MRI and CT. Eur Radiol 20(6):1492–1501. https://doi.org/10.1007/s00330-009-1668-z

George O, Hope BT (2017) Cortical and amygdalar neuronal ensembles in alcohol seeking, drinking and withdrawal. Neuropharmacology 122:107–114. https://doi.org/10.1016/j.neuropharm.2017.04.031

Glass L, Ware AL, Mattson SN (2014) Neurobehavioral, neurologic, and neuroimaging characteristics of fetal alcohol spectrum disorders. Handb Clin Neurol 125:435–462. https://doi.org/10.1016/b978-0-444-62619-6.00025-2

Halliday G, Ellis J, Harper C (1992) The locus coeruleus and memory: a study of chronic alcoholics with and without the memory impairment of Korsakoff's psychosis. Brain Res 598(1–2):33–37

Halliday G, Ellis J, Heard R, Caine D, Harper C (1993) Brainstem serotonergic neurons in chronic alcoholics with and without the memory impairment of Korsakoff's psychosis. J Neuropathol Exp Neurol 52(6):567–579

Harding AJ, Wong A, Svoboda M, Kril JJ, Halliday GM (1997) Chronic alcohol consumption does not cause hippocampal neuron loss in humans. Hippocampus

7(1):78–87. https://doi.org/10.1002/(SICI)1098-1063(1997)7:1<78::AID-HIPO8>3.0.CO;2-3

Harper C (1998) The neuropathology of alcohol-specific brain damage, or does alcohol damage the brain? J Neuropathol Exp Neurol 57(2):101–110

Harper C (2009) The neuropathology of alcohol-related brain damage. Alcohol Alcohol 44(2):136–140. https://doi.org/10.1093/alcalc/agn102

Harper C, Kril J (1985) Brain atrophy in chronic alcoholic patients: a quantitative pathological study. J Neurol Neurosurg Psychiatry 48(3):211–217

Harper CG, Kril JJ (1990) Neuropathology of alcoholism. Alcohol Alcohol 25(2–3):207–216

Harrison NL, Skelly MJ, Grosserode EK, Lowes DC, Zeric T, Phister S, Salling MC (2017) Effects of acute alcohol on excitability in the CNS. Neuropharmacology 122:36–45. https://doi.org/10.1016/j.neuropharm.2017.04.007

Hermens DF, Lagopoulos J, Tobias-Webb J, De Regt T, Dore G, Juckes L, Latt N, Hickie IB (2013) Pathways to alcohol-induced brain impairment in young people: a review. Cortex 49(1):3–17. https://doi.org/10.1016/j.cortex.2012.05.021

Hoyme HE, Kalberg WO, Elliott AJ, Blankenship J, Buckley D, Marais AS, Manning MA, Robinson LK, Adam MP, Abdul-Rahman O, Jewett T, Coles CD, Chambers C, Jones KL, Adnams CM, Shah PE, Riley EP, Charness ME, Warren KR, May PA (2016) Updated clinical guidelines for diagnosing fetal alcohol spectrum disorders. Pediatrics 138(2). https://doi.org/10.1542/peds.2015-4256

Hurley RA, Filley CM, Taber KH (2011) Central pontine myelinolysis: a metabolic disorder of myelin. J Neuropsychiatry Clin Neurosci 23(4):369–374. https://doi.org/10.1176/appi.neuropsych.23.4.369

Jain R, Balhara YP (2010) Impact of alcohol and substance abuse on adolescent brain: a preclinical perspective. Indian J Physiol Pharmacol 54(3):213–234

Kleinschmidt-Demasters BK, Rojiani AM, Filley CM (2006) Central and extrapontine myelinolysis: then… and now. J Neuropathol Exp Neurol 65(1):1–11

Kohler CG, Ances BM, Coleman AR, Ragland JD, Lazarev M, Gur RC (2000) Marchiafava-Bignami disease: literature review and case report. Neuropsychiatry Neuropsychol Behav Neurol 13(1):67–76

Korbo L (1999) Glial cell loss in the hippocampus of alcoholics. Alcohol Clin Exp Res 23(1):164–168

Kril JJ, Halliday GM (1999) Brain shrinkage in alcoholics: a decade on and what have we learned? Prog Neurobiol 58(4):381–387

Kril JJ, Halliday GM, Svoboda MD, Cartwright H (1997) The cerebral cortex is damaged in chronic alcoholics. Neuroscience 79(4):983–998

Kumar S, Fowler M, Gonzalez-Toledo E, Jaffe SL (2006) Central pontine myelinolysis, an update. Neurol Res 28(3):360–366. https://doi.org/10.1179/016164106x110346

Lampl C, Yazdi K (2002) Central pontine myelinolysis. Eur Neurol 47(1):3–10

Marshall SA, McClain JA, Kelso ML, Hopkins DM, Pauly JR, Nixon K (2013) Microglial activation is not equivalent to neuroinflammation in alcohol-induced neurodegeneration: the importance of microglia phenotype. Neurobiol Dis 54:239–251. https://doi.org/10.1016/j.nbd.2012.12.016

Mead EA, Sarkar DK (2014) Fetal alcohol spectrum disorders and their transmission through genetic and epigenetic mechanisms. Front Genet 5:154. https://doi.org/10.3389/fgene.2014.00154

Memo L, Gnoato E, Caminiti S, Pichini S, Tarani L (2013) Fetal alcohol spectrum disorders and fetal alcohol syndrome: the state of the art and new diagnostic tools. Early Hum Dev 89(Suppl 1):S40–S43. https://doi.org/10.1016/s0378-3782(13)70013-6

Montoliu C, Sancho-Tello M, Azorin I, Burgal M, Valles S, Renau-Piqueras J, Guerri C (1995) Ethanol increases cytochrome P4502E1 and induces oxidative stress in astrocytes. J Neurochem 65(6):2561–2570

Morisot N, Ron D (2017) Alcohol-dependent molecular adaptations of the NMDA receptor system. Genes Brain Behav 16(1):139–148. https://doi.org/10.1111/gbb.12363

Moselhy HF, Georgiou G, Kahn A (2001) Frontal lobe changes in alcoholism: a review of the literature. Alcohol Alcohol 36(5):357–368

Nguyen VT, Chong S, Tieng QM, Mardon K, Galloway GJ, Kurniawan ND (2017) Radiological studies of fetal alcohol spectrum disorders in humans and animal models: an updated comprehensive review. Magn Reson Imaging 43:10–26. https://doi.org/10.1016/j.mri.2017.06.012

Oscar-Berman M, Shagrin B, Evert DL, Epstein C (1997) Impairments of brain and behavior: the neurological effects of alcohol. Alcohol Health Res World 21(1):65–75

Pearce JM (2009) Central pontine myelinolysis. Eur Neurol 61(1):59–62. https://doi.org/10.1159/000175124

Pfefferbaum A, Sullivan EV (2005) Disruption of brain white matter microstructure by excessive intracellular and extracellular fluid in alcoholism: evidence from diffusion tensor imaging. Neuropsychopharmacology 30(2):423–432. https://doi.org/10.1038/sj.npp.1300623

Ravan S, Martinez D, Slifstein M, Abi-Dargham A (2014) Molecular imaging in alcohol dependence. Handb Clin Neurol 125:293–311. https://doi.org/10.1016/b978-0-444-62619-6.00018-5

Roberto M, Varodayan FP (2017) Synaptic targets: chronic alcohol actions. Neuropharmacology 122:85–99. https://doi.org/10.1016/j.neuropharm.2017.01.013

Roszel EL (2015) Central nervous system deficits in fetal alcohol spectrum disorder. Nurse Pract 40(4):24–33. https://doi.org/10.1097/01.NPR.0000444650.10142.4f

Sachdeva A, Chandra M, Choudhary M, Dayal P, Anand KS (2016) Alcohol-related dementia and neurocognitive impairment: a review study. Int J High Risk Behav Addict 5(3):e27976. https://doi.org/10.5812/ijhrba.27976

Senturias YS (2014) Fetal alcohol spectrum disorders: an overview for pediatric and adolescent care providers. Curr Probl Pediatr Adolesc Health Care 44(4):74–81. https://doi.org/10.1016/j.cppeds.2013.12.012

Senturias Y, Asamoah A (2014) Fetal alcohol spectrum disorders: guidance for recognition, diagnosis, differential diagnosis and referral. Curr Probl Pediatr Adolesc Health Care 44(4):88–95. https://doi.org/10.1016/j.cppeds.2013.12.008

Silveri MM, Dager AD, Cohen-Gilbert JE, Sneider JT (2016) Neurobiological signatures associated with alcohol and drug use in the human adolescent brain. Neurosci Biobehav Rev 70:244–259. https://doi.org/10.1016/j.neubiorev.2016.06.042

Squeglia LM, Jacobus J, Tapert SF (2014) The effect of alcohol use on human adolescent brain structures and systems. Handb Clin Neurol 125:501–510. https://doi.org/10.1016/b978-0-444-62619-6.00028-8

Sullivan EV, Harding AJ, Pentney R, Dlugos C, Martin PR, Parks MH, Desmond JE, Chen SH, Pryor MR, De Rosa E, Pfefferbaum A (2003) Disruption of frontocerebellar circuitry and function in alcoholism. Alcohol Clin Exp Res 27(2):301–309. https://doi.org/10.1097/01.alc.0000052584.05305.98

Tang Y, Pakkenberg B, Nyengaard JR (2004) Myelinated nerve fibres in the subcortical white matter of cerebral hemispheres are preserved in alcoholic subjects. Brain Res 1029(2):162–167. https://doi.org/10.1016/j.brainres.2004.09.035

Victor M, Adams RD, Collins GH (1971) The Wernicke-Korsakoff syndrome. A clinical and pathological study of 245 patients, 82 with post-mortem examinations. Contemp Neurol Ser 7:1–206

Weil ZM, Karelina K (2017) Traumatic brain injuries during development: implications for alcohol abuse. Front Behav Neurosci 11:135. https://doi.org/10.3389/fnbeh.2017.00135

Wong EL, Stowell RD, Majewska AK (2017) What the spectrum of microglial functions can teach us about fetal alcohol spectrum disorder. Front Synaptic Neurosci 9:11. https://doi.org/10.3389/fnsyn.2017.00011

Zahr NM (2014) Structural and microstructural imaging of the brain in alcohol use disorders. Handb Clin Neurol 125:275–290. https://doi.org/10.1016/b978-0-444-62619-6.00017-3

Zahr NM, Kaufman KL, Harper CG (2011) Clinical and pathological features of alcohol-related brain damage. Nat Rev Neurol 7(5):284–294. https://doi.org/10.1038/nrneurol.2011.42

Zuccoli G, Siddiqui N, Cravo I, Bailey A, Gallucci M, Harper CG (2010) Neuroimaging findings in alcohol-related encephalopathies. AJR Am J Roentgenol 195(6):1378–1384. https://doi.org/10.2214/ajr.09.4130

Intoxication: Street Drugs 50

50.1 Introduction

50.1.1 General Aspects

The major substances abused include:

- Cannabis
- Opiates
- Cocaine
- Amphetamine
- Methamphetamine
- XTC

The classification of street drugs can be done as follows (Karch and Drummer 2015):

Class	Examples
Cocaine	
Natural stimulants	• Absinthe • Caffeine • Ephedrine • Khat
Synthetic stimulants	• Amphetamine and methamphetamine • Methylphenidate • Phenylpropanolamine • Fenfluramine
Hallucinogens	
Opiates	• Morphine • Heroin • Codeine • Methadone • Propoxyphene • Fentanyl • Other
Dissociative anesthetics	• Phencyclidine (PCP) • Ketamine • Gamma-hydroxybutyrate
Anabolic steroids	
Solvents	

50.1.2 Clinical Signs and Symptoms

Clinical signs due to drug toxicity include:
- Cardiovascular complications
  - Infarction
  - Subarachnoidal hemorrhage
- Psychiatric symptoms
- Neurologic symptoms
  - Resulting from cerebral ischemia and cerebrovascular diseases
- Sudden paraparesis, or paraplegia of the thoracolumbar region leading to death in some cases due to transverse myelitis/myelopathy
- Motor disorders
  - Akathisia
  - Choreoathetosis
  - Dystonia
  - Parkinsonism

50.1.3 Neuroimaging Findings

Neuroradiology Findings
- Subtle changes in cerebral blood flow (CBF)
- Glucose metabolism
- Receptor densities or metabolite profiles

Nuclear Medicine Imaging Findings
- CBF-SPECT and FDG-PET show disseminated cerebral blood flow defects and hypometabolism especially in cocaine and methamphetamine abusers, but also in heroine addicted patients.
- Most frequently perfusion deficits were described (in descending frequency) in the frontal cortex, temporal cortex, inferior parietal cortex, and basal ganglia. Affected are the neocortex, basal ganglia, limbic system, and midbrain.
- Some reports state an improvement or disappearance of the changes after withdrawal of the drugs, suggesting that some of these defects could be caused by vasoconstrictor effects of the drugs (particularly in cocaine abusers). These hypoperfused and hypometabolizing areas show no correlation in CT or MRI.
- D2 receptor decrease in the striatum has been reported in cocaine, methamphetamine, and heroine abusers.
- F-DOPA uptake has been reported to be significantly lower in cocaine abusers, too.
- DAT binding was found to be reduced in cocaine high in some studies (blocked by cocaine). After acute abstinence, DAT binding was elevated in cocaine abusers. After withdrawal of cocaine, D2 receptor binding improves.
- In methamphetamine abusers (and abstinent methamphetamine abusers), DAT binding was found to be decreased correlating with alterations in motor tests and the severity of psychiatric symptoms. After withdrawal of the drug, reports state an improvement in D2 receptors and DAT binding with the least improvement in methamphetamine addicted patients.
- Increases in opioid receptor binding tracers were described in abstinent cocaine abusers between 1 and 12 weeks. Uptake in these patients correlated with craving.
- Cannabinoid receptors (CB1) have been monitored in cannabis abusers and they were found to be downregulated in correlation with the duration of cannabis abuse with a return to normal levels after 4 weeks of withdrawal.
- Studies dealing with craving have been done (i.e., perfusion PET and FDG-PET) which demonstrated perfusion and metabolizing increases in the frontal cortex, amygdala, and insula. Dopaminergic function seems to play a role in craving, but further studies have to be done to assess the significance of these findings.
- It has to be mentioned that other diseases with reduction of CBF or glucose metabolism have to be taken into account and that drug consumption can mimic changes due to other diseases (vascular, psychiatric, medication).

50.2 Opiates

Fatalities in opioid abusers are a major public health issue worldwide. Significant risk factors include loss of tolerance after a period of abstinence and concomitant use of alcohol and other CNS depressants. Moreover, systemic disease, e.g., pulmonary and hepatic disease as well as HIV-infection, may increase susceptibility to a fatal overdose.

50.2.1 Neuroimaging Findings

Computed Tomography (CT) (Fig. 50.1a)
- No gross abnormalities
- Cerebral atrophy might be seen in chronic heroin abusers

Magnetic Resonance Imaging (MRI) (Fig. 50.1b–f)
- No specific changes
- Areas of demyelination in the deep white matter

50.2 Opiates

Magnetic Resonance Spectroscopy (MRS)
- Reduction of *N*-acetylaspartate in the frontal cortex in long-term heroin abusers

Nuclear Medicine Imaging Findings
- SPECT: perfusion deficits
- PET: perfusion deficits

50.2.2 Neuropathology Findings

Macroscopic Features (Fig. 50.2a–d)
- Cerebral edema
- Vascular congestion
- Increased brain weight

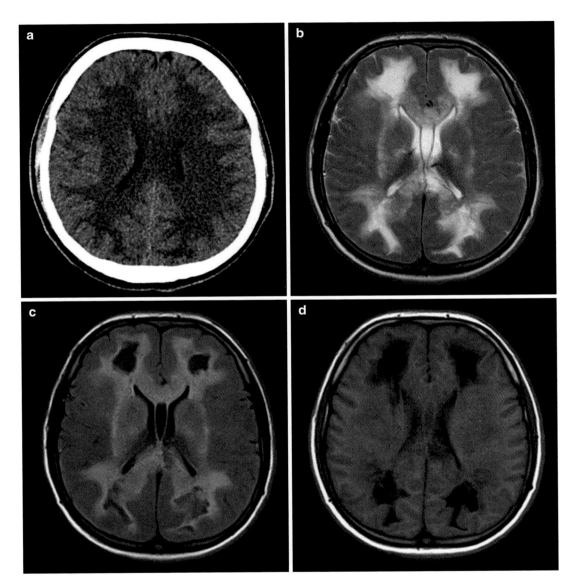

Fig. 50.1 Multi-drug abuse in a 25-year-old patient with toxic encephalopathy CT (**a**), T2 (**b**), FLAIR (**c**), T1 (**d**), DWI (**e**), and ADC (**f**)

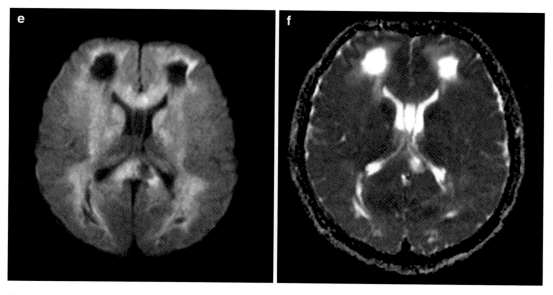

Fig. 50.1 (continued)

- Bilateral, symmetrical ischemic lesions/necrosis of the globus pallidus can be found in 5–10% of heroin addicts (Fig. 50.2a–d)
- Infections including:
  - Brain abscess
  - Meningitis
  - Ventriculitis

Microscopic Features (Figs. 50.2e–n and 50.3a–v)
- No morphological evidence of cellular injury in rapid death after heroin injection
- Hypoxic nerve cell damage in cases of delayed death
- Ischemic nerve cell damage after a survival period of 5 h or longer
- Neuronal loss in the globus pallidus (hypodensities on CT scans)
- Morphine has been selectively demonstrated in neurons, axons, and dendrites of the hippocampus by immunohistochemistry
- Transverse myelitis/myelopathy
- Perivascular pigment-laden macrophages
- Infections include:
  - Brain abscess
  - Meningitis
  - Ventriculitis
- Lymphocytic meningitis is indicative of an early stage of HIV-1 infection
- Edema
- *Hypoxic-ischemic leukoencephalopathy*
  - Loss of neurons in the hippocampal formation and/or Purkinje cell layer
  - Enhanced expression of glial fibrillary acidic protein by astrocytes and/or a proliferation of microglia
- *Spongiform leukoencephalopathy (nonspecific toxic demyelination)*
  - Occurs worldwide almost exclusively after inhalation of pre-heated heroin ("chasing the dragon," "Chinese blowing")
  - The clinical features progress from motor restlessness and cerebellar signs to pyramidal and pseudobulbar signs and, in some patients, to a terminal stage with spasms, paraparesis, and death
  - Diffuse spongiosis of the white matter
  - Loss of oligodendrocytes
  - Reduction of axons
  - Astrogliosis
  - Gray matter is usually unremarkable

50.2 Opiates

- Brain stem, spinal cord, and peripheral nerves are spared
- DD: The presence of spongiosis with astrogliosis and the absence of typical hypoxic lesions distinguish these cases from those with delayed leukoencephalopathy following severe hypoxia

50.2.3 Molecular Neuropathology

- Cerebrovascular diseases:
  - Global cerebral hypoxia due to:
    ○ Hypoventilation and/or hypotension during heroin intoxication
    ○ Focal decrease of the perfusion pressure

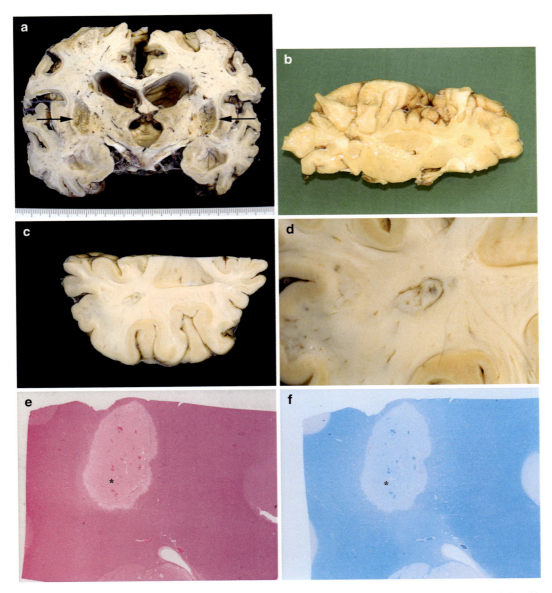

Fig. 50.2 Bilateral necroses of the putamen (**a**), focal necroses in the white matter (**b–d**). The focal necrosis at low magnification (**e**: H&E), (**f**: LFB), (**g**: GFAP), (**h**: CD68). The area of necrosis is well delineated from the unaffected brain tissue (**i–l**: H&E). The luxol fast blue stain shows loss of myelin with only very few myelinated fibers within the lesion (**m, n**)

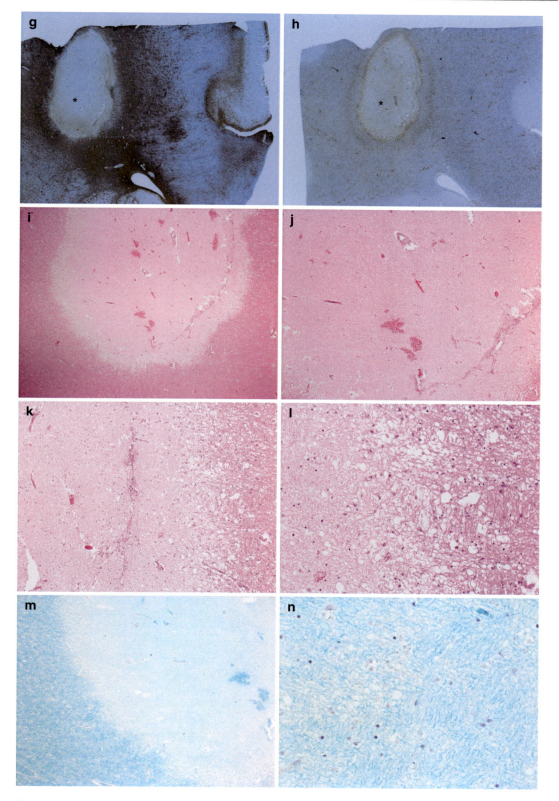

Fig. 50.2 (continued)

50.2 Opiates

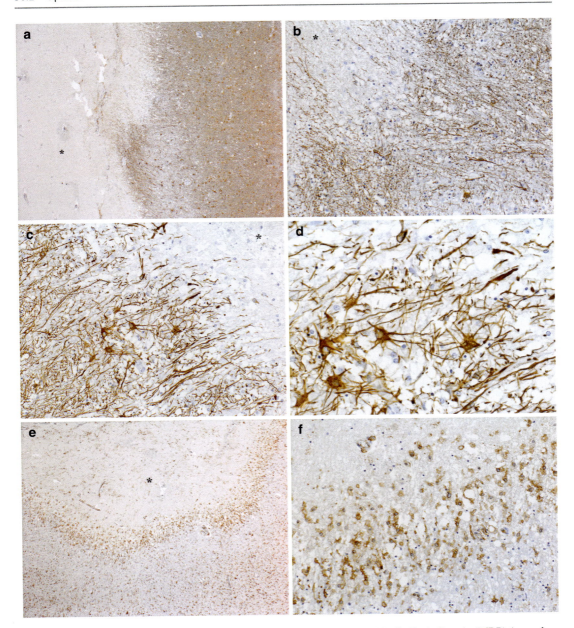

Fig. 50.3 Immunophenotype: strong rim of GFAP-positive astrocytes between the lesion and brain tissue (**a–d**), of HLA-DRII positive microglial cells with macrophage phenotype (**e–h**), rarefaction of myelin proteins: proteolipid protein (PLP) (**i, j**: border zone, **k**: unaffected brain, **l**: lesion), Myelin Basic Protein (MBP) (**m, n**: border zone, **o**: unaffected brain, **p**: lesion), Myelin-Associated Glycoprotein (MAG) (**q, r**: border zone, **s**: unaffected brain, **t**: lesion), Myelin Oligodendrocyte Glycoprotein (MOG) (**u, v**), (*lesion)

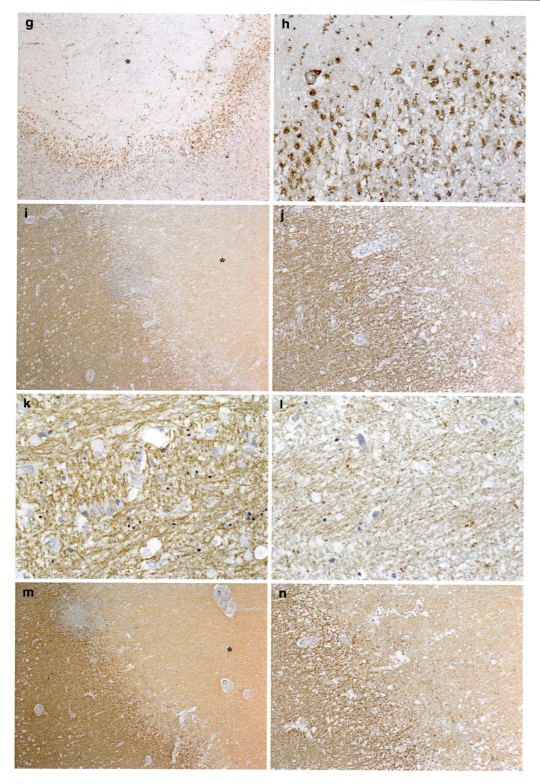

Fig. 50.3 (continued)

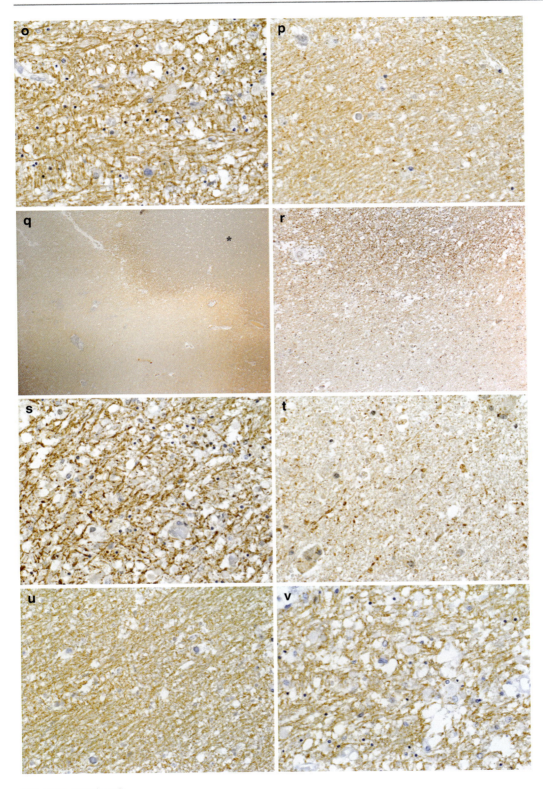

Fig. 50.3 (continued)

- Vascular hypersensitivity reaction to heroin in persons who were reexposed to the drug after a period of abstinence
- Cerebral arteritis, necrotizing angiitis, or vasculitis
- Embolism from adulterants
- Positional vascular compression
- μ-Opioid receptors on human erythrocytes are significantly elevated in chronic opiate abusers and showed high deformability
- Marked sudden hypotension leads to necrosis in the arterial boundary zones between the major arteries
• Hypoxic-ischemic leukoencephalopathy
  - Hypoxia secondary to respiratory depression affects the cerebral white matter
  - Loss of neurons in the hippocampal formation and/or Purkinje cell layer is frequently seen and is attributable to primary respiratory failure
  - Enhanced expression of glial fibrillary acidic protein by astrocytes and/or a proliferation of microglia are found in the hippocampus. Since such reactive processes are the result of primary neuronal damage, it can be assumed that chronic intravenous drug abuse obviously results in ischemic nerve cell loss
  - Perivascular macrophages are sometimes observed and are attributed to repeated intravenous injections of impure heroin
• Spongiform Leukoencephalopathy (nonspecific toxic demyelination)
  - A lipophilic toxin related to contaminants in conjunction with cerebral hypoxia is considered to be the cause, but a definite toxin has not yet been identified
  - Spongiform leukoencephalopathy may be the outcome of a complex mechanism directly triggered by heroin which causes mitochondrial as well as hypoxic injury in specific and limited areas of the cerebral white matter
  - The mitochondrial respiratory chain complexes IV, III, and V are unchanged

• Neurotransmitters, receptors, and second messengers
  - All opiate effects are mediated via several specific types of opioid receptors
  - The μ-receptors mediate analgesia, euphoria, respiratory depression, hypothermia, bradycardia, and miosis
  - Long-term opiate abuse is not associated with a reduced density of CNS μ- and δ-opioid receptors
  - Increased density of μ-opioid receptor-immunoreactive neurons has been demonstrated in Brodmann Area 11 of the human cerebral cortex and is associated with a state of functional hypersensitivity in acute heroin intoxication
  - The second messenger signaling system seems to play a crucial role
    ○ The coupling of opioid receptors to their effectors is mediated by guanosine triphosphate binding (G-) proteins that transmit extracellular, receptor-detected signals across the cell membrane to intracellular effectors
    ○ Opiates acutely inhibit adenylyl cyclase activity (that converts ATP to cAMP) via G-proteins resulting in decreased cellular cAMP levels
    ○ Chronic opiate exposure induces an upregulation in this adenylyl cyclase-cAMP system, which is interpreted to be a compensatory response to the sustained inhibition of the opioid receptor system in order to maintain homeostasis
    ○ The long-term effect of opiates on the cAMP pathway is mediated via the transcription factor CREB (cAMP response element-binding protein), with the locus coeruleus, the mesolimbic dopaminergic system, and the extended amygdala being the major target areas
    ○ Autopsy studies revealed that long-term heroin abuse causes an increase in certain G-proteins in different regions of the brain of heroin addicts:

- The Gβ subunit in the temporal cortex
- The subunits Gαi$_{1/2}$, Gαo, Gαs, and Gβ in the frontal cortex
- Opiate addiction is associated with abnormalities in second messenger and signal transduction systems involving G-proteins
  o A decreased level of Ca^{2+}-dependent protein kinase C (PKC)-α in the frontal cortex of opiate addicts
  o An increased level of a membrane-associated G-protein-coupled receptor kinase
  o Downregulation of the PKC-α enhances the upregulation of Gαi$_{1/2}$ proteins for compensating the opiate-induced desensitization of the μ-opioid receptor system
  o Further findings:
    - A significant downregulation of the adenylyl cyclase subtype I in the temporal cortex, which may play an important role in the molecular mechanism of chronic opiate addiction
    - A significant decrease in the density of alpha 2-adrenoreceptors in the frontal cortex, hypothalamus, and caudate nucleus without changes in affinity values
    - A marked decrease in the immunoreactivity of PKC-αβ in the frontal cortex
  o Markedly decreased levels of immunoreactive neurofilament proteins in the frontal cortex of chronic opiate addicts might represent a specific long-term effect indicating neuronal damage after chronic abuse
  o No reduction in the density of dopaminergic nerve terminals in the striatum
  o Reduction of tyrosine hydroxylase (TH) protein and of the dopamine (DA) metabolite homovanillic acid in the nucleus accumbens and decreased DA concentration reflect either a compensatory downregulation of DA biosynthesis in response to prolonged dopaminergic stimulation caused by heroin, or reduced axoplasmic transport of tyrosine hydroxylase
  o Striatal levels of serotonin (5-hydroxytryptamine or 5-HT) were either normal or elevated, whereas the concentration of the 5-HT metabolite 5-hydroxyindoleacetic acid was decreased
  o The density of I2-imidazoline receptors and the immunoreactivity of the related receptor protein were decreased in astrocytes of the frontal cortex, indicating that chronic opiate abuse induces downregulation of I2-imidazoline receptors in astrocytes and presumably downregulates the functions associated with these receptors, e.g., reduced growth of astrocytes

50.3 Cocaine

Cocaine abuse represents the third most common addiction disorder next to alcohol and cannabis.

50.3.1 Clinical Signs and Symptoms

- Seizures
  - In 2–10% of cocaine users
  - Self-limiting generalized tonic-clonic seizures
  - Status epilepticus and consecutive death have been reported in single cases
- Movement disorders observed in cocaine users, especially in "crack" abusers include:
  - Akathisia
  - Choreoathetosis
  - Dystonia
  - Parkinsonism

50.3.2 Neuroimaging Findings

- The following changes are mainly found in chronic cocaine abusers.

CT Scans
- Diffuse cerebral atrophy which was positively correlated with the duration of cocaine abuse

MRI
- Age-related hyperintense areas in the white matter attributed to ischemic lesion
- Evidence of caudate nucleus and putamen enlargement
- No significant differences in the total brain volume or the presence of white matter lesions in cocaine abusers
- MR angiography: a dose-dependent cerebral vasoconstriction after cocaine administration in healthy human volunteers
- Reduction of global CBF and cerebral perfusion deficits in human cocaine users receiving a single intravenous cocaine dose
- Angiography: segmental stenoses and dilatations
- A cocaine-induced cerebral vasculitis considered to be the cause of the ischemic and hemorrhagic lesions

Nuclear Medicine Imaging Findings
- A global reduction in cerebral glucose metabolism
- Focal perfusion deficits in different brain regions
- Perfusion deficits are partially reversible after abstinence

50.3.3 Neuropathology Findings

Macroscopic Features
- Intracerebral and subarachnoidal hemorrhages
- Due to arteriovenous malformations or aneurysms
- Ischemic infarctions
  - Can be found in every brain region, and nearly half of the patients presented with neurological deficits within the first 3 h after cocaine intake

50.3.4 Molecular Neuropathology

- Cocaine crosses the blood-brain barrier rapidly due to its high lipophilic properties
- Cocaine is mainly metabolized to form the inactive metabolites ecgonine methyl ester (EME) and benzoylecgonine (BE), which do not significantly cross the blood-brain barrier
- Although the uptake of BE into the brain is very low, the enzyme butyrylcholine esterase that catalyzes the metabolism of cocaine to BE is abundantly present in the cerebral white matter
- In the presence of alcohol, cocaine is metabolized to cocaethylene (CE), which crosses the blood-brain barrier rapidly. With a longer half-life time, CE accumulates to a four times higher concentration and possesses a similar pharmacologic profile to cocaine
- Cocaine and its major metabolites are widely distributed and receptors with varying affinities for cocaine are found throughout the brain
- The striatum is the region with the highest density of cocaine receptors, which is also the region containing the receptors with the greatest affinity for cocaine
- Lower levels of activity are found in the frontal and occipital cortex
- Most of the CNS effects of cocaine are mediated through alterations of the neurotransmitters
  - Dopamine (DA)
  - Norepinephrine (NE)
  - Serotonin (5-HT)
  - Acetylcholine (Ach)
  - γ-Aminobutyric acid (GABA)
- Cocaine
  - Blocks the presynaptic reuptake of neurotransmitters resulting in their accumulation in the synaptic cleft, thus producing a sustained action on the receptor system followed by neurotransmitter depletion
  - Enhances DA neurotransmission by interacting with the dopamine transporter (DAT), inhibiting the clearance of DA and stimulating the enzyme tyrosine hydroxylase

- The interactions of cocaine in the mesocorticolimbic "reward" system constitute the basis for its reinforcing properties
- Marked reductions in the levels of:
  - Enkephalin mRNA
  - μ-opioid receptor binding
  - DA uptake site binding
  - Elevation in levels of dynorphin mRNA
  - κ opioid receptor binding
  - In the striatum of human cocaine-related deaths
- In chronic cocaine abusers
  - A decrease in the levels of DA was seen in the caudate nucleus and frontal cortex, but not in the putamen, nucleus accumbens, and cerebral cortex.
  - An increase of DA D_1 and D_2 gene expression in the nucleus accumbens, caudate nucleus, putamen, or substantia nigra.
  - Increase of cocaine binding sites on the DAT with a decrease of the DA D_1-receptor density in the striatum and of D_1 and D_3 receptor density in the nucleus accumbens.
  - Reduction in vesicular monoamine transporter-2 (VMAT-2) immunoreactivity and of the transcription factor NURR1 in autopsy samples of human cocaine abusers might reflect damage to dopaminergic system.
  - Overexpression of α-synuclein in midbrain DA neurons in chronic cocaine abusers may occur as a protective response to changes in DA turnover and increased oxidative stress resulting from cocaine abuse.
  - Upregulation of κ_2-opioid receptors in the limbic system and of CREB in the ventral tegmental area.
  - An increase of the serotonin transporter in the striatum, substantia nigra, and limbic system.
  - Decreased activity of phospholipase A_2 and phosphocholine cytidylyltransferase in the putamen, a DA-rich brain area.

Experimentally, cocaine enhances

- leukocyte migration across the cerebral vessel wall
- opens the blood-brain barrier to HIV-1 invasion by a direct effect on brain endothelial cells and by the induction of pro-inflammatory cytokines and chemokines

Seizures:

- The pathogenetic mechanisms are believed to be due to a reduction of the seizure threshold or by induction of cardiac arrhythmia

Motor disorders:

- Disturbances in the dopaminergic transmission in the nigrostriatal motor system

50.4 Cannabis

Cannabis abuse is the most common illicit drug in use today. Δ^9-tetrahydrocannabinol (THC), the major psychoactive component of cannabis, has a high abuse potential and leads to psychological dependency.

50.4.1 CNS Complications of Cannabis

- Cardiovascular complications
  - Cerebral infarction
  - Transitory ischemic attacks
  - Cannabis-induced vasospasm or a cannabis-induced hypotension
- CNS complaints
  - Psychiatric symptoms
  - Panic attacks
  - Anxiety
  - Depression
  - Psychosis
  - Affect cognition
  - Impair verbal and memory skills
- THC
  - Increases the depressive effect of alcohol, sedatives and opiates
  - Its interactions with stimulants, e.g., amphetamines or cocaine, are complex and can be either additive or antagonistic

50.4.2 Neuroimaging Findings

- Subtle CNS alterations
- MRI studies failed to detect morphological brain changes in long-term cannabis abusers

Nuclear Medicine Imaging Findings
- PET and SPECT studies showed:
- Transient vasodilatation with an increase of CBF and metabolism after acute cannabis abuse
- In chronic cannabis abusers, a decreased cerebral metabolism and CBF in the frontal lobe and cerebellum
- The age at which exposure to cannabis begins seems to be important for the existence of CBF changes, with the early adolescence as a critical period
- The cessation of chronic cannabis abuse is believed to lead to a decrease in the functional level of the frontal lobes

50.4.3 Neuropathology Findings

Macroscopic and Microscopic Findings
- Infarcts (see Chap. 18)

50.4.4 Molecular Neuropathology

- THC is:
- Distributed heterogeneously
- Highest concentrations in neocortical, limbic, sensory, and motor areas
- THC and other cannabinoids exert their effects by the interaction with specific cannabinoid (CB)-receptors
    - Two cannabinoid receptors, CB1 and CB2, have been pharmacologically characterized and anatomically localized
        o CB1 receptors are found predominantly in the central and peripheral nervous system, where they have been implicated in presynaptic inhibition of transmitter release
        o CB2 receptors are present on immune cells, where they may be involved in cytokine release
    - Both receptors are coupled through G-proteins to signal transduction mechanisms
        o Inhibition of adenylyl cyclase
        o Activation of mitogen-activated protein kinase
        o Regulation of calcium and potassium channels (CB1 only)
        o Other signal transduction pathways
    - Endogenous cannabinoid agonists ("endocannabinoids")
        o Mediate the effects of cannabinoids
        o These lipid mediators of the eicosanoid class, notably arachidonoylethanolamide (anandamide), 2-arachidonoylglycerol and 2-arachidonylglyceryl ether (noladin ether), bind to both cannabinoid receptor types
        o They have been implicated in a variety of physiological functions, e.g., pain reduction, motor regulation, learning, memory, appetite stimulation, and reward

The CB1 receptors are:
- Distributed heterogeneously within the brain
    - The highest density in the substantia nigra, basal ganglia, hippocampus, and cerebellum
    - In the neocortex, they are present with the highest density in the frontal cortex, dentate gyrus, mesolimbic dopaminergic system, and temporal lobe
    - This specific distribution of CB1-receptors correlates well with the effects of cannabinoids on memory, perception, and the control of movement
- Chronic exposure to THC fails to irreversibly alter brain cannabinoid receptors
    - The very low density of CB1 receptors in the brain stem and medulla oblongata explains the low acute toxicity and lack of lethality of cannabis

- THC-induced neuronal death
  - THC has a time- and concentration-dependent toxic effect on cultured hippocampal, cortical, and neonatal neurons
  - THC-induced generation of free radicals could lead to lipid peroxidation and subsequent neuronal apoptosis

At the cellular level:

- Abnormalities in the expression of transcription factors
- NO formation
- Alterations in the brain dopaminergic system

50.5 Amphetamine and Methamphetamine

Over the past years, the illicit use of amphetamine and methamphetamine has significantly risen worldwide.

50.5.1 Clinical Signs and Symptoms

Adverse CNS events include:
- Seizures
- Agitation
- Psychosis
- Aggressive behavior
- Suicidality

Amphetamines are the second-most-common cause (after cocaine) of:
- Ischemic stroke
- Hemorrhagic stroke occurring largely in persons younger than 45 years
- Subarachnoidal hemorrhages
- Intracerebral hemorrhages

50.5.2 Neuroimaging Findings

- Ischemic stroke (see Chap. 18)
- Hemorrhagic stroke (see Chap. 19)

50.5.3 Neuropathology Findings

Macroscopic and Microscopic Findings
- Ischemic stroke (see Chap. 18)
- Hemorrhagic stroke (see Chap. 19)

50.5.4 Molecular Neuropathology

- Amphetamine, methamphetamine
- are a subclass of psychostimulants
  - share a molecular site of action at monoamine transporters, in particular the dopamine transporter (DAT)
- bind to the three major monoamine transporters
  - Dopamine (DA)
  - Serotonin (5-HT)
  - Norepinephrine (NE)
- its actions at DATs are most central to both the motor activating and reinforcing (rewarding) properties of these substances, but there are differences in the molecular mechanisms by which these drugs interact with DATs
- Acute administration of psychostimulants enhances synaptic concentrations of DA and other monoamines
- The potent sympathomimetic effects of amphetamine and methamphetamine include:
  - Elevation of pulse rate and blood pressure
  - Increased level of alertness
  - Decreased fatigue
  - Suppression of appetite
- The euphoric action and the reinforcing effect are related to their ability to release DA in the mesocorticolimbic "reward" system and ACh in the cerebral cortex

The neurotoxic effects of amphetamine and methamphetamine

- on the dopaminergic system
  - desensitization of DA receptor function
  - marked reduction of DA levels
  - dopaminergic axonal markers, e.g., tyrosine hydroxylase, DATs, and VMAT-2 levels

- alterations in the serotonergic system
- methamphetamine-induced loss of dopaminergic cell bodies in the substantia nigra
- predispose methamphetamine users to develop parkinsonism as they age, at least the ones that survive their abuse
- mediated by multiple mechanisms including
  - generation of free radicals and NO
  - excitotoxicity
  - disruption of mitochondria
  - induction of immediate early genes as well as transcription factors
  - hyperthermia

The *pathophysiology of cerebrovascular complications* related to amphetamine and methamphetamine abuse may involve several mechanisms.

- A sudden elevation in blood pressure
- Cerebral vasculitis
  - Necrotizing angiitis closely resembling periarteritis nodosa
  - Hemorrhages
  - Infarctions
  - Microaneurysms
  - Perivascular cuffing occurring in small-to-medium-sized arteries
- Induce inflammatory genes in human brain endothelial cells
- The vasoconstrictive effect of both substances may also lead to the development of ischemic stroke

50.6 Designer Drugs

The abuse of amphetamine, methamphetamine, and amphetamine derivatives such as 3,4-methylenedioxymethamphetamine (MDMA) and 3,4-methylenedioxyamphetamine (MDA) is an important issue in current forensic medicine.

50.6.1 Substances

Common substances include:

- DOM (4-methyl-2,5-dimethoxyamphetamine)
- DOB (4-bromo-2,5-dimethoxyamphetamine)
- MDA (3,4-methylenedioxyamphetamine)
- MDEA
- MDE (3,4-methylenedioxyethylamphetamine, "Eve")
- MDMA (3,4-methylenedioxymethamphetamine, "Ecstasy," "Adam," "XTC"), 4-MTA (4-methylthioamphetamine, "Flatliners")
- PMA (4-para-methoxyamphetamine)
- The street name "Ecstasy" subsumizes different hallucinogenic amphetamine derivatives with MDMA and MDEA being the main components

50.6.2 Modes of Action

MDMA

- acts mainly
  - on the serotonergic system
  - peripheral and central nervous system (CNS)
- has sympathomimetic properties
- modulates psychomotor and neuroendocrine functions
- The unique effect of MDMA is the feeling of intimacy and closeness, designated as "entactogenic"
- MDMA acts as an
  - indirect monoaminergic agonist
  - displays relatively high, similar affinities for α-adrenoceptors, 5-HT$_2$ receptors, M-1 muscarinic receptors, and H-1 histamine receptors
  - binds with less affinity to DA and NE uptake sites, M-2 muscarinic receptors, α$_1$-adrenoceptors, beta-adrenoceptors, 5-HT$_1$ receptors, and D1 and D2 DA receptors. MDMA blocks 5-HT reuptake and induces 5-HT release and, to a lesser extent, also causes DA and NE release
  - The 5-HT release appears to be related to MDMA action on the 5-HT transporter (5-HTT)
  - In addition to its inhibition of monoamine reuptake, MDMA might also increase extracellular levels of monoamines by inhibiting brain monoamine oxidase activity

In human postmortem tissue

- a distinct immunopositive reaction of MDMA and MDA was observed
  - in the white matter

- in all cortical brain regions
- the neurons of the basal ganglia
- the hypothalamus
- the hippocampus
- the cerebellar vermis
- but in the brain stem relatively weak staining of neurons is seen

50.6.3 Molecular Neuropathology

Mechanisms of MDMA-induced neurotoxicity

- Nonhuman primates have been shown to be more sensitive to the neurotoxic effects of MDMA than rats
- The serotonergic system seems to be mostly affected, i.e.,
  - serotonergic neurodegeneration and axonal loss
- Current hypotheses of its damaging mechanisms include:
  - Formation of toxic MDMA metabolites
  - Generation of free radicals
  - Disturbances in neurotransmitter systems
    - Serotonergic
    - Dopaminergic
    - GABA-ergic
    - Glutamatergic
  - Nitric oxide system
  - Hyperthermia

50.6.4 Outcome

Acute and long-term neurotoxic effects include:

- Impaired cognitive performance
- Increased incidence of neuropsychiatric disorders

Fatalities
The cause of death may be due to:
- Cardiovascular collapse
- Hyponatremia
- Hepatic failure

- Exertional hyperthermia or serotonin syndrome may lead to disseminated intravascular coagulation
- Rhabdomyolysis
- Acute renal failure
- Traumatic injuries, e.g., traffic accidents

Central Nervous System Complications
- Ischemic stroke.
- Hemorrhagic cerebral infarction of unknown etiology.
- Intracranial hemorrhage.
- Subarachnoidal hemorrhage.
- Sinus vein thrombosis.
- Hypersensitivity vasculitis.
- Leukoencephalopathy.
- In the globus pallidus, bilateral hyperintense lesions can be found.
  - Necrosis of the globus pallidus
  - Diffuse astrogliosis
  - Spongiform changes of the white matter
- Other neuropathological findings in deaths after "ecstasy" consumption encompass:
  - Complications of hyperthermia
  - Disseminated intravascular coagulopathy
  - Cerebral edema
  - Focal hemorrhages
  - Nerve cell loss evident in the locus coeruleus

Selected References

Bachtell R, Hutchinson MR, Wang X, Rice KC, Maier SF, Watkins LR (2015) Targeting the toll of drug abuse: the translational potential of toll-like receptor 4. CNS Neurol Disord Drug Targets 14(6):692–699

Beardsley PM, Thomas BF, McMahon LR (2009) Cannabinoid CB1 receptor antagonists as potential pharmacotherapies for drug abuse disorders. Int Rev Psychiatry 21(2):134–142. https://doi.org/10.1080/09540260902782786

Benavides DR, Bibb JA (2004) Role of Cdk5 in drug abuse and plasticity. Ann N Y Acad Sci 1025:335–344. https://doi.org/10.1196/annals.1316.041

Bodea S (2017) CNS metabolism in high-risk drug abuse: insights gained from (1)H-, (31)P-MRS and PET. Radiologe. https://doi.org/10.1007/s00117-017-0255-6

Buttner A (2011) Review: The neuropathology of drug abuse. Neuropathol Appl Neurobiol 37(2):118–134. https://doi.org/10.1111/j.1365-2990.2010.01131.x

Chang L, Haning W (2006) Insights from recent positron emission tomographic studies of drug abuse and dependence. Curr Opin Psychiatry 19(3):246–252. https://doi.org/10.1097/01.yco.0000218594.46431.2f

Egleton RD, Abbruscato T (2014) Drug abuse and the neurovascular unit. Adv Pharmacol 71:451–480. https://doi.org/10.1016/bs.apha.2014.06.019

Engleman EA, Rodd ZA, Bell RL, Murphy JM (2008) The role of 5-HT3 receptors in drug abuse and as a target for pharmacotherapy. CNS Neurol Disord Drug Targets 7(5):454–467

Ernst M, Kimes AS, Jazbec S (2003) Neuroimaging and mechanisms of drug abuse: interface of molecular imaging and molecular genetics. Neuroimaging Clin N Am 13(4):833–849

Fonseca AC, Ferro JM (2013) Drug abuse and stroke. Curr Neurol Neurosci Rep 13(2):325. https://doi.org/10.1007/s11910-012-0325-0

Gatley SJ, Volkow ND, Wang GJ, Fowler JS, Logan J, Ding YS, Gerasimov M (2005) PET imaging in clinical drug abuse research. Curr Pharm Des 11(25):3203–3219

Goforth HW, Murtaugh R, Fernandez F (2010) Neurologic aspects of drug abuse. Neurol Clin 28(1):199–215. https://doi.org/10.1016/j.ncl.2009.09.010

Ham S, Kim TK, Chung S, Im HI (2017) Drug abuse and psychosis: new insights into drug-induced psychosis. Exp Neurobiol 26(1):11–24. https://doi.org/10.5607/en.2017.26.1.11

Heinbockel T, Wang ZJ (2015) Cellular mechanisms of action of drug abuse on olfactory neurons. Int J Environ Res Public Health 13(1):ijerph13010005. https://doi.org/10.3390/ijerph13010005

Karch SB, Drummer OH (2015) Karch's pathology of drug abuse, 5th edn. CRC Press, Boca Raton

Lindsey KP, Gatley SJ, Volkow ND (2003) Neuroimaging in drug abuse. Curr Psychiatry Rep 5(5):355–361

Lundqvist T (2010) Imaging cognitive deficits in drug abuse. Curr Top Behav Neurosci 3:247–275. https://doi.org/10.1007/7854_2009_26

Miczek KA, Nikulina EM, Takahashi A, Covington HE 3rd, Yap JJ, Boyson CO, Shimamoto A, de Almeida RM (2011) Gene expression in aminergic and peptidergic cells during aggression and defeat: relevance to violence, depression and drug abuse. Behav Genet 41(6):787–802. https://doi.org/10.1007/s10519-011-9462-5

Miguel-Hidalgo JJ (2009) The role of glial cells in drug abuse. Curr Drug Abuse Rev 2(1):72–82

Neiman J, Haapaniemi HM, Hillbom M (2000) Neurological complications of drug abuse: pathophysiological mechanisms. Eur J Neurol 7(6):595–606

Nikulina EM, Johnston CE, Wang J, Hammer RP Jr (2014) Neurotrophins in the ventral tegmental area: role in social stress, mood disorders and drug abuse. Neuroscience 282:122–138. https://doi.org/10.1016/j.neuroscience.2014.05.028

Noble F, Lenoir M, Marie N (2015) The opioid receptors as targets for drug abuse medication. Br J Pharmacol 172(16):3964–3979. https://doi.org/10.1111/bph.13190

Raffa RB (2009) The M5 muscarinic receptor as possible target for treatment of drug abuse. J Clin Pharm Ther 34(6):623–629. https://doi.org/10.1111/j.1365-2710.2009.01059.x

Revitsky AR, Klein LC (2013) Role of ghrelin in drug abuse and reward-relevant behaviors: a burgeoning field and gaps in the literature. Curr Drug Abuse Rev 6(3):231–244

Rodriguez MJ, Pugliese M, Mahy N (2009) Drug abuse, brain calcification and glutamate-induced neurodegeneration. Curr Drug Abuse Rev 2(1):99–112

Sanchez AB, Kaul M (2017) Neuronal stress and injury caused by HIV-1, cART and drug abuse: converging contributions to HAND. Brain Sci 7(3). https://doi.org/10.3390/brainsci7030025

Sanna PP, Repunte-Canonigo V, Guidotti A (2012) Gene profiling of laser-microdissected brain regions and individual cells in drug abuse and schizophrenia research. Methods Mol Biol 829:541–550. https://doi.org/10.1007/978-1-61779-458-2_34

Urbano FJ, Bisagno V, Garcia-Rill E (2017) Arousal and drug abuse. Behav Brain Res 333:276–281. https://doi.org/10.1016/j.bbr.2017.07.013

Volkow ND, Fowler JS, Wang GJ, Swanson JM (2004) Dopamine in drug abuse and addiction: results from imaging studies and treatment implications. Mol Psychiatry 9(6):557–569. https://doi.org/10.1038/sj.mp.4001507

Volkow ND, Fowler JS, Wang GJ, Baler R, Telang F (2009) Imaging dopamine's role in drug abuse and addiction. Neuropharmacology 56(Suppl 1):3–8. https://doi.org/10.1016/j.neuropharm.2008.05.022

Zhang K, Jing X, Wang G (2016) MicroRNAs as regulators of drug abuse and immunity. Cent Eur J Immunol 41(4):426–434. https://doi.org/10.5114/ceji.2016.65142